MOTOR
SPEECH
DISORDERS

SUBSTRATES,
DIFFERENTIAL DIAGNOSIS,
AND MANAGEMENT

MOTOR SPEECH DISORDERS

SUBSTRATES, DIFFERENTIAL DIAGNOSIS, AND MANAGEMENT

JOSEPH R. DUFFY, PHD
Head, Section of Speech Pathology
Department of Neurology, Mayo Clinic
and
Professor, Mayo Medical School
Rochester, Minnesota

with 76 illustrations

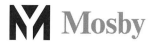

An Imprint of Elsevier Science
St. Louis   London   Philadelphia   Sydney   Toronto

Mosby

An Imprint of Elsevier Science

Publisher: Don Ladig
Executive Editor: Martha Sasser
Associate Developmental Editor: Kellie F. White
Project Manager: Linda Clarke
Production Editor: Veda King
Manufacturing Supervisor: Tim Stringham
Designer: Nancy McDonald
Cover: Carolyn O'Brien

Printed in the United States of America

Mosby, Inc.
11830 Westline Industrial Drive
St. Louis, MO 63146

Library of Congress Cataloging-in-Publication Data

Duffy, Joseph R.
  Motor speech disorders : substrates, differential diagnosis, and
management / Joseph R. Duffy. — 1st ed.
    p.   cm.
  Includes bibliographical references and index.
  ISBN 0-8016-6944-8 (alk. paper)
  1. Speech disorders.   I. Title.
  [DNLM: 1. Dysarthria—diagnosis.   2. Dysarthria—therapy.
3. Speech Disorders—diagnosis.   4. Speech Disorders—therapy.   WL
340.2 D858m   1995]
RC423.D84   1995
616.85'5—dc20
DNLM/DLC   95–3081

02 03 04 18 17 16 15 14 13 12 11 10

To

My parents

and to

Ella Duchaine, Many Plans, and Bean.

You know who you are.

You know what you mean.

Preface

At the midpoint of this decade of the brain, neuroscientists can point with pride to significant advances in what we know about the brain's structure and function, and with humility to how much remains unknown. Similarly, healthcare providers who work with people suffering from neurologic disease know that the services provided are better today than ever before but not as good as they would like them to be.

Clinicians who diagnose and help care for people with neuropathologies of speech are no strangers to gains and gaps in knowledge and clinical services. This book addresses the neurologic underpinnings of speech, the speech disorders that can develop when the nervous system goes awry, and the ways in which motor speech disorders can be assessed, diagnosed, and managed. Its contents reflect what we think we know about these things. Within and between the lines of each page, the lacunae will be apparent.

The book is intended primarily for graduate students, practicing clinicians, and researchers in the discipline of speech-language pathology. The topics addressed here should also be of interest to people in related disciplines—such as neurology, neuropsychology, and rehabilitation medicine—who are interested in speech disorders as an index of neurologic disease and its localization, and the differential diagnostic value of speech disorders to medical diagnosis and care.

The book is divided into three major parts that address (1) the substrates of motor speech and its disorders, (2) the disorders and their diagnoses, and (3) management. The relationship of the information covered within each of the three parts to each other hopefully conveys the importance of knowing something about each of them if one is to be "good" at any of them.

Part One, Chapters 1 through 3, addresses substrates. Chapter 1 provides basic definitions of motor speech disorders (the dysarthrias and apraxia of speech) and discusses their distinction from other speech abnormalities. Data from the Mayo Clinic speech pathology practice are reviewed, providing a sense of the prevalence and distribution of motor speech disorders in multidisciplinary medical practices. The chapter also provides an overview of perceptual, acoustic, and physiologic methods for studying motor speech

disorders. Finally, it reviews approaches to characterizing the disorders and introduces the categorization scheme developed by Darley, Aronson, and Brown as the book's vehicle for discussing the dysarthrias.

Chapter 2 reviews the neurologic bases of motor speech and its pathologies. It focuses on structures and functions that are important to speech, the pathologies that may produce motor speech disorders, and some of the physical and behavioral deficits that may accompany motor speech disorders. Its discussion of the relationship of motor speech to the nervous system's final common pathway, direct and indirect activation pathways, and control circuits provides a foundation for understanding the distinctions among the major categories of motor speech disorders that are addressed in subsequent chapters.

Chapter 3 addresses the examination of motor speech disorders. It reviews the purposes of examination, particularly as it relates to differential diagnosis. Clinical examination is reviewed in detail, including history taking, evaluation of each component of the speech mechanism during nonspeech activities, the perceptual analysis of speech, intelligibility assessment, and acoustic and physiologic assessment.

Part Two, Chapters 4 through 15, focuses on the disorders and their diagnoses. Chapters 4 through 11 address the major types of dysarthria (including flaccid, spastic, ataxic, hypokinetic, hyperkinetic, unilateral upper motor neuron, and mixed dysarthrias) and apraxia of speech. Each chapter begins with a brief review of relevant neurologic and neuropathologic underpinnings and reviews some of the conditions that are commonly or relatively uniquely associated with the motor speech disorder under discussion. This is followed by a review of the etiology, localization, associated cognitive problems, and intelligibility for 56 to 300 quasirandomly selected cases with each type of motor speech disorder. Each chapter then discusses common patient perceptions and complaints, reviews confirmatory oral mechanism and related findings, and discusses in detail salient perceptual speech characteristics as well as associated acoustic and physiologic findings. Each chapter ends with 4 to 7 case studies that illustrate some of the major points made in the text. The case studies provide a sense of the clinical reality of the disorders, the ways in which knowledge is applied in clinical practice, and the value and shortcomings of the enterprise.

Chapter 12 addresses forms of neurogenic mutism that reflect severe motor speech disorders, aphasia, or nonaphasic cognitive and affective deficits. Chapter 13 addresses several neurogenic speech disturbances (acquired neurogenic stuttering, palilalia, echolalia, cognitive and affective disturbances, aphasia, pseudoforeign accent, and aprosodia) that have close or distant relationships to motor speech disorders. Both Chapters 12 and 13 end with several illustrative case studies.

One of the most challenging diagnostic problems in medical speech pathology practices involves the distinction between problems that reflect neuropathology and those that reflect psychopathology. Chapter 14 addresses acquired psychogenic speech disorders. It discusses their common etiologies and, on the basis of a review of 215 cases, describes their most common speech characteristics. The important aspects of history taking and the observations that contribute to diagnosis are reviewed. The variety of speech characteristics associated with psychogenic voice and fluency disorders, as well as less frequently occurring psychogenic articulation, resonance, and prosodic abnormalities are described. Several case studies show how people with these disorders sometimes present in clinical practice.

Chapter 15 provides general guidelines for differential diagnosis. It synthesizes and summarizes the information in Chapters 4 through 14 that is most important to differential diagnosis. It emphasizes distinctions among the dysarthrias, between dysarthrias and apraxia of speech, between motor speech disorders and aphasia, among different forms of mutism, between motor speech disorders and other neurogenic speech disorders, and between neurogenic and psychogenic speech disorders.

Part 3, Chapters 16 through 20, addresses management. Chapter 16 provides an overview of general principles for managing motor speech disorders. It discusses broad management goals, factors that influence management decisions, and the medical, prosthetic, behavioral, augmentative and alternative communication, and counseling and support aspects of management. It reviews in some detail principles and guidelines for behavioral treatment that can be applied to all motor speech disorders.

Chapter 17 focuses on management of the dysarthrias. It discusses speaker-oriented approaches that include medical, prosthetic, and behavioral interventions for improving respiration, phonation,

resonance, articulation, rate, and prosody. It also examines management in relation to specific types of dysarthria, highlighting the fact that differential diagnoses among the dysarthrias can influence management, and that some approaches are well suited to certain dysarthrias whereas other approaches are not. The chapter also addresses communication-oriented strategies that may be used by dysarthric speakers or their listeners to facilitate communication, independent of dysarthria type and changes in speech production per se. Chapter 18 follows a format similar to that of Chapters 16 and 17, but focuses specifically on apraxia of speech. It makes clear that dysarthrias and apraxia of speech share a number of management attributes but, because their underlying natures are fundamentally different, their management differs in a number of important ways.

Chapter 19 briefly discusses the management of the other neurogenic speech disturbances that are discussed in Chapter 13. In keeping with the primary focus of the book, it emphasizes treatment (or the inappropriateness of treatment) of the speech characteristics associated with them, rather than the affective, cognitive, or linguistic disturbances that may underlie some of them.

Chapter 20 addresses the management of acquired psychogenic speech disorders. Although verging on being tangential to the purposes of the book, this chapter is included because the frequent dramatically and rapidly successful management of psychogenic speech disorders can make a valuable contribution to diagnosis in cases where there is uncertainty about neurogenic versus psychogenic etiology. It is hoped that the chapter contributes to clinicians' differential diagnostic skills as well as their treatment skills.

The impetus for this book grew out of my desire to integrate what is known about the bases of motor speech disorders with the realities of my clinical practice in which differential diagnoses and management are the order of the day. I have learned a great deal while writing this book and have become a wiser and better clinician because of it, but I am more certain than ever that there is a lot to learn. Some of what I don't know can be found in the minds and daily practices of other clinicians, scientists, and scholars, and some of it represents unanswered or unformulated questions. I do hope that the facts and clinical observations and thoughts that are reflected in these pages provide a friendly learning vehicle for clinicians and researchers in training, a source of useful information for practicing clinicians and researchers, and some seeds of interest in increasing our understanding of these disorders and our ability to help people who have them.

Acknowledgments

Many people deserve recognition and my gratitude for their contributions to this book. The contributions have included mentorship, encouragement, feedback, sympathy, infusions of humor, and friendship that in some circles might be called psychotherapy. It is for others to judge the value of this work. It is for me to say thank you to those who helped me with it and to absolve them from responsibility for its shortcomings.

A number of people read drafts of portions of this book and made comments that I know have made it better. I thank Hugh Morris and Steven Leder, and especially Julie Liss and Vicki Hammen, for their helpful comments on drafts of the first 10 or 11 chapters. My colleague Jack Thomas deserves special thanks for his comments and suggestions on Chapter 6 and several of the management chapters. Richard Dewey provided useful comments and help with portions of Chapter 8. Several rating scales in Chapter 3 are better because of comments from my colleagues Bob Keith, Jack Thomas, Virginia Scardino, Marita Douglas, Bill McGann, and Gerry Werven. I thank Arnie Aronson for his comments on Chapter 9 and especially for his wise advice about how to think about writing a book and how best to communicate important information.

A number of people have served as my mentors over the years and the very special influences of Bob Duffy, Fred Darley, and Arnie Aronson float among these pages. The thousands of patients who have taught me about motor speech disorders, my colleagues in the Department of Neurology at the Mayo Clinic, and my colleagues and very good friends in my CAC family have all helped shape this book.

I also thank the staff at Mosby–Year Book for their help and support, especially Kellie White, Associate Developmental Editor. I greatly appreciate the valuable anatomic illustrations that were prepared by Bob Benassi; his pictures are worth many words. Jacque Trefz, secretary extraordinaire, has my eternal gratitude and respect for her competence, speed, spirit and endurance in the preparation of the book amidst the chaos of her regular responsibilities.

This book might not have been started or finished without the support, enthusiasm, and patience of my wife, friend, and colleague, Penny Myers. Her intangible gifts to me were matched by her comments and editorial suggestions for more chapters than anyone else could be coerced to read. My thanks also to Matt and Melanie for understanding my absence on weekends and for their frequent and enthusiastic "How's the book?"

Contents

PART ONE

Substrates

1 Defining, Understanding, and Categorizing Motor Speech Disorders

Chapter Outline

Speech is a unique, complex, dynamic motor activity through which we express our thoughts and emotions and respond to and control our environment. It is among the most powerful tools possessed by our species, and the degree to which we employ it effectively contributes to the character and quality of our lives.

Under most circumstances, the form and content of adults' speech is achieved with an ease that belies the complexity of the operations underlying them. Studying normal speech processes helps establish the enormity of the act. Unfortunately, neurologic disease can also unmask the complex underpinnings of speech by disturbing its expression in a wide variety of predictable ways. These disturbances, the mechanisms that help to explain them, the signs and symptoms that define them, and their management are the subjects of this book.

THE NEUROLOGIC PROCESS OF SPEECH PRODUCTION

Normal speech requires the integrity and integration of a number of cognitive, neuromuscular, and musculoskeletal activities. These activities can be summarized, in a very basic way, as follows:

1. Thoughts, feelings, and emotions must generate an intent to communicate and then be organized and converted to verbal symbols in a manner that abides by the rules of language. These activities will be referred to as *cognitive-linguistic processes*.

2. The intended verbal message must be organized for neuromuscular execution. This activity includes the selection and organization of sensorimotor "programs" that will activate the speech muscles at appropriate coarticulated times, durations, and intensities. This process will be referred to as *motor speech programming*.

3. Central and peripheral nervous system activity must execute speech motor programs by innervating the respiratory, phonatory, resonatory, and articulatory muscles in a manner that generates an acoustic signal that faithfully reflects the goals of the programs. The neuromuscular transmission and subsequent muscle contractions and movements of speech structures will be referred to as *neuromuscular execution*.

The combined processes of speech motor programming and neuromuscular execution will be referred to as *motor speech processes*.

THE NEUROLOGIC BREAKDOWN OF SPEECH PRODUCTION

When the nervous system becomes disordered, so may the production of speech. In fact, changes in speech may announce the presence of neurologic disease. The effects of neuropathology on speech are often lawful, predictable, and clinically unique and recognizable. The recognition and understanding of predictable patterns of speech disturbance and their underlying neurophysiologic bases are valuable for at least three reasons

1. *Understanding nervous system organization for speech motor control.* The predictable association of patterns of speech deficit with localizable nervous system pathology can contribute to our understanding of the nervous system's anatomic and physiologic organization for motor speech control and its relationship to the control of other motor activities. Just as the study of aphasia has taught us something about the organization and localization of cognitive-linguistic processes associated with language behavior, the study of motor speech disorders informs us about the physiology and localization of speech production.

2. *Differential diagnosis and localization of neurologic disease.* The correlation of speech deficits with pathology in different portions of the nervous system can contribute to the identification and localization of neurologic disease. The importance of this has been traditionally undervalued. Aronson (1987) called the contribution of speech diagnosis to medical diagnosis "one of the best-kept secrets of our time" (p. 36), something usually ignored by both speech pathology and medicine. Because speech changes can be the *first* or *only* manifestation of both organic and psychiatric disease, recognition of these changes can have a significant impact on medical diagnosis and care. This necessitates modification of the attitude that speech diagnosis should always follow medical/neurologic diagnosis, and that speech-language pathology diagnosis is always isolated from medical diagnostic and management efforts. Our knowledge has reached a point where the clinical diagnosis of motor speech disorders can be considered valuable to *neurologic localization and diagnosis.* This value will hopefully be made clear in many of the succeeding chapters, especially within the context of some illustrative case histories.

3. *Management.* The identification of deviant speech characteristics, their localization to respiration, phonation, resonance, articulation, or prosody, and an understanding of their likely neuropathophysiology can provide important clues for management. For example, knowing that an individual's articulatory distortions are primarily related to incoordination, and not to weakness, might lead to efforts to facilitate coordination (for example, by modifying rate and prosody), rather than attempts to increase strength through exercise.

BASIC DEFINITIONS

It is necessary to define some terms that will be used throughout this book to refer to certain neurologically based disturbances of speech. For those learning about these disorders for the first time, the definitions will provide a framework for beginning to think about them. For those more familiar with the topic, the definitions will establish boundaries of meaning that are sometimes blurred in the medical and speech pathology literature.

Dysarthria

The work of Darley, Aronson, and Brown (1969a & b; 1975) provided the modern refinement of the definition of dysarthria and is nearly universally accepted by speech-language pathologists and many neurologists. They defined dysarthria as:

... a collective name for a group of speech disorders resulting from disturbances in muscular control over the speech mechanism due to damage of the central or peripheral nervous system. It designates problems in oral communication due to paralysis, weakness, or incoordination of the speech musculature (1969a, p. 246).

This definition explicitly recognizes or implies that the disorder:

1. is neurologic in origin, and associated with pathology of central and/or peripheral nervous system structures involved in motor activities.

2. is a disorder of movement due to abnormal neuromuscular execution that may affect the speed, strength, range, timing, or accuracy of speech movements. It can affect respiration, phonation, resonance, articulation, and prosody, either singly or in combination.

3. often can be categorized further. Because dysarthria is a collective label, it can be subdivided into different types, each type characterized by distinguishable auditory perceptual characteristics and, presumably, by different underlying neuropathophysiology. The ability to categorize the dysarthrias, therefore, has implications for the localization of the lesion leading to the particular dysarthria type.

The definition of dysarthria used here is considerably more narrow and refined than common medical dictionary definitions. For example, some physicians use the term dysarthria generically to refer to any disturbance of articulation or speech (for example, Metter, 1985). Others use it to refer to any neurogenic disturbance of speech or language, failing to distinguish it from aphasia, apraxia of speech, and other neurogenic communication disorders. Such broad, vague definitions weaken the differential diagnostic and conceptual value of the term, and should be avoided in research and clinical practice.

Apraxia of speech

Darley (1965) was a major force in developing the modern concept of apraxia of speech. His work, and that of many others, have helped establish an accepted definition for the disorder. Apraxia of speech can be defined as *a neurogenic speech disorder resulting from impairment of the capacity to program sensorimotor commands for the positioning and movement of muscles for the volitional production of speech. It can occur without significant weakness or neuromuscular slowness, and in the absence of disturbances of conscious thought or language.* This definition is largely consistent with those used by Darley, Aronson, and Brown (1975) and Wertz, LaPointe, and Rosenbek (1984).

Unlike dysarthria, apraxia of speech rarely is too broadly defined. In fact, its existence as a distinct clinical entity is often ignored outside the speech pathology literature. Consequently, its clinical manifestations are frequently buried within categories of aphasia or under the generic heading of dysarthria. This is unfortunate for a number of reasons, but especially because the localization of apraxia of speech is different than that for most types of dysarthria, and because its management is different from that for dysarthria and aphasia.

Motor speech disorders

Motor speech disorders can be defined as *disorders of speech resulting from neurologic impairment affecting the motor programming or neuromuscular execution of speech. They encompass apraxia of speech and the dysarthrias.*

SPEECH DISTURBANCES THAT ARE DISTINGUISHABLE FROM MOTOR SPEECH DISORDERS
Other neurologic disorders

Other neurogenic speech disturbances. There are several forms of disturbed speech that neither clearly represent nor traditionally have been defined as motor speech disorders. They are nonetheless neurologic in origin and distinct in their clinical characteristics. These deficits include but are probably not limited to: acquired neurogenic stuttering-like behavior; palilalia; echolalia; certain forms of mutism; pseudo-foreign dialect; and so-called "aprosodia" associated with right hemisphere dysfunction. These disorders will be discussed in Chapter 13, which focuses on neurogenic speech disturbances not typically categorized under the headings of dysarthria or apraxia of speech.

Cognitive, linguistic, and cognitive-linguistic disturbances. Changes in speech resulting from linguistic and other cognitive deficits (for example, aphasia, akinetic mutism, other cognitive and affective disturbances that attenuate or inhibit speech) are sometimes difficult to distinguish from motor speech disorders. In addition, because they often co-occur with motor speech disorders, they

may make the speech examination and diagnosis of the motor speech disorder difficult. Chapter 15 will address the distinctions among motor speech disorders, aphasia, and other neurogenic speech and cognitive-linguistic disturbances that may influence the perceptual characteristics of speech and complicate differential diagnosis.

Sensory deficits. The emphasis on the motor aspects of speech in this book is not intended to minimize the importance of sensory processes in speech production or the potential impact of sensory disturbances on speech. The effect of congenital deafness, for example, on the development of speech is devastating; even deafness acquired in adulthood can result in some degradation of speech. The effects of hearing loss on speech production, however, are distinguishable in a number of ways from motor speech disorders and will not be discussed further in this book.

Tactile, kinesthetic, and proprioceptive sensation are also important to the development and maintenance of normal speech, and their malfunction has been implicated in certain motor speech disorders (the role of sensation in movement control will be discussed in Chapter 2). It is, therefore, important to think of motor speech processes and disorders as sensorimotor and not just motor in character. Although it is not the intent of this book to discuss speech deficits resulting from primary tactile, kinesthetic, or proprioceptive disturbances, there will be some brief discussion of "sensory dysarthria" in Chapters 4 (Flaccid Dysarthria) and 6 (Ataxic Dysarthria), and the possible influence of sensory disturbances on apraxia of speech in Chapter 11 (Apraxia of Speech).

Non-neurogenic disturbances

There are influences on speech production that are not encompassed by cognitive-linguistic or motor speech processes. Some are clearly localized outside of the nervous system. Others reside in the "mind" but are neither neuromotor nor specifically cognitive-linguistic in character. These influences are discussed briefly in the following paragraphs.

Musculoskeletal defects (for example, laryngectomee, cleft lip and palate, fractures, abnormal variants in cavity size and shape). The integrity of muscle, cartilage, and bone is crucial to normal speech; injury, disease, congenital absence, loss to aging or poor care (for example, teeth) or surgical removal of muscle, cartilage, and bone can alter speech. Other physical influences, such as abnormal variations in the size and shape of the primary speech structures or the effects of systemic illness, can also alter speech in ways that exceed, mask, or exacerbate the effects of focal neuropathologies on speech. The reader's awareness of these factors is assumed and will not be discussed further in any detail.

Non-neurogenic/non-psychogenic voice disorders. Certain voice disorders could actually be subsumed under the musculoskeletal defects described in the preceding section. They are given separate recognition here, however, because they are often more difficult to distinguish from motor speech disorders and sometimes are misinterpreted as reflecting neuropathology. These include, for example, dysphonias associated with vocal cord bowing, hormonal disturbances, head/neck neoplasms, and vocal abuse. The diagnosis may be established by history or during physical examination, and the experienced clinician can often hear that the dysphonia is not neurogenic. These disorders will not be addressed in detail in this book but will receive some recognition in Chapter 3.*

Psychogenic disorders. Speech can undergo change as a result of abnormal psychological states (for example, schizophrenia, depression, conversion disorder). The speech manifestations of these psychogenic disorders are often difficult to distinguish from those stemming from neurologic disease. Because psychological disorders reside in the mind, arguably they are fundamentally neurologic (if one believes that the mind and brain are inextricably linked). Because they are not primarily neuromotor in nature, however, it is important to distinguish them from motor speech disorders.

Psychogenic voice and speech disorders are commonly encountered in neurologic practice and they not infrequently accompany neurologic disturbance. They will be discussed in some detail in Chapters 14 (Acquired Psychogenic Speech Disturbances) and 20 (Managing Acquired Psychogenic Speech Disorders).

Normal variations in speech production

Age-related changes in speech. Normal aging is associated with changes in speech that are physiologically, acoustically, and perceptually detectable. These include, at the least, changes in pitch, voice quality, rate, and prosodic variations (see Beaseley and Davis, 1981, for a review of age related speech changes). Some of these changes can be similar to the salient features of some forms of dysarthria; therefore, the identification of a speech characteristic as "deviant," and possibly indicative of dysarthria, often may depend on an awareness of the range of normal for the patient's age, sex, and general physical condition. Unfortunately, many of these judgments are dependent on

subjective clinical experience because objective measures and life span norms are either not available or are associated with extreme variability of normative data.

Variations in style. The qualitative character of speech varies as a function of normal differences in personality, assumed speaking roles, and emotional state. Such variations often and justifiably go unnoticed by clinicians and researchers intent upon recognizing pathology, but they sometimes must be identified explicitly for accurate diagnosis.

PREVALENCE AND DISTRIBUTION OF MOTOR SPEECH DISORDERS

The incidence and prevalence of motor speech disorders in the population are uncertain. Based on the prevalence of stroke alone, and their common association with stroke and certain other neurologic diseases, motor speech disorders are undoubtedly common in neurologic practice. It has been estimated, for example, that about 60% of noncomatose people who have had strokes suffer from some kind of speech or language impairment (Weinfeld, 1981). Therefore, motor speech disorders probably represent a significant proportion of the communication disorders seen in medical speech-language pathology practices (Yorkston, Beukelman, & Bell, 1988).

The representation of motor speech disorders among acquired communication disorders can be estimated by examining their proportionate distribution in a speech-language pathology practice within a large inpatient and outpatient medical institution. Figure 1–1 summarizes the distribution of acquired communication disorders seen in the Section of Speech Pathology in the Department of Neurology at the Mayo Clinic between 1987–90.* The data indicate that motor speech disorders

---

*See Aronson (1990) for a comprehensive review of all varieties of voice disorders.

---

*The data base is derived from speech pathology diagnostic consultations for outpatients and patients in two acute care hospitals and a rehabilitation unit. The diagnostic categories represent patients' primary communication disorder (many patients had more than one type of communication problem). The sample from which the data are derived is probably not representative of that seen in many speech pathology practices. That is, the majority of outpatient evaluations were conducted as part of patients' medical diagnostic evaluations and not necessarily as part of a rehabilitation program; this was also true for a substantial proportion of individuals in the acute hospital settings. Patient referrals came from many medical subspecialties, but most from neurology, otorhinolaryngology, neurosurgery, physical medicine, and internal medicine. Some outpatients were self-referred. The sample is probably fairly representative of the distribution of acute, progressive, and chronic acquired communication disorders (with the exception of those related to hearing loss) in large combined primary and tertiary care inpatient and outpatient medical practices.

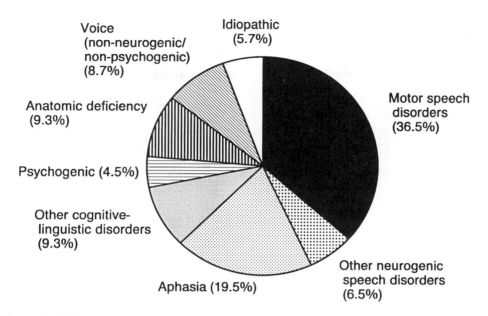

Figure 1–1 Distribution of acquired communication disorders, Speech Pathology, Dept. of Neurology, Mayo Clinic, 1987–90. Based on 4,756 evaluations of people with a primary speech pathology diagnosis of acquired communication disorder. Referrals were derived primarily from neurology, otorhinolaryngology, neurosurgery, physical medicine, internal medicine, and self-referred patients. Numbers reflect diagnostic consultations and not number of patients receiving treatment.

Motor speech disorders include dysarthrias and apraxia of speech. *Aphasia* includes all types of acquired aphasia. *Other neurogenic speech disorders* include: stuttering-like behavior; aprosodia; spastic dysphonia associated with tremor and other movement disorders; central nervous system mutism, aphonia and reduced loudness; and speech deficits associated with sensory disturbances. *Other cognitive-linguistic disorders* include: dementia; confusion; cognitive communication deficits associated with traumatic brain injury; alexia with or without agraphia; specific memory loss; ictal speech arrest; neurogenic language disorder of undetermined type. *Anatomic deficiency* includes laryngectomy and glossectomy. *Voice (non-neurogenic/non-psychogenic)* disorders include etiologies of: vocal abuse; papilloma; intubation and tracheostomy; vocal cord bowing; hormonal imbalance; neoplasm; acromegaly; and surgery. *Psychogenic* includes speech disorders characterized by: mutism; aphonia and dysphonia; spastic dysphonia; dysprosody; stuttering-like behavior; infantile speech; articulation disturbance; foreign accent; high pitch; and abnormal loudness. Idiopathic disorders (i.e., of unknown etiology) include: dysphonias; stridor; palilalia; monopitch; pseudoforeign accent; stuttering-like behavior.

represent a substantial proportion of the acquired speech, voice, language, and cognitive-communication disturbances referred for diagnostic assessment. However, these figures may not represent the "true" distribution of these disturbances in a large medical practice. For example, it is possible that the distribution in Figure 1–1 represents only those cases in which a speech-language pathology evaluation was considered necessary for medical diagnosis or for clinical management recommendations.

Figure 1–2 isolates from Figure 1–1 the acquired neurogenic communication disorders. Motor speech disorders (dysarthrias and apraxia of speech) account for about 50% of the primary

diagnoses, far more prevalent than any other category, including aphasia. Again, this distribution probably reflects the relative importance or value placed upon accurate differential diagnosis of motor speech disorders plus recommendations for management, as opposed to referral for management recommendations alone.

These data testify to the prominence of motor speech disorders among acquired communication disorders encountered in comprehensive medical speech pathology practices and, probably, neurology practices. They justify ongoing laboratory and applied research and the development of clinical diagnostic and management expertise in the area of motor speech disorders.

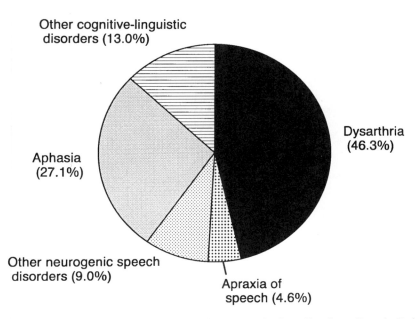

Figure 1–2 Distribution of acquired neurogenic communication disorders, Speech Pathology, Dept. of Neurology, Mayo Clinic, 1987–90. Based on 3,417 evaluations of people whose primary speech pathology diagnosis was an acquired neurogenic communication disorder.

    Dysarthria includes all dysarthria types. *Apraxia of speech* includes acquired apraxia of speech. *Other neurogenic speech disorders* include: stuttering-like behavior; aprosodia; spastic dysphonia associated with tremor and other movement disorders; central nervous system mutism, aphonia, and reduced loudness; and speech deficits associated with sensory disturbances. *Aphasia* includes all types of acquired aphasia. *Other cognitive-linguistic disturbances* include: dementia; confusion; cognitive communication deficits associated with traumatic brain injury; alexia with or without agraphia; specific memory loss; ictal speech arrest; and neurogenic language disorder of undetermined type.

METHODS FOR STUDYING AND CATEGORIZING MOTOR SPEECH DISORDERS

Motor speech disorders can be studied in a number of ways, all of which contribute to their characterization. The methods can be categorized under three broad headings: perceptual, acoustic, and physiologic.

Perceptual methods

Perceptual methods are based primarily on the auditory-perceptual attributes of speech. They are the "gold standard" for clinical differential diagnosis, judgments of severity, many decisions about management, and the assessment of functional change. At the same time, they are subject to unreliability of judgments among clinicians, they may be difficult to quantify, and they cannot directly test hypotheses about the pathophysiology underlying perceived speech abnormalities. In the hands (ears, eyes, and hands, actually) of experienced clinicians, however, the auditory-perceptual

classification of motor speech disorders is a valid and valuable diagnostic and clinical decision-making tool. It is unlikely that it ever will be replaced by other methods, however sophisticated, because the evaluation of a speech disorder always begins with the perceptual judgment by someone that speech is abnormal or different in some way.

    Darley, Aronson, and Brown (1969a & b; 1975) pioneered the modern use of auditory perceptual assessment to characterize the dysarthrias and to identify the clusters of salient perceptual characteristics that are associated with lesions in different portions of the central and peripheral nervous system. It is their approach to classifying the dysarthrias that is used today by most clinicians charged with differential diagnosis. It is also used by many researchers investigating the underlying acoustic and physiologic bases of motor speech disorders. In fact, one outcome of the work of Darley, Aronson, and Brown was the generation of a number of hypotheses about the physiological bases of the dysarthrias. Their hypotheses grew out of an integration of the perceptual characteristics identified in their studies with what was known (or believed) about the general role played by damaged portions of the nervous system in movement control. They have helped set the direction of acoustic and physiologic studies, the results of which are often interpreted in reference to the clinical hypotheses. With remarkable frequency, acoustic and physiologic studies have confirmed and further refined the perceptually based hypotheses of Darley, Aronson, and Brown.

The auditory modality has been the focus of research into the perceptual characteristics of the dysarthrias, but the value of visual and tactile observations in clinical assessment should not be ignored. Although dysarthria is a speech phenomenon, and therefore cannot be diagnosed solely on the basis of visual or tactile observation, such observations can provide valuable confirmatory evidence for diagnosis. For example, unilateral upper and lower facial weakness, tongue atrophy and fasciculations, and inability to puff the cheeks without occluding the nares all are suggestive of lower motor neuron weakness; they help support a diagnosis of flaccid dysarthria when deviant speech characteristics are logically associated with them. If the patient's speech does not reflect a flaccid dysarthria, the visual observations nonetheless need explanation, both for their lack of relevance to the speech diagnosis and for their relevance to neurologic diagnosis. Therefore, visual and tactile observations of the speech mechanism at rest, during nonspeech movement, and during speech are an important component of the motor speech examination.

Acoustic methods

Acoustic analyses have proven valuable to the more complete understanding of motor speech disorders. They can contribute to the acoustic quantification and description of clinically perceived deviant speech. They provide confirmatory support for perceptual judgments that speech rate is slow, voice is breathy or contains tremor or interruptions, pitch and loudness variability are reduced, resonance is hypernasal, articulation is imprecise, speech diadochokinetic rates are irregular, and so on. Their capacity to make visible and quantify the speech signal can be used as baseline data and an index of stability, improvement, or deterioration over time, and may serve a useful role in providing feedback during management activities. Specific acoustic attributes of speech associated with motor speech disorders will be addressed in those chapters dealing with each of

the dysarthrias and apraxia of speech.

State-of-the-art instrumentation for acoustic analysis has become increasingly affordable and accessible to practicing clinicians in recent years. Use of instrumentation no longer need be restricted to research laboratories, and it is likely that the direct clinical relevance and applicability of acoustic analysis will increase in the future. Acoustic analysis has obvious descriptive value for the assessment and monitoring of motor speech disorders. Whether or not it will eventually add to or modify diagnoses based on auditory-perceptual judgments has yet to be determined.

Physiologic methods

Auditory-perceptual and acoustic analyses, by definition, are focused on the signal emitted from the vocal tract. Physiologic analyses move "upstream" toward the source of activity that generates the speech signal and, therefore, represent another level of explanation. They focus on the movements of speech structures and air, the muscle contractions that generate movement, the relationships among movements and muscle contractions at different levels of the musculoskeletal speech mechanism, the temporal parameters and relationships among central and peripheral neural activity and biomechanical activity, and the temporal relationships among central nervous system structures that are active during the planning and execution of speech. Physiologic studies have addressed whether certain speech characteristics reflect weakness, spasticity, incoordination, reduced range of movement and the like, and on the specific muscles and dynamics of movement in which those characteristics are reflected.

Physiologic analyses have increased our understanding of speech motor control and its various pathophysiologic breakdowns. They have refined and sometimes challenged perceptually based explanations for the pathophysiology of certain motor speech disorders. Physiologic analyses have also been valuable in examining whether certain disorders reflect linguistic, motor programming, or neuromuscular deficits, distinctions that can be very difficult or impossible on the basis of clinical perceptual assessment alone. Similar to acoustic methods, they may represent an important source of feedback during management efforts. Finally, Putnam (1988) has argued that physiologic measurements "will insure that treatment is based on evidence of, rather than inferencing about, underlying pathophysiology" (p. 109). Specific physiologic measures of speech used to study motor speech disorders will be addressed in those chapters dealing with the dysarthrias and apraxia of speech.

The physiological study of motor speech disorders has much to offer the quantification, description, understanding, and perhaps management of motor speech disorders. Similar to acoustic analyses, however, its contribution to clinical diagnosis beyond that which can be derived from clinical perceptual assessment is not yet established.

The clinical salience of the perceptual analysis of motor speech disorders

The emphasis in this book will be on clinical perceptual assessment and the auditory perceptual and pragmatic outcomes of management for motor speech disorders. This emphasis does not reflect a conclusion that acoustic and physiologic approaches are unimportant to understanding motor speech disorders, or that they cannot be valuable to clinical practice. In fact, frequent reference will be made to the contributions of those methods and their relationship to perceptual observations and hypotheses. The emphasis on perceptual assessment derives from several beliefs:

1. The evaluation of the person with a suspected motor speech disorder *begins* with a perceptually based assessment of speech. Any acoustic or physiologic assessment that may follow is motivated and directed by the results of the perceptually based assessment. If descriptive or diagnostic errors are made at this entry point, whatever follows may be misguided and misleading, both to diagnosis and management.

2. The usefulness of perceptually based differential diagnosis, relative to its contribution to localization and diagnosis of neurologic disease, has been established. The degree to which other methods add to, modify, contradict, or contribute equally to that effort is not yet clear. Again, this does not minimize the contribution of acoustic and physiologic methods to the description, understanding, and quantification of motor speech disorders. It does, however, argue for perceptually based methods as the *foundation of clinical practice*.

3. The standard for judging the functional outcome of management of motor speech disorders is based primarily on judgments of auditory-perceptual and communicative effectiveness.

CATEGORIZING MOTOR SPEECH DISORDERS
Characterizing motor speech disorders

Motor speech disorders vary along a number of dimensions and this variance has generated different categorization schemes. Darley, Aronson, and Brown (1975) and Yorkston, Beukelman, and Bell (1988) identified dimensions that characterize motor speech disorders and are important to both diagnosis and management. Some dimensions reflect a neurologic and etiologic approach to classification. Others are specifically tied to the signs and symptoms of the speech disorders themselves.

Variables relevant to neurologic and etiologic perspectives include:

1. *Age at onset.* Motor speech disorders can be congenital or acquired. This distinction can be reflected in patient behaviors and can impact on management decisions and prognosis. Time of onset in acquired disorders is almost always clear in adults, usually (but not always) obvious in children, and rarely challenges clinical diagnosis beyond a careful history and neurologic examination. It is important for clinicians to recognize the distinction, but not usually a challenge to establish.

   The focus of this book will be on acquired rather than congenital disorders. This reflects: (a) an orientation to the contribution of differential diagnosis of motor speech disorders to medical diagnosis and localization (a challenge more pervasive for acquired than congenital disorders), and (b) the greater wealth of information on differential diagnosis and management in adults. However, it is likely that many of the principles of classification, diagnosis, and management discussed in this book can be applied or adapted to children with congenital and acquired motor speech disorders.

2. *Course.* Motor speech disorders can usually be characterized as: *congenital* (for example, as in cerebral palsy); *chronic* or *stationary* (for example, cerebral palsy in adults, after plateauing has occurred in stroke); *improving* (for example, during spontaneous recovery from stroke or closed head injury); *progressive* or *degenerative* (for example, amyotrophic lateral sclerosis or Parkinson's disease); or *exacerbating-remitting* (for example, multiple sclerosis). Monitoring motor speech disorders over time may actually establish the course of disease or help eliminate diagnoses incompatible with a particular course. In many cases, the course is already established. Nonetheless, knowledge of the course of a problem has an important influence on management decisions.

3. *Site of lesion.* Lesions associated with motor speech disorders can occur in many locations. They include such diverse loci as the neuromuscular junction, the peripheral and cranial nerves, the brainstem, the cerebellum, the pyramidal and extrapyramidal pathways, and the

cerebral cortex. Establishing site of lesion is a primary goal of neurologic evaluation and one to which differential diagnosis of motor speech disorders can contribute. Knowledge of site of lesion can predict certain speech deficits. Incompatability of speech findings with known or postulated lesion sites can raise doubts about presumed localization or suggest the presence of additional lesions or even different diseases. (For example, the presence of a mixed hypokinetic-spastic-ataxic dysarthria in someone with a diagnosis of Parkinson's disease should raise questions about the neurologic diagnosis or suggest the presence of neurologic dysfunction beyond that explainable by Parkinson's disease alone).

4. *Neurologic diagnosis*. Broad categories of neurologic disease include vascular, degenerative, inflammatory, neoplastic, toxic-metabolic, traumatic, and congenital-developmental etiologies. Within each of the broad categories, more specific diagnoses often can be applied.

A motor speech disorder, by itself, usually is not diagnostic of a particular broad neurologic etiology or specific disease. Because many diseases can affect multiple and variable portions of the nervous system, it is neither valid nor feasible to classify motor speech disorders by disease (for example, "the dysarthria of multiple sclerosis"). At the same time, some dysarthria types are found very commonly in some neurologic diseases and rarely or never in others. Therefore, identification of a specific motor speech disorder may provide confirmatory (compatible) evidence for disease diagnosis or cast doubt on other diagnostic possibilities.

5. *Pathophysiology*. Presumably, it is the underlying pathophysiology (weakness, spasticity, etc.) that determines the deviant perceptual features of speech in motor speech disorders. Therefore, the presence of certain abnormalities of speech suggest one or more pathophysiologic disturbance and vice versa.

Factors relevant to the speech disorders themselves include:

1. *Speech components involved*. Motor speech disorders can be categorized on the basis of the components of the speech system that are affected. Knowing whether respiration, phonation, resonance, or articulation are affected can make important contributions to speech diagnosis and nearly always has an impact on management decisions.

2. *Severity*. Severity usually does not differentiate among motor speech disorders because all of them vary along the severity continuum. Severity can raise questions about diagnosis, however. For example, deviant speech characteristics suggestive of profound weakness leading to severe reduction in intelligibility are usually accompanied by physical findings that confirm the weakness; if the physical examination is incompatible with underlying weakness, it may be necessary to consider psychogenic etiology.

Determining severity is always crucial to management decisions. Severity, coupled with information about diagnosis and course of disease, helps determine when management is necessary, whether it will be short- or long-term, whether it should focus on improving speech or developing augmentative forms of communication, and so on.

3. *Perceptual characteristics*. The perceptual characteristics of speech have already been discussed as factors crucial to differential diagnosis and management. Because it has a firm grounding in clinical research, because it has been so heuristically valuable to the acoustic and physiologic study of motor speech disorders, and because it is so salient to daily clinical activity, the perceptually based classification scheme of Darley, Aronson, and Brown (1975) will form the framework around which motor speech disorders will be discussed in this book.

The perceptual method of classification

Table 1–1 summarizes the classification scheme that will be used in this book. It was developed by Darley, Aronson, and Brown in their influential studies of the dysarthrias (1969a & b) and in their now classic book *Motor Speech Disorders* (1975).

Darley, Aronson, and Brown studied six major types of dysarthria (flaccid, spastic, ataxic, hypokinetic, hyperkinetic, and mixed), with the implication that the category of mixed dysarthria could include a large number of different combinations of single dysarthria types. This is certainly the case in a number of combinations that were described by the above mentioned and subsequent investigators (they will be discussed in Chapter 10, Mixed Dysarthrias).

Two categories have been added since earlier versions of Table 1–1. Unilateral upper motor neuron dysarthria was alluded to by Darley, Aronson, and Brown (1975) but not specifically studied by them in their 1969 work. It does, however, occur commonly in patients with unilateral hemispheric lesions, often co-occurs with aphasia and apraxia of speech, and is considered a sign (sometimes the only sign) of unilateral stroke by neurologists. It has, therefore, been added as a dysarthria type and will be discussed as such in Chapter 9.

The category of type Undetermined has also been added. It is included to recognize explicitly

Table 1–1 Major types of motor speech disorders (dysarthrias and apraxia of speech).

Type	Localization	Neuromotor basis
Dysarthria		
Flaccid	Lower motor neuron (final common pathway, motor unit)	Weakness
Spastic	Bilat. upper motor neuron (direct & indirect activation pathways)	Spasticity
Ataxic	Cerebellum (cerebellar control circuit)	Incoordination
Hypokinetic	Basal ganglia control circuit (extrapyramidal)	Rigidity/reduced range of movement
Hyperkinetic	Basal ganglia control circuit (extrapyramidal)	Involuntary movements
Unilateral upper motor neuron	Unilateral upper motor neuron	Weakness/? incoordination
Mixed	More than one	More than one
Undetermined	?	?
Apraxia of Speech	Left (dominant) hemisphere	Motor programming

Adapted from the work of Darley FL, Aronson AE, and Brown JR: Differential diagnostic patterns of dysarthrias, J Speech Hear Res 12:246, 1969a; Clusters of deviant speech dimensions in the dysarthrias, J Speech Hear Res 12:462, 1969b; and Motor Speech Disorders, Philadelphia, 1975, WB Saunders.

that perhaps not all perceptually distinct dysarthria types have been recognized, and that further subcategorization of already recognized dysarthrias may someday be justified (in fact, it is currently appropriate to subcategorize certain of the hyperkinetic dysarthrias). The category also recognizes that although a speech disorder may be recognized as a neurogenic motor speech disorder, its manifestations may be sufficiently subtle, complicated, or unusual to lead to a diagnosis of "motor speech disorder, type undetermined," perhaps with qualifiers that rule out what the clinician is certain the nature of the disorder is not. Figure 1–3 summarizes the distribution of motor speech disorders seen in the Section of Speech Pathology in the Department of Neurology at the Mayo Clinic between 1987 and 1990.

SUMMARY

1. Neurologic disease can affect motor speech processes in a manner that reflects the localization and underlying pathophysiology of the neurologic disturbance. These speech disturbances can be perceptually distinct, and their recognition can contribute to the localization and diagnosis of neurologic illness. Their recognition can also contribute to our knowledge about the neural organization and control of normal speech and to clinical management decisions.

2. The breakdown of motor speech can reflect disturbances in motor programming or neuromuscular execution. They are designated apraxia of speech and dysarthria, respectively. These disorders are distinct from one another and also distinct from speech abnormalities attributable to sensory deficits, other neurogenic disturbances that affect communication, musculoskeletal defects, psychopathology, age-related speech changes, and variations attributable to style and personality.

3. Motor speech disorders are not unusual in medical practice and are probably common in neurologic practice. They probably represent a substantial proportion of the communication disorders seen in medical speech pathology practices, especially practices in which differential diagnosis is valued as a measure of the presence and localization of disease.

4. Motor speech disorders may be studied perceptually, acoustically, and physiologically. Each method contributes to our understanding of the disorders. The perceptual analysis of salient speech characteristics currently is the first and

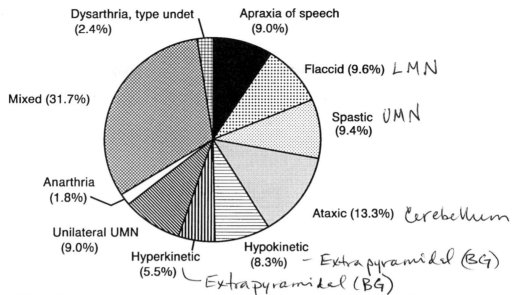

Figure 1–3 Distribution of motor speech disorders, Speech Pathology, Dept. of Neurology, Mayo Clinic, 1987–90. Based on 1,738 evaluations of people whose primary speech pathology diagnosis was a neurogenic motor speech disorder.

most important contributor to diagnosis and measures of functional change in response to management.

5. The perceptual method for classifying motor speech disorders developed by Darley, Aronson, and Brown reflects presumed underlying pathophysiology and it correlates with nervous system localization of lesion. It has clinical utility and considerable heuristic value for clinical and laboratory research. It will form the framework for the discussion of diagnosis and management in the remainder of this book.

REFERENCES

Aronson AE: Clinical voice disorders, New York, 1990, Thieme.

Aronson AE: The clinical Ph.D.: implication for the survival and liberation of communicative disorders as a health care profession, Asha Nov:35, 1987.

Beaseley DS and Davis GA: Aging: communication processes and disorders, New York, 1981, Grune and Stratton.

Darley FL: Lacunae and research approaches to them. In Milliken C and Darley FL, editors: Brain mechanisms underlying speech and language, New York, 1967, Grune and Stratton.

Darley FL, Aronson AE, and Brown JR: Clusters of deviant speech dimensions in the dysarthrias, J Speech Hear Res 12:462, 1969b.

Darley FL, Aronson AE, and Brown JR: Differential diagnostic patterns of dysarthria, J Speech Hear Res 12:246, 1969a.

Darley FL, Aronson AE, and Brown JR: Motor Speech Disorders, Philadelphia, 1975, WB Saunders.

Metter EJ: Speech disorders, New York, 1985, WB Saunders.

Putnam AHB: Review of research in dysarthria. In Winitz H, editor: Human communication and its disorders: a review— 1988, Norwood, NJ, 1988, Ablex Publishing.

Weinfeld F: The 1981 national survey of stroke, Stroke 1:1, 1981.

Wertz RT, LaPointe LL, and Rosenbek JC: Apraxia of speech in adults: the disorder and its management, New York, 1984, Grune and Stratton.

Yorkston KM, Beukelman D, and Bell K: Clinical management of dysarthric speakers, San Diego, 1988, College-Hill Press.

2 Neurologic Bases of Motor Speech and its Pathologies

Knowledge of neuroanatomy and neurophysiology is the foundation for differential diagnosis and management of motor speech disorders. An examination of that foundation, together with a brief overview of neuropathologies, is the purpose of this chapter.

It is not the intent here to present an in-depth view of neuroanatomy, neurophysiology, or the neuroscience of speech. Instead, this broad overview will be clinically oriented and applicable to information in subsequent chapters on specific motor speech disorders. The structures and functions that will be emphasized are those that: (1) are directly implicated in motor speech activity; (2) are relevant to understanding the mechanisms by which motor speech disorders may be produced; and (3) are relevant to physical and behavioral deficits that may accompany motor speech disorders and that are supportive of certain motor speech diagnoses.*

Before grappling with the content of this chapter, a caveat and a comfort are in order. The caveat

---

*Much of the organization of this chapter relies heavily on the conceptualization of nervous system organization, function, and pathology used in *Medical Neurosciences* by Daube, Reagan, Sandok, and Westmoreland (1986).

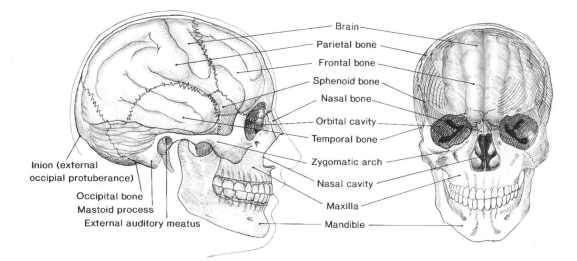

Figure 2–1 Lateral and anterior views of the major bones of the skull.

is for readers who are not familiar with the neurologic bases of speech or who are just beginning to integrate such information into clinical practice. It is likely that the number of terms and concepts that will be encountered here will be overwhelming and not obviously relevant to the understanding, diagnosis, and management of motor speech disorders. And, there may well be a sense that even when the facts are grasped, they will not be understood in a way that makes their application easy or automatic. These feelings are natural when learning how to think about problems with which one has little or no experience. The basic fact is that this material will not, and perhaps cannot, be understood rapidly. The first encounter with it will probably be somewhat of a struggle.

The comfort is that, in time, much of this will make sense and be valuable, if not essential, to clinical practice and research in the area of motor speech disorders. An increased depth of understanding of the material presented here may best be achieved by referring back to it when reading each chapter on specific motor speech disorders. It may be better still to refer back to this chapter in the course of evaluating and working with people with motor speech disorders. The opportunity to integrate this didactic information with patients' medical histories, laboratory and neuroimaging findings, and, most important, the sights and sounds of their disordered speech, is probably the best way to understand this material. In fact, it can be argued that this information cannot be integrated as a foundation for clinical practice until clinical practice has actually begun.

GROSS NEUROANATOMY AND MAJOR NEUROLOGIC SYSTEMS

In this section, we will first address the bony boundaries of the nervous system—the skull and spinal column. The major anatomic levels and relevant structural landmarks of the nervous system will then be introduced. This will be followed by a review of the nervous system's coverings (meninges and associated spaces), its internal cavities (the ventricles), its source of nutrients (vascular supply), and, finally, by a brief introduction to the visceral, consciousness, sensory, and motor systems.

The skull and spinal column

The brain is housed in the skull, the spinal cord within the spinal column. Our primary focus will be on the skull because it contains most of the central nervous system (CNS) structures that subserve speech. It also contains the nuclei (origin) of the cranial nerves that innervate all of the speech muscles, except those of respiration.

The bones of the skull (Figure 2–1) form a fused nonyielding covering for the adult brain, which serves a protective function against trauma. This protection is offset somewhat by the inability of the adult brain to expand in response to pressure from certain internal pathologic processes (e.g., hemorrhage, hydrocephalus, tumor), a situation that can produce diffuse neurologic abnormalities as a result of mass effects and increased intracranial pressure.

Viewed from above (Figure 2–2), three distinct shallow cavities areas are apparent at the base of the skull: the *anterior, middle, and posterior fos-*

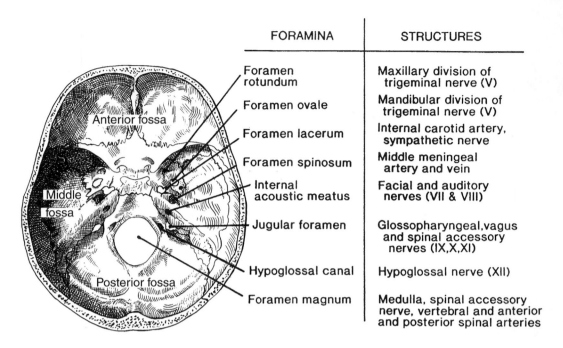

FORAMINA	STRUCTURES
Foramen rotundum	Maxillary division of trigeminal nerve (V)
Foramen ovale	Mandibular division of trigeminal nerve (V)
Foramen lacerum	Internal carotid artery, sympathetic nerve
Foramen spinosum	Middle meningeal artery and vein
Internal acoustic meatus	Facial and auditory nerves (VII & VIII)
Jugular foramen	Glossopharyngeal,vagus and spinal accessory nerves (IX,X,XI)
Hypoglossal canal	Hypoglossal nerve (XII)
Foramen magnum	Medulla, spinal accessory nerve, vertebral and anterior and posterior spinal arteries

Figure 2–2 Base of the skull, viewed from above, illustrating the major cranial fossae and foramina through which some vascular structures and the cranial nerves supplying speech muscles exit.

sae. The posterior and middle fossae contain symmetrically placed foramina (holes) through which the paired cranial nerves exit to innervate peripheral structures, most notably the head and neck speech muscles. These fossae help define two of the major levels of the CNS, the posterior fossa level and the supratentorial level (anterior and middle fossae). Discussions of localization of neuropathology often refer to lesions as supratentorial or posterior fossa in origin (Figure 2–3).

Major anatomic levels of the nervous system

The major anatomic levels of the nervous system can be related to the boundaries of the skull and spinal column. They are also roughly demarcated by the meninges and components of the ventricular and vascular systems, which will be discussed later. The major levels and their skeletal, meningeal, ventricular, and vascular characteristics, as well as their relationship to the major types of motor speech disorders, are summarized in Table 2–1.

Supratentorial level. The supratentorial level is located above a rigid, nearly horizontal membrane known as the *tentorium cerebelli* (Figure 2–3), which forms the upper border of the posterior fossa, covers the dorsal surface of the cerebellum, and separates the anterior and middle fossae from the posterior fossa. The supratentorial level includes externally visible paired *frontal, temporal,*

parietal, and *occipital lobes* of the *cerebral hemispheres* (Figure 2–4). It also includes the *basal ganglia, thalamus, hypothalamus,* and *cranial nerves I (olfactory)* and *II (optic),* which are buried within the depths of the hemispheres.

Posterior fossa level. The major structures of the posterior fossa are the *brainstem* (the pons, medulla, and midbrain), the *cerebellum,* and the *origins of the paired cranial nerves III through XII* (Figure 2–4).

The area of the posterior fossa dorsal to the aqueduct of Sylvius (Figure 2–5) is known as the *tectum;* its major structures are the *inferior and superior colliculi* (known collectively as the *corpora quadrigemina*), which are major relay stations for the auditory and visual systems, respectively. The area ventral to the aqueduct of Sylvius and fourth ventricle is known as the *tegmentum;* it contains many nuclei, including the *reticular formation* and *white matter pathways.* The large cerebral and cerebellar pathways in the most ventral region below the tegmentum form the base region of the midbrain and pons.

The cerebellum lies dorsal to the fourth ventricle, pons, and medulla. It is comprised of a *right and left hemisphere* and a midline *vermis.*

Ten of the twelve paired cranial nerves (all but I and II) have their origin in and emerge from the brainstem. Several of them represent the last link

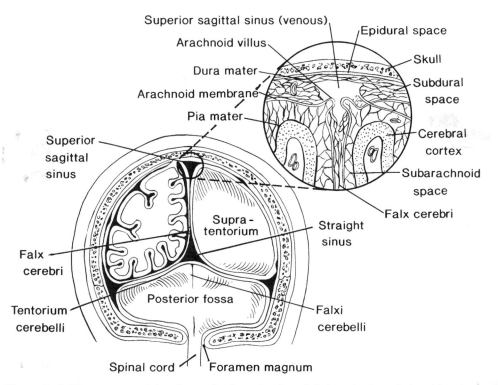

Figure 2–3 The supratentorial and posterior fossa levels and their major boundaries. Also shown (*inset*) are the meninges and their associated spaces.

or *final common pathway* from the nervous system to the speech muscles. Their names, their origins, and their general functions are summarized in Table 2–2.

Although the cranial nerves serving speech have their origin within the skull, they are actually part of the peripheral nervous system. This distinction is important to understanding the pathophysiology of flaccid dysarthria and its differences from the other dysarthrias, all of which result from CNS dysfunction.

Spinal level. The adult *spinal cord* begins at the lower end of the medulla at the level of the *foramen magnum,* the large, centrally located opening in the posterior fossa at the lower end of the medulla (Figures 2–2 and 2–3). It is surrounded by the bony *vertebral column,* which includes 7 cervical, 12 thoracic, and 5 lumbar vertebrae. The spinal cord terminates at the level of the first lumbar vertebra. Thirty-one pairs of spinal nerves are attached to it via *dorsal* (posterior) and *ventral* (anterior) *nerve roots.* The dorsal roots are sensory in function, the ventral roots are motor.

Peripheral level. The peripheral level, or *peripheral nervous system (PNS),* consists of the *cranial and spinal nerves.* As already noted, most of the cranial nerves originate in the brainstem, exit from the skull through paired foramina, and

travel to and from the structures they innervate. The spinal nerves, which contain the joined dorsal and ventral roots, enter the peripheral level as they emerge from the vertebral column to travel to and from the structures they innervate. The course, innervation, and function of the cranial and spinal nerves subserving speech functions are discussed later in this chapter.

The meningeal coverings and associated spaces

The *meninges* (coverings) of the CNS consist of three layers—the dura, arachnoid, and pia mater (Figure 2–3).

The *dura mater* is the outermost membrane. It consists of two layers of fused tissues that separate in certain regions to form the *intracranial venous sinuses,* areas where venous blood drains from the brain. The folds of the dura in the cranial cavity form two barriers: the *falx cerebri,* which is located between the two hemispheres, and the *tentorium cerebelli.*

The arachnoid lies beneath the dura and is applied loosely to the surface of the brain. The pia mater, the thin innermost layer, is closely attached to the brain's surface. The pia mater and arachnoid are collectively known as the *leptomeninges.*

The spaces around the meninges are functionally important and relevant to certain pathologies.

Table 2–1 Relationships among the major anatomic levels of the nervous system, skeleton, meninges, ventricular system, vascular system, and major motor speech disorder types

Anatomic level	Skeleton	Meninges	Ventricular system	Vascular system	Motor speech disorder
Supratentorial (hemispheres, lobes, basal ganglia, hypothalamus, cranial nerves I & II)	Skull (anterior & middle fossae)	Above tentorium cerebelli Lateral to falx cerebri	Lateral & third ventricles Subarachnoid space	Carotid arterial system Ophthalmic arteries Middle cerebral arteries Anterior cerebral arteries Vertebrobasilar system Posterior cerebral arteries	Apraxia of speech Dysarthria Spastic Unilateral UMN Hypokinetic Hyperkinetic
Posterior Fossa Brainstem (pons, medulla, midbrain) & cerebellum	Skull Posterior fossa	Below falx cerebelli	Fourth ventricle Subarachnoid space	Vertebrobasilar system Vertebral arteries Basilar artery	Dysarthria Spastic Unilateral UMN Hyperkinetic Ataxic Flaccid
Spinal	Veretebral column (below foramen magnum)	Spinal meninges	Spinal subarachnoid space	Anterior spinal artery Posterior spinal arteries	Dysarthria Flaccid
Peripheral (cranial & spinal nerves)	Face & skull Noncranial & nonspinal bones	None	None	Branches of major extremity vessels	Dysarthria Flaccid

UMN, upper motor neuron.

The *epidural space* is located between the inner bone of the skull and the dura. The *subdural space* is beneath the dura. Blood and pus from injury or infection can accumulate in the epidural and subdural spaces. The *subarachnoid space,* beneath the arachnoid, surrounds the brain and spinal cord and is filled with *cerebrospinal fluid;* it is connected to the interior of the brain through the *ventricular system* (Figure 2–5).

Most pathologies capable of producing motor speech disorders that involve the meninges and meningeal spaces stem from infection, venous vascular disorders, hydrocephalus, and trauma with associated hemorrhage and edema.

The ventricular system (cerebrospinal fluid system)

The ventricular system lies within the depths of the brain (Figure 2–5). The ventricles are cavities that contain *cerebrospinal fluid (CSF),* most of which is produced by *choroid plexuses* located in each ventricle. Each cerebral hemisphere contains a *lateral ventricle,* which is connected by way of the *foramen of Monro* to the midline-located *third ventricle.* The third ventricle narrows into the *aqueduct of Sylvius,* which leads to the *fourth ventricle* between the brainstem and cerebellum. The *foramen of Luschka* and the *foramen of Magendie* in the fourth ventricle link the ventricular system to the subarachnoid space.

Together, the ventricular system and the subarachnoid space make up the *CSF system.* CSF circulates throughout the ventricles and subarachnoid space and is absorbed in the *arachnoid villi* in the brain or *leptomeninges* within the subarachnoid space in the spinal cord. The CSF system thus can be found within several of the major anatomic levels of the nervous system, including the supratentorial, posterior fossa, and spinal levels. Its primary functions are to *cushion and buffer the CNS from physical trauma* and to help maintain a stable environment for neural function.

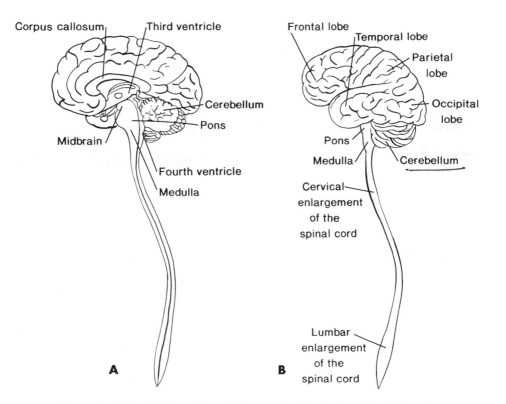

Figure 2–4 Mesial, **A**, and lateral, **B**, aspects of the brain and spinal cord.

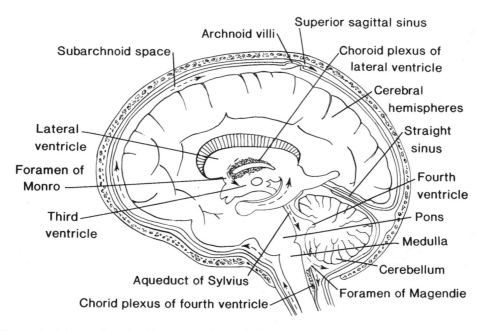

Figure 2–5 The subarachnoid space and ventricular system in which cerebrospinal fluid is produced and circulates.

Table 2–2 Location and general function of the cranial nerves

	Nerve	Anatomic origin	Function
I	Olfactory	Cerebral hemispheres	Smell
II	Optic	Diencephalon	Vision
III	Oculomotor	Midbrain	Eye movement; pupil constriction
IV	Trochlear	Midbrain	Eye movement
V	Trigeminal*	Pons	Jaw movement; face, mouth, jaw sensation
VI	Abducens	Pons	Eye movement
VII	Facial*	Pons	Facial movement; hyoid elevation; stapedius reflex; salivation; lacrimation; taste
VIII	Cochleovestibular	Pons, medulla	Hearing, balance
IX	Glossopharyngeal*	Medulla	Pharyngeal movement; pharynx and tongue sensation; taste
X	Vagus*	Medulla	Pharyngeal, palatal, and laryngeal movement; pharyngeal sensation; control of visceral organs
XI	*Spinal* Accessory*	Medulla, spinal cord	Shoulder and neck movement
XII	Hypoglossal*	Medulla	Tongue movement

*Involved in speech production

The vascular system (Figures 2–6, 2–7, 2–8)

The vascular system is literally the lifeblood of the nervous system and is found at all of the major anatomic levels of the nervous system. It provides oxygen and other nutrients to neural structures and removes metabolic wastes from them. It is also a major source of lesions that can lead to motor speech disorders.

All of the vessels that supply the brainstem and cerebral hemispheres arise from the *aortic arch* in the chest. Blood enters the brain by way of the *carotid system* and the *vertebrobasilar system.* These two systems are capable of some communication with each other through connecting anastomotic channels in the brainstem, known as the *circle of Willis* (Figure 2–6).

The carotid system originates with the paired *internal carotid arteries* that arise in the neck from the common carotid arteries at the level of the thyroid cartilage (Figure 2–6). They enter the skull through the carotid canal located in the petrous portion of each temporal bone. They pass through the cavernous sinus lateral to the sphenoid bone, and eventually to the circle of Willis.

Each internal carotid artery separates at the circle of Willis into two of the major cerebral arteries, the *anterior cerebral artery* and the *middle cerebral artery.* The anterior cerebral arteries are connected to each other by the *anterior communicating artery;* they course upward in the midline and supply the medial surface of the cerebral hemispheres and the superior portion of the frontal and parietal lobes. The middle cerebral arteries course laterally and their branches supply much of the lateral surfaces of the cerebral hemispheres and the deep structures of the frontal and parietal lobes (Figure 2–8).

Vascular disturbances in the left or right carotid artery, and in the left or right anterior and middle cerebral arteries, can produce dysarthrias. Left middle cerebral artery disturbances are a very common cause of apraxia of speech.

The vertebrobasilar system begins with the paired *vertebral arteries,* which enter the brainstem through the foramen magnum and join at the lower border of the pons to form the *basilar artery.* Branches from these arteries supply the midbrain, pons, medulla, cerebellum, and portions of the cervical spinal cord. The *posterior cerebral arteries,* branches of the vertebrobasilar system, supply the occipital lobe, the thalamus, and the inferior and medial portions of the temporal lobe in each hemisphere (Figures 2–7 and 2–8).

Vascular disturbances in the vertebrobasilar system often lead to motor speech disorders. Table 2–3 summarizes the vascular supply to the brain, the anatomic regions supplied by its components, and some of the neurologic signs and symptoms associated with vascular disturbances.

The visceral system

The visceral system is represented at all of the major anatomic levels of the nervous system, including: the hypothalamus and parts of the limbic lobe supratentorially; the reticular formation and portions of some cranial nerves in the posterior fossa; longitudinal pathways in the brainstem and spinal cord; and many ganglia, receptors, and effectors at the peripheral level. It contains afferent and efferent components that interact to *maintain a balanced internal environment (homeostasis) through the regulation of visceral glands and organs.*

The consciousness system

Structures in the consciousness system are found only at the supratentorial and posterior fossa levels.

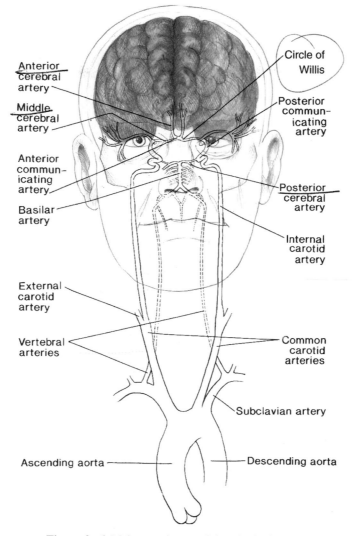

Figure 2–6 Major arteries supplying the brain.

They include: the reticular formation and ascending projection pathways; portions of the thalamus; pathways to widespread areas of the cerebral cortex; and portions of all lobes of the cerebral cortex. This system is *crucial to maintaining wakefulness, consciousness, awareness of the environment and, on a higher level, selective and sustained attention.* Malfunctions within it can contribute to cognitive deficits, including language and communication, and can also affect the adequacy of motor behavior, including speech.

The sensory system

The sensory system is found at all of the major anatomic levels of the nervous system. It includes: peripheral receptor organs; afferent fibers in cranial, spinal, and peripheral nerves; dorsal root ganglia (spinal level); ascending pathways in the spinal cord and brainstem; portions of the thala-

mus; and thalamocortical connections, primarily to sensory cortex in the temporal, parietal, and occipital lobes. Special sensory systems, such as hearing and vision, are also located at the peripheral, posterior fossa, and supratentorial levels.

The motor system

The motor system is present at all of the major anatomic levels of the nervous system and is directly *responsible for all motor activity involving striated muscle.* It includes: efferent connections of the cortex, especially the frontal lobes; the basal ganglia, cerebellum, and related CNS pathways; descending pathways to motor nuclei of cranial and spinal nerves; efferent fibers within cranial and spinal nerves; and striated muscle. It is *essential to normal reflexes, to maintaining normal muscle tone and posture, and to the planning, initiation, and control of voluntary movement, including speech.*

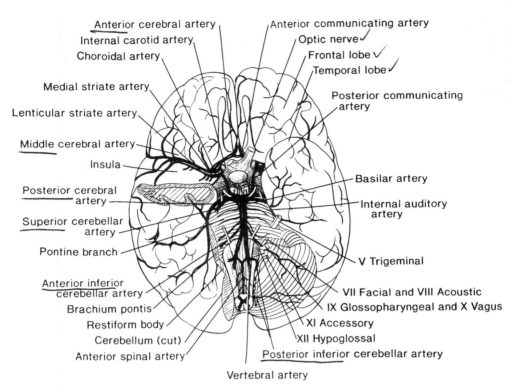

Figure 2–7 Inferior view of the carotid, vertebral, and basilar arteries and some of their major branches and their relationship to major brainstem and cerebral structures.

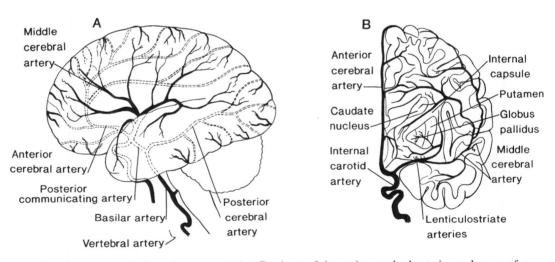

Figure 2–8 Lateral, **A,** and anteroposterior, **B,** views of the major cerebral arteries and some of their penetrating branches to subcortical structures.

Lesions in nonmotor areas of the nervous system may produce alterations in motor speech, but they do so only indirectly through their effects on the motor system. For example, a lesion in the vascular system does not, in and of itself, produce motor speech disorders; any resulting motor speech disorder would derive from the effect of that lesion on portions of the motor system involved in speech production.

PRIMARY STRUCTURAL ELEMENTS OF THE NERVOUS SYSTEM

The nervous system is composed of *neurons* and *supporting cells* (see Table 2–4). The structure

Table 2-3 Vascular supply to the brain, some of the major anatomic regions supplied, and some of the primary neurologic and motor speech deficits that result from vascular disturbance. Motor speech disorders and other deficits affecting spoken communication are highlighted in bold.

Main vessels	Anatomic region supplied	Signs and symptoms*
I. Carotid system		
A. Branches of internal carotid	Most of the cerebral hemispheres	Contralateral hemiplegia
		Contralateral hemianesthesia
		Hemianopsia or ipsilateral blindness
		Aphasia (left)
		Apraxia of speech (left)
		Unilateral UMN dysarthria
		Spastic dysarthria (if bilateral)
		Hypokinetic dysarthria
		Hyperkinetic dysarthria
1. Anterior choroidal	Optic tract	Hemianopsia or upper quadrant defect
	Cerebral peduncle	
	Lateral geniculate body	Contralateral hemiplegia
	Portions of internal capsule	Thalamic sensory changes
		Unilateral UMN dysarthria?
		Spastic dysarthria (if bilat)?
2. Ophthalmic	Orbit and surrounding tissue	Unilateral blindness
	Muscles and bulb of the eye	Optic atrophy
3. Anterior cerebral	*Cortical branches*	Contralateral lower extremity weakness
	Anterior ¾ of medial surface of cerebral hemispheres; frontal lobe, medial-orbital surface; frontal pole; superior lateral border of hemispheres; anterior ⅘ of corpus callosum	Paraplegia (if bilateral)
		Cortical sensory defects, foot and leg
		Contralateral forced grasping and groping, sucking reflex
	Deep branches	Incontinence
	Internal capsule, anterior limb; part of head of caudate nucleus	Gait & limb apraxia
		Aphasia?
		Abulia, akinetic mutism, cognitive impairments
		Apraxia of speech (left)?
		Unilateral UMN dysarthria?
		Spastic dysarthria (if bilateral)?
		Hypokinetic dysarthria?
		Hyperkinetic dysarthria?
4. Middle cerebral	*Cortical branches*	Contralateral hemiplegia
	Cortex & white matter of parietal lobe and lateral and inferior frontal lobe; superior parts of temporal lobe & insula	Contralateral cortical sensory deficit
		Homonymous hemianopsia
		Paralysis of conjugate gaze to side opposite lesion
		Aphasia (left)
		Apraxia of speech (left)
		Unilateral UMN dysarthria
		Spastic dysarthria (if bilat)
		Limb apraxia
	Penetrating branches	Contralateral hemiplegia or hemiparesis

Continued.

Table 2-3—cont'd

Main vessels	Anatomic region supplied	Signs and symptoms*

I. Carotid system
  A. Branches of internal carotid
    4. Middle cerebral
	Putamen; part of head & body of caudate nucleus; outer part of globus pallidus; internal capsule; posterior limb; corona radiata	Contralateral hemisensory deficits
		Contralateral movement disorders
		Aphasia (left)
		Apraxia of speech (left)
		Unilateral UMN dysarthria
		Spastic dysarthria (if bilateral)

II. Vertebrobasilar system A. Posterior cerebral	Red nucleus; substantia nigra; cerebral peduncles; reticular formation; oculomotor and trochlear nuclei; superior cerebellar peduncles; hippocampus; portions of thalamus; inferomedial temporal lobe; occipital lobe	Contralateral hemiparesis Oculomotor palsy Ataxia & tremor Memory & attention deficits Unilateral sensory loss Homonymous hemianopsia Movement disorders Variety of visual deficits Dyslexia without agraphia **Aphasia (left)** **Unilateral UMN dysarthria** **Spastic dysarthria (if bilateral)** **Ataxic dysarthria** **Hyperkinetic dysarthria**
B. Basilar artery	Pons; middle & superior cerebellar peduncles; cerebellar hemispheres; upper midbrain & subthalamus	Quadriplegia (if bilateral) Hemiplegia Coma (if bilateral) Somnolence Oculomotor deficits Visual defects Nystagmus Ipsilateral cerebellar ataxia Nausea and vomiting Cranial nerve involvement (III–XII) **Spastic dysarthria (if bilateral)** **Anarthria (if bilateral)** **"Locked-in" syndrome (if bilateral)** **Ataxic dysarthria** **Unilateral UMN dysarthria** **Flaccid dysarthria** **Palatal myoclonus**
C. Vertebral artery	Medulla; cerebellum (posterior inferior)	Contralateral hemiplegia & sensory loss Ptosis Ipsilateral weakness of IX, X, XI, XII nerves (LMN) Nystagmus, vertigo Ipsalateral ataxia Ipsilateral loss of facial sensation (Vth nerve) & taste Hiccups Nausea & vomiting **Spastic dysarthria (if bilateral)** **Ataxic dysarthria** **Unilateral UMN dysarthria** **Flaccid dysarthria**

*Signs and symptoms occur with vascular disturbance on the right or left, unless otherwise specified in parentheses.
UMN, upper motor neuron.
LMN, lower motor neuron.

Table 2-4 Structural elements of the nervous system

Structure	Locus	Function
Neurons	CNS & PNS	Drive all neurologic functions
Nerves	Brainstem/spinal cord to end organs (PNS)	PNS motor & sensory functions
Tracts/pathways	CNS	Communication among groups of neurons
Commissural	Between cerebral hemispheres	
Association	Within cerebral hemispheres	
Projection	To & from higher & lower centers within CNS (for example, cortex & thalamus)	
Supporting cells		
Oligodendroglia	Surround CNS axons (myelin)	Insulation; speed neuronal transmission
Schwann cells	Surround PNS axons (myelin)	Insulation; speed neuronal transmission
Astrocytes	Relate to CNS blood vessels & neurons	Transport substances from blood vessels to neurons
		Blood-brain barrier
Ependymal cells	Lining of ventricles	Separate ventricles from parenchyma
	Choroid plexuses	Produce CSF
Microglia	Scattered in CNS	
	Form macrophages	Ingest/remove damaged tissue
Connective tissue	Form meninges	Covering of CNS
	Sheaths on PNS nerve fibers & nerves	Cover & bind fibers together in PNS nerves

CNS, central nervous system.
PNS, peripheral nervous system.
CSF, cerebrospinal fluid.

and function of these cells have been studied extensively and are reviewed here only superficially.* An understanding of the physiology of neuronal function is important because it forms the foundation for understanding the actions of the speech motor system. The cursory summary given here reflects the more global focus of this book, and an assumption that the reader already has an understanding of this relatively molecular topic.

The neuron

The neuron is the most important structural element of the nervous system. Its electrochemical activities drive all neurologic functions. Its numbers in humans are astounding, on the order of 100 billion, give or take a factor of 10 (Hubel, 1979). In the adult, most disease processes affecting neurons result in their degeneration and loss.

Neurons in different parts of the nervous system vary in size and shape, but they all contain a *cell body, dendrites*, and an *axon* (Figure 2-9). The cell body is the central processing unit and is responsible for the neuron's metabolic functions.

Dendrites and an axon extend from the cell body into surrounding tissue. Their length and structure vary greatly across different types of neurons. Dendrites are often numerous but short, with many branches; they are responsible for gathering information transmitted from surrounding neurons. Neurons have only one axon that may extend away from the cell body for a few millimeters or for several feet, its diameter generally varying with its length. Neurons with axons that travel extended distances are generally specialized for conducting information. Neurons whose axons terminate near their own dendrites and cell body are more involved in complex interactions within pools or networks of neurons, and are involved in "information processing."

The axon conducts electrical energy away from the cell body to the next neuron in a chain or circuit, or to muscle or glands. Communication among neurons or between neurons and muscles takes place at regions known as *synapses* (Figures 2-9 and 2-10). In neuronal synapses, the axon usually forms a synapse with the cell body or dendrites of another neuron. In most instances the axon and dendrite (or muscle fibers) are separated by a *synaptic cleft*. At the tip of the axon are tiny *synaptic vessicles,* which contain a chemical neurotransmitter that carries the axon's signal to a

*Excellent reviews of basic neuronal structure and function can be found in many sources, such as Brown (1980), Kennedy and Abbs (1982), Larson (1989), Perkins & Kent (1986), and Stevens (1979).

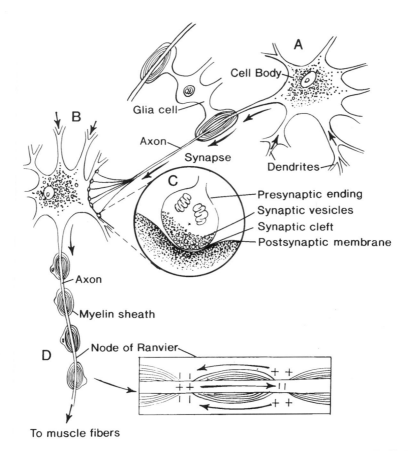

Figure 2–9 The neuron, **A,** and the anatomy of neuron-to-neuron communication, **B, C.** Dendrites receive information while the axon transmits information to other neurons. The action potential in **D** is moving through saltatory conduction in the direction of the arrow inside the axon.

receiving dendrite or to muscle fibers. In neuromuscular synapses, *acetylcholine* is the crucial neurotransmitter substance. If released in sufficient quantity at the neuromuscular junction it leads to movement through contraction of muscle fibers.

The "message" carried by a single axon to another neuron is simple; it either facilitates or inhibits the neuron receiving it from firing a message of its own. All that varies in the message of a single neuron is the rate at which it is sent. This "go" or "no go" form of communication leads to a limited set of simple, stereotypic behavioral outcomes in organisms with limited numbers of neurons. In the human nervous system, however, axons branch repeatedly, forming anywhere from 1,000 to 10,000 synapses, and their cell bodies and dendrites receive information from in the order of 1,000 other neurons. (The number of synapses in the brain may be in the order of 100 trillion!) As a result, the "decision" of a neuron to fire or not is a product of the sum of the messages it receives from multiple sources.

Nerves, tracts, and pathways

The activity of a single neuron is of little consequence to people's observable behavior. Only through the activity of many neurons does "meaningful" sensory, motor, and cognitive activity occur. For example, voluntary movement can result only from the integrated activity of astounding numbers of neurons conducting impulses at many levels of the CNS motor system plus the final influence of impulses carried by many axons travelling in nerves to many muscle fibers. Because our focus here is on motor behavior, we are most interested in the *collected activities* of groups of neurons that join forces to accomplish particular goals.

The major PNS structure is the *nerve* (Figure 2–10), which is a *collection of nerve fibers (axons)* bound together by connective tissue. Peripheral nerves (cranial and spinal nerves) travel between the CNS (where their cell bodies reside) and peripheral *end organs,* which are the sensory, motor, and visceral structures that they innervate.

A nerve contains up to thousands of nerve fibers of varying sizes. Fibers relevant to speech motor

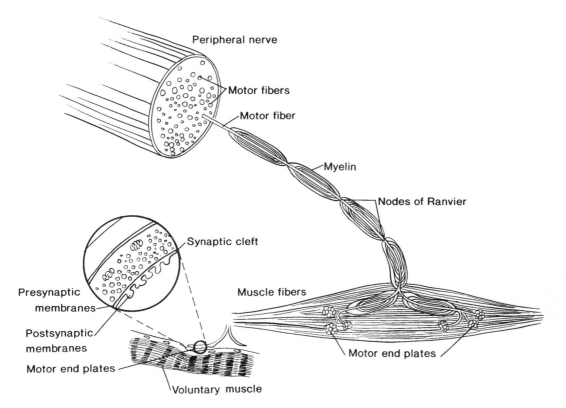

Figure 2–10 The motor unit. A myelinated axon (motor fiber) carries an action potential that results in the release of acetylcholine from synaptic vesicles across the neuromuscular junction (*inset*) to trigger muscle fiber contraction. The final common pathways innervating muscles for speech contain many thousands of such motor units.

and sensory functions are generally relatively large and *myelinated* (myelin is defined in the following section). They conduct impulses relatively quickly.

The term "nerve" is reserved for groups of fibers that travel together in the PNS. Groups of fibers that travel together in the CNS are called *tracts* or *pathways* and are similar to nerves. The major distinction is that CNS tracts and pathways transmit impulses to other neurons, rather than from nerve to end organs.

Fiber tracts in the CNS are categorized according to the areas that they connect. *Commissural fiber tracts* connect homologous areas in the two cerebral hemispheres. *Association fiber tracts* connect cortical areas within a hemisphere to one another. *Projection fiber tracts* contain afferent and efferent fibers that connect higher and lower centers in the CNS. Their specific names usually reflect the areas that they connect. For example, afferent projection fibers from the thalamus to the cortex are known as thalamocortical fibers; efferent fibers from the cortex to the cranial nerves are known as corticobulbar fibers; efferent fibers from the cortex to the *red nucleus* in the midbrain are known as corticorubral fibers ("rubral," meaning

red, refers to the red nucleus). Afferent and efferent projection fibers are crucial components of the circuits that direct motor activities.

Supporting cells

Oligodendroglia and Schwann cells. These cell types form the insulation or *myelin* that surrounds axons in the CNS and PNS. Myelin is formed by *Schwann cells* in the PNS. It can be found wrapped around most peripheral nerves. Small gaps between each myelinated segment of peripheral nerve are known as *nodes of Ranvier.* Electrical signals travelling down axons skip from node to node with a resulting increased speed of transmission, a process known as *saltatory conduction* (Figures 2–9 and 2–10). *Oligodendroglia cells* are the source of myelin in the CNS.

Astrocytes. Astrocytes are found in the CNS. They are anatomically and functionally related to blood vessels. They abut on the walls of capillaries but also relate to neurons. Evidence suggests that astrocytes help transport substances between the blood and neurons (*parenchyma*) of the CNS. They are an important part of the *blood-brain barrier,* a mechanism that prevents the passage of many metabolites from the blood into the brain, thereby protecting it from toxic compounds and variations in blood composition.

Ependymal cells. Ependymal cells line the ventricular system and form a barrier between ventricular fluid and the parenchyma. They also form the choroid plexuses, which produce ventricular and cerebrospinal fluid.

Microglia. Microglia are small in number and are scattered throughout the nervous system. They function in response to destructive CNS processes by proliferating rapidly to become *macrophages* (scavenger cells) that ingest and remove damaged tissue.

Connective tissues. Connective tissues make up the meninges. There is little fibrous connective tissue within the CNS parenchyma. In the PNS, connective tissues form thin layers on myelinated nerve fibers, help bind fibers together within nerves, and can be found covering areas at the trunks of nerves. They are analogous to the meninges that surround the CNS.

Pathologic reactions of structural elements

Nervous system cells change in response to neurologic disease. In some disorders, the change is physiologic. In others, there is a structural response that reflects the specific effects of damage or a response to the pathologic process. Some structural responses are nonspecific whereas others are specific to a particular disease.

Neuronal reactions. Neuronal loss occurs in response to many disease states. In response to *ischemia* (*deprivation of oxygen and cessation of oxidative metabolism, as occurs in stroke*), there may be acute swelling of the neuron, with shrinkage occurring within 12 hours, and eventual cell loss.

In response to severe injury to axons, cell bodies may swell and lose some of their internal components, a process known as *central chromatolysis* or *axonal reaction*. These changes can be seen a few days after injury and peak at 2 to 3 weeks. Unlike ischemic cell change, this process is reversible, with normal appearance re-emerging in a few months.

Axons and their myelin sheaths cannot survive when they are separated from their cell bodies by injury or disease. Degeneration of the axon distal to the point of separation is known as *Wallerian degeneration*. In the PNS, however, regeneration of the nerve is possible if the cell body survives. This happens through sprouting of the portion of the axon still connected to the cell body. If the sprouts find their way to the degenerating distal nerve trunk, function eventually may be restored. This sprouting may occur at a rate of approximately

3 mm per day. *Functionally significant regeneration of nerve tracts does not occur in the CNS.*

Neurofibrillary degeneration is characterized by the formation of clumps of neurofibrils in the cytoplasm of CNS neurons. It is the most common form of degeneration associated with clinical dementia, particularly Alzheimer's disease. *Senile plaques* are a related pathologic change. They are characterized by deposits of *amyloid* (a fibrous protein) in cell bodies, as well as by degenerated nerve processes.

Inclusion bodies are abnormal, discrete deposits in nerve cells. Their presence may identify specific diseases (for example, Parkinson's disease, Pick's disease, certain viral infections).

Abnormal accumulation of metabolic products in nerve cells are known as *storage cells*. Several metabolic diseases can produce such accumulation. Because of the degree of swelling that may take place in the cell body, they are referred to as "balloon" cells.

When the lower motor neuron innervation of a muscle is destroyed, the muscle will waste away or *atrophy*. In contrast, injury to a CNS axon usually does not result in death of postsynaptic neurons. However, the activities of postsynaptic neurons may be altered by *diaschisis—a process in which neurons function abnormally because influences necessary to their normal function have been removed by damage to neurons to which they are connected.* This process may explain abnormalities in neuronal function at sites distant from a lesion within the CNS. *Positron emission tomography (PET)* has demonstrated that neuronal cell death in one region of the brain can be associated with changes in metabolic functions of adjacent and even distant neuronal regions to which the damaged area has important anatomic connections.* These findings highlight the functional importance of interrelationships among groups of neurons in the CNS and the inadequacies inherent in any attempt to attribute normal or pathologic behavior—including motor speech disorders—solely to activity or pathology in any single structure or pathway.

Supporting cell reactions. Myelin may shrink or break down in response to nonspecific injuries. There are also groups of diseases that specifically affect myelin.

In *demyelinating disease,* myelin is attacked by some exogenous agent, broken down, and absorbed. The axons covered by the affected myelin

---

*For discussions of PET and remote metabolic effects of lesions, see Dobkin and others (1989), Metter and others (1984), Mlcoch and Metter (1994), and Powers and Raichle (1985).

are usually left intact. The most common demyelinating disease is *multiple sclerosis,* but demyelinization also occurs in other CNS and PNS diseases, such as *Guillain-Barrè syndrome.*

Other diseases that specifically affect myelin are *leukodystrophies* or *dysmyelinating diseases.* In them, myelin is abnormally formed in response to inborn errors in metabolism. The abnormality leads to the eventual breakdown of myelin.

Astrocytes react to many CNS injuries by forming scars in injured neural tissue. *Gliosis, astrocytosis,* and *astrogliosis* are terms that refer to this nonspecific process. Astrocytes may also react more specifically to certain diseases, especially metabolic diseases, such as those that may occur in hepatic (liver) failure. They may also form *inclusion bodies* in cell nuclei in response to certain viral infections.

CLINICOPATHOLOGIC CORRELATIONS

It is appropriate to diverge briefly to discuss a general approach for categorizing the localization, course, and general nature of neurologic disease. Along with the subsequent discussion of the motor system and the neurology of motor speech, this will set the stage for addressing the assessment of motor speech disorders in the next chapter.

Localizing nervous system disease and determining its course

Neurologic signs and symptoms reflect the location of a lesion and not necessarily its specific cause. Disease often can be localized on the basis of history and clinical examination. Broad categories for describing the localization and history of disease are summarized in Table 2–5.

In broad terms, the *localization* of neurologic disease can be:
1. *Focal,* involving a single circumscribed area or contiguous group of structures (for example, left frontal lobe).
2. *Multifocal,* involving more than one area or more than one group of contiguous structures (for example, cerebellar and cerebral hemisphere plaques associated with multiple sclerosis).
3. *Diffuse,* involving roughly symmetric portions of the nervous system bilaterally (for example, generalized cerebral atrophy associated with dementia).

Determining specific pathology depends partly on establishing the course or temporal profile of disease. The *development* of symptoms can be:
1. *Acute,* within minutes.
2. *Subacute,* within days.
3. *Chronic,* within months.

The *evolution* or course of disease after symptoms have developed can be:
1. *Transient,* when symptoms resolve completely after onset.
2. *Improving,* when severity is reduced but symptoms are not resolved.
3. *Progressive,* when symptoms continue to progress or new symptoms appear.
4. *Exacerbating-remitting,* when symptoms develop, then resolve or improve, then recur and worsen, and so on.
5. *Stationary,* when symptoms remain unchanged for a period of time after they have reached maximum severity.

Motor speech disorders can appear at any point during the development and evolution of neurologic disease. As a result, their pres-

Table 2–5 Common localization, development, and evolutionary characteristics for various etiologies of neurologic disease

	Etiology					
	Degenerative	Inflammatory	Toxic/metabolic	Neoplastic	Traumatic	Vascular
Localization	Diffuse	Diffuse Focal	Diffuse	Focal	Diffuse Multifocal Focal	Focal Multifocal Diffuse
Development	Chronic	Subacute	Acute Subacute Chronic	Chronic Subacute	Acute	Acute
Evolution	Progressive	Progressive Exacerbate/ remit	Progressive Stationary	Progressive	Improving Stationary	Improving Stationary Transient Progressive

ence may be very informative to localization and diagnosis.

Broad etiologic categories

Categorizing types of pathologic changes is useful for understanding neurologic disease. Each category can produce motor speech disorders, although the distribution of the various types of motor speech disorders varies across various etiologies. Specific diseases associated with each of the following broad etiologic categories are defined and discussed in chapters on the motor speech disorders with which they are most commonly encountered.

(1) *Degenerative diseases.* These are characterized by a gradual decline in neuronal function of unknown cause. In some cases, neurons atrophy and disappear whereas in others neuronal changes may be more specific (for example, neurofibrillary tangles in Alzheimer's disease). Degenerative diseases are most often *chronic, progressive,* and *diffuse,* but they sometimes begin with focal manifestations. When causes for them are found, they are usually shifted to a more specific disease category.

(2) *Inflammatory diseases.* These are characterized by an inflammatory response to microorganisms, toxic chemicals, and immunologic reactions. Their pathologic hallmark is an outpouring of white blood cells. The development of clinical signs and symptoms is usually *subacute.*

Many inflammatory diseases are progressive and diffusely located in the leptomeninges and cerebrospinal fluid (*meningitis*) or in the brain parenchyma (*encephalitis*). Inflammation in the PNS may occur in single nerves or in multiple nerves.

Some CNS inflammatory diseases are focal. When focal, there may be *abscess formation,* a process in which astrocytes proliferate to form a wall of glial fibers that limits spread of infection, eventually leaving a cavity that reflects loss of the enclosed brain tissue.

(3) *Toxic-metabolic diseases.* Vitamin deficiencies, genetic biochemical disorders, complications of kidney and liver disease, and drug toxicity are examples of toxic and metabolic diseases that can alter neuronal function. Their effects are usually diffuse, but sometimes focal. Their development and course can be *acute, subacute, or chronic.*

(4) *Neoplastic diseases.* Any cell type in the nervous system can become neoplastic. However, neurons in the adult nervous system do not normally undergo cell division and, therefore, neuronal neoplasms (*neurocytomas*) are rare. In contrast, astrocytes are very reactive and, consequently, *astrocytomas* are the most common primary CNS tumor. *Oligodendrogliomas, ependymomas,* and *microgliomas* can arise from their constituent cell types. Cells of the leptomeninges

give rise to *meningiomas,* and Schwann cells give rise to *schwannomas.* Nervous system tumors rarely *metastasize* (spread) outside the CNS but systemic cancer can metastasize to the CNS. Tumors usually create focal signs and symptoms and are *chronic* or *progressive* in temporal profile.

Not all focally progressive mass lesions represent neoplasm. Blood clots (*hematomas*) and *edema* are examples of mass lesions that are non-neoplastic in character.

(5) *Traumatic diseases.* Traumatic injury usually has an identifiable precipitating event (for example, automobile accident, fall, gunshot wound). Onset is almost always *acute,* with maximum damage at onset.

PNS traumatic injuries can be focal or multifocal. CNS traumatic injuries are often diffuse initially, as in *concussion* (an immediate and transient loss of consciousness or other neurologic function following head injury). The course is usually one of *resolution or improvement;* residual focal signs and symptoms tend to reflect areas of severe anatomic damage (often associated with contusions, lacerations, and hematomas).

An exception to the general rule of acute onset of signs and symptoms from trauma can occur in *subdural hematoma.* The bleeding in this case is under low pressure because it occurs in veins crossing from the brain to the dural sinuses, where blood is then drained from the brain. Blood accumulates slowly and symptoms may not emerge for days or even months.

Traumatic brain injuries (TBI) can be subdivided into penetrating and *closed head injuries (CHI).* Penetrating head wounds (for example, bullets, shrapnel) may produce relatively focal neurologic abnormalities. CHI occurs much more frequently and is the principal cause of death and disability in Americans under age 35 (Salazar, 1990). Motor vehicle accidents, falls, and sports injuries represent some of the major causes of CHI.

Although cognitive deficits are the most common and perhaps persistent neurologic deficits associated with CHI, motor impairments are not uncommon. Some studies suggest that one third of CHI survivors are dysarthric (Rusk, Block, and Lowman, 1969; Sarno, Buonagura, and Levita, 1986).

It is appropriate to discuss briefly the pathogenesis of CHI because it is complex and applicable to understanding the mechanisms by which it may produce diverse motor speech disorders. Injuries from CHI can create focal lesions, diffuse axonal injury, and superimposed hypoxia/ischemia and microvascular damage (Salazar, 1990). Focal contusions often occur at the site of impact and result in focal neurologic deficits. They are known as *coup injuries.* If the injury is associated with acceleration, the motion of the brain may also cause trauma at sites opposite the point of impact, causing a *contrecoup* lesion. The most common site of these focal injuries are the orbitofrontal region and the anterior temporal lobes. These are locations where the brain abuts on edges of the skull (see Figures 2–1 and 2–2) and, therefore, is subject to trauma when the head rapidly decelerates (as in falls or sudden impacts). This often causes rupture (tearing) of veins in the area of the trauma, although hemorrhage in CHI can be extradural, subdural, subarachnoid, or intracerebral.

Diffuse axonal injury is viewed as the principle cause of persistent severe neurologic deficit in CHI (Salazar, 1990). It can occur even after mild concussion. It results from shearing of axons, commonly in the centrum semiovale, corpus callosum, and brainstem. The trauma generates a physiologic response in the affected axons that eventually leads to their being severed. Diffuse axonal injuries occur more frequently when trauma is associated with rotational forces (Gordon, 1990).

Hypoxia and ischemia (see next section on vascular disease) can occur in response to trauma, as can more subtle microvascular damage. These vascular sequelae can result from stretch and strain on blood vessels, from effects on vascular regulatory systems (for example, decreased vascular system response to changes in CO_2), from transient hypertension, from increased intracranial pressure, and from a transient breakdown in the blood-brain barrier. The most frequent sites of ischemic damage in CHI include the hippocampus, basal ganglia, cortex, and cerebellum (Jennett and Teasdale, 1981).

The effects of CHI are therefore the result of the direct effects of trauma (coup and contrecoup damage) as well as delayed secondary injury by biochemical events in response to the trauma. These processes include, but are not limited to ischemia, altered vascular reactivity, brain swelling, and the creation of conditions that lead to secondary infection. The complex pathophysiology of CHI can obviously lead to a wide variety of focal, multifocal, and diffuse nervous system lesions.

Vascular diseases. Vascular disease is the most common cause of neurologic disease and, in all likelihood, motor speech disorders. The most common type of cerebrovascular disease is *stroke* (or *infarct* or *cerebrovascular accident*), in which neurons are deprived of oxygen and glucose because of an interruption in blood supply. This deprivation is known as *ischemia.*

Within seconds of an ischemic event neurons cease to function. Pathologic changes occur within minutes. Infarcts are nearly always *sudden in onset* and usually focal. The course of symptoms is usually one of *stabilization and improvement.* When progression of symptoms occurs, it usually reflects the development of cerebral edema (common in the aftermath of ischemia) or continuing infarction of adjacent tissue.

Ischemic infarcts have several sources. The most common cause is *embolism,* in which a fragment of material (an embolus) travels through a blood vessel to a point of arterial narrowing sufficient to block its further passage, with subsequent occlusion of the flow of blood behind it. Embolic strokes tend to develop suddenly and without warning. Emboli most commonly come from the heart, but they may also derive from the aortic arch and carotid and vertebral arteries. Embolic material can be a blood clot, atherosclerotic plaque, clump of bacteria, piece of tumor or lining from an artery, or other solid materials that may travel in the bloodstream.

Ischemia can also be caused by *thrombosis,* or the narrowing and occlusion of an artery at a fixed point. Thrombosis frequently reflects a build-up of *atherosclerotic plaque,* made up of lipids (fatty deposits) and fibrous material, on the inner lumen of a vessel wall. Such thromboses usually occur in the internal carotid, vertebral, or basilar arteries. Thrombotic strokes are sometimes preceded by *transient ischemic attacks (TIAs),* characterized by neurologic symptoms that last for seconds to minutes. Motor speech and language deficits are among the most common symptoms of TIAs. TIAs are warning signs of underlying cerebrovascular disease and impending stroke.

Not all thrombotic strokes are associated with atherosclerosis. Some other sources of thrombotic occlusion include: spontaneous or traumatically induced dissections of the carotid, vertebral, or intracranial arteries at the base of the skull; certain hematologic disorders; and mass effects exerted on arteries by tumors or by *aneurysms.* Aneurysms are *balloonlike malformations in weakened areas of arterial walls.* They are most commonly found in the internal carotid, anterior, or middle cerebral arteries.

Infarcts may also be *hemorrhagic.* In *cerebral hemorrhage,* a vessel ruptures into the brain, with accumulation of blood in neural tissue (*intraparenchymal* or *intracerebral hemorrhage*). These events are often associated with elevated blood pressure and chronic hypertension. Symptoms appear abruptly and are focal, but progression of symptoms can occur because of mass effects from blood accumulation. The thalamus, basal ganglia, brainstem, and cerebellum are common sites of intracerebral hemorrhage.

The most common extracerebral hemorrhage is *subarachnoid hemorrhage,* in which a vessel ruptures on the surface of the brain and blood spreads over its surface and throughout the subarachnoid space. Onset is *abrupt,* but symptoms and pathologic changes are often *diffuse.* Ruptured aneurysms are a common cause of subarachnoid hemorrhage. They may also result from rupture of an *arteriovenous malformation (AVM),* which is an abnormally formed collection of veins and arteries. AVMs can become enlarged by expansion of weak vessel walls and create neurologic symptoms through mass effects. Subarachnoid hemorrhage may eventually occur if the weakened walls rupture. Finally, *subdural* and *extradural hemorrhage* may occur, often from CHI in which dural blood vessels are torn open.

THE SPEECH MOTOR SYSTEM

The motor system contains the complex network of structures and pathways that control movement. It resides at all levels of the nervous system and mediates many activities of striated and visceral muscles. An appreciation of its organization and basic operating principles is necessary for understanding normal speech production and motor speech disorders. The remainder of this chapter will lay the foundation for that understanding.

The motor system can be subdivided in a number of ways. Unfortunately, categorizing the components of an integrated, complex, and incompletely understood system inevitably produces some ambiguity, overlap, and confusion. Nonetheless, it would be impossible to develop an understanding of the speech motor system without parsing it in some way.

The motor system can be organized according to its functions as well as its anatomy. Functional labels contribute to understanding what the components do rather than simply where they are. On this basis, four major divisions of the motor system can be delineated (based on Daube and others, 1986):

1. The final common pathway
2. The direct activation pathway
3. The indirect activation pathway
4. The control circuits

These divisions have identifiable anatomic correlates, and both anatomic and functional designations will be used here in an effort to tie them together in the reader's mind. The major divisions, their broad functions and primary structures, and some common related designations are summarized in Table 2–6. The relationships among the four major divisions, and with programming, sensation, and movement, is illustrated in Figure 2–11.

Although the discussion of the motor system naturally emphasizes *efferent pathways,* the role of sensory or *afferent pathways* cannot be ignored. Sensorimotor integration is necessary for normal movement, and lesions of sensory portions of the sensorimotor system can result in abnormal motor behavior.

The final common pathway—basic structures and functions

The *final common pathway (FCP)* is often referred to as the *lower motor neuron (LMN) system.* The words "final common" identify it as the *peripheral mechanism through which all motor activity is mediated;* that is, all other components of the motor system must act through it. It is *the last link in the chain of neural events that lead to movement.*

To understand the role of the FCP in movement requires an appreciation of its interaction with muscle. The FCPs involved in speech generate activity in *skeletal* or *somatic* muscles, which are muscles that can be subjected to voluntary control with relative ease. Skeletal muscles, with their constituent muscle fibers, move body parts by exerting forces on muscles, tendons, and joints. It is important to remember that individual muscles can only relax, stretch, or contract. By themselves, they cannot produce complex movements. However, they can be involved in complex motor activities when integrated with the actions of larger groups of contiguous or distant muscles. The following subsections review some of the basic nerve and muscle functions and interactions that are involved in skeletal muscle movements.

The motor unit, alpha motoneurons, and extrafusal muscle fibers. The contractile elements of skeletal muscles are known as *extrafusal muscle fibers.* They are under the direct control of LMNs, or *alpha motoneurons,* whose origins are in the brainstem or the anterior horns of the spinal cord. LMNs control the activities of groups of muscle fibers. An LMN and the muscle fibers innervated by it are known as a *motor unit* (Figure 2–10). Although this discussion will focus on the activities of single neurons, it must be kept in mind that functional neuromuscular activity involves the combined effects of many neurons acting together in nerves.

The axon of an alpha motoneuron leaves the brainstem or spinal cord within a cranial or spinal nerve and travels to a specific muscle. There it subdivides into a number of terminal branches that make contact with muscle fibers. Because they branch, *each axon in a nerve may innervate several muscle fibers.* At the same time, *each muscle fiber may receive input from branches of several different alpha motoneurons.* This redun-

Table 2–6 Functional and anatomic divisions of the motor system that are relevant to speech production

Major division	Basic function	Major structures	Related designations
Final common pathway	Stimulates muscle contraction & movement. Other motor divisions must act through it to influence movement.	Cranial nerves Spinal nerves	Lower motor neuron system
Direct activation pathway	Influences consciously controlled, skilled voluntary movement	Corticobulbar tracts Corticospinal tracts	Upper motor neuron system, direct motor system, pyramidal tracts
Indirect activation pathway	Mediates subconscious, automatic muscle activities including posture, muscle tone, & movement that support & accompany voluntary movement	Corticorubral tracts Corticoreticular tracts Rubrospinal, reticulospinal, vestibulospinal tracts & related tracts to relevant cranial nerves	Upper motor neuron system, indirect motor system, extrapyramidal system
Control circuits	Integration/coordination of sensory information & activities of direct & indirect activation pathways to control movement		
Basal ganglia	Plans & programs postural & supportive components of motor activity	Basal ganglia, substantia nigra, subthalamus, cerebral cortex	Extrapyramidal system
Cerebellar	Integrates & coordinates execution of smooth, directed movements	Cerebellum Cerebellar peduncles, reticular formation, red nucleus, pontine nuclei, inferior olive, thalamus, cerebral cortex	Cerebellum

dancy permits flexibility in the amplitude and frequency at which muscles are stimulated to contract in spite of the fact that individual neuronal impulses are stereotyped in amplitude and duration.

The size of a motor unit is determined by the number of extrafusal muscle fibers innervated by a single motoneuron. The number of muscle fibers per axon is known as the *innervation ratio.* Muscles concerned with fine, discrete movements have smaller innervation ratios than those that perform cruder movements. Therefore, proximal limb muscles may have ratios of over 500:1, in contrast to some facial muscles in which one neuron may supply only about 25 extrafusal muscle fibers (Darley, Aronson, & Brown, 1975).

In addition to innervating extrafusal muscle fibers, alpha motoneurons also innervate interneurons, or *Renshaw cells,* through collateral fibers from the axons of alpha motoneurons. Renshaw cells are capable of inhibiting alpha motoneurons, in effect producing a negative feedback response, which can immediately turn off the alpha motoneuron after it fires and prepare it to fire again.

Gamma motoneurons, intrafusal muscle fibers, the gamma motor system, and the stretch reflex. In addition to alpha motoneurons, motor nerves contain gamma motoneurons. Unlike alpha motoneurons, gamma motoneurons innervate *muscle spindle*s or *intrafusal muscle fibers* which are located parallel to extrafusal muscle fibers. Gamma motoneurons are smaller in diameter and slower conducting than alpha motoneurons. Their activity is strongly influenced by the cerebellum, basal ganglia, and indirect activation pathways of

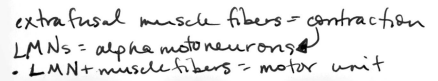

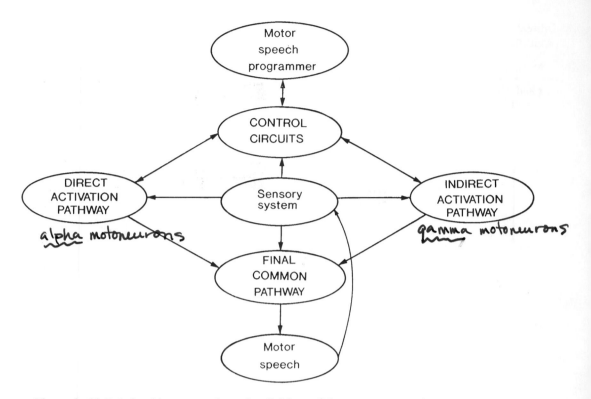

Figure 2–11 Relationships among the major divisions of the motor system, the sensory system, the motor speech programmer, and motor speech.

the CNS. The activities of alpha motoneurons are more strongly tied to the direct activation pathways.

Gamma motoneurons, their role in a functional unit known as the *gamma loop,* and their relationship to alpha motoneurons and the activities of the direct and indirect activation pathways of the CNS are important to movement control. They are crucial to maintaining *muscle tone,* a normal property of muscle that establishes its appearance as neither too taut nor too flabby. Muscle tone results from a mild degree of resistance that occurs in a muscle in response to its being stretched; it is actually a manifestation of a basic but crucial normal reflex known as the *stretch reflex.* The stretch reflex represents the "desire" of muscle to maintain its original length whenever it is stretched. Normal muscle tone is a sustained phenomenon because muscles are never completely relaxed; in a sense they are always maintained in a state of readiness for movement. The sustained nature of muscle tone makes it an ideal support mechanism upon which quick, unsustained skilled movements may be superimposed. This support system is mediated through the *gamma motor system.*

The gamma motoneuron is the efferent component of the gamma motor system. Its firing causes muscle spindles to contract (shorten). This shortening is detected by sensory receptors (*annulospi-*

ral endings) in the spindles that trigger impulses through sensory neurons back to the spinal cord or brainstem where they synapse with alpha motoneurons. The alpha motoneuron, in turn, directs impulses back to extrafusal muscle fibers, stimulating them to contract until they are the same length as the muscle spindles. Once this equalization has taken place, the sensory receptor no longer detects shortening and the "loop" is inactivated. During movement this process is, for practical purposes, continuous.

The gamma loop therefore consists of the gamma motoneuron, muscle spindle, stretch receptor and sensory neuron, the LMN, and extrafusal muscle fibers. It has been described here as a mechanism through which muscle length adjusts reflexively to the relative length of muscle spindles. This mechanism can be used by the indirect activation pathways of the CNS to preset the desired length of the muscle spindle for static postures (for example, extending the arm and holding it stable; possibly for moving the arytenoid cartilages into position for sustained phonation). It can also be used to prepare for and anticipate the degree of muscle contraction required for intended ongoing movement. The relationship between the alpha and gamma motoneurons, muscle spindles, and the gamma loop are illustrated in Figure 2–12.

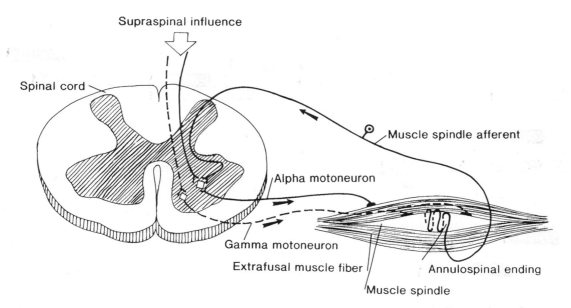

Figure 2–12 The motor unit, gamma loop, and stretch reflex. Extrafusal muscle fibers and muscle spindles are stimulated to contract by alpha and gamma motoneurons, respectively. When relaxed, the muscle spindle's sensory receptor (annulospiral ending) is silent. When muscle is stretched by movement, so is the spindle. This is detected by the sensory ending and transmitted to the spinal cord (or brainstem) where the alpha motoneuron is led to fire, producing extrafusal muscle fiber contraction that, in effect, resists the stretch on muscle. The stretch reflex is the basis for normal muscle tone.

Supraspinal (and suprabulbar) influences can use this same mechanism to "preset" movement. For example, the indirect activation pathway may stimulate the gamma motoneuron to produce muscle spindle contraction, which is detected by sensory endings and transmitted to alpha motorneurons that then stimulate extrafusal muscle contraction that is sufficient to balance the relationship between the extrafusal muscle and the muscle spindle. The movement "target" is reached when this balance is achieved.

Influences upon the FCP. As implied in the preceding discussion, the LMN integrates activity from several sources, including the peripheral sensory system, the direct activation pathway, and the indirect activation pathway. The integrated activity of LMNs results in movement.

The sensory system's *direct* relationship with alpha motoneurons involves synapses at the level of the spinal cord and brainstem. These synapses produce simple, stereotyped, involuntary *reflexes* (for example, the gag reflex) that are limited to specific muscles and body parts. Damage to the peripheral sensory pathways will abolish or reduce reflexes by removing or weakening the trigger for them. Reflexes can also be lost or diminished by damage to the FCP.

Voluntary movement emerges through the activity of the FCP, but it is considerably more complex than the sensory-motor reflexes just described. True volitional or even relatively automatic complex movements depend on the influence of direct and indirect activation pathways and control circuits in the CNS. Nonetheless, such activities can be brought to fruition only through the FCP.

Effects of damage. Damage to the motor unit prevents the normal activation of muscle fibers. However, because each muscle fiber may be innervated by several alpha motoneurons, damage to a single alpha motoneuron does not eliminate the possibility of muscle fiber contraction. As a result, damage to a nerve may lead only to *weakness* or *paresis* if all of the alpha motoneurons supplying the muscle are not damaged. Paralysis results if a muscle is deprived of all of its input from LMNs.

With a loss of innervation, muscles eventually lose bulk and undergo atrophy. In addition, excess or spontaneous motor unit activity and a lowered firing threshold may occur in motor unit disease. These spontaneous motor unit discharges may be seen on the surface of the skin as brief localized twitches known as *fasciculations*. Finally, muscles deprived of LMN input will also generate slow repetitive action potentials and contract regularly. This process, which cannot be seen through the skin, is known as *fibrillation.*

To summarize, the action of the FCP is both simple and profound. On the one hand, its role in complex and voluntary movement is only as a conduit to muscle of messages "written" and controlled elsewhere. Without it, however, muscle cannot be activated and movement is impossible. *Damage at this level of the motor system is responsible for the speech characteristics of flaccid dysarthria.*

The final common pathway and speech

The FCP for speech includes: the paired cranial nerves that supply muscles involved in phonation, resonance, articulation, and prosody; and the paired spinal nerves involved in respiratory activities. Following is an overview of the origin, course, and function of the cranial and spinal nerves that are most important for motor speech production.

Trigeminal nerve (Vth cranial nerve). The trigeminal nerve is the largest of the cranial nerves. Its sensory functions include: the transmission of pain; thermal and tactile sensation from the face and forehead; mucous membranes of the nose and mouth; the teeth; and portions of the cranial dura. It also conveys deep pressure and kinesthetic

information from the teeth, gums, hard palate, and temperomandibular joint, as well as sensation from stretch receptors in the jaw. Its motor components are responsible for innervating the muscles of mastication, the tensor tympani, and the tensor veli palatini.

The nerve emerges on the midlateral surface of the pons as a large sensory and smaller motor root (Figure 2–13). It is divided into *ophthalmic, maxillary,* and *mandibular branches,* all of which arise from the trigeminal ganglion where most of the sensory nerve cell bodies are located. The ophthalmic branch is concerned with sensation in the upper face and will not be discussed further.

The *maxillary branch* is complex in its distribution. Its multiple branches carry sensation from the maxilla and maxillary sinus; the mucous membranes of the mouth; the nasal cavity, palate, and nasopharynx; the teeth; the inferior portion of the auditory meatus; the face; and the meninges of the anterior and middle cranial fossa. Its fibers origi-

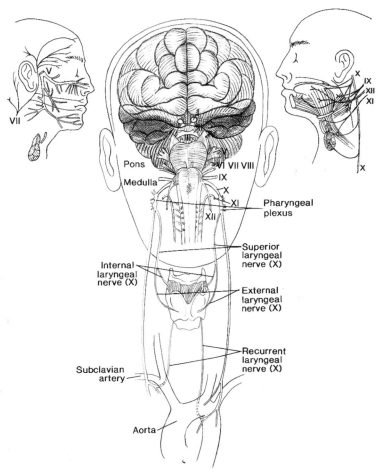

Figure 2–13 The primary cranial nerves for speech.

nate in the *trigeminal ganglion** (also called the *semilunar* or *gasserian ganglion*) that is located in a depression in the petrous bone on the floor of the middle cranial fossa. They travel from the ganglion out to the periphery through the *foramen rotundum* in the middle fossa (Figure 2–2). They travel inward from the ganglion to the brainstem, entering the midlateral aspect of the pons. From there, fibers carrying touch sensation from the face synapse with the chief sensory nucleus of the nerve within the pons.

Like all peripheral sensory fibers, the primary sensory neurons of the maxillary branch have CNS connections. Some fibers synapse with the adjacent reticular formation. Information is also transmitted in crossed and uncrossed fibers of the *trigeminothalamic tracts* that synapse in the thalamus. Neurons from the thalamus project through the internal capsule to the lower third of the ipsilateral postcentral gyrus in the cortex, where conscious perception of sensation occurs.

Pain and temperature fibers of the maxillary branch descend in the brainstem to various points along the medulla and the upper segment of the cervical spinal cord. These axons synapse with cell bodies in the nucleus of the *spinal tract of the trigeminal nerve;* along the way, small sensory components of cranial nerves IX and X also join the nerve's spinal tract. After these synapses, fibers cross at various levels to the opposite side and ascend in the trigeminothalamic tract to the thalamus. From there, thalamocortical neurons transmit sensory information to the parietal lobe.

The *mandibular branch,* the nerve's largest branch, contains both sensory and motor fibers. Its motor nucleus is located in the midpons, close to the nerve's chief sensory nucleus. As it leaves the skull through the *foramen ovale* (Figure 2–2), it branches repeatedly to send fibers to the tensor veli palatini, tensor tympani, and jaw muscles.

The sensory branches of the mandibular branch carry sensation from the mucous membrane of the mouth, from the side of the head and scalp, from the lower jaw, and from the anterior two-thirds of the tongue. They also carry proprioceptive information from muscles involved in jaw movement to the *mesencephalic nucleus* in the midbrain, adjacent to the fourth ventricle. There is evidence for the presence of muscle spindles in the muscles of mastication, and evidence of Golgi tendon organs in the temporalis and masseter muscles (Larson and Pfingst, 1982); these may play an important role in the sensorimotor control of jaw movement during speech.

The central connections of mandibular sensory neurons project to the masticatory nucleus of the nerve to provide reflex control of bite. The motor nucleus also receives sensory input from other cranial nerves (for example, input from the acoustic nerve influences the part of the motor nerve that innervates the tensor tympani, so that tension on the tympanic membrane can be adjusted for loudness variations).

LMN lesions of the masticatory nucleus or its axons lead to *paresis or paralysis and to eventual atrophy of masticatory muscles on the paralyzed side.* Unilateral Vth nerve lesions do not have major effects on speech. Bilateral lesions are devastating because the jaw hangs open, cannot be closed, or moves slowly and with limited range, thereby preventing facial, bilabial, and lingual articulatory movements from achieving accurate place and manner of articulation.

(2) *Facial nerve (VIIth cranial nerve).* The paired facial nerve is a mixed motor and sensory nerve. Its motor component supplies the stapedius muscle and muscles of facial expression. Its sensory components provide innervation to the submandibular, sublingual, and lacrimal glands, as well as to taste receptors on the anterior two-thirds of the tongue. Only the motor component has a clear role in speech (Figure 2–13).

Motor fibers that innervate the muscles of facial expression constitute the largest part of the nerve. They arise in the facial nucleus located in the lower third of the pons. Fibers of the nerve pass medially and arch dorsally, forming a loop around the abducens nucleus, before reaching the lateral surface of the pons and emerging as the facial nerve.

As they leave the pons, the motor fibers travel adjacent to the nerve's sensory fibers. Accompanied by fibers of the VIIIth (auditory) nerve, motor and sensory divisions of the facial nerve leave the cranial cavity through the *internal auditory meatus* (Figure 2–2). Motor fibers travel through the facial canal and exit at the stylomastoid foramen below the ear and pass through the parotid gland. From there, the buccal and mandibular branches of the nerve innervate the muscles of facial expression. Motor fibers of the nerve also give off branches to supply the stapedius, the platysma, and other submental muscles.

LMN lesions of the nerve can *paralyze muscles on the entire ipsilateral side of the face.* Such lesions affect all voluntary, emotional, and reflex movements, and atrophy occurs, resulting in *facial asymmetry. Fasciculations* may be seen in the perioral area and chin.

(3) *Glossopharyngeal nerve (IXth cranial nerve).* The glossopharyngeal nerve is a mixed motor and sensory nerve. Of relevance for speech are its

---

*Primary sensory neuron cell bodies of cranial nerves are usually located just outside of the CNS in sensory ganglia.

motor supply to the stylopharyngeus muscle of the pharynx and its transmission of sensory information from the pharynx, tongue, and eustachian tube (Figure 2–13).

Motor fibers to the stylopharyngeus muscle originate in the rostral portion of the *nucleus ambiguus,* which is located within the reticular formation in the lateral medulla. The nucleus ambiguus is a complex grouping of cell bodies, containing fibers of the IXth, the Xth, and portions of the XIth cranial nerves.

The motor component of the nerve emerges from the medulla just above the rootlets of the vagus nerve. It passes through the *jugular foramen* (Figure 2–2) with the vagus and accessory nerves to innervate the stylopharyngeus, which elevates the pharynx during swallowing and speech.

The afferent fibers of the nerve, which carry sensation from the pharynx and tongue, arise from cell bodies in the *inferior (petrosal) ganglion* in the jugular foramen. They terminate in the nucleus of the *tractus solitarius,* which lies ventrolateral to the dorsal motor nucleus of the vagus and extends along the length of the medulla. The tractus solitarius also receives visceral afferent fibers from the facial and vagus nerves.

Within the medulla there are reflex connections between pharyngeal sensory and motor neurons that mediate the *gag reflex.* CNS neurons carrying pain, temperature, and probably touch and pressure sensation leave the medulla, cross the midline, and ascend to the contralateral thalamus. From there, thalamocortical neurons pass to the postcentral sensory cortex where sensation reaches conscious awareness.

Glossopharyngeal nerve lesions are usually accompanied by damage to the vagus nerve. Damage to the nerve is most predictably associated with *reduced pharyngeal sensation and a decrease in the gag reflex.* Lesions of the glossopharyngeal nerve sometime lead to pain of unknown etiology known as *glossopharyngeal neuralgia.*

Vagus nerve (Xth cranial nerve). The paired vagus nerve is a complex and lengthy mixed motor and sensory nerve (Figure 2–13) that plays a crucial role in speech production. Its relevant motor functions include the innervation of the striated muscles of the soft palate, pharynx, and larynx. Its relevant sensory role includes transmission of sensation from those same structures. Among its additional functions are parasympathetic innervation to and sensation from the thorax and abdominal viscera, and sensory innervation from the external auditory meatus and taste receptors in the posterior pharynx. Only those branches of the vagus nerve relevant to speech production will be discussed here.

Motor fibers of the vagus nerve supplying muscles of the soft palate, pharynx, and larynx arise from the *nucleus ambiguus* in the lateral medulla (along with motor fibers of the IXth and portions of the XIth nerves). Motor neurons innervating the soft palate and pharynx are located in the most caudal region of the nucleus. Those innervating the larynx are located most rostrally. Sensory fibers from the soft palate, pharynx, and larynx have their cell bodies in the *inferior (nodose) ganglion,* located in or very near the *jugular foramen;* communication with the hypoglossal, accessory, glossopharyngeal, and facial nerves can take place at this level. The central processes of the sensory fibers terminate in the nucleus of the *tractus solitarius.*

The vagus nerve emerges from the lateral aspect of the medulla between the *inferior cerebellar peduncle* and the *inferior olive.* It exits the skull through the jugular foramen with the IXth and XIth nerves (Figure 2–2). Near its exit from the skull three branches become identifiable. The *pharyngeal branch* travels down the neck between the internal and external carotid arteries and enters the pharynx at the upper border of the middle pharyngeal constrictor muscle. There it breaks up and joins with branches from the glossopharyngeal and external laryngeal nerves to form the *pharyngeal plexus.* From there it distributes fibers to all the muscles of the pharynx and soft palate except the stylopharyngeus (IX) and the tensor veli palatini (innervated by the mandibular branch of the Vth nerve). It also supplies the palatoglossus muscle of the tongue. The pharyngeal branch is primarily responsible for pharyngeal constriction and for retraction and elevation of the soft palate during velopharyngeal closure for speech and swallowing.

The *superior laryngeal nerve* branch of the vagus descends adjacent to the pharynx, first posterior and then medial to the internal carotid artery. About 2 cm below the inferior ganglion it divides into the internal and external laryngeal nerves.

The *internal laryngeal nerve* is purely sensory. It carries sensation from mucous membrane lining the larynx down to the level of the vocal folds, the epiglottis, the base of the tongue, aryepiglottic folds, and the dorsum of the arytenoid cartilages. It also transmits information from muscle spindles and other stretch receptors in the larynx.

The *external laryngeal nerve* supplies the inferior pharyngeal constrictor and the cricothyroid muscles. Its innervation of the cricothyroid is especially important for phonation, because the cricothyroid lengthens the vocal cords for pitch adjustments.

The third major branch of the vagus, the *recurrent laryngeal branch,* is so-called because it doubles back on itself before reaching the larynx. The right and left recurrent laryngeal nerves take different paths. The right recurrent laryngeal nerve branches from the vagus nerve anterior to the subclavian artery, then loops below and behind the artery and ascends behind the common carotid artery in the groove between the trachea and the esophagus. It enters the larynx between the inferior horn of the thyroid and cricoid cartilage. The left recurrent laryngeal nerve is longer than the right, arising from the vagus at the aortic arch. It hooks under the arch near the heart and ascends in the groove between the trachea and esophagus and enters the larynx between the inferior horn of the thyroid and cricoid cartilage. Both the right and left recurrent laryngeal nerves innervate all of the intrinsic muscles of the larynx except the cricothyroid. General sensation from the vocal cords and larynx lying below them is carried by sensory fibers of the recurrent laryngeal nerves. Thus, the *superior and recurrent laryngeal nerves are responsible for all laryngeal motor activities involved in phonation and swallowing.*

The effects of vagus nerve lesions depend on the particular branch of the nerve that has been damaged. Damage to all of its branches will produce *weakness of the soft palate, pharynx, and larynx.* Unilateral LMN lesions can affect resonance, voice quality, and swallowing, but usually affect phonation more prominently than resonance. Bilateral LMN lesions can have devastating effects on resonance and phonation, with significant secondary effects on prosody and clarity of articulation; swallowing may be severely impaired. The specific effects of unilateral and bilateral lesions to each of the nerve's branches will be discussed in Chapter 4.

Accessory nerve (XIth cranial nerve). The paired accessory nerve has a cranial and spinal portion (Figure 2–13). The cranial portion arises from the nucleus ambiguus, emerges from the side of the medulla, and passes through the jugular foramen (Figure 2–2). Branches from the nerve join the jugular ganglion of the vagus nerve and the remaining fibers become part of the pharyngeal and superior and recurrent laryngeal branches of the vagus nerve. The cranial portion contributes fibers to the uvula, levator veli palatini, and intrinsic laryngeal muscles, but does so while intermingled with the fibers of the vagus nerve. Although most texts discuss the cranial portion of the accessory nerve, others (*Clinical Examinations in Neurology,* 1991) discuss its fibers as part of the inferior portion of the vagus nerve, arguing that it is confusing to consider them part of the accessory nerve just because they mingle for a short distance

in the cranium with the spinal portion of the accessory nerve.

Cell bodies of the spinal portion of the nerve reside in the ventral horn of the first five or six cervical segments of the spinal cord. Its axons ascend in the spinal canal lateral to the spinal cord and enter the posterior fossa through the *foramen magnum.* They then leave the skull through the *jugular foramen* (with the glossopharyngeal, vagus, and cranial portion of the accessory nerve) to innervate the sternocleidomastoid and trapezius muscles.

Lesions in the region of the foramen magnum (where the ascending nerve enters the skull) or in the region of the jugular foramen (where it exits the skull) *can weaken head rotation* toward the side opposite the lesion (sternocleidomastoid weakness). It can also *reduce the ability to elevate or shrug the shoulder* on the side of the lesion.

Hypoglossal nerve (XIIth cranial nerve). The paired sensory and motor hypoglossal nerve (Figure 2–13) innervates all intrinsic and all but one of the extrinsic muscles of the tongue (the exception is the palatoglossus, supplied by the vagus nerve). Its long, thin nucleus extends through most of the medulla and lies in the floor of the fourth ventricle. Its fibers travel ventrally to exit from the medulla as a number of rootlets between the medullary pyramids and inferior olive. The rootlets then converge and pass through the *hypoglossal foramen* in the posterior fossa (Figure 2–2). After leaving the skull, the nerve lies medial to cranial nerves IX, X, and XI and travels in the vicinity of the common carotid artery and internal jugular vein. It eventually loops anteriorly above the greater cornu of the hyoid bone and passes to the intrinsic and extrinsic muscles of the tongue.

The hypoglossal nucleus receives taste and tactile information from the nucleus of the tractus solitarius and the sensory trigeminal nucleus. These sensory processes are important for speech as well as chewing, swallowing, and sucking.

Damage to the hypoglossal nucleus or its axons can lead to *atrophy, weakness, and fasciculations of the tongue on the side of the lesion.* Unilateral weakness causes the tongue to deviate to the side of the lesion when protruded.

***The* spinal nerves.** Upper cervical spinal nerves supply neck and shoulder muscles that are indirectly implicated in voice, resonance, and articulation. For practical purposes, however, the discussion of spinal nerve contributions to speech will be confined to respiratory activities.

The discussion of respiratory activity will be largely confined to *external respiration,* or the exchange of air between the lungs and outside atmosphere; *internal respiration,* or the process of

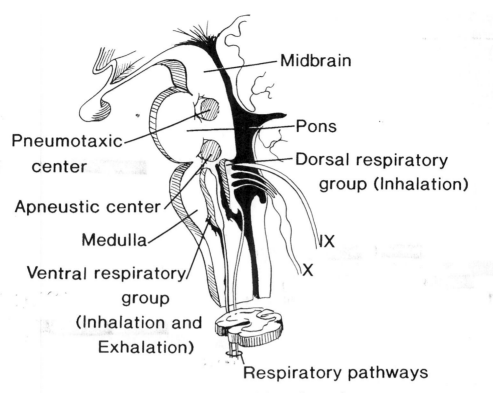

Figure 2–14 Respiratory centers and descending respiratory tracts.

exchanging oxygen and carbon dioxide between the lungs and blood and cells of the body, is only indirectly relevant to respiratory functions for speech. Similarly, the spinal nerves will be discussed as they relate to forced respiration, as opposed to quiet respiration, because forced respiration is the process used for speech production.*

LMNs subserving respiration are spread from the cervical through the thoracic divisions of the spinal cord. Those supplying the diaphragm arise from the 3rd, 4th, and 5th cervical segments of the spinal cord. Those supplying the intercostal and abdominal muscles of respiration are spread throughout the thoracic portion of the spinal cord. Accessory muscles of respiration, certain neck and shoulder girdle muscles (for example, sternocleidomastoid and trapezius) are spread through the upper and middle cervical cord down to the sixth cervical segment.

Fibers from the 3rd, 4th, and 5th cervical nerves combine in the *cervical plexus* to form the paired *phrenic nerves.* Each phrenic nerve innervates one

half of the *diaphragm,* the most important muscle of inhalation, and the most important respiratory muscle for speech. The remaining muscles of inhalation (external and internal intercostal, sternocleidomastoid, scalene, and pectoralis muscles) are innervated by motor neurons from branches of the lower cervical nerves, the intercostal nerves, the phrenic nerve, and the anterior and medial thoracic nerves.

Quiet exhalation occurs primarily through passive forces that bring the rib cage and inhalatory muscles to their resting position. Abdominal muscles are active in forced exhalation, however, and are innervated by the 7th through 12th intercostal nerves, branches of the iliohypogastric and ilioinguinal nerves, and the lower six thoracic and upper two lumbar nerves.

The CNS is responsible for matching respiratory rate to the variety of metabolic demands that arise from various activities, including speech. The respiratory center is made up of several widely distributed bilaterally located groups of neurons in the medulla and pons (Figure 2–14).

Dorsal respiratory neurons are located along the length of the medulla in its reticular formation and the nucleus of the tractus solitarius (also the termination point of sensory neurons from the vagus and glossopharyngeal nerves). Stimulation of these

---

*Detailed discussion of the neuroanatomy and physiology of respiratory functions for speech can be found in Aronson (1990), Barlow and Farley (1989), Hixon (1987), and Kennedy and Kuehn (1989).

Table 2–7 Distinctions among the lower motor neuron and upper motor neuron divisions of the nervous system

	Lower motor neuron *FCP*	Upper motor neuron	
		Direct activation pathway	Indirect activation pathway
Origin **Destination**	Brainstem & spinal cord Muscle	Cerebral cortex Cranial & spinal nerve nuclei	Cerebral cortex Cranial & spinal nerve nuclei
Function	Produce muscle actions for reflexes & muscle tone Carry out UMN commands for voluntary movements & postural adjustments	Direct voluntary, skilled movements	Control posture, tone, & movements supportive of voluntary movement
Distinctive signs of lesions	Weakness of all movements (voluntary & automatic) Diminished reflexes Decreased muscle tone Atrophy Fasciculations	Loss of skilled movement Hyporeflexia Babinski sign Decreased muscle tone *Uni UMN*	Spasticity *Bi UMN* Clonus -*inapp. mvmt c̄ continuous contraction* Hyperactive stretch reflexes Increased muscle tone Decorticate or decerebrate posture

UMN, upper motor neuron.

neurons produces inhalation and is important to maintaining the smooth rhythm of respiration.

Ventral respiratory neurons are located along the length of the medulla, in its ventrolateral portion. They can stimulate exhalation or inhalation but are primarily responsible for providing force during exhalation.

The *apneustic center* is located in the lower pons. It seems to serve as an additional drive to inspiration. The *pneumotaxic center* is located in the upper pons. It helps regulate inspiratory volume by inhibiting inspiration.

Because LMNs supplying the respiratory muscles are distributed widely, diffuse impairment is required to interfere significantly with respiration, especially respiration for speech. The exception to this is damage to the 3rd, 4th, and 5th cervical segment of the spinal cord, where damage can paralyze the diaphragm bilaterally and seriously affect breathing. Significant *weakness of respiratory function can affect voice production, loudness, phrase length, and prosody.*

The direct activation pathway and speech

The direct activation pathway has a rather direct connection and major activating influence on the FCP. It is also known as the *pyramidal tract* or *direct motor system*. It can be divided into the *corticobulbar tract,* which influences the activities of the cranial nerves, and the *corticospinal tract,* which influences the activity of the spinal nerves. Together, they form part of the *upper motor neuron (UMN) system.*

The distinction between the UMN and LMN systems is a basic cornerstone of clinical neurology and is crucial to understanding the distinctive effects of lesions within each system on motor behavior, including speech. The anatomic and physiologic differences between the two systems are fairly straightforward. They are summarized in Table 2–7.

The concept of the UMN system can be confusing. One source of confusion lies in the degree to which the direct and indirect activation pathways and the control circuits are encompassed by the concept of the UMN. According to Gilman and Winans (1982), UMNs include neurons that regulate LMNs and that are controlled directly or indirectly by the cortex, cerebellum, or basal ganglia; "in the strictest sense, the neurons in all such pathways should be referred to as upper motoneurons" (p. 26). From this standpoint, the direct and indirect activation pathways, and perhaps the control circuits, are all part of the UMN system. In practice, however, most clinicians use the term "upper motor neuron" only when referring to the corticospinal and corticobulbar tracts. These pathways are traditionally defined as pyramidal or direct activation pathways. For our purposes, it is probably best to think of the UMN system as that part of the motor system that (1) is contained entirely within the CNS and is distinctly different from the location and functions of the LMN system; (2) does not include the basal ganglia and cerebellar control circuits; (3) does include the corticospinal and corticobulbar tracts; and (4) is predominantly a direct activation pathway. These distinctions will be clarified further during discussion of the indirect activation pathway and the control circuits.

The direct activation pathway for speech has a major influence on the cranial and spinal nerves that form the FCP for speech production, and it is connected *directly* from the cortex to them. The effect of the direct activation system on the FCP is primarily facilitory. Thus, the direct system leads to movement (not inhibition of movement), presumably finely controlled, discrete movement, such as that required for speech.

Cortical components. The direct activation pathway, including its components that are related to speech production, originates in the cortex of *each* cerebral hemisphere. From this standpoint, it is appropriate to think of the direct activation pathway*s* (*right* and *left*).

The main launching platform for the direct motor system is the *primary motor cortex* (also commonly called the *precentral gyrus, motor strip,* or *Brodmann's area 4*) (Figure 2–15). It is located just anterior to the *central sulcus,* or *rolandic fissure,* the dividing line between the frontal and parietal lobes. Although the primary motor cortex is the cortical focal point of the pyramidal tracts for speech, only about one third of the direct system originates in it. Its fibers also arise from the *premotor cortex,* located just anterior to the primary motor area in the frontal lobe. The *supplementary motor area,* a portion of the premotor area also of importance for speech, is located on the medial aspect of each hemisphere. Finally, UMN fibers also originate in the postcentral gyrus in the parietal lobe (sometimes called the *secondary motor area*), which overlaps with the primary sensory area. In addition to sending fibers through the direct activation pathways, these cortical motor areas are also believed to contribute to other motor pathways (that is, the indirect activation or extrapyramidal pathways).

Three characteristics of motor cortex organization further define the cortical anatomic and physiologic organization of the direct activation pathway:

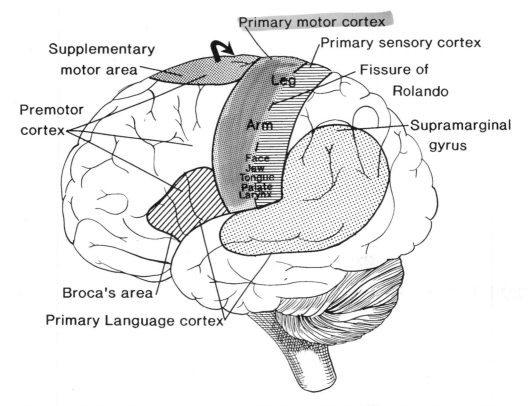

Figure 2–15 The major cortical components of the direct and indirect activation pathways and the motor speech programmer.

1. Striated muscles are represented in an upside down fashion along the length of the motor strip. For example, cell bodies sending axons to LMNs that innervate muscles of the face, tongue, and larynx are influenced by neurons in the lowest portion of the strip, whereas the hand, arm, abdomen, leg and foot, in ascending sequence, are represented at its more upper and superior medial aspects.

2. The number of motoneurons devoted to striated muscle is allocated according to the degree to which fine control of voluntary movement is required, and not according to muscle size. Therefore, the relatively small muscles of the face, tongue, jaw, palate, and larynx are allocated a disproportionately large number of primary motor cortex neurons. This distribution reflects the primary function of the direct activating system for speech—the discrete control of precise movements.

3. The motor cortex is organized in columns of neurons extending vertically from the surface to deeper layers of the cortex. These columns seem to represent functional entities that direct groups of muscles that act on a joint (this organization presumably includes groups of muscles that work together, even if they do not act on joints, such as the face, tongue, lips, and palate). It therefore seems that movements, rather than muscles, are represented in the cerebral cortex because "individual muscles are represented repeatedly, in different combinations, among the columns" (Gilman and Winans, 1982, p. 182). This conclusion receives some support from the results of cortical stimulation studies in people undergoing neurosurgery for control of seizures. Stimulation of motor cortex in such patients has produced results including vocalization, tongue protrusion, palatal elevation (Penfield & Roberts, 1959). Although not skilled, these behaviors require the activity of groups of muscles, not just single muscles. It is equally important, however, to recognize that stimulation of motor cortex does not yield words or "meaningful" utterances, suggesting that words or phrases are not stored in discrete areas of the motor cortex (or any other cerebral location, for that matter).

The organization of the *primary sensory cortex* (commonly called the *sensory strip*) located in the postcentral gyrus, is similar to that of the primary motor cortex. This similarity, particularly the rich allocation of cortical sensory neurons to the relatively small cranial speech muscles, attests to the importance of sensory processes in speech control.

Tracts. Axons of the direct activation pathway for speech travel in the *corticobulbar* and *corticospinal tracts.* Fibers with direct connections to the brainstem nuclei of cranial nerves V, VII, IX, X, XI, and XII travel in the corticobulbar tracts. Fibers with direct connections to the spinal nerves in the anterior horns of the spinal cord that serve respiratory muscles travel in the corticospinal tracts (Figure 2–16).

The corticobulbar and corticospinal tracts are arranged in a fanlike mass of fibers that converges from the cortex toward the brainstem. They are collectively known as the *corona radiata.* In the vicinity of the basal ganglia and thalamus, the corona radiata converges into a compact band known as the *internal capsule.* The internal capsule is an important region because it contains all afferent and efferent fibers that project to and from the cortex. Afferent fibers in the internal capsule arise mainly from the thalamus and project as *thalamocortical radiations* to nearly all regions of the cerebral cortex.

A horizontal section of the internal capsule (see Figure 2–17) reveals its three major divisions: the *anterior limb,* located between the caudate nucleus and putamen, contains anterior thalamic radiations, prefrontal corticopontine fibers, and fibers from the orbital cortex that project to the hypothalamus; the *posterior limb,* flanked by the thalamus and globus pallidus, contains corticospinal fibers, frontopontine fibers, the superior thalamic radiation (which projects general somatosensory information to the postcentral gyrus), and some corticotectal, corticorubral, and corticoreticular fibers; and the *genu,* which lies between the anterior and posterior limbs, contains corticobulbar and corticoreticular fibers.

Because thalamocortical, corticobulbar, and corticospinal fibers occupy such a compact area in the internal capsule, even small capsular lesions can produce widespread motor deficits. Lesions in the genu and posterior limb produce greater effects on speech than lesions elsewhere in the internal capsule.

Destination. In general, the UMN system innervates LMNs on both sides or predominantly the opposite side of the body (for example, the direct activation system originating in the left hemisphere innervates cranial and spinal nerves on the right (*contralateral*) side, or on both sides of the body).

The direct activation pathway innervation of the speech cranial nerves is primarily bilateral (see Table 2–8). However, there are some important exceptions, including the tongue and, to a greater degree, the lower face; the lower facial muscles (supplied by the VIIth nerve) are innervated predominantly by contralateral corticobulbar fibers.

Corticobulbar pathways to cranial nerve motor nuclei involved in speech do not all project directly from the cortex to motor nuclei of cranial nerves.

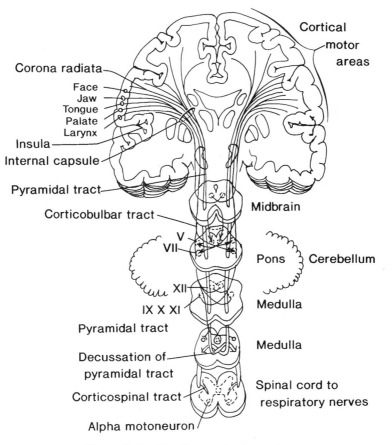

Figure 2–16 The direct activation pathways.

Many so-called corticobulbar fibers are actually corticoreticular fibers whose influence on cranial nerve nuclei is through synapses in the reticular formation (Carpenter, 1978), technically making them part of the indirect rather than the direct activation system. The direct corticobulbar system is a phylogenetically newer system, likely developed for its primary purpose of controlling finely coordinated skilled movements such as speech.

Further increasing the complexity of the direct activation system is the fact that the corticobulbar and corticospinal tracts are not purely motor. They also send fibers to synapse on interneurons that can influence local reflex arcs and nuclei in ascending sensory pathways. In the brainstem, these sensory nuclei include, but are not limited to, the trigeminal sensory nucleus and the nucleus of the tractus solitarius, both of which are relevant to speech and other oromotor activities. These synapses illustrate how descending cortical motor impulses can influence sensory input to the cortex, including that from speech structures.

Function. The direct activation pathways are crucial to voluntary motor activity, especially consciously controlled skilled, discrete-and-often-rapid movements. Movements generated through the system can be triggered by specific sensory stimuli, but they are not considered reflexes because they are voluntary and not stereotyped. Movements are also generated by cognitive activity that intervenes between sensation and movement and may involve complex planning. Speech clearly falls into the types of movements mediated through the direct activation system.

Effects of damage. Lesions produce a loss or reduction of voluntary skilled movements, although weakness is usually not as profound as that that can occur with LMN lesions. When the UMN lesion is unilateral, weakness is on the opposite side of the body. Because the FCP and peripheral sensation are not part of the direct activation pathways, normal reflexes are preserved.

Because of the predominantly bilateral UMN supply to cranial nerves V, IX, X, and XI, the effects of unilateral UMN lesions on jaw movement and the velopharyngeal, laryngeal, and respi-

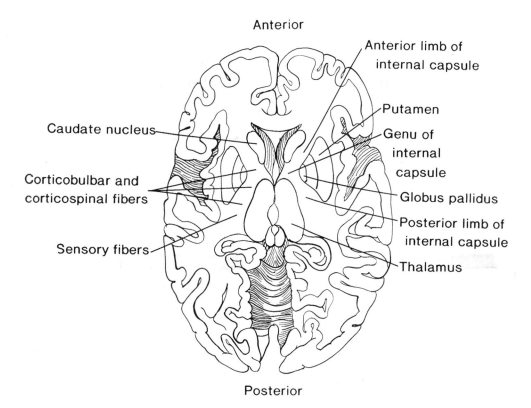

Figure 2–17 Internal capsule, thalamus, and basal ganglia (*horizontal section*).

Table 2–8 Direct and indirect activation pathway (UMN) innervation of cranial nerves related to speech

Cranial nerve	UMN innervation
Trigeminal (V) = *bi*	Bilateral*
Facial (VII) = *bi*	
Upper face = *bi*	Bilateral
Lower face = *contralateral*	Predominantly contralateral[†]
Glossopharyngeal (IX) = *bi*	Bilateral
Vagus (X, all branches) = *bi*	Bilateral
Accessory (XI) = *bi*	Bilateral
Hypoglossal (XII) = *contralateral*	Contralateral > bilateral[‡]

*Right and left cranial nerves receive input from UMNs coming from both the right and left cerebral hemispheres.
[†]Right and left cranial nerves receive input mostly from UMN fibers coming from the opposite cerebral hemisphere.
[‡]UMN supply may be bilateral but with greater input from the contralateral cerebral hemisphere.

ratory functions for speech are minor. UMN innervation of the hypoglossal nerve seems to vary in the degree to which it is bilateral, but unilateral UMN lesions will frequently cause some tongue weakness on the side opposite the lesion. Contralateral lower facial weakness can be quite prominent after unilateral UMN lesions.

Unilateral UMN lesions can produce a relatively mild dysarthria that seems primarily to reflect weakness and loss of skilled movement. It is called *unilateral UMN dysarthria*. Its neuropatho-

logic underpinnings and clinical characteristics will be discussed in Chapter 9.

Bilateral UMN lesions affecting speech can have mild-to-devastating effects on speech, and they usually reflect the combined effects of direct and indirect activation pathway dysfunction. The resulting speech disorder can reflect bilateral weakness and loss of skilled movement, as well as alterations in muscle tone (spasticity). This dysarthria is known as *spastic dysarthria*. It will be discussed in detail in Chapter 5.

The indirect activation pathway and speech

The indirect activation pathway is complex and its functions for speech are poorly understood. Its anatomy and activities are difficult to separate completely from those of the basal ganglia and cerebellar control circuits. However, the indirect activation pathway is a source of input to LMNs, whereas the control circuits are not. In addition, separating the control circuits from the indirect activation pathway is clinically valuable because some dysarthrias are specifically tied to control circuit pathology whereas others are associated with pathology in portions of the indirect activation pathways that do not include major control circuit structures.

The indirect activation pathway is often referred to as the *extrapyramidal tract* or *indirect motor system.* Its designation as "indirect" derives from

the multiple synapses between its origin in the cerebral cortex and its arrival and activation of the FCP. In a sense, it follows a "local" route with stops en route to the FCP, in contrast to the "express" or nonstop route followed by the direct activation pathway. Technically, it can be considered part of the UMN system, at least in so far as it is contained entirely within the CNS and is distinct from the LMN system.

Cortical components and tracts. The indirect activation pathway is complex (Figure 2–18). It is made up of a number of short pathways and interconnected structures between its origin in the cerebral cortex and its final interaction with the cranial nerve nuclei and anterior horn cells of the spinal cord.

Corticoreticular tracts, projecting from the cortex to the reticular formation, arise mostly from

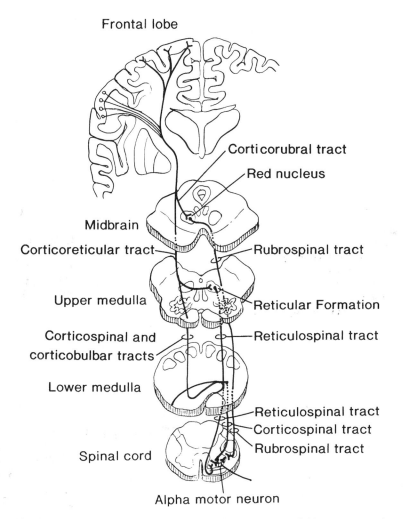

Frontal lobe

Corticorubral tract
Red nucleus

Midbrain
Corticoreticular tract — — Rubrospinal tract

Upper medulla — Reticular Formation

Corticospinal and corticobulbar tracts — Reticulospinal tract

Lower medulla

— Reticulospinal tract
— Corticospinal tract
— Rubrospinal tract

Spinal cord

Alpha motor neuron

Figure 2–18 The indirect activation pathway. Note that the tracts of this system are intermingled with those of the corticobulbar and corticospinal tracts (the direct activation pathway).

the motor, premotor, and sensory cortex. They are intermingled with corticospinal and corticobulbar fibers of the direct activation pathways. They descend to enter the reticular formation in the medulla and pons where their fibers are distributed bilaterally, but with a contralateral predominance. Regions of the reticular formation receiving these fibers have ascending and descending projections, as well as projections to the cerebellum and cranial nerve nuclei. The indirect system also sends fibers from the cortex to the red nucleus through the *corticorubral tracts,* another indirect path from the cortex to the LMNs.

Motor function roles of the reticular formation, vestibular, and red nucleus. The *reticular formation* is a field of scattered cells lying between large nuclei and fiber tracts in the medulla, pons, and midbrain. It mediates consciousness and ascending sensory information and has complex effects on LMNs.

Portions of the reticular formation excite extensor motoneurons and inhibit flexor motoneurons, a process that contributes to muscle tone. Fibers in these *reticulospinal tracts* terminate mainly on gamma motoneurons (recall the role of the gamma motoneuron and gamma loop in the stretch reflex and maintenance of normal muscle tone). Other portions of the reticular formation inhibit extensor motoneurons and excite flexors. To exert their influence, these inhibitory reticular fibers must be excited by supratentorial motor pathways. The fibers of these pathways terminate in the spinal cord in the same general areas where corticospinal tracts (direct activation pathway) terminate. The influence of the reticular formation on cranial nerve motor function is not well understood, although *collateral fibers from the reticular formation do project to the cranial nerve nuclei* (Carpenter, 1978).

Responses of the reticular formation to stimulation help identify the influence it may have on motor activities that are relevant to speech. Stimulation can: facilitate and inhibit reflex activity and cortically induced voluntary movement; influence muscle tone; affect phasic respiratory activities; facilitate and inhibit ascending sensory information (Carpenter, 1978).

The *vestibular nuclei,* located in the floor of the fourth ventricle in the pons and medulla, receive sensory input from the vestibular apparatus of the ear and from the cerebellum. They project to the brainstem, cerebellum, and spinal cord. Ascending and descending brainstem projections of the vestibular nuclei run in the *medial longitudinal fasciculus.* They modulate the activities of the eye and neck muscles.

Vestibular and certain cerebellar influences upon the spinal cord are mediated through the *vestibulospinal tract,* which terminates on both alpha and gamma motoneurons. This tract is thought to facilitate reflex activities and spinal mechanisms that control muscle tone. Although the vestibular system projects to cranial nerve motor nuclei, its specific role in speech is uncertain.

The *red nucleus* is an oval mass of cells in the midbrain tegmentum. It receives cortical projections through the *corticorubral tracts.* It also serves as a relay station between a pathway from the cerebellum to the ventrolateral nucleus of the thalamus and, ultimately, the cortex. Input from the cerebellum and the basal ganglia can also modify descending activity in the red nucleus. The *rubrospinal tract* facilitates flexor and inhibits extensor alpha and gamma motoneurons, but its major influence is on flexor muscle groups in the limbs. Its specific influence on cranial motor nerves involved in speech is unclear, but a role can be assumed because it is implicated in certain disorders affecting speech (for example, palatopharyngolaryngeal myoclonus).

Destination. The indirect activation pathway ultimately influences the activities of both gamma and alpha motoneurons of the FCP. Gamma motoneurons have a lower response threshold than alpha motoneurons, however, so they are more sensitive—respond more readily—to indirect motor system input.

Function. The indirect activation pathway helps regulate reflexes and maintain posture, tone, and associated activities that provide a framework on which the direct activation pathway can accomplish skilled, discrete actions. Its activities are subconscious and typically require the integration of activities of many supporting muscles. It ensures that specific speech movements occur without constant or variable interference with their speed, range, and direction.

Effects of damage. Diseases affecting the indirect activation pathways are manifest in a variety of ways. In general, lesions affect muscle tone and reflexes.

The effects of indirect activation pathway lesions are different for flexor and extensor muscles. Lesions damaging corticoreticular fibers above the midbrain and red nucleus produce increased extensor tone in the legs and increased flexor tone in the arms (that is, the legs tend to be extended and resist bending; the arms tend to flex and resist extension). This occurs because all descending pathways are uninhibited; such a state is known as *decorticate posturing.* Lesions at the level of the midbrain below the red nucleus remove arm flexor excitation and result in excitation of all extensor muscles and a generalized increase in extensor tone; this state is known as *decerebrate posturing*. Lesions below the medulla result in a loss of all descending input and produce generalized flaccidity in muscles supplied by spinal nerves.

Lesions of the brainstem that damage the reticular formation often lead to death. Damage to the indirect activation pathways above that level, however, will produce certain predictable deficits, including decorticate posturing. When cortical controls become nonfunctional, the unchecked reticular system makes extensor muscles hyperexcitable, a condition manifest clinically as increased muscle tone or *spasticity*. The specific muscles that become spastic depend on the level of the lesion, but the effects are usually particularly strong in axial and proximal muscles (toward the center of the body).

Lesions of motor pathways from the cerebral hemispheres are common and are usually referred to as *UMN lesions*. They tend to affect both direct and indirect pathways. Consequently, the clinical picture may include spasticity and increased muscle stretch reflexes as a result of indirect pathway involvement, as well as a loss of skilled movements resulting from direct pathway involvement. Weakness can result from damage to direct or indirect pathways. The effects of indirect versus direct activation pathway lesions are summarized in Table 2–7.

Clinical findings in UMN lesions may change over time. When descending CNS pathways to alpha and gamma motoneurons are destroyed, motor activity is initially greatly diminished, as are muscle tone and reflexes. However, because alpha and gamma motoneurons may still be influenced by other input (for example, peripheral sensory input), they may eventually recover their excitability and even become hyperexcitable. Therefore, even though voluntary activity may be absent or diminished, reflexes may become hyperactive because inhibitory influences from central pathways are lost.

The effects of spasticity on speech, in general, are to slow movement and to cause hyperadduction of the vocal cords during phonation. These effects tend to be minimal when UMN lesions are unilateral, but they can range from mild to severe when lesions are bilateral. Bilateral UMN lesions affecting speech that include indirect activation pathways are often accompanied by hyperactive reflexes, pathologic reflexes, dysphagia, and disinhibition of physical expression of emotion.

The dysarthrias resulting from indirect activation pathway involvement are usually encountered in combination with direct pathway involvement.

They include *unilateral UMN dysarthria* when lesions are unilateral, and *spastic dysarthria* when lesions are bilateral. They will be discussed in Chapters 9 and 5, respectively.

Control circuits

Control circuits are so-called because they integrate or help control the diverse activities of the many structures and pathways involved in motor performance. Unlike the direct and indirect activation pathways, the *control circuits do not have direct contact with LMNs.*

Considering the different roles played by the direct and indirect activation pathways in movement, it makes sense that there are mechanisms within the CNS that coordinate or integrate their activities. For example, the skilled movements activated through the direct activation pathways need to be planned and executed with knowledge about the posture, orientation in space, tone, and physical environment in which movement will occur (aspects of movement mediated through the indirect activation pathways). At the same time, the creation of appropriate posture and tone must be done with some information about the goals to be achieved by voluntary movements that are mediated through the direct activation pathways. This integration and coordination are accomplished through the activities of the *basal ganglia control circuit* and the *cerebellar control circuit*. These circuits influence movement through their input to the cerebral cortex and, from there, via the direct and indirect activation pathways.

The basal ganglia control circuit and speech

Location and course. The basal ganglia include the caudate nucleus, putamen, and globus pallidus (Figures 2–17 and 2–19). The term *striatum* refers to the caudate nucleus and putamen, which act together as a functional unit. The putamen and globus pallidus are known collectively as the *lentiform nucleus*. The *substantia nigra* and the *subthalamic nucleus* are anatomically and functionally closely related to the basal ganglia and its activities as a control circuit.

The basal ganglia are often considered part of, or synonymous with, the indirect motor system or extrapyramidal system. This is technically correct because the basal ganglia lie outside the pyramids of the medulla, have strong functional ties to the extrapyramidal pathways, and are not part of the direct activation pathways. Daube and others (1986), however, point out that the cerebellum is also "extrapyramidal" but is never considered as part of the extrapyramidal system. Therefore, it seems conceptually simpler to view the basal ganglia as one of two major motor control circuits

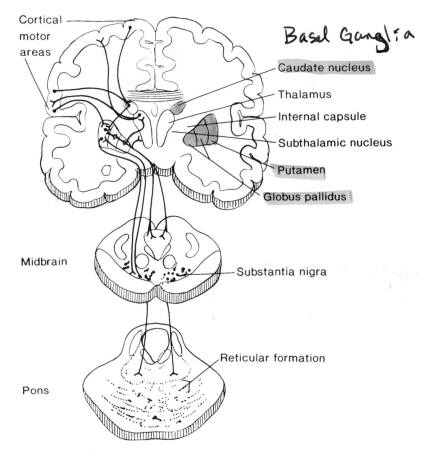

Figure 2–19 The basal ganglia control circuit.

and not as a major descending pathway for motor activity.

The striatum is the receptive portion of the basal ganglia. It receives major projections from the frontal cortex as well as input from certain thalamic nuclei and the substantia nigra. The cortical-putamen pathway may be especially important to motor control because its fibers originate in the premotor cortex; the caudate nucleus receives fibers from the more anterior portions of the frontal lobe (McClean, 1988). The striatum sends efferent fibers to the substantia nigra and is the major source of input to the globus pallidus.

The major efferent pathways of the basal ganglia originate in the globus pallidus. Most of these efferent fibers go to the ventrolateral nucleus of the thalamus for relay back to the cortex. They also go to the subthalamic nucleus, the nearby red nucleus, and the reticular formation in the brainstem. Basal ganglia pathways are thus made up of several loops: striatum to globus pallidus to thalamus to cortex to striatum; striatum to substantia nigra to striatum; globus pallidus to subthalamus to globus pallidus.

The striatum is rich in two important neurotransmitters, *acetylcholine (ACh)* and *dopamine.* The balance between these neurotransmitters is important to motor control, and imbalance is implicated in movement disorders associated with several basal ganglia diseases. ACh is the synaptic transmitter for most of the neurons with axonal terminations within the striatum. Dopamine is manufactured in the substantia nigra and transmitted by way of *nigrostriatal tracts* to the striatum where it acts as a neurotransmitter. Therefore, if neurons in the substantia nigra are destroyed, the dopamine content in the striatum will be lowered. In addition to ACh and dopamine, most efferent fibers from the striatum to the globus pallidus and from the globus pallidus to the substantia nigra release an inhibitory neurotransmitter called *gamma-aminobutyric acid (GABA).*

Function. The functions of the individual components of the basal ganglia for movement control are not well understood. As a group, however, they seem important for maintaining normal posture and static muscle contraction upon which voluntary, skilled movements are superimposed. They also seem important to regulating the amplitude, velocity and, possibly, the initiation of movements (Adams and Victor, 1991).

The basal ganglia control circuit is probably important to generating components of motor programs for speech, particularly those that help maintain a stable musculoskeletal environment in which discrete speech movements can occur. In general, its activities seem to have a damping effect on cortical discharges. That is, it appears that the cortex initiates impulses for movement that are in excess of those required to accomplish movement goals, and that one role of the basal ganglia is to damp or modulate those impulses to an appropriate degree.

To summarize, the basal ganglia control circuit seems to be an important participant in regulating muscle tone; movements associated with goal-directed activities such as the armswing during walking; automatic activities such as chewing and walking; postural adjustments during skilled movements such as stabilizing the shoulders and arms during typing; the relationship of required movement to the environment, such as speaking with restricted jaw movement; and the learning of new movements (Brown, 1980).

Effects of damage. The effect of basal ganglia control circuit lesions on movement can be manifest in one of two ways: reduced mobility or *hypokinesia;* and involuntary movements or *hyperkinesia.*

Hypokinesia is often associated with disease of the substantia nigra, which results in a deficiency of dopamine supply to the basal ganglia. The effect is an increase in muscle tone, with subsequent increased resistance to passive movements, a condition known as *rigidity*. In rigidity, movements are slow and stiff, and may be initiated or stopped with difficulty. This excessive restriction of movement is reflected in the reduced range of movement underlying many of the deviant speech characteristics of *hypokinetic dysarthria.*

It is relevant to note here that there seems to be a speech counterpart to the basal ganglia's contribution to some of the automatic aspects of movement. For example, in certain basal ganglia diseases (most notably, Parkinson's disease), the face becomes "masked" or expressionless. The hypokinetic dysarthria of such patients can be affectively expressionless as well, even when linguistic content may convey emotionally laden thoughts. These abnormalities highlight the important functional role of the basal ganglia control circuit in the physical expression of affect. Similarly, its speech pathology demonstrates that dysarthria affects the character of much more than the segmental-phonemic-linguistic messages conveyed in speech; it also can affect the suprasegmental-prosodic-emotional components of messages.

Hyperkinesia can result from excessive activity in dopaminergic nerve fibers, thereby reducing the circuit's damping effect on cortical discharges. This results in involuntary movements, which can vary considerably in their locus, speed, constancy, regularity and predictability, and the conditions that promote or inhibit their occurrence. These excessive and often unpredictable variations in muscle tone and movement underly many of the deviant speech characteristics associated with the *hyperkinetic dysarthrias.*

Lesions of the basal ganglia control circuit that involve its subcortical components (that is, the basal ganglia and their related subcortical nuclei) generally produce more profound speech disturbances than do lesions to its cortical components. This is usually the case for all of the dysarthrias, a fact that underscores the importance of attending to more than the cortical contributions to movement when studying motor speech disorders.

The variety of movement disorders that may be encountered in disease of the basal ganglia will be discussed in Chapters 7 and 8, which deal with hypokinetic dysarthria and hyperkinetic dysarthria, respectively.

The cerebellar control circuit and speech

Location and course. The cerebellum and its connections constitute the cerebellar control circuit. The cerebellum can be divided into anterior, posterior, and flocculonodular lobes. From side to side, the midportion of the cerebellum is the *vermis,* which forms the midline of the anterior and posterior lobes. The right and left cerebellar hemispheres are to the side of the vermis (Figure 2–20). Each cerebellar hemisphere is connected to the contralateral thalamus and cerebral hemisphere, and each controls movements on the ipsilateral side of the body.

The *flocculonodular lobe* has primary connections to the vestibular mechanism for modulating equilibrium and the orientation of the head and eyes. The *anterior lobe* is a projection area for spinocerebellar proprioceptive information. It is important for regulating posture, gait, and truncal tone. The *posterior lobe* is a recent phylogenetic development. Its lateral cerebellar hemispheres are particularly important as a servomechanism for coordinating skilled, voluntary muscle activity and muscle tone.

Fiber tracts enter or leave the cerebellum through three structures: the inferior, middle, and superior cerebellar peduncles. The *inferior cerebellar peduncle,* or *restiform body,* contains mostly afferent fibers but also has efferent flow to

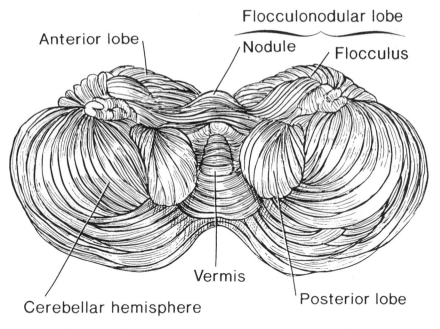

Figure 2-20 Major anatomic subdivisions of the cerebellum.

vestibular mechanisms and to the reticular formation. The *middle cerebellar peduncle,* or *brachium pontis,* is an afferent pathway whose fibers decussate in the pons. The *superior cerebellar peduncle,* or *brachium conjunctivum,* is mostly efferent.

The sole output neurons of the cerebellar cortex are *Purkinje cells,* which comprise the middle layer of cells in the cerebellar cortex. The axons of Purkinje cells synapse in the deep cerebellar nuclei, structures from which cerebellar output departs through the superior or inferior cerebellar peduncles. These nuclei include the *dentate, globose, emboliform,* and *fastigial nuclei* (Figure 2-21). The dentate nucleus may be particularly important for speech control because it seems to be active in initiating movement, executing preplanned motor tasks, and regulating posture (Gilman, Gloedel, & Lechtenberg, 1981).

The areas of the cerebellum that appear most involved in speech control are the vermis and the cerebellar hemispheres. This conclusion is based on the sites of cerebellar damage most frequently encountered in dysarthria resulting from cerebellar lesions. The importance of the cerebellar hemispheres for speech control can also be inferred from their known importance for coordinating skilled, voluntary muscle activity.

The primary and necessary cerebellar pathways for speech production probably include: reciprocal connections with the cerebral cortex; auditory feedback and proprioceptive input from speech muscles, tendons, and joints; reciprocal connections with brainstem components of the indirect

activation pathways; and cooperative activity with the basal ganglia control circuit through interactions in the thalamus, cortex, and various components of the indirect motor system.

Two cortical-cerebellar pathways appear important for speech control. One is from the primary motor and premotor regions of the cortex to the lateral cerebellar hemispheres via pontine nuclei, with a return pathway to the same cortical areas through deep cerebellar nuclei and ventral thalamic nuclei. This loop seems important to planning and programming learned movements. The second pathway is from descending corticospinal and corticobulbar fibers to the intermediate aspects of the cerebellar hemispheres, with a return pathway to the primary motor cortex through deep cerebellar nuclei and ventral thalamic nuclei. This loop provides the cerebellum with immediate (relatively direct) information about cortical output (McClean, 1988), presumably about cortical intentions for skilled movement. The intermediate portions of the cerebellar hemispheres also project to brainstem and spinal motor centers via the red nucleus. The existence of these pathways suggests that the intermediate cerebellum uses sensory input to influence cortical motor output during movement, including speech.

Function. The cerebellar control circuit probably functions for speech control in ways that are similar to its contributions to movement in general. Similar to the basal ganglia control circuit, we know it has a specialized role in speech motor

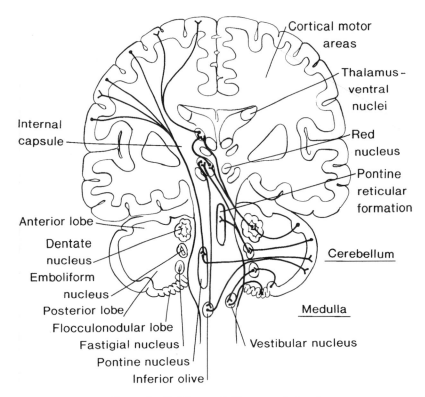

Figure 2–21 The cerebellar control circuit.

control because distinctive speech disturbances result from damage to it.

The cerebellum's functional role in speech can be conceptualized in the following way (relying heavily on discussions by Allen and Tsukahara (1974), Eccles (1977), Kent and Netsell (1975), Kent, Netsell and Abbs (1979), and Netsell and Kent (1976)).

1. Preliminary information from the cortex about intended speech goals activates the cerebellum's role in long-range movement planning. This role is mostly anticipatory in character and is based on learning and experience, and on preliminary sensory information. Input from the cortex also prepares the cerebellum to check the adequacy of speech output as feedback from muscles, tendons, and joints arrives from the periphery.

2. Initial cortical motor speech commands are probably provisional, imprecise, and in excess of those necessary to accomplish movement goals. The exclusive inhibitory output of the cerebellum's Purkinje cells subsequently results in smooth, coordinated speech movements, perhaps, as Eccles (1977) described, in a manner analogous to chiseling away from a block of stone to achieve form in a sculpture.

3. The cerebellum can bias or tune muscle spindles to optimize sensory feedback about the state of speech muscles. It interprets this sensory information and integrates it with ongoing input from the cortex about upcoming movement goals. This updating function can influence subsequent cortical motor output and ultimately smooth the actions of agonist and antagonist muscles within and among different speech subsystems (phonation, articulation, etc).

To summarize, the cerebellum receives advance notice about intended speech from the cortex so that it will be prepared to check the adequacy of the outcome when feedback from speech muscles, tendons, and joints arrives from the periphery. With its input to the cortex it is capable of influencing subsequent cortical motor speech output based on feedback it has received and ongoing information from the cortex about upcoming speech goals. These corrective modifications help to smooth the coordination of contracting muscles and the opposing activity of antagonistic muscles, resulting in smoothly flowing, well-coordinated speech.

Effects of damage. Damage to cerebellar control mechanisms produces signs that can be associated with the functions of its lobes. Its effects can be summarized as follows:

1. Flocculonodular lesions are associated with *truncal ataxia* (inability to stand or sit without

swaying or falling), disturbances in gait, and *nystagmus* (abnormal eye movements).

2. Anterior lobe lesions are associated with gait ataxia.

3. Posterior lobe lesions, especially in the cerebellar hemispheres, are associated with *limb ataxia* and *hypotonia, intention tremor,* and *incoordination* ipsilateral to the side of lesion.

The effects on speech of cerebellar or cerebellar pathway lesions generally can be attributed to incoordination and hypotonia and are classified as *ataxic dysarthria.* Damage to the vermis or the cerebellar hemispheres bilaterally generally has more serious consequences for speech than damage to portions of the circuit that lie outside the cerebellum. Ataxic dysarthria will be discussed in Chapter 6.

THE CONCEPTUAL-PROGRAMMING LEVEL AND SPEECH

How and where in the nervous system are ideas and the content of speech messages formulated? How and where is this content transformed into neural impulses that generate muscle contractions and movements that result in meaningful intelligible speech? What specifies the goals and the sequence of skilled movements for speech that are transmitted through the direct activation pathways? How is the indirect activation pathway informed about motor goals and what is it that the control circuits are told to control? What is the role of sensation in speech production? How can normal speech be produced so quickly? What are the criteria by which the motor system determines that goals have been achieved?

These questions are relevant to the understanding of motor speech control and some of its pathologies. The answers lie partly within the activities of the direct and indirect activation pathways, the control circuits, and the FCP, but they also lie at a level of function that has not yet been addressed. Darley, Aronson, and Brown (1975) called this the *conceptual-programming level* of motor organization for speech.

The conceptual-programming stage represents the highest level of motor organization. The designation "highest" is conferred because neural activity at this level establishes the meaning or goals of the speech act and the essentials of the program for achieving them. The designation does not necessarily mean that the most severe motor speech disorders occur with lesions at this level.

The conceptual-programming stage is concerned with establishing an idea or plan for activity and with specifying the movements that must occur for the plan to be realized. The term *teleopraxis* has been used to refer to this process. It is derived from the Greek words *telos,* meaning that which is shaped by a purpose or goal, and *praxis,*

meaning action or the performance of movement (Darley, Aronson, and Brown, 1975). The combination of these roots implies that the process straddles the boundaries between an internal, nonmotor, thought-related process and a sensorimotor programming process that results in movement. Where these central processes take place is only partly understood. How they take place is far less certain.

Darley, Aronson, and Brown (1975) discussed five stages that characterize activities that occur at the conceptual-programming level.* The ensuing discussion of these stages will emphasize speech motor control, but it is important to recognize that many of the assumptions about conceptual-programming mechanisms are based on general concepts and principles of motor behavior. The five stages, summarized in Table 2–9, include:

1. conceptualization
2. spatial-temporal planning (linguistic planning)
3. motor planning
4. performance
5. feedback

The first three stages are most relevant to this discussion. The performance and feedback stages have already been addressed during discussion of other components of the motor system.

Although it can be assumed that conceptualization precedes speech initiation, it would be incorrect to assume that the five stages operate in a fixed repetitive sequence during natural speech. It is more likely that the relationships among them reflect parallel and temporally overlapping activities rather than sequential activities.

Conceptualization

This stage involves developing a desire to do something and establishing a purpose or goal for action. These nonlinguistic "thoughts," "ideas," and "feelings," and the desire to act on them, fall into the "sphere of conscious awareness and intentional action" (Kent, 1990, p. 370). These attributes are cognitive and affective in nature. They do not necessarily involve the specific words that ultimately may be uttered; in fact, the thought may remain internal and never emerge as speech.

Localization. The neural bases for this conceptual or general cognitive process cannot be

---

*Much has been done in recent years to modify, refine, and more completely specify what may go on at the conceptual-programming level, and a number of specific models have been proposed. However, the broad stages outlined by Darley, Aronson, and Brown will serve our purpose of outlining the general processes and requirements that lead to the planning and programming of speech. Readers desiring an introduction to more detailed information on this topic are referred to Kent (1990) for a comprehensive but concise summary of models of speech formulation and production and their relation to various motor speech disorders.

Table 2–9 The conceptual-programming level of speech production

Process	Components	Neural substrate	Disorders affecting speech
Conceptualization	Cognitively & affectively generated thoughts, feelings, & emotions, & a sense of desire to express them to achieve a goal	Widespread	General intellectual impairment (for example, dementia) Confusion
Spatial-temporal (linguistic) planning	Highly interactive semantic & syntactic processing, ultimately taking a phonologic form	Left hemisphere perisylvian cortex (especially temporal-parietal), with less specific contributions from subcortical structures (thalamus & basal ganglia)	Aphasia
Motor planning/ programming	The compiling of motor commands for the production of phonetic segments & syllables at particular rates & with particular patterns of stress & prosody, based on acoustic (& other modality) goals & feedback	1. Dominant hemisphere → somatosensory cortex, premotor cortex (Broca's area), supplementary motor cortex, motor cortex, insula	Apraxia of speech
		2. Control circuits →	Dysarthrias (? apraxia of speech)
		3. Limbic system →	Altered affect/prosody
		4. Right hemisphere →	?"aprosodia"
		5. Thalamus & reticular formation →	Dysarthrias
Performance	Motor execution	Direct activation pathway Indirect activation pathway Control circuits LMNs	Dysarthrias
Feedback	Multimodality feedback to the above components	Peripheral & central sensory pathways	Dysarthrias & peripheral sensory-based speech disturbances

localized. Cortical activity is crucial, but it is probably bilateral and widespread. In fact, conceptualization is best viewed as involving the brain as a whole because alertness, affect, attention, and the sensory and motor processes that frequently acquire the "data" that drive or motivate thought and action are " . . . supported, empowered, and even urged by subcortical systems, including the ascending activating system of the brainstem, the hypothalamus, the limbic system, and various thalamic nuclei" (Darley, Aronson, and Brown, 1975, p. 62).

Effects of damage. Deficits in conceptualization often reflect diffuse impairment of cognitive or affective functions and are commonly associated with dementia, confusion, or other disturbances of affect or thought. Speech associated

with such impairments can be motorically normal. The disorders are reflected in message content, organization, or affective tone, but not in motor planning or execution. This indicates that the conceptual stage is essential to normal, appropriate, and meaningful communication but that it is not essential to normal motor speech production.

Spatial-temporal planning (linguistic planning)

To accomplish a motor act, it is necessary to know the body parts to be used, the space in which the action will take place, and the temporal sequence of its various components. In other words, a plan must be formulated.

For propositional speech, *linguistic units* form the content of the plan. Once an idea and the intention to express it develop (perhaps even before that), the language system must be activated to formulate the verbal message.

Linguistic planning involves cognitive operations on abstract rules. In its early stages, there are strong interactions between semantic and syntactic processes, and the message may be without phonological form. Once semantic and syntactic interactions begin to yield an adequately formulated expression, the utterance takes phonological shape (abstract phonemes are identified and ordered). Linguistic planning also requires attention, retrieval, and working memory processes, and the ability to discard from active processing utterances that have already been formulated and executed. Once these linguistic processes have been completed, a mental image of the verbal goal can be said to exist.

Localization. Linguistic planning seems centered in the *dominant hemisphere perisylvian cortex,* most importantly the temporoparietal and posterior frontal cortex. In a less definitive way, the dominant hemisphere's thalamus and basal ganglia may also be involved in linguistic planning. Other cortical areas may be recruited as well, depending on the source of the stimulus to speak (for example, the occipital lobes when speaking involves reading aloud). The *left hemisphere* is the dominant hemisphere for linguistic planning (and motor speech programming) in the great majority of individuals.

Effects of damage. Impairment in linguistic planning reflects dominant hemisphere pathology and is called aphasia or *dysphasia.* Signs of aphasia include difficulties with word retrieval, reduced auditory retention span, and other errors and inefficiencies associated with the semantic, syntactic, morphemic, and phonologic aspects of language. These impairments are usually observable in all verbal and nonverbal propositional modalities (that is, speech, verbal comprehension, reading, writing, pantomime, sign language) because the damaged processes are central or common to normal symbolic function for all input and output modalities. These problems (particularly phonologic ones) will be discussed in more detail in Chapter 15, which focuses on differential diagnosis.

Motor planning (programming)

Motor speech programming is at the heart of the conceptual-programming level for the motor organization for speech. Once a phonologic representation of a verbal message is developed, a plan for neuromuscular execution can be organized and activated. At this point an important transition is made between cognitive-linguistic functions and motor functions. Phoneme selection and ordering during linguistic planning are closely related to and difficult to separate from the motor programming required for their phonetic emergence as

speech. However, the separation of phonologic processes from motor programming does have theoretical, anatomic, physiologic, and clinical support. This will be addressed further in Chapters 11 and 15.

The requirements and goals of motor speech programming. Speech programming involves translation of the abstract linguistic-phonologic representation into a code that can be used by the motor system to generate movements that result in speech. This requires the selection of movements and the programming of their sequential and durational properties. More basically, the process must account for: identification of muscles; sequences for muscle contraction and relaxation; speed, strength, and duration of muscle excitation and inhibition; and coordination of speech muscle activities with other muscles involved in the act.

The task of speech programming is enormously complex. Darley, Aronson, and Brown (1975) pointed out that about 100 different muscles, each containing about 100 motor units, are involved in speaking. Therefore, about 140,000 neuromuscular events are generated per second at an average speaking rate of 14 phonemes per second. It would be impossible to plan consciously each of these neuromuscular events in such a time frame. Normal adults have little awareness of their speech muscles when they speak, unless they are learning how to pronounce a difficult multisyllabic word or sequence of words or are trying to correct an inadvertent error of articulation. Most of the time, we decide what to say and simply set the activity in motion. It is assumed, therefore, that once speech has been learned, programming usually involves the selection, sequencing, activation and fine tuning of *preprogrammed movement sequences* that are considerably more comprehensive than those represented by the contractions of individual muscle fibers, muscles, or even groups of muscles.

What must the motor speech programmer accomplish for successful communication? Ultimately, and that is what counts, spoken language must meet a condition of *perceptual or motor equivalence rather than acoustic or motor invariance* (motor equivalence refers to the capacity to achieve a movement goal in a variety of ways) (Lindblom, 1982). In other words, specific linguistic messages can be produced in neuromuscularly variable ways as long as the acoustic result generates a reliably accurate perception by the listener. This flexibility reduces the demands on the motor system for perfection, promotes efficiency and speed, and is analogous to what apparently happens during many nonspeech skilled movements (for example, throwing a ball to a target need not be accomplished in an unvarying way; distance, posture, requirements for speed, etc. vary in nearly infinite ways and the neural program to accomplish the goal must be modified accordingly).

This goal-oriented or listener-oriented organization of speech programming highlights a fundamental difference between linguistic and motor mechanisms. An unspoken sentence (language) can be viewed as discrete and context-free, separable sequentially into phonemes, morphemes, words, and phrases. In contrast, motor speech is a continuous and context-dependent activity in which articulators reach targets reliably despite considerable variability in their starting positions. In addition, the acoustic correlates of sequences of abstract phonemes do not reflect a sequence of discrete events. This is because of *coarticulation, the temporal-spatial overlap of movements necessary for the production of more than one sound occurring at a single point in time.* Nonetheless, the apparent "noise" generated by these coarticulatory movements are recognized as sequenced phonemes; in fact, the noise is crucial to their recognition. In a sense, the speech signal is a partial temporal hologram, in which multiple pieces of information—that is, information about more than one sound—can be found at single points in time. This redundancy greatly increases the speed at which speech can be produced and still be understood. These characteristics suggest that the motor commands for successive phonemes are processed simultaneously or that plans for moving the articulators from one position to the next are established in advance. The neural apparatus is apparently organized so that distinctions that can be heard are linked closely to distinctions that can be produced (Perkins and Kent, 1986).

Localization of cortical components (Figure 2–15). Motor speech programming is an important function of the *premotor* and *supplementary motor areas* of the dominant hemisphere's frontal lobe, but those areas do not represent the only structures involved in motor programming.

The premotor area appears to specify movements at a relatively abstract level. It receives input from multiple sensory modalities, is linked to the basal ganglia and cerebellum, and has reciprocal connections with the primary motor cortex. The influence of the premotor cortex on the primary motor cortex may be mostly indirect, involving a route through the basal ganglia and their related structures, and the thalamus (Adams and Victor, 1991). The premotor area's multiple connections with sensory and motor structures suggests that it may use sensory information to organize and guide motor behavior. Lesions of the premotor cortex are associated with deficits in complex skilled limb movements and problems with coordination of lip, tongue, and jaw movements for chewing and swallowing in primates (Square and Martin, 1994).

Broca's area, a part of the premotor cortex, appears intimately tied to speech programming. Its role is suggested by its connections to portions of the temporal and parietal lobes that are intimately involved in language processes, as well as its proximity to the primary motor cortex. It is located at the foot of the third frontal convolution in the dominant hemisphere, just anterior to the portion of the primary motor area in which the orofacial and neck muscles are richly represented.

It is often assumed that Broca's area is *the* location of the motor speech programmer. This is incorrect. On clinical grounds alone, it is clear that damage to other areas of the dominant hemisphere can result in deficits that appear to reflect a disturbance of motor speech programming. It is noteworthy, however, that these other areas represent loci of interface between Broca's area and language formulation areas or between Broca's area and other portions of the motor system.

The *supplementary motor area* is also associated with motor speech programming. It is located on the mesial surface of the hemispheres. It receives projections from the primary motor and premotor cortex and from the basal ganglia by way of the thalamus. It projects fibers to the primary motor, premotor, cingulate, and parietal cortex. Its strong connections to the limbic system implicate it in mechanisms that "drive" or motivate action. It is thought to play a role in the initiation of propositional speech and the control of rhythm, phonation, and articulation (Jonas, 1981). Cortical stimulation studies indicate that stimulation of the area can evoke or arrest vocalization, slow speech, or induce dysfluencies and distortions (Penfield and Roberts, 1974).

The parietal lobe *somatosensory cortex* and the *supramarginal gyrus* also appear to play a role in motor speech planning and programming, especially in the integration of sensory information in preparation for motor activity. Finally, the *insula* (Figure 2–16) has been implicated in disorders of motor speech programming (Dronkers, Redfern, and Shapiro, 1993).

The role of sensation. The initial motor program seems designed to initiate speech movements, but completion of the act may require proprioceptive feedback about muscle activity. Abbs and Kennedy (1982) have pointed out that the role of afferent control mechanisms in speech has been underemphasized, even though "speech motor control is almost certainly more than simply transmitting the contents of a predetermined motor tape over existing descending pathways . . ."

(p. 94). There is wide agreement that speech motor control is an acquired skill that is learned through the imitation of acoustic patterns provided by normal speakers.

There is little doubt that sensation contributes in some way to speech motor control. How this contribution is made, however, is not clear. The following points address some characteristics of motor control that seem to require sensory assistance and some facts about the sensory system that permit that assistance.

1. Auditory and sensory input from muscles have diverse input to the speech motor system. They have direct, rapid (that is, short latency) input to motoneurons supplying speech muscles at the brainstem and spinal levels. These afferent influences also exist in longer latency multisynaptic pathways through the cortex, basal ganglia, and cerebellum.

2. Intelligible speech can be produced by structures that are continuously changing position, in the presence of structural roadblocks (for example, objects in the mouth) and when structures that normally move are blocked from doing so (for example, a bite block restricting jaw movement). This means that commands leading to the production of specific sounds cannot be invariant because the actions depend on the phonetic and physical environment (recall the previous discussion of coarticulation and motor equivalence). Only through knowledge about these states can the system produce a reliable acoustic signal that matches the linguistic intent. Because intelligible speech does require the relatively reliable achievement of articulatory targets, knowledge about where structures (for example, the tongue) will come from and their movement velocity seems essential. Integration of sensory information from peripheral mechanoreceptors may form a primary source of this knowledge.

3. An important concept in motor physiology is that descending pathways from higher brain centers can influence sensory processing at the brainstem and spinal levels. This permits sensory pathways to be pretuned or sensitized by the motor system so optimal use can be made of sensory information. This mechanism is exemplified in the gamma motoneuron system in which muscle spindle sensitivity and readiness to respond can be influenced by UMNs (direct and indirect activating pathways). At the cortical level, primary motor area neurons are most responsive to sensory input from regions to which they provide motor innervation. Finally, the speech system's ability to produce what is able to be perceived is perhaps the strongest argument for a role of sensory processes in speech motor control.

4. Abnormal processing of sensory information may have an impact on certain dysarthrias (McClean, 1987). For example, disordered movement in individuals with cerebral palsy may result from damage to sensory pathways projecting to the ventrolateral thalamic nucleus, the major relay from the cerebellum and basal ganglia to the motor and premotor cortex. The thalamus is also the primary input relay for somatosensory information to the postcentral gyrus, including mechanoreceptor input from tongue, perioral, jaw, laryngeal, and respiratory systems. Relatedly, surgical lesions are sometimes successfully placed in the ventrolateral nucleus of the thalamus to control movement disorders. This is accomplished by interrupting the central afferent component of cortical, basal ganglia, and cerebellar loops that generate and control movement. These observations reflect strong interactions between the sensory and motor systems in movement control.

Reflexes, learning, and automaticity of movement. It is likely that higher levels of the nervous system, such as dominant hemisphere cortical motor areas, determine overall movement targets and sequences. It is also likely that noncortical pathways are involved in programming the details and execution of speech movements (Abbs and Kennedy, 1982). Many aspects of these lower level reflexlike processes are dependent on afferent information from the periphery about movement and the movement environment. These lower level actions are stereotyped, have the advantage of speed, and do not require conscious effort. Higher level regulation of movement by sensorimotor cortex and the control circuits is slower because of increased pathway length and number of synapses; because it is less automatic, more sophisticated and purposeful output geared to accomplishing goal-oriented movement is possible. Speech-motor behavior may reflect the cooperation of short latency automatic sensory-motor pathways, longer latency relatively more consciously mediated pathways, and intermediate pathways between those extremes.

It is likely that the allocation of resources for motor-speech programming and control among high, low, and intermediate levels of the motor system vary as a function of experience, learning, task complexity, and speaker intentions. It is reasonable to assume that higher levels of the system carry a heavier programming and control responsibility when the speech task is motorically complex or novel, when demands for accuracy and precision are greater than average, and when the speaker intends to be precise, emphatic, intelligible without ambiguity, or impressive. Conversely, higher-level control may be less vigilant when the utterance is highly overlearned and stereotypic, understood easily in the physical and social context, considered insignificant, or is poorly attended to. It is possible that some aspects of speech are directed by preprogrammed groups of motor commands that are released upon presentation of an appropriate stimulus, as long as the relationship between stimulus and response has been established by learning and practice.

Finally, speech structures are probably not homogeneous relative to degree of motor control. For example, the speed and discreteness and diversity of tongue, lip, and jaw movements during speech appear different and greater than those associated with velopharyngeal and respiratory movements. It is quite possible that the programming and control requirements among various speech structures are different.

Control circuit influences. The roles of the basal ganglia and cerebellar control circuits in motor system activities, almost by definition, involve them in motor speech planning and programming. This is because, as already noted, the primary influence of control circuits is through their input to the cortical areas involved in programming speech movements.

It is reasonable to assume that cortical motor speech programming areas play a crucial role in establishing acoustic and motor targets and sequences and the preliminary movement program prior to the initiation of speech. It is also likely that the control circuits are informed of the program prior to the initiation of speech so they may provide a proper tonal and postural environment as well as information to the cortex about how program goals can be achieved. Once speech is initiated, they probably play an ongoing role in modifying cortical programming activity and subsequent direct and indirect activation pathway signals to speech muscles.

The basal ganglia control circuit is probably important to the preprogramming and regulation of the slower components of speech movements, those that provide postural support for rapid speech movements such as those involved in articulation (Abbs and Kennedy, 1982; Kornhuber, 1975). The cerebellar control circuit is probably involved in programming and regulating more rapid speech movements.

Limbic system influences. The limbic system is a supratentorally located group of nuclei and pathways comprised of the olfactory areas, hypothalamic and thalamic nuclei, and the limbic lobe of the cortex. The limbic lobe is located on the medial surface of the cortex and includes the orbital frontal region, the cingulate gyrus, and medial portions of the temporal lobe. The limbic system plays a crucial role in visceral and emotional activity and mediates information about internal states such as thirst, hunger, fear, rage, pleasure, and sex. The limbic areas of the cortex play an important role in regulating memory and learning, modulating drive or motivation, and influencing the affective components of experience (Mesulam, 1985).

Nowhere more than in speech are emotions and propositional meaning combined. It is likely that limbic system influences are present prior to or during the conceptualization stage and that emotional content influences and modifies what happens during linguistic planning, particularly the semantic component. Its influence goes beyond its impact on linguistic content, however, because speech conveys emotions and meanings beyond those that can be attributed to words. Emotions are conveyed in speech primarily through prosody or suprasegmental variations in pitch, loudness, and duration. The limbic system probably represents a primary drive to the prosodic-emotional character of speech, particularly when the emotion conveyed is involuntary, unintentional, or automatic. Primitive reflexive examples are laughter and crying, nonspeech prosodic vocal activities that often cannot be inhibited by voluntary effort. Therefore, the emotional components of prosody are mediated less by linguistic activity than by the influence of the limbic system and other cortical areas, most notably in the right hemisphere (see next section).

Cognitive and emotional disorders can affect speech, usually by attenuating or exaggerating prosody in a manner that accurately reflects the individual's general cognitive or emotional state. Conversely, many motor speech disorders result in prosodic disturbances that prevent, exaggerate, or distort the individual's capacity to convey vocally their true inner emotional state.

Right hemisphere influences. It is generally believed that the cortical programming of speech undertaken in the left hemisphere is transmitted across the corpus callosum to the right hemisphere where its motor pathways carry out the program in coordination with the left hemisphere. However, the right hemisphere is not entirely passive regarding speech production, even though its role is not well delineated. Evidence indicates that it contributes to the perception and motor organization of the prosodic components of speech, especially those that express graded or subtle attitudes and emotions (Mesulam, 1985).

People with right hemisphere lesions sometimes display "flattened" or reduced prosodic speech variations, a problem that has been called "*aprosodia*" (Ross, 1981). There is some dispute about whether the attenuated prosody reflects hypoarousal, depression, or difficulty programming prosodic features for speech (Myers, 1994). Nonetheless, the deficits are important to recognize and distinguish from the better understood dysarthrias and apraxia of speech, as well as from prosodic disturbances reflecting other abnormalities of cognition and affect. The role of the right hemisphere in speech production and motor speech deficits associated with right hemisphere damage will be discussed in Chapter 13.

Reticular formation and thalamic influences. The role of the reticular formation in the activities of the indirect and direct activation pathways, the control circuits, and the sensory system has been discussed. In fact, its multiple functions have led to its significance being buried in discussions of the more "dedicated" portions of the motor system. It is highlighted here simply to emphasize that its multiple roles, connections, and central location give it a significant integrative role in nervous system activities. Its contribution to maintaining alertness, monitoring sensory input, maintaining and helping to focus attention, and refining motor activity influence the emotional and propositional content and neuromuscular adequacy of speech.

The thalamus deserves recognition for the same reasons. Its role in the activities of the control circuits, its primary importance as a sensory processor, its direct ties to cortical language and motor speech systems, its integrative role in attention and vigilance, and its role within the limbic system make it very difficult to assign it a single role. However, its diverse activities include an important role in the circuitry necessary for normal speech production.

Effects of damage. The motor programming role of the dominant hemisphere for speech is never more dramatically illustrated than when it becomes damaged. In fact, such a disturbance helped give birth to modern behavioral neurology in the mid-1800s as part of attempts to localize diseases affecting "higher level" motor and cognitive disturbances. The problem, which is distinguishable from aphasia and dysarthria, is known by many labels. For reasons that will be explained later, the disturbance of speech motor programming associated with dominant hemisphere pathology will be called *apraxia of speech*. Its clinical features and additional discussion of its nature will be addressed in Chapter 11.

Performance

Performance is the level of motor control that activates motoneurons, muscle contractions, and movement. This is accomplished by the combined activities of the direct and indirect activation pathways, the control circuits, the final common pathway, feedback from sensory pathways, and ongoing contributions from the motor speech programmer. It has already been discussed within the context of the functions of all other levels of the speech motor system (see Figure 2–11).

Feedback

This involves the use of sensory information about the ongoing and completed movements that have been generated and the subsequent modification of ongoing and future movements based upon that information. This activity may take place at the spinal and brainstem level, in the cerebellum, thalamus, basal ganglia, and cortex. These mechanisms have already been discussed.

SUMMARY

This chapter has presented a broad overview of neuroanatomy and neurophysiology and some basic information about neuropathology. The goal has been to provide a foundation for understanding motor speech activity and its neuropathologies. The major points that have been addressed can be summarized as follows:

1. Most of the crucial components of the speech-motor system have their origins within the skull. They are surrounded by meningeal coverings and spaces for cerebrospinal fluid and vascular structures and are nourished and protected by the ventricular and vascular systems.

2. The major anatomic levels of the nervous system include the supratentorial, posterior fossa, spinal, and peripheral levels, all of which contain components of the motor system.

3. The functional systems of the brain include the cerebrospinal fluid, visceral, vascular, consciousness, sensory, and motor systems. The cerebrospinal and vascular systems support neurologic functions but have no direct role in speech because they are not neural in structure. The visceral and consciousness systems have important but indirect influences on motor speech activities, and damage to them does not necessarily produce specific motor speech disorders. The sensory system is strongly and rather directly linked to the reflexive and volitional activities of the motor system, including speech. The motor system is directly involved in motor speech production.

4. The nervous system is made up of neurons and supporting cells. Supporting cells facilitate neuronal function and pathologic reactions

in them can be a cause or reaction to neurologic disease. The neuron is the functional unit of the nervous system. Movement of muscles, tendons, and joints require activity of many neurons which, in the PNS, are grouped together in nerves and in the CNS are grouped together in tracts and pathways. Death, injury, degeneration, and other malfunctions of neurons are directly responsible for behavioral disturbances, including motor speech disorders.

5. Neurologic disease can be focal, multifocal, or diffuse in localization, and its development can be acute, subacute, or chronic. The evolution of disease can be transient, improving, progressive, exaccerbating-remitting, or stationary. Neurologic etiologies can be categorized as degenerative, inflammatory, toxic-metabolic, neoplastic, traumatic, or vascular. Motor speech disorders can be associated with any pattern of localization, temporal course, or etiology.

6. The motor system is present at all anatomic levels of the nervous system. Its major divisions include the final common pathway, the direct activation pathway, the indirect activation pathway, the basal ganglia control circuit, and the cerebellar control circuit. Each division plays a specific role in motor activity, but there is overlap among the anatomy and functions of the divisions and they must operate together to produce normal motor behavior. Damage to any of the divisions can produce relatively distinct neurologic deficits whose recognition is helpful to the localization of disease.

7. The motor system for speech is part of the motor system in general. Speech system activities are manifest through movements triggered by cranial and spinal nerves that innervate respiratory, phonatory, resonatory, and articulatory muscles. Cranial nerves V, VII, IX, X, XI, and XII, and the phrenic nerves from the cervical level of the spinal cord, are the nerves of the final common pathway that are most important for speech production.

8. The direct activation pathways originate in the cortex and pass directly as corticobulbar and corticospinal tracts to control skilled speech movements carried out through the final common pathway.

9. The indirect activation pathway also originates in the cortex but influences alpha and gamma motoneurons of the LMN system only after synapses at multiple points in the CNS. It regulates reflex activities of LMNs, and maintains posture, tone, and associated activities

that provide a stable framework on which skilled actions can be imposed.

10. The basal ganglia control circuit, consisting of the basal ganglia and related structures, affects motor activities primarily through its influence on cortical motor functions. It assists in generating motor speech programs, especially those program components that maintain a stable musculoskeletal environment in which skilled movements can occur; its ultimate influence on LMNs is primarily through indirect pathways.

11. The cerebellar control circuit, consisting of the cerebellum and related pathways, influences motor activity primarily through its influence on the cortex. It also receives proprioceptive information from the periphery. The circuit's role is to coordinate speech through its knowledge of cortically set goals and its access to results at the periphery.

12. The conceptual-programming level establishes speech goals and the programs for achieving them. Conceptualization—the thoughts and ideas that drive a desire to speak—require cortical activity, but they are not easily localizable and are best thought of as a function of many cortical and subcortical areas of the brain.

13. The language system, with crucial contributions from left (dominant) hemisphere perisylvian cortex, organizes and sequences the linguistic content of spoken language that a speaker intends a listener to perceive.

14. Motor speech programming and planning is at the interface between the language formulation and neuromuscular execution stages of verbal expression. It is responsible for coding linguistic content into neuronal impulses that are compatible with the operations of the motor system. The goal of motor programming for speech is the generation of movement patterns that result in an acoustic signal that matches the speaker's message. Motor speech programs are not and cannot be invariant because of the infinite number of possible utterances, the variability of directions and distances from which articulatory targets must be reached, and because speech gestures overlap in time. The complexity of the movements, and the speed at which they are normally accomplished, make it probable that many aspects of speech movements in mature speakers are preprogrammed.

15. The left (dominant) hemisphere is very important to speech programming. The control circuits also play an important role in speech programming and control.

16. Sensory processing at the brainstem and spinal levels, as well as higher levels of the sensory system, probably plays an important role in the programming and ongoing control of speech movements.
17. It is likely that the responsibilities of the various components of the speech programming and execution system vary as a function of learning, experience, complexity, and speaker intent. If so, this is a further caution against strict localization of speech motor programming and control to single structures.
18. The limbic system, right hemisphere, reticular formation, and thalamus contribute to the programs that are generated to produce emotional and intended linguistic meanings conveyed in speech.
19. Deficits at the conceptualization and linguistic planning levels can impair the content of speech. They can exist independently of motor speech impairments.
20. Deficits in the dominant hemisphere's speech programming activities and deficits in the motor system's neuromuscular execution of the speech program are known as apraxia of speech and dysarthria, respectively. The assessment of these disorders is the subject of the next chapter.

REFERENCES

Abbs JH and Kennedy JG: Neurophysiological processes of speech movement control. In Lass NJ, McReynolds LV, Northern JL, and Yoder DE, editors: Speech, language, and hearing, vol. 1, normal processes, Philadelphia, 1982, WB Saunders.

Adams RD and Victor M: Principles of neurology, New York, 1991, McGraw-Hill.

Allen GI and Tsukahara N: Cerebrocerebellar communication systems. Physiol Rev 54:957, 1974.

Aronson AE: Clinical voice disorders, New York, 1990, Thieme Inc.

Barlow SM and Farley GR: Neurophysiology of speech. In Kuehn DP, Lemme ML, and Baumgartner JM, editors: Neural bases of speech, hearing, and language, Boston, 1989, College-Hill.

Brown DR: Neurosciences for allied health therapies, St. Louis, 1980, Mosby–Year Book.

Carpenter MB: Core text of neuroanatomy, Baltimore, 1978, Williams and Wilkins.

Clinical examinations in neurology, ed 6, St. Louis, 1991, Mosby–Year Book.

Darley FL, Aronson AE, and Brown JR: Motor speech disorders, Philadelphia, 1975, Saunders.

Daube JR, Reagan TJ, Sandok BA et al: Medical neurosciences, Boston, 1986, Little, Brown, and Co.

Dobkin JA, Levin RL, Lagreze HL et al: Evidence for transhemispheric diaschisis in unilateral stroke, Arch Neurol 46:1333, 1989.

Dronkers NF, Redfern B, and Shapiro JK: Neuroanatomic correlates of production deficits in severe Broca's aphasia, J Clin Exp Neuropsychol 15:59, 1993 (abstract).

Eccles JC: The understanding of the brain, New York, 1977, McGraw-Hill.

Gilman S, Gloedel JR, and Lechtenberg R: Disorders of the cerebellum, Philadelphia, 1981, FA Davis.

Gilman W and Winans SS: Manter & Gatz's essentials of clinical neuroanatomy and neurophysiology, Philadelphia, 1982, FA Davis.

Gordon B: Postconcussional syndrome. In Johnson RT, editor: Current therapy in neurologic disease, ed. 3, Philadelphia, 1990, BC Decker.

Hixon TJ: Respiratory functions in speech and song, Boston, 1987, College-Hill Press.

Hubel DH: The brain. In The brain, a Scientific American book, San Francisco, 1979, WH Freeman and Co.

Jennett B and Teasdale G: Management of head injuries, Philadelphia, 1981, FA Davis.

Jonas S: The supplementary motor region and speech emission, J Commun Disord 14:349, 1981.

Kennedy JG and Abbs JH: Basic neurophysiological mechanisms underlying oral communication. In Lass NJ, McReynolds LV, Northern JL, and Yodor DE, editors: Speech, language, and hearing, vol. 1, Normal processes, Philadelphia, 1982, WB Saunders.

Kennedy JG and Kuehn DP: Neuroanatomy of speech. In Kuehn DP, Lemme ML, and Baumgartner, editors: Neural bases of speech, hearing, and language, Boston, 1989, College-Hill.

Kent RD: The acoustic and physiologic characteristics of neurologically impaired speech movements. In Hardcastle WJ and Marchal A, editors: Speech production and speech modelling, The Netherlands, 1990, Kluwer Academic Publishers.

Kent R and Netsell R: A case study of an ataxic dysarthric: cineradiographic and spectrographic, J Speech Hear Disord 40:115, 1975.

Kent R, Netsell R, and Abbs JH: Acoustic characteristics of dysarthria associated with cerebellar disease, J Speech Hear Res 22:627, 1979.

Kornhuber HH: Cerebral cortex, cerebellum, and basal ganglia: an introduction to their motor function. In Evarts EV, editor: Central processing of sensory input leading to motor output, Cambridge, 1975, MIT Press.

Larson CR: Basic neurophysiology. In Kuehn DP, Lemme ML, and Baumgartner JM, editors: Neural bases of speech, hearing and language, Boston, 1989, College-Hill.

Larson CR and Pfingst BE: Neuroanatomic bases of hearing and speech. In Lass NJ, McReynolds LV, Northern JL, and Yoder DE, editors: Speech, language, and hearing, vol. 1, Normal processes, Philadelphia, 1982, WB Saunders.

Lindblom B: The interdisciplinary challenge of speech motor control. In Grillner S et al, editors: Speech motor control, New York, 1982, Pergamon Press.

McClean MD: Neuromotor aspects of speech production and dysarthria. In Yorkston KM, Beukelman DR, and Bell KR, editors: Clinical management of dysarthric speakers, Boston, 1988, College-Hill.

Mesulam MM: Principles of behavioral neurology, Philadelphia, 1985, FA Davis.

Metter EJ et al: Local cerebral metabolic rates of glucose in movement and language disorders from positron tomography, Am J Physiol 246:R897, 1984.

Mlcoch AG and Metter EJ: Medical aspects of stroke rehabilitation. In Chapey R, editor: Language intervention strategies in adult aphasia, Baltimore, 1994, Williams and Wilkins.

Myers PS: Communication disorders associated with right hemisphere brain damage. In Chapey R, editor: Language intervention strategies in adult aphasia, Baltimore, 1994, Williams and Wilkins.

Netsell R and Kent RD: Paroxysmal ataxic dysarthria, J Speech Hear Disord 41:93, 1976.

Penfield W and Roberts L: Speech and brain mechanisms, New York, 1974, Athenium.

Perkins WH and Kent RD: Functional anatomy of speech, language, and hearing, San Diego, 1986, College-Hill Press.

Powers JW and Raichle ME: Positron emission tomography and its application to the study of cerebrovascular disease in man, Stroke 16:361, 1985.

Ross ED: The aprosodias, Arch Neurol 38:561, 1981.

Rusk H, Block J, and Lowman E: Rehabilitation of the brain-injured patient: a report of 157 cases with long-term follow-up of 118. In Walker E, Caveness W, and Critchley M, editors: The late effects of head injury, Springfield, 1969, Charles C. Thomas.

Salazar AM: Closed head injury. In Johnson RT, editor: Current therapy in neurologic disease, Philadelphia, 1990, BC Decker.

Sarno MT, Buonaguro A, and Levita E: Characteristics of verbal impairment in closed head injured patients, Arch Phys Med Rehabil 67:1986, 400.

Stevens CF: The neuron: a Scientific American book, San Francisco, 1979, WH Freeman and Co.

Square PA and Martin RE: The nature and treatment of neuromotor speech disorders in adphasia. In Chapey R, editor: Language intervention strategies in adult aphasia, Baltimore, 1994, Williams and Wilkins.

Examination of Motor Speech Disorders

The process of identifying a speech problem as neurologic and then localizing it within the nervous system is similar to a neurologist's efforts to localize disease and establish a neurologic diagnosis. The differences between the speech pathology and neurology efforts are that speech may be only one of the person's neurologic problems and that speech diagnosis is usually not diagnostic of specific neurologic disease. But these differences do not always exist. Speech difficulty sometimes is the presenting complaint and the only detectable neurologic abnormality, and its diagnosis may permit localization and a tentative disease diagnosis. Speech examination is therefore an important component of many neurologic examinations.

This chapter discusses the examination of speech in people with suspected motor speech disorders. It is not the intent here to discuss the interpretation or application of examination findings to diagnosis or management, beyond a few illustrative examples. The association of examination results with specific speech diagnoses will be addressed in each chapter on the motor speech disorders (Chapters 4–14) and the chapter on differential diagnosis (Chapter 15).

PURPOSES OF MOTOR SPEECH EXAMINATION

The motor speech examination is characterized by several activities and goals that are relevant to diagnosis. Different goals are often pursued simultaneously but they can be isolated and sequenced in a way that helps organize the activities that make up the examination. These goals include description, problem detection, establishing diag-

nostic possibilities, establishing a diagnosis, and specifying severity.

Description and problem detection

Description, which *characterizes the features of speech*, represents the data base upon which diagnostic and treatment decisions are made. In some cases, the diagnostic process ends with description because findings are insufficient to establish a diagnosis or even a limited list of diagnostic possibilities. The bases for description derive from: the patient's history and description of the problem; oral mechanism examination; the perceptual characteristics of speech and results of standard clinical tests; and acoustic and physiologic analyses of speech.

Description and diagnosis are not synonymous. Diagnosis depends upon sufficient, valid, and reliable data (description) but *description without establishing the meaning of the data is of little value when the goal is diagnosis*. An attempt to establish meaning should always be made. If the attempt fails, it can be concluded that a diagnosis cannot be made, and the reasons for it can be explained. It is reasonable to state as principle that *when the results of the speech examination cannot go beyond description, the reasons why should be stated explicitly*.

Once speech can be described, the clinician asks if the characteristics are normal or abnormal. This is the first step in diagnosis—and an important one. If all aspects of speech are within the range of normal, the diagnosis is normal speech. If some aspects of speech are abnormal, then their meaning must be interpreted. *The process of narrowing the diagnostic possibilities and arriving at a specific diagnosis is known as differential diagnosis.*

Establishing diagnostic possibilities

If speech is abnormal, then a list of diagnostic possibilities can be generated. Because the emphasis here is on motor speech disorders, the list can grow out of answers to questions such as the following:

1. Is the problem neurologic?
2. If the problem is not neurologic, is it nonetheless organic? For example, is it due to dental/occlusal abnormality, mass lesion of the larynx, or is it psychogenic?
3. If the problem is or is not neurologic, is it recently acquired or longstanding? For example, might it reflect unresolved developmental stuttering, articulation disorder, or language disability?
4. If the problem is neurologic, is it a motor speech disorder or another neuropathology that is affecting verbal expression (for example, aphasia, dementia, akinetic mutism)?
5. If a motor speech disorder is present, is it a dysarthria or apraxia of speech?
6. If a dysarthria is present, what is its type?

Establishing a diagnosis

Once all reasonable possibilities have been addressed, a single diagnosis may emerge or, at the least, the possibilities may be ordered from most to least likely. For example, concluding that speech is not normal, that it is not psychogenic in origin, and that it is a dysarthria but of undetermined type, is of diagnostic value. It implies the existence of an organic process, places the lesion in the nervous system, and localizes it to the motor system. If it also can be concluded that the dysarthria is not flaccid, then the lesion is further localized to the central and not the peripheral nervous system, and certain neurologic diagnoses can be eliminated or considered unlikely. If the characteristics of the disorder are unambiguous and compatible with only a single diagnosis, then a single speech diagnosis can be given along with its implications for localization.

Establishing implications for localization and disease diagnosis

When a motor speech disorder is identified, its implications for neurologic localization should be addressed explicitly, especially if the referral source is unfamiliar with the method of classification. For example, if spastic dysarthria is the diagnosis, it is appropriate to state that the disorder is associated with bilateral involvement of upper motor neuron (UMN) pathways. If a tentative neurologic diagnosis has already been made, it is

appropriate to address the compatibility of the speech diagnosis with it. For example, if the working neurologic diagnosis is Parkinson's disease but the patient has a mixed spastic-ataxic dysarthria, it is important to report that this mixed dysarthria is atypical in Parkinson's disease. Finally, if neurologic diagnosis is uncertain or if speech is the only sign of disease, it is appropriate to identify possible diagnoses that specific motor speech disorders are "classically" tied to. For example, a flaccid dysarthria that emerges only with speech stress testing and recovers with rest has a very strong association with myasthenia gravis.

Specifying severity

The severity of a motor speech disorder should always be estimated. This estimate is important for at least three reasons: (1) subjective or objective measures of severity can be matched against the patient's complaints; gross mismatches between patient and clinician judgment may introduce, for example, the possibility of psychogenic contributions to the disorder, poor insight, or limited concern about speech on the patient's part; (2) it influences prognosis and management decision making; (3) severity estimates at the time of initial examination represent baseline data against which future changes can be compared.

Specifying severity is actually part of the descriptive process. It is discussed here because of its relevance to determining disability and handicap, as opposed to determining the presence of impairment, which is more properly a component of the diagnostic process. Disability and handicap are more relevant to decisions about management than diagnosis.

Once severity is established, it is appropriate to address the implications of the examination for prognosis and management. These will be considered in Chapters 16–20.

GENERAL GUIDELINES FOR EXAMINATION

The motor speech examination has three essential components: (1) history, (2) identification of salient speech features, and (3) identification of confirmatory signs. With this information, a diagnosis is made, recommendations formulated, and results communicated to the patient, referring physician, and others.

History

An anonymous sage has said that 90% of neurologic diagnosis depends on the patient's history (Rowland, 1989). A wise neurology colleague of the author has said that nearly all clinical neurologic diagnosis is based on speech, either its content or its manner of expression. It would be difficult to argue that the spoken history told by the patient is less important to motor speech evaluation and diagnosis.

Experienced clinicians often reach a diagnosis by the time greetings and amenities have been exchanged and a history obtained. Subsequent formal examination confirms, documents, refines, and, sometimes, revises the diagnosis. The history reveals the time course and the patient's observations of the disorder. It also puts contextual speech on display at a time when anxiety is generally less than during formal examination, and when physical effort, task comprehension, and cooperation are not essential.

Salient features

Salient features are those features that contribute most directly and influentially to diagnosis. They include the speech characteristics themselves and their presumed neuromuscular substrates. Darley, Aronson, and Brown (1975) discussed six salient neuromuscular features that influence speech production. They form a useful framework for integrating observations made during examination. They include strength, speed of movement, range of movement, accuracy, steadiness, and tone. Abnormalities associated with these features are summarized in Table 3–1.

Strength. Muscles have sufficient strength to perform their normal functions, plus a reserve of

Table 3–1 Salient neuromuscular features of speech and associated abnormalities commonly encountered in motor speech disorders

Feature	Abnormality associated with motor speech disorders
Strength	Reduced, usually consistently but sometimes progressively
Speed	Reduced or variable (increased only in hypokinetic dysarthria)
Range	Reduced or variable (predominantly excessive only in hyperkinetic dysarthria)
Steadiness	Unsteady, either rhythmic or arrhythmic
Tone	Increased, decreased, or variable
Accuracy	Inaccurate, either consistently or inconsistently

excess strength. Reserve strength allows extended periods of contraction without excessive fatigue, as well as contraction against resistance.

When a muscle is weak it cannot contract to a desired level, sometimes even for brief periods. It may fatigue more rapidly and dramatically than normal. Sometimes a desired level of contraction can be obtained but ability to sustain it decreases dramatically after a short time.

Muscle weakness can affect all three of the major speech valves (laryngeal, velopharyngeal, and articulatory) and it can be present in all components of speech production (respiration, phonation, resonance, articulation, and prosody). It is most apparent and dramatic in lower motor neuron (LMN)/final common pathway (FCP) lesions and, therefore, in flaccid dysarthria. Its presence can be inferred from perceptual and acoustic analyses of speech, observed visually at rest and during speech, detected on oral mechanism examination, or measured physiologically.

Speed. Muscle activity during speech is rapid, especially the laryngeal, velopharyngeal, and articulatory movements that valve expired air to produce the approximately 14 phones per second that characterize conversational speech. These quick, unsustained, and discrete movements are known as *phasic movements*. Phasic movements can occur as single contractions or repetitively. They begin promptly, reach targets quickly, and relax rapidly. Phasic speech movements are mediated primarily through direct activation UMN pathway input to alpha motor neurons (see Chapter 2).

Excessive speed is uncommon in motor speech disorders, although it may occur in hypokinetic dysarthria. Excessive speech rate in dysarthria is nearly always also associated with decreased range of movement.

Slow movements are common in neuromuscular disorders. Movements may be slow to start, slow in their course, or slow to stop or relax. Single as well as repetitive movements may be slow. Reduced speed can occur at all major speech valves and during all components of speech production. Slow movement strongly affects the prosodic features of speech because normal prosody is so dependent on quick muscular adjustments that influence rate of sound production and pitch and loudness variability. The effects of reduced speed are most apparent in spastic dysarthria but also are present in other dysarthria types. The effects of altered speed can be perceived in speech, can be visibly apparent during speech and oral mechanism examination, and may be measured physiologically and acoustically.

Range. The distance traveled by speech structures is precise for single and repetitive movements. Variations in the range of repetitive movements are usually small.

Consistent, inappropriately excessive range of movement during voluntary speech is not common in neurologic disease. In contrast, decreased range is common and may occur in a context of slow, normal, or excessively rapid rate; for example, hypokinetic dysarthria is often characterized by decreased range of movement and excessively rapid rate. In other instances, range may be variable and unpredictable. Variability in range is common in ataxic and hyperkinetic dysarthrias.

Abnormalities in range of movement often have a major influence on the prosodic features of speech, sometimes resulting in restricted or excessive prosodic variations. Such abnormalities can occur at all of the major speech valves and all components of speech production. They can be inferred from acoustic and perceptual analyses of speech, visible during speech and nonspeech movements of the articulators, and measured physiologically.

Steadiness. At rest, there is a measurable 8 to 12 Hz oscillation of body muscles. During normal movement there are usually no visible interruptions or oscillations of body parts, although amplitude sometimes increases to visibly detectable levels in healthy people. This *physiologic tremor* can occur in extreme fatigue, under emotional stress, or during shivering.

When motor steadiness breaks down in neurologic disease, the results can be broadly categorized as *involuntary movements or hyperkinesias. Tremor* is the most common involuntary movement. It consists of alternating, repetitive, relatively rhythmic oscillations of a body part, generally ranging in frequency from 3 to 12 Hz. It may occur at rest (*resting tremor*), when a structure is maintained against gravity (*postural tremor*), during movement (*action tremor*), or it may be accentuated toward the end of a movement (*terminal tremor*).

Tremor may have no perceptible effect on speech respiration, resonance, or articulation. It commonly affects phonation and, when severe, it can affect prosody. Its effects are most easily detected during sustained vowel production. The effects of tremor can be perceived during speech, seen during speech or oral mechanism exam, and measured physiologically and acoustically.

Another major category of involuntary movement consists of random, unpredictable, adventitious movements that may vary in their speed, duration, and amplitude. These movements are often labeled *dystonia, dyskinesia, chorea* or *athetosis.* They may be severe enough to interrupt or alter the direction of intended movement. They

may be present at rest, during sustained postures, or during movement.

Unpredictable hyperkinesias can affect movement at all of the major speech valves and all components of speech production. They can affect accuracy and often produce major alterations in prosody. They are the primary cause of abnormal speech in hyperkinetic dysarthria. The effects of unpredictable hyperkinesias can be perceived during speech, seen during speech and oral mechanism examination, measured physiologically, and inferred from acoustic measurements.

Tone. Muscle tone was discussed in Chapter 2. The gamma loop and indirect activation pathway are crucial for proper maintenance of tone, which creates a stable framework upon which rapid voluntary movements can be superimposed.

In pathology, muscle tone may be excessive or reduced. It may fluctuate in regular fashion, or wax and wane unpredictably, slowly or rapidly. Alterations in tone may occur at all speech valves and at all levels of speech production.

Abnormal tone is associated with flaccid dysarthria when consistently reduced, with spastic or hypokinetic dysarthria when consistently increased, and with hyperkinetic dysarthria when variable. The effects of abnormal tone can be inferred from perceptual speech characteristics, seen during speech and oral mechanism examination, measured physiologically, and inferred from acoustic measurements.

Accuracy. Individual, repetitive, and complex sound sequences are normally executed with enough precision to ensure intelligible and efficient transmission of linguistic and emotional meaning. They result from precision in the tone, strength, speed, range, steadiness, and timing of muscle activity. From this standpoint, accuracy reflects the outcome of the well-timed and coordinated activities of all other neuromuscular features. If strength, speed, range, steadiness, and tone have been properly planned, modulated, coordinated, and timed, then speech movements will be accurate. If speech sounds or words are inaccurate and neuromuscular performance is normal, it is possible that the linguistic plan or the ideational content are defective, placing the source of the problem outside of the motor system; an alternative explanation is that the problem lies in the programming and control components of the motor system and not in the neuromuscular execution apparatus.

Inaccurate movements can result in a variety of speech errors. For example, if force and range of movement are excessive, structures may overshoot targets. If force and range of movement are decreased, target undershooting may result. If timing is poor, the direction and smoothness of movements may be faulty and the rhythm of repetitive movements may be poorly maintained.

Inaccurate movements resulting from constantly present defects in strength, speed, range, and tone may result in predictable degrees of articulatory imprecision or other speech abnormalities. If the source of inaccuracy lies in timing or unpredictable variations in other neuromuscular components, errors may be unpredictable, random, or transient.

Inaccurate movements may occur at all of the major speech valves and at all levels of speech production, but are generally perceived most easily in articulation and prosody. Inaccuracy can occur in all dysarthrias, but when it is the result of inadequate timing or coordination, it is usually a manifestation of ataxic dysarthria or apraxia of speech. When associated with random or unpredictable variations in movement, it often reflects hyperkinetic dysarthria.

It should be apparent that the various neuromuscular features of movement interact and influence each other during speech. For example, reduced strength is usually associated with reduced accuracy, tone, and range of movement. Increased or variable tone is usually associated with reduced or variable speed, range of movement, steadiness, and accuracy. Reduced range of movement may be associated with variations in speed, tone, or accuracy. It is rare that only a single abnormal neuromuscular feature will be present in someone with a motor speech disorder.

Confirmatory signs

Confirmatory signs are additional clues about the location of pathology. In the context of speech examination, they are *signs other than deviant speech characteristics and the salient neuromuscular features that characterize them* that help confirm the speech diagnosis. Therefore, observations of a nonspeech nature, even of the speech muscles, must be considered circumstantial (confirmatory) evidence and not salient. Nonetheless, such observation can be helpful in establishing a diagnosis.

Confirmatory signs can be found in speech or nonspeech muscles. Examples of confirmatory signs within the speech system are atrophy, reduced tone, fasciculations, poorly inhibited laughter or crying, reduced normal reflexes or the presence of pathologic reflexes, and the strength of the cough and coup de glotte. It is important to keep in mind that such signs are not *diagnostic* of dysarthria or apraxia of speech. For example, atrophy of the tongue without any perceivable

impairment of lingual articulation would not warrant a diagnosis of dysarthria. It might reflect a XIIth nerve lesion, but to diagnose dysarthria would require a *speech* deficit to be present. Confirmatory signs confirm or support conclusions about the nature of a speech disorder, but *a particular motor speech diagnosis does not require that confirmatory signs be present.*

Confirmatory signs from the nonspeech motor system come from observations of gait and station, direct muscle observation, muscle stretch reflexes, superficial and pathologic reflexes, hyperactive limb reflexes, limb atrophy and fasciculations, loss of automatic movements associated with activities like walking, and difficulty initiating limb movements. In the context of the speech examination, they also include observations of strength, speed, accuracy, tone, steadiness, and range of movements at rest or during nonspeech tasks.

Confirmatory signs will be discussed within each chapter on the specific dysarthrias and apraxia of speech and also briefly during the overview of the motor speech examination that follows.

Integration of findings

Once the history has been obtained, and speech features and confirmatory signs examined, they are integrated to formulate an impression about their meaning. This constitutes diagnosis. Diagnosis may range from a conclusion that a diagnosis cannot be made, to a formulation of the most likely possibilities, to a formulation about what the disorder is not, to a clearly stated diagnosis, or to a combination of several of these possibilities (for example, "The patient has a spastic dysarthria, perhaps with an ataxic component. There is no evidence of apraxia of speech."). The process of differential diagnosis will be discussed in detail in Chapter 15.

THE MOTOR SPEECH EXAMINATION

The motor speech examination can be divided into five parts: (1) history, (2) examination of the oral mechanism during nonspeech activities, (3) assessment of perceptual speech characteristics, (4) assessing intelligibility, and (5) acoustic and physiologic analyses.

History

The history provides basic facts about the onset and course of the problem, an index of the patient's awareness of impairment, and the degree to which the problem is disabling or handicapping. It also puts on display the salient features, confirmatory signs, and severity of the speech problem.

No history is the same and the specific questions that elicit it will vary considerably. Factors affecting how history-taking is approached include the patient's cognitive abilities and personality, whether or not the patient perceives a problem, what has already been clearly established by other professionals, and the severity of the speech deficit. If patients have cognitive limitations, significantly reduced intelligibility, and inadequate augmentative means of communication, or if they do not perceive a speech deficit, then the history from them will be limited. If the etiology and time course are already clear, they need not be pursued beyond confirmation. The history sometimes must be provided or supplemented by someone who knows the patient well. History-taking should be controlled by the clinician and not the patient, with questions and their sequence strongly influenced by the facts provided by the patient and by their manner of doing so.

The format of history-taking will often include the following.

Introduction and goal setting. Once basic amenities have been exchanged, the examination often can begin with a simple but important question, *"Why are you here?"* Some representative responses include: "to find out what's wrong with me"; "to find out what's wrong with my speech"; "to find out if you can help me with my speech"; "because my doctor told me to come here"; "there's nothing wrong with me and I don't know why they brought me here." The answers are an index of the patient's orientation, awareness, and concern about their speech, the priority they place on their speech versus other aspects of their illness, the relative importance to them of diagnosis versus clinical management, their ability to provide a history, and the depth and manner in which the history will have to be taken. This introduction also allows the clinician to inform the patient about the purposes and procedures of examination, and its place in their overall evaluation and management.

Basic data. Age, education, occupation, and marital and family status should be noted. It may be important to establish if there was a history of childhood speech, language, or hearing deficit, if treatment for those problems was necessary, and if they had resolved before the current medical condition developed. This is essential when abnormalities are inconsistent with other medical findings but could be developmental in nature. The most common longstanding speech deficits encountered in adults with suspected neurologic disease are persisting developmental articulation errors, articulatory distortions associated with dental or occlusal abnormalities, and developmental stuttering.

Onset and course. Information about the onset and course of the speech deficit is useful to neurologic diagnosis, prognosis, and management decisions. It also reveals something about the patient's perception of the problem. Relevant questions include:

1. Do you have any difficulty with your speech? If not, has anyone else commented on a change or problem with your speech?

2. When did the speech problem begin? Did it begin suddenly or gradually? Who noticed it first, you or someone else?

3. Did you develop any other difficulties when your speech problem began? Were other problems present before the speech problem began? Did other problems develop after the speech problem began?

4. Has the speech problem changed? Better, worse, stable, better-then-stable, fluctuating?

5. Has your speech ever returned to normal? If so, when and for how long?

Associated deficits. Information about associated deficits that may represent confirmatory signs includes:

1. Have you had any difficulty with chewing? Drooling?

2. Is it difficult to move food around in your mouth? Why?

3. Does food get stuck in your cheeks or on the roof of your mouth? Do you have to remove it with your finger or a fork?

4. Do you have trouble moving food back in your mouth to get a swallow started?

5. Do you have trouble with swallowing? Food or liquid? Do you have trouble getting a swallow started? Do you lose food or liquid out of your mouth? Does food or liquid ever go into or out of your nose when you swallow? Does food or liquid go down before you swallow and cause coughing or choking? Do you gag or choke when swallowing? Do you choke or cough after completing a swallow? Have you had to modify your diet because of these problems? Have you lost weight?

6. Have you had any change in your emotional expression? Do you cry or laugh more easily or less easily than in the past?

7. Are you taking any medications that seem to affect your speech?

The patient's perception of deficit. It is important to establish the patient's perception of the problem. This can provide useful confirmatory information.

1. What did your speech sound like when the problem began? Did anything feel different when you spoke?

2. Describe your current speech difficulty. How does it sound to you? How does it feel to speak? Is

it faster or slower? Louder or softer? Less precise? Is speaking effortful?

3. Have you noticed any change in the appearance or feeling in your face or mouth?

Consequences of the disorder. This information is useful for determining disability and handicap.

1. Do people ever have trouble understanding you? When? What do you do if that happens?

2. Do you ever have to write to make yourself understood? Has your speech problem affected your work? Does it prevent you from doing anything?

Management. This provides information about what the patient and others have done to manage the speech disorder. It is useful for determining prognosis and future management recommendations.

1. What have you done to compensate for your speech difficulty? Have you had any help for your speech? When? For how long? What was done? Did it help?

2. Do you think you need help with your speech now?

Awareness of diagnosis and prognosis. It is important to know what patients understand about their medical diagnosis and prognosis. This helps determine the manner in which the speech diagnosis and management issues will be discussed. For example, patients who are in the process of evaluation to determine the nature of their disease may not be interested or emotionally ready to discuss management of their speech problem.

1. What have you been told is the cause of this problem?

2. In view of this diagnosis, what is going to happen?

Examination of the speech mechanism during nonspeech activities

The speech mechanism examination can be very informative, although moreso for some motor speech disorders than others. In general, it provides information about the size, strength, symmetry, range, tone, steadiness, speed, and accuracy of orofacial movements, particularly the jaw, face, tongue, and palate. The observations are primarily visual and tactual, but also rely on auditory information. The milieu in which the observations are made include: at rest, during sustained postures, during movement, and reflexes. Evidence from the examination may help confirm conclusions drawn about speech. Even if not confirmatory of a speech deficit, the observations may nonetheless be salient to neurologic evaluation.

The face at rest. At rest, the normal face is grossly symmetric and exhibits normal tone and little spontaneous movement. It is neither droopy nor fixed in a posture associated with strong emotion (for example, smiling, on the verge of tears).

To observe the face at rest, patients should be instructed to relax, look forward, and let their lips part so they can breathe quietly through their mouth. Some patients can maintain this relaxed posture more easily with their eyes closed.

The following questions should then be addressed.

1. *Is the face symmetric?* Are the angles of the mouth symmetric? Is asymmetry due to a drooping of the entire face on one side, a droop at the corner of the mouth, or a flattening in the angle of the nasolabial fold? Recognize that some asymmetry is the rule rather than the exception; a difference in the length and prominence of the nasolabial fold is especially common. Some asymmetry often can be seen at rest or during voluntary and spontaneous or emotional responses (see Figure 3–1).

It has been suggested that the left side of the face is more expressive emotionally than the right; a frequent explanation is that the right hemisphere (which has predominant control over innervation of the lower left face) has a specialized role in emotional expression. Although some evidence supports this observation, data from neurologically intact people show that asymmetries can be seen in favor of the right or left side of the face and that differences are not necessarily compatible with hypotheses about hemispheric specialization (Hager and Ekman, 1985; Thompson, 1985). Differences in facial morphology may explain some of the differences observable in people without neurologic disease. What is important for clinical examination is that mild facial asymmetries are not uncommon and that the direction of the asymmetry is not very predictable.

Clinical evidence suggests that the motor control of voluntary facial expression is different than control of spontaneous expression. For example, Monrad-Krohn (1924) observed that patients with lower facial paresis resulting from central nervous system (CNS) lesions would sometimes smile symmetrically in response to a joke, but asymmetry would be evident when they were asked to smile voluntarily; he observed the opposite in some patients with postencephalitic parkinsonism. These observations indicate that it is of value to elicit a spontane-

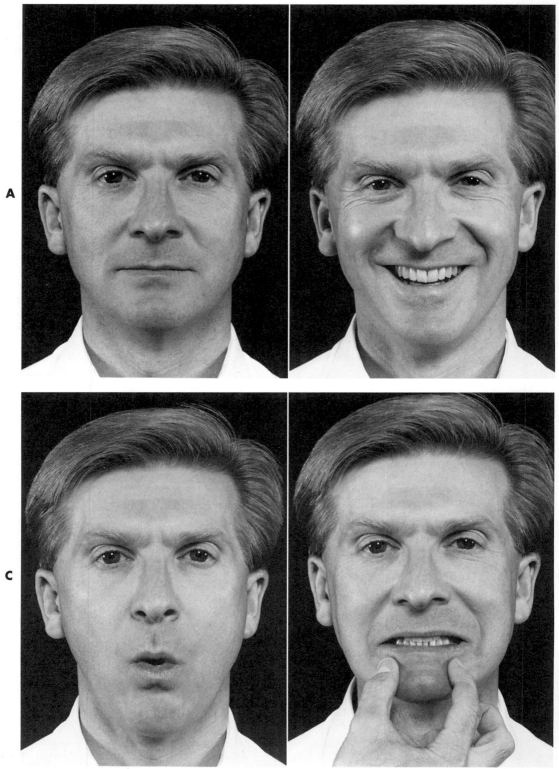

Figure 3–1 A, the normal face at rest; **B,** during spontaneous smiling; **C,** lip rounding; **D,** lip retraction against pressure.

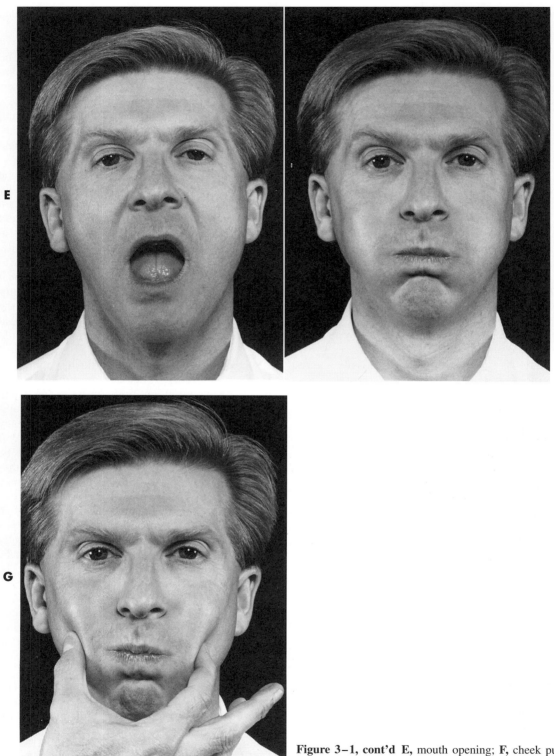

Figure 3–1, cont'd E, mouth opening; **F,** cheek puffing; and **G,** cheek puffing against pressure.

ous emotional smile and to compare the extent of facial movement during it to that of a voluntary smile or lip retraction.

2. Is the face expressionless, masklike, and unblinking? Is it held in a fixed expression of smiling, astonishment, or perplexity? Does the upper lip appear stiff?

3. Are abnormal spontaneous, involuntary movements present? Do the eyes shut tightly and uncontrollably? Is there quick or slow symmetric or asymmetric pursing or retraction of the lips? Are there spontaneous smacking noises of the lips? Can the patient inhibit these movements on request? If so, do they reappear when inhibitory efforts cease?

4. Are the lips tremulous or are there tremor-like rhythmic movements of the lips? Are *fasciculations* present, especially around the mouth or chin?

The face during sustained postures. Observing the face during sustained postures allows additional observations of symmetry, range of movement, strength and tone, and the ability to maintain a sustained posture.

Useful sustained facial postures include: retraction of the lips; rounding or pursing of the lips; puffing the cheeks; and sustained mouth opening. The patient should be asked to sustain each posture after it is demonstrated by the examiner (Figure 3–1).

The following questions should be addressed.

1. Are the lips' retraction, rounding, and puffing symmetric? Is their range of movement normal or restricted? When opening the mouth, is the configuration of the lips symmetric or does one side lag?

2. Is the patient able to resist the examiner's attempt to push the upper or lower lip toward the midline when the lips are retracted, or resist the examiner's attempt to spread the lips when they are rounded? Does air escape through the lips when the patient puffs the cheeks or can the seal be broken with less than normal pressure when the examiner squeezes the cheeks?

3. Does *tremulousness* appear or disappear during sustained facial postures? Are additional movements present that distort or alter the ability to maintain the sustained posture?

4. Can the patient maintain the posture for several seconds or is the effort discontinued even when the patient is instructed to maintain it?

The face during movement. The face should be observed during speech, emotional responses, and volitional nonspeech tasks. During speech and emotional responses, range and symmetry of facial movement and expressiveness should be noted. Mild asymmetry in the range of facial movement is normal during speech and nonverbal emotional responses.

Nonspeech tasks can include rapid repetitions of lip pursing, lip retraction, and cheek puffing. The patient should be instructed to repeat the movements as rapidly and steadily as possible. Observations of rate, range, and regularity of movement should be made. Observations of symmetry and the occurrence of regular or irregular involuntary movements should be made during speech and emotional responses.

The patient's emotional responses should be observed. The congenial clinician can usually elicit a spontaneous smile from the patient. When this does not happen naturally, asking "If I told you a joke would you smile?" while smiling at the patient often is sufficient to trigger a smile. The symmetry of smiling and the degree to which the angles of the mouth elevate to normal height (again, recognizing that some asymmetry is normal) should be noted. More important, the degree of movement asymmetry relative to that observed during voluntary lip retraction should be observed.

Does the patient have difficulty inhibiting laughter or crying? This loss of inhibition can become apparent at any time during examination, but one of the simplest ways to trigger disinhibition is to ask the patient "Do you have any difficulty controlling laughter or crying?" It should be recognized, however, that it can be difficult to distinguish crying that reflects a pathologic loss of motor control from crying that may occur as a result of the psychological distress, sorrow, and depression that can be expected in patients who are coping with disease.

The jaw at rest. The mandible is usually lightly closed or slightly open at rest. The jaw can be observed when the face is observed at rest. The following questions can be asked:

1. Does the jaw hang lower than normal?

2. Are there spontaneous, apparently involuntary quick or slow movements of the jaw, such as clenching, opening or pulling to one side, or tremor-like up and down movements? Has the patient learned any postural adjustments or tricks that tend to inhibit sustained involuntary movements (for example, clenching the jaw, holding a pipe in the mouth, touching a hand to the side of the jaw or neck)?

The jaw during sustained posture (Figure 3–2). The jaw can be observed during sustained facial posture tasks, especially during mouth opening (Figure 3–1, E). The following questions should be asked.

1. Does the jaw deviate to one side when the patient attempts to open it as widely as pos-

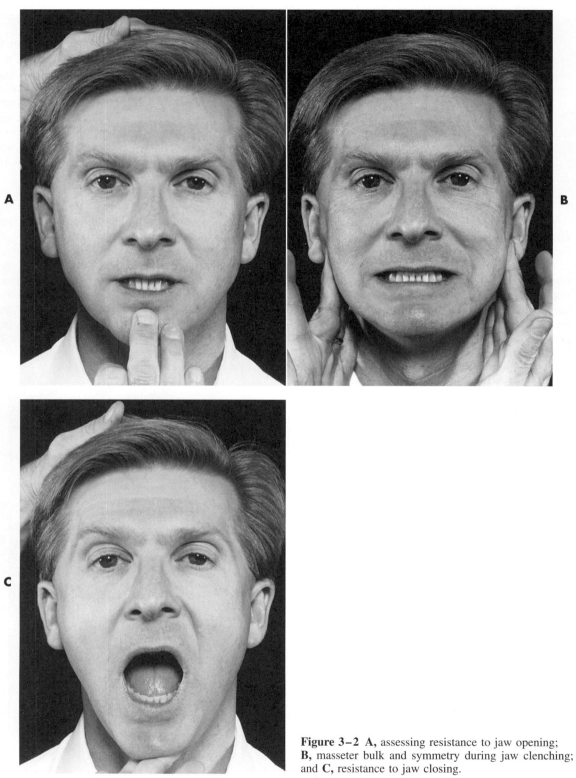

Figure 3–2 A, assessing resistance to jaw opening; **B,** masseter bulk and symmetry during jaw clenching; and **C,** resistance to jaw closing.

sible? Is the patient able to open the mouth widely or is excursion limited?

2. Can the patient resist the examiner's attempt to open the jaw when told to clench the teeth? Can they close the jaw against resistance from the examiner (either by holding the midline of the jaw with the hand or by placing a tongue blade on the lower teeth and resisting closure)? Do the masseter and temporalis muscles have normal bulk and bulge when the patient bites down?

3. Can the patient resist the examiner's attempt to close the jaw when they are told to hold it open?

The jaw during movement. The jaw should be observed for symmetry of opening and closing and for range of movement during speech and spontaneous movements. The patient should be asked to rapidly open and close the mouth; the speed and regularity of movements, as well as involuntary movements that may interrupt the course of the jaw alternating motion rates (AMRs) should be noted.

The tongue at rest. The tongue should be examined at rest (Figure 3–1, E). The patient should be told to open the mouth and let the tongue relax on the floor of the mouth. The degree to which the normal tongue lies at rest varies considerably and some low amplitude spontaneous movement is common. With this in mind, the following questions can be addressed.

1. Is the tongue full and symmetric? If symmetric, is its size normal? If small, are there symmetric or unilateral grooves or furrowing in the tongue representing atrophy? (Indentations along tongue's lateral side edges may represent teeth marks and not atrophy.) Are *fasciculations* present (repetitive dimpling or highly localized twitchlike movements of the tongue)? Fasciculations should be looked for only when the tongue is at rest inside the mouth; with the tongue protruded, normal spontaneous movements can be confused with fasciculations.

2. Does the tongue remain quiet on the floor of the mouth? Are quick, slow, or sustained movements of large portions of the tongue apparent in the form of protrusion, retraction, lateralization, or writhing?

The tongue during sustained postures (Figure 3–3). The patient should be asked to protrude the tongue and sustain the posture. Mild deviation toward one side or the other is not unusual in normal tongues, but the direction of deviation usually is inconsistent. The meaningfulness of deviation, when subtle, can be determined by having the patient repeat the task several times; consistent deviation to one side may reflect weak-

ness. The following questions should be addressed.

1. Can the patient protrude the tongue to a normal degree? Does the tongue consistently deviate to one side or the other? Deviation should be judged by the relationship of the tongue to the midline of the chin, especially when unilateral facial weakness is present; an alternative is to hold up the corner of the mouth so that it is roughly symmetric with the unimpaired side, so that tongue deviation can be judged more validly.

2. Can the patient resist the examiner's attempt to push the tongue back into the mouth? (A tongue blade placed against the tip of the tongue can be used for this purpose.)

3. Can the patient push out the cheek on each side with their tongue? If so, can they resist pressure from the examiner's finger to push the tongue inward? With the tongue outside of the mouth, can the patient resist the examiner's attempt to push the tongue to one side with the tongue blade? Does the tongue resist pressure at first and then suddenly give way completely?

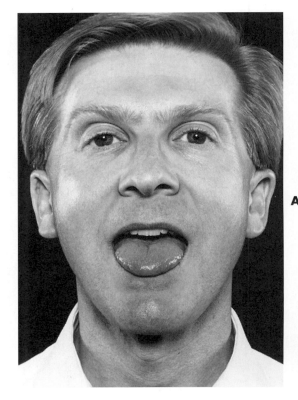

A

Figure 3–3 A, the tongue during protrusion; **B,** resisting pressure to push it inward with a tongue blade; **C,** lateralizing to the cheek; **D,** resisting inward pressure when lateralized; **E,** lateralize outside the mouth, as for lateral lingual AMRs.

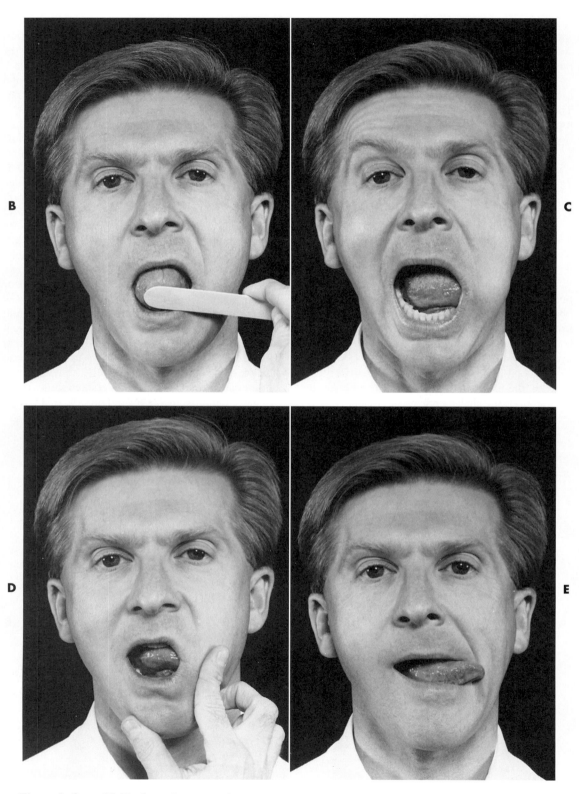

Figure 3–3 cont'd For legend see opposite page.

The tongue during movement. The patient should be asked to move the tongue from side to side as rapidly as possible. Speed, regularity, and range of motion should be noted.

The velopharynx at rest. The patient should be asked to open the mouth as widely as possible. The tongue should then be depressed with a tongue blade (Figure 3–4). The following questions should be addressed.

1. Does the palate hang low in the mouth? Does it rest on the tongue?
2. Are the palatal arches symmetric or does one side hang lower than another? (Normal palates are often asymmetric, especially after tonsillectomy or palatal surgery.)
3. Are there spontaneous rhythmic or arhythmic beating movements of the palate (that is, myoclonus)?

The velopharynx during movement. The patient should be asked to prolong "ah." Important observations relate to the presence, absence, and symmetry of palatal movement. Inferences about the adequacy of palatal movement for speech should be avoided. The following questions should be asked.

1. Is palatal movement symmetric? If asymmetric, does the palate elevate more strongly to the side opposite that which was lower at rest?

2. Is there evidence of nasal airflow on a mirror held at the nares during vowel prolongation (Figure 3–4), prolongation or repetition of pressure sounds (/s/, /p/), or words or phrases with nonnasal sounds? Does resonance change during vowel prolongation with the nares occluded versus unoccluded?

The integrity of velopharyngeal closure also can be addressed indirectly by having the patient puff the cheeks and protrude the tongue simultaneously. This *modified tongue-anchor test* (Dalston, Warren, and Dalston, 1990; Fox and Johns, 1970) may not be valid if there is significant tongue or facial weakness. Patients with palatal weakness sometimes impound intraoral pressure by assisting velopharyngeal closure with the back of the tongue. Tongue protrusion during cheek puffing prevents this compensation, so the cheeks cannot be puffed and nasal escape of air will occur if the palate is significantly weak. It sometimes helps for the examiner to occlude the nares while the patient puffs and protrudes the tongue and then to release the nares, observing whether or not air is then nasally emitted. It is important to demonstrate this task to the patient because some normal individuals have difficulty understanding or coordinating the movements for it. Only the inability to

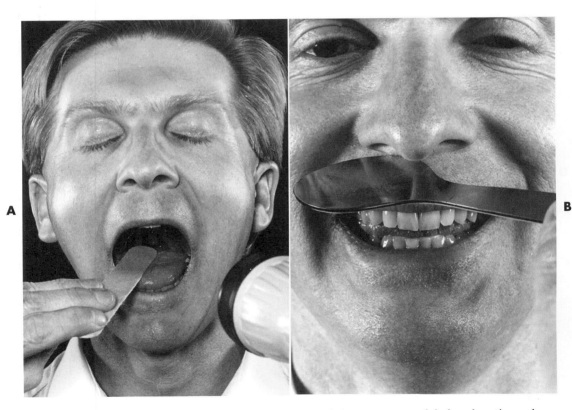

Figure 3–4 A, position for examining the soft palate and pharynx at rest and during phonation and gagging; and **B,** examining for nasal airflow during prolongation of /i/ or production of pressure consonants.

puff the cheeks because of nasal air escape when the tongue is actually protruded is meaningful to the assessment of velopharyngeal weakness.

To directly observe the extent of velopharyngeal activity during speech, videofluoroscopy or nasendoscopy is necessary. Lateral, frontal, and basal view videofluoroscopy provide good information about palatal, lateral pharyngeal wall, and sphincteric activity of the velopharyngeal mechanism during speech, as does nasendoscopy. Lateral view videofluoroscopy may be sufficient if documentation of palatal weakness is of primary concern.

The larynx. The gross integrity of vocal cord adduction can be inferred from two tasks. First, the patient should be asked to cough; the important observation is the *sharpness of the cough*, not its loudness. A weak or "mushy" or breathy cough may reflect vocal cord adductor weakness, poor respiratory support, or both. Second, the patient should be asked to produce a *"coup de glotte" (glottal coup),* which is a sharp glottal stop or grunting sound; this maneuver does not require much respiratory force or sustained airflow. Again, the *sharpness of the coup* is the important observation. A weak cough but sharp glottal coup may reflect respiratory weakness. A weak coup but normal cough, or equally weak cough and coup, tend to be associated with laryngeal weakness or combined laryngeal and respiratory weakness.

Weakness of vocal cord abduction can be inferred from the presence of *inhalatory stridor* (noisy or phonated inhalation). This sometimes can be detected during quiet breathing, but is more readily detected during inhalation for speech or when the patient takes a quick, deep breath.

Laryngeal examination should be pursued when structural lesions or LMN lesions of the laryngeal branches of the vagus nerve are a possibility. Supranuclear lesions do not result in clearly visible asymmetry of the vocal cords (although systematic study to confirm this observation is lacking). Laryngeal exam, however, can be useful in documenting abnormalities of laryngeal movements in certain CNS movement disorders that affect the larynx. The most common ways to view vocal cord activity are through indirect mirror laryngoscopy and direct laryngoscopy. Structural abnormalities (for example, neoplasms, nodules, polyps, inflammation) that alter the mechanical properties of the vocal cords, weakness or paralyses that impair vocal cord mobility, and significant abnormal involuntary movements of the vocal cords can be observed. More sophisticated visualization of the larynx with optically precise rigid laryngoscopes and visualization of laryngeal activity during connected speech with flexible fibreoptic laryngoscopy are possible. Videostroboscopy

permits visualization of vocal cord motion (the mucosal wave) during the phonatory vibratory cycles and, therefore, the analysis of much more subtle abnormalities of vocal cord function. Electroglottography, photoglottography, and acoustic analyses permit the quantification and analysis of various correlates of vocal cord activity during phonation.

Respiration. Some valuable information about respiratory adequacy for speech can be derived from observations of the patient during quiet breathing and a few nonspeech activities. During quiet breathing the following questions can be asked.

1. Is posture normal? If not, is the patient slouched in the chair or bent forward or to the side? Does the patient tend to gravitate over time toward abnormal posture in a chair or wheelchair, and does it require effort or assistance to resume a more normal posture? Is the head drooped forward? Does it rest on the chest? Is the patient braced in the wheelchair in order to maintain normal posture? All of these abnormal postures may restrict abdominal and thoracic movements and reduce respiratory support for speech.

2. Does the patient complain of shortness of breath at rest, during physical exertion, or during speech? Is breathing rapid, shallow, or labored? (Rate of quiet breathing during wakefulness is about 16 to 18 cycles/minute with each inspiratory and exhalatory cycle taking 2 to 3 seconds.) Are abdominal and thoracic movements limited in range? Is breathing accompanied by shoulder movement, neck extension, retraction of the neck just above the upper sternum on inhalation, or flaring of the nares on inhalation? Rapid, shallow breathing and excessive assistive shoulder or neck movement during breathing may reflect respiratory weakness and predict reduced loudness or phrase length.

3. Is breathing rate irregular? Are there any abrupt or slower abdominal, thoracic, or torso movements that alter or interrupt normal cyclical breathing? Such irregularities may reflect a movement disorder and predict abnormalities in loudness, prosody, and phrasing.

Sophisticated pulmonary function tests may document and explain sources of abnormal respiratory function for speech. However, in most situations where respiratory weakness may be present, a few simple tasks can help determine if respiratory support is sufficient for speech.

1. As already noted, when weakness is suspected, contrasting the sharpness of the cough versus glottal coup may help separate respiratory from laryngeal contributions to reduced loudness or

short phrases. A weak cough with limited abdominal and thoracic excursion may reflect respiratory weakness.

2. Hixon, Hawley, and Wilson (1982) described a simple water glass manometer that can be used to estimate the ability to generate respiratory driving pressure sufficient for speech (Figure 3–5). It requires a drinking glass (12 cm or more in depth) filled with water and calibrated in centimeters and a drinking straw that is affixed by a paper clip to the glass at a given depth. To maintain a stream of bubbles through the straw, a person must sustain breath pressure equal to the depth of the straw in the water. The ability to maintain a stream of bubbles for 5 seconds with the straw at a depth of 5 cm suggests that breath support is sufficient for most speech purposes. For this test to be valid as a measure of respiratory support, the patient must be able to maintain velopharyngeal closure (or have the nares occluded) and achieve a tight lip seal around the straw.*

Reflexes. Reflexes can provide confirmatory clues about the presence of neuropathology and its localization in the CNS versus peripheral nervous system (PNS). Those that can be tested in the context of the speech mechanism examination include normal reflexes and primitive reflexes. *Normal reflexes are those whose presence is a reflection of normal nervous system function.* Their absence can reflect PNS pathology. *Primitive reflexes are those which are present during infancy but tend to disappear during nervous system maturation.* Their presence in adults is often associated with CNS pathology, especially in frontal lobe cortical and subcortical regions. They appear to represent a "release phenomena" or a reduction of cortical inhibitory influence on lower centers of the brain.

Normal reflexes vary greatly among individuals in the ease with which they are elicited and in their response amplitude. Primitive reflexes are present in a certain percentage of normal adults and tend to reappear with normal aging, so cautious interpretation of them is required.

1. Gag reflex. The gag or pharyngeal reflex is a normal reflex elicited by stroking the back of the tongue, posterior pharyngeal wall, or faucial pillars on both sides with a tongue blade. The afferent

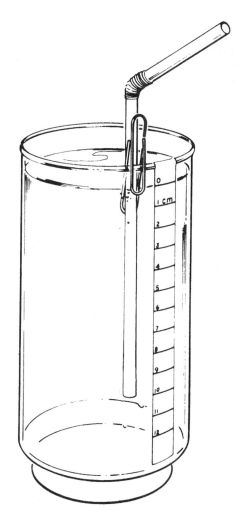

Figure 3–5 Water glass manometer for determining ability to generate and sustain respiratory driving pressure sufficient for speech. (From Hixon TJ, Hawley JL, and Wilson KJ: An around-the-house device for the clinical determination of respiratory driving pressure: a note on making the simple even simpler, J Speech Hear Disord 47:413, 1982.)

pathway for the stimulus is through the glossopharyngeal nerve (IX); the motor response is through the glossopharyngeal and vagus (X). The reflex is characterized by elevation of the palate, retraction of the tongue, and sphincteric contraction of the pharyngeal walls. Normal responses vary greatly and range from no response to a vigorous gag that may be elicited merely by touching the tongue.

In general, the gag reflex is clinically significant only if it is asymmetrically elicited. If absent on one side but not the other, it is probably abnormally hypoactive on the less responsive side. When asymmetric it is useful to ask the patient if the stimulus feels different between the two sides; if so, reduced sensation may be responsible for the

---

*A slightly more complex but nonetheless simple U-tube manometer for measuring intraoral breath pressure has been described by Netsell and Hixon (1978). Their article explains the rationale for the device, and provides an illustration and specifications for it. Hixon, Hawley, and Wilson (1982) point out, however, that its successor, the water glass manometer, is simpler to construct and probably easier to use.

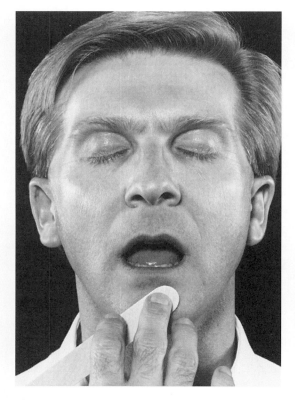

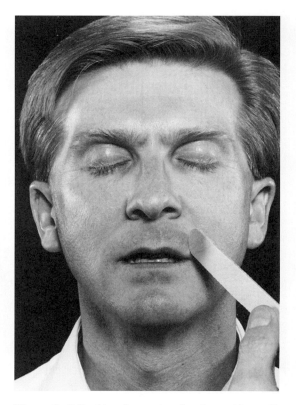

Figure 3–6 Position for testing for the jaw jerk reflex (procedure and response described in text).

Figure 3–7 Position for testing for the sucking reflex (procedure and response described in text).

decreased reflex response. If reported sensation is not different, the motor component of the reflex may be deficient.

2. Jaw jerk. The jaw jerk (maxillary reflex) is a primitive deep muscle stretch reflex that may be pathologic when present in adults. To test for it, the patient should be relaxed, with the lips parted and the jaw about halfway open. A tongue blade (or fingertip) is placed on the patient's chin and the blade is then tapped with a reflex hammer or a finger of the other hand (Figure 3–6). A positive or pathologic response is a quick closing of the jaw in response to the quick stretch on the masseter muscles caused by the tapping.

The jaw jerk is present in about 10% of normal adults (Walton, 1982). In general, however, its presence may be confirmatory of bilateral UMN disease above the level of the midpons (that is, above the nuclei of the trigeminal nerve, whose sensory and motor branches are involved in the reflex).

3. Sucking reflex. The sucking reflex is a primitive reflex. It is tested by stroking the upper lip with a tongue blade, beginning at the lateral aspect of the upper lip and moving medially toward the philtrum (Figure 3–7). This should be done on both sides. There is no response to the stimulus in

adults. The positive or pathologic response is a pursing of the lips. When present it can be confirmatory of UMN disease, especially diffuse damage to the premotor cortex. The reflex is frequently elicited in patients with dementia (Brazis, Masdeu, and Biller, 1985; Walton, 1982).

When the sucking reflex is very exaggerated, the patient may purse the lips as an object approaches the mouth, or may turn the mouth toward a tactile stimulus to the corner of the mouth or cheek. When this occurs, it is called a *rooting reflex.*

4. Snout reflex. The primitive snout reflex is similar to the sucking reflex in its characteristics and meaning. It can be elicited by a light tap of the finger on the philtrum or tip of the nose (Gilroy and Meyer, 1979). The reflex is a puckering or protrusion and elevation of the lower lip and depression of the lateral angles of the mouth (Figure 3–8). It can also be elicited by backward pressure of the examiner's index finger on the midline of the patient's upper lip and philtrum (Jacobs and Gossman, 1980).

Voluntary versus "automatic" nonspeech movements of speech muscles. Differences can exist between nonspeech volitional movements of speech muscles and movements during relatively

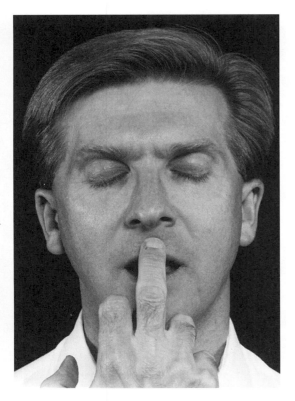

Figure 3–8 Position for testing for the snout reflex (procedure and response described in text).

automatic or overlearned responses. Differences between movements of the face during emotional responding and voluntary performance have already been discussed.

Just as speech programming ability can be stressed or facilitated, so too can nonspeech programming ability. Whenever supratentorial lesions (particularly dominant hemisphere lesions) or apraxia of speech or aphasia are suspected, the ability to imitate or follow commands for nonspeech movements of the speech muscles should be examined. The goal is to test for *nonverbal oral apraxia*.

The tasks are simple and several of them are identical to those in routine oral mechanism examination. They are best elicited by verbal command, but if comprehension problems exist (as is often the case when aphasia is present), or if the patient comprehends but has difficulty performing a task, imitation should also be used.

The observations are different than those during routine oral mechanism examination. They focus on the ability to perform without off-target approximations, frank errors, or a frustrating awareness that performance is incorrect with accompanying attempts at self-corrections. For example, asked to cough, patients with nonverbal oral

apraxia will sometimes say "cough, cough" or "huh, huh," then recognize the response's inadequacy and attempt to self-correct. They often improve on imitation but may be inaccurate if tested again a few moments later. Such patients often reflexively perform the acts they are unable to do when requested (for example, unable to cough on command, they may later cough reflexively). These discrepancies reflect a nonverbal oral apraxia and dominant hemisphere pathology and are very often associated with apraxia of speech and aphasia. Some tasks that are useful for assessing for the presence of nonverbal oral apraxia are provided in the box on page 81.

Assessment of perceptual speech characteristics

Motor speech disorders can be assesssed in many ways. What is important is that the examination capture those observations that are most critical to diagnosis and management. It is also important to recognize that what must be done for diagnostic purposes may not be identical to what is done to establish recommendations and a plan for management. The focus at this point will be on methods for identifying the perceptually salient deviant dimensions of speech that lead to diagnosis.

The most useful method for describing deviant perceptual characteristics of speech derives from the work of Darley, Aronson, and Brown. Because their work has been so influential to the understanding of the dysarthrias, and because it remains relevant, a brief summary of the foundation on which the clinical differential diagnosis of the dysarthrias is based is appropriate.

The Mayo Clinic dysarthria studies. The classic text, *Motor Speech Disorders* (Darley, Aronson, and Brown, 1975), was the outgrowth of extensive clinical research and two important articles that summarized those research efforts (Darley, Aronson, and Brown, 1969a & b).

Darley, Aronson, and Brown (1969a & b) analyzed speech samples from 212 patients. A minimum of 30 patients fell into seven groups: (1) bulbar palsy, (2) pseudobulbar palsy, (3) cerebellar lesions, (4) parkinsonism, (5) dystonia, (6) choreoathetosis, and (7) amyotrophic lateral sclerosis (ALS). These groups are equivalent to the categories of flaccid, spastic, ataxic, hypokinetic, hyperkinetic (dystonia and choreoathetosis), and mixed dysarthria, respectively, discussed by the authors in their 1975 book and by many subsequent clinicians and investigators. Each patient had unequivocal neurologic signs and symptoms that placed them into one and only one of the seven groups. Speech was abnormal in all cases but speech characteristics were not used to establish neurologic diagnoses.

TASKS FOR ASSESSING NONVERBAL ORAL MOVEMENT
CONTROL AND SEQUENCING

Instructions: Ask the patient to perform the following tasks. If failed in response to command, use imitation. The following scale can be used to score responses.

4. Accurate, immediate, effortless
3. Accurate but awkwardly or slowly produced
2. Accurate after trial and error searching movements
1. Inaccurate or only partially accurate, important component missing or off-target
NR = **N**o **r**esponse
V = **A**ccompanying or substituted **v**ocalization/**v**erbalization (for example, patient says "cough" instead of coughing)
P = **P**erseverative response

Item	Command	Imitation
1. Cough	_____	_____
2. Click your tongue	_____	_____
3. Blow	_____	_____
4. Bite your lower lip	_____	_____
5. Puff out your cheeks	_____	_____
6. Smack your lips	_____	_____
7. Stick out your tongue	_____	_____
8. Lick your lips	_____	_____
9. Bite your lower lip and then click your tongue	_____	_____
10. Smack your lips and then cough	_____	_____

Adapted and modified from Spriesterbach, Morris, and Darley (1978).

Audio recorded samples of reading and, in some cases, conversation and sentence imitation, were reviewed. A list of 38 speech and voice dimensions that seemed pertinent to the range of speech disorders was compiled. The dimensions were related to pitch, loudness, voice and resonance, respiration, prosody, and articulation. Two overall dimensions, intelligibility and bizarreness, were also included.

The authors listened to each sample within each neurologic diagnostic category up to 38 times, each time rating one of the 38 dimensions on a 7-point equal-appearing interval scale (certain economies were adopted so that 38 repetitions were not always necessary). Temporal and inter-judge reliability were good. The mean of the three judges' ratings was used for statistical analyses.

The deviant speech characteristics for each of the seven groups were analyzed in a manner that allowed comparisons among groups and identification of the most distinctive features within each group. "Clusters" of deviant speech characteristics were also identified. *Clusters represented the tendency for certain deviant speech dimensions to co-appear in certain groups of patients.* Each group had a unique pattern of clusters that were logically related to the presumed underlying neuromuscular substrate of the particular neurologic disorder. The analysis also permitted certain inferences about the neuromuscular bases for individual deviant speech characteristics.

Darley, Aronson, and Brown expressed the hope that their conclusions would serve as hypotheses for "more accurate physiologic and neurophysiologic measurements to further delineate the problems of dysarthria" (1969b, p. 462). The hope was realized, and many subsequent acoustic and physiologic studies have related their findings to the hypotheses of Darley, Aronson, and Brown. In addition, numerous subsequent perceptual studies of dysarthria associated with specific neurologic diseases have relied on Darley, Aronson, and Brown's methods or the deviant dimensions identified by them. Finally, many clinicians who must differentiate among the dysarthrias rely on their ability to recognize the deviant characteristics and clusters of deviant speech characteristics identified in the work of Darley, Aronson, and Brown, and subsequent investigators.

Distinctive speech characteristics. The distinctive speech characteristics encountered in each of the dysarthrias will be addressed in chapters dealing with each dysarthria type. Appendix A lists the 38 dimensions and their definitions. It also contains some additional characteristics that seem relevant to the description of dysarthric speech. The reader should become familiar with all of these terms because they form the foundation for all subsequent discussion of the dysarthrias.

The box on page 82 shows a rating form that may be useful for identifying and rating deviant speech dimensions. It contains all of the character-

RATING SCALE FORM FOR DEVIANT SPEECH CHARACTERISTICS

Name: _____   Speech diagnosis: _____
                                  Neurologic diagnosis: _____
Age: _____   Date of examination: _____

Dysarthria Rating Scale

Rate speech by assigning a value of 0–4 to each of the dimensions listed below (0 = normal; 1 = mild; 2 = moderate; 3 = marked; 4 = severely deviant). A + should be used to indicate excessive or high; − should be used to indicate reduced or low when appropriate.

Pitch	Pitch level (+/−) _____	**Respiration**	Forced inspiration-expiration _____
	Pitch breaks _____		Audible inspiration _____
	Monopitch _____		Inhalatory stridor _____
	Voice tremor _____		Grunt at end of expiration _____
	Myoclonus _____		
	Diplophonia _____		
Loudness	Monoloudness _____	**Prosody**	Rate _____
	Excess loudness variation _____		Short phrases _____
	Loudness decay _____		Increased rate in segments _____
	Alternating loudness _____		Increased rate overall _____
	Overall loudness (+/−) _____		Reduced stress _____
			Variable rate _____
			Prolonged intervals _____
			Inappropriate silences _____
			Short rushes of speech _____
			Excess & equal stress _____
Voice quality	Harsh voice _____	**Articulation**	Imprecise consonants _____
	Hoarse (wet) _____		Prolonged phonemes _____
	Breathy voice (continuous) _____		Repeated phonemes _____
	Breathy voice (transient) _____		Irregular articulatory breakdowns _____
	Strained-strangled voice _____		Distorted vowels _____
	Voice stoppages _____		
	Flutter _____		
Resonance (& intraoral pressure)	Hypernasality _____	**Other**	Slow AMRs _____
	Hyponasality _____		Fast AMRs _____
	Nasal emission _____		Irregular AMRs _____
	Weak pressure consonants _____		Simple vocal tics _____
			Palilalia _____
			Coprolalia _____

Intelligibility _____

Bizarreness _____

Based on the dimensions used in Mayo Clinic dysarthria studies (Darley, Aronson, and Brown, 1969a&b), plus additional features that may help characterize dysarthria.

istics listed and defined in Appendix A. Several of the features added to the 38 characteristics of Darley, Aronson, and Brown are task-specific (AMRs, vowel prolongation).

In our clinic, we rate speech dimensions on a 0–4 scale (0 = normal, 1 = mild, 2 = moderate, 3 = marked, 4 = severe). This departure from the 7-point scale used by Darley, Aronson, and Brown is not important because the *presence* of a deviant speech characteristic is generally more important to differential diagnosis than its severity. The reason for the 0–4-point scale is its correspondence to commonly used terms for severity (normal, mild, moderate, marked, severe) and its correspondence to the 0–4 scale used by many neurologists to rate motor and sensory examination results. It should be noted, however, that the 0–4 scale can be expanded by 4 points by using ratings between categories if necessary (for example: 0,1 = equivocally present; 2,3 = moderate-marked impairment). Certain dimensions can also be rated plus or minus. For example, rating of reduced loudness can be modified by a minus, increased loudness modified by a plus; when pitch is high it is rated plus, when low minus; when rate is slow it is rated minus, when fast plus. With training and experience, clinicians achieve acceptable reliability making severity ratings with this scale. The difficult challenge to the clinician's ear for diagnostic purposes is learning to detect the presence of deviant dimensions. This is met by experience and the opportunity to check one's perceptions with an experienced clinician (see Kearns and Simmons, 1988).

Once the ratings have been compiled, they can be used to describe the patient's speech. Experienced clinicians reading an accurate description of deviant speech characteristics can recognize the important clusters and arrive at an accurate diagnosis without hearing the speech sample. This is not advisable for clinical practice but it does demonstrate the usefulness of describing speech in this manner.

"Styles" used for perceptual analysis. A symphony can be parsed and its complex underpinnings understood through a careful analysis of its notes, cadence, instruments, and the interactions and temporal relationships among them. Its theme, moods, and message, on the other hand, are best appreciated simply by "taking in" its performance, associating its emotional message with past experience, and appreciating its unique character.

Distinguishing among the dysarthrias can be approached in similar ways. Less experienced clinicians often must be analytic in their approach to diagnosis because they do not yet have an internalized perceptual representation of the dysarthrias for reference. As a result they carefully identify and list speech characteristics and match them against the characteristics associated with various dysarthria types. This process is valuable because it trains the ears to recognize the salient speech features and is essential to documenting the presence and severity of deviant speech features. What can be missed in this analytic process, however, is the message conveyed by the constant and temporally varying interactions among all of the individual's normal and abnormal speech char-

acteristics. This appreciation of gestalt cannot always be obtained by a checklist approach alone.

Experienced clinicians often arrive at a diagnosis by synthesis. They may recognize the speech pattern as a familiar tune, the category of tune represented by a specific dysarthria type. When this occurs, the purpose of a listing of speech characteristics is to document their presence and severity, and to summarize some of the reasons for the diagnosis. The risk of this synthesizing approach is that unique and important characteristics may be missed or dismissed, with resultant misdiagnosis. The "taking in" of the pattern of speech, however, can be the most sensitive, reliable, and efficient route to diagnosis.

Tasks for speech assessment. A small number of well-selected speech tasks can elicit most of the information necessary for a description and interpretation of abnormal speech. The most important tools for doing this are the ears and eyes of the clinician and an audio or audio-video recorder for repeated analyses of the speech sample when necessary.

The following tasks are designed to isolate as well as possible the respiratory-phonatory, the velopharyngeal, and the articulatory systems for independent assessment and then to permit observation of them in simultaneous natural operation.

1. Vowel prolongation. Phonation cannot be assessed independent of respiratory function, and disorders at one level can affect function at the other. Fortunately, speech is relatively resistant to respiratory disturbance and phonation is implicated in dysarthrias far more frequently than are respiratory disturbances. As a result, most abnormalities of voice implicate the laryngeal mechanism rather than the respiratory system.

The simplest task for isolating the respiratory-phonatory system for speech is vowel prolongation. The patient should be instructed to "*take a deep breath and say 'ah' for as long and as steadily as you can, until you run out of air.*" This should be followed by a short example by the clinician. It is best not to specify pitch or loudness level because most patients will respond at their conversational pitch and loudness level. If the pitch or loudness produced is noticeably different from conversational levels, the patient should be reinstructed to repeat the task at more natural levels; it may be necessary to instruct them to be higher or lower, quieter or louder, and it is often necessary to ask them to persist in duration. Sometimes the patient will ask, "Should I breathe when I do this?" A simple "yes" generally suffices and ensures that the clinician will not find evidence for task-specific muteness!

The dimensions to be attended to are those categorized under pitch, loudness, and voice quality

Table 3–2 Maximum phonation duration in seconds for the vowel /a/, representing averages across studies of young and elderly (generally over age 65) male and female adults summarized in Kent, Kent and Rosenbek's (1987) review of maximum performance tests of speech production. Standard deviations are given in parentheses.

	Median*	Minimum†	Maximum‡
Young males	28.5 (8.4)	22.6 (5.5)	34.6 (11.4)
Young females	22.7 (5.7)	15.2 (4.1)	26.5 (11.3)
Elderly males	13.8 (6.3)	13.0 (5.9)	18.1 (6.6)
Elderly females	14.4 (5.7)	10.0 (5.6)	15.4 (5.8)

* Median value of the means and standard deviations reported across studies.
† Lowest mean and lowest standard deviation reported across studies.
‡ Highest mean and highest standard deviation reported across studies.
Note: The median of the minimum values in the ranges reported for young males = 15.0; for young females = 11.8; for elderly males = 8.5; for elderly females = 6.5.

in the box on page 82. Monopitch and monoloudness should not be rated because they represent the goal and not deviant features during vowel prolongation. The maximum duration of the vowel also should be recorded. Maximum vowel duration varies widely among normal speakers; in general, in the absence of other evidence of respiratory or laryngeal abnormality, not much can be made of durations that exceed 7 or 8 seconds (see Table 3–2 for a summary of expected vowel duration values). Nonetheless, vowel duration can be used as baseline data against which future comparisons can be made, especially when the examiner is convinced that a maximum effort has been made.

The examiner should observe the jaw, face, tongue, and neck during vowel prolongation. Patients may display adventitious movements of those structures during what should be a fixed posture task. Quick or slow adventitious movements could represent an underlying movement disorder.

2. *Alternating motion rates. Alternating motion rates* (AMRs), or *diadochokinetic rates,* are very useful for determining the speed and regularity of reciprocal movements of the jaw, lips, and anterior and posterior tongue. They also permit assessment of precision of articulatory movements, the adequacy of velopharyngeal closure, and respiratory and phonatory support for sustaining the task. These latter observations are usually secondary; the primary value of AMRs is for assessing speed and regularity of rapid repetitive articulatory movements.

The patient should be instructed to *"take a breath and repeat 'puh-puh-puh-puh-puh' for as long and steadily as you can."* This should be followed by a 2 to 3 second example by the clinician. Although the task is to perform for as long as possible, a 3 to 5 second sample usually

suffices. Patients can be told to stop when the sample is sufficient for clinical judgments.

When repetitions of /p∧/ are completed, the patient should be asked to repeat the task for /t∧/ and /k∧/. AMRs for other consonant-vowel (CV) syllables can also be pursued if other places and manners of articulation are of interest.

Inability to sustain speech AMRs for more than a few seconds often reflects inadequacies at the respiratory-phonatory or velopharyngeal levels. When patients adopt a repetitive rhythm or peculiar cadence or have difficulty producing regular repetitions, they should be reinstructed or even allowed to practice at a slowed rate before being asked to produce maximum rates. Some patients will produce very rapid AMRs at the expense of precision; they should be instructed to go as fast as they can without being imprecise.

Speech AMRs for /p∧/, /t∧/, and /k∧/ usually can be produced precisely at maximum rates of 5 to 7 repetitions per second, with repetition of /k∧/ usually somewhat slower than /p∧/ or /t∧/. Approximate expected values for speech AMRs are summarized in Table 3–3. Rates can be adequately estimated with a stopwatch or can be measured instrumentally. Experienced clinicians can make judgments of speed and regularity without computing rate and variability, and the same 0–4 scale used for rating perceptual speech characteristics of speech can be employed. For example, mildly slowed AMR rate would be rated −1, severely slowed rate (approximately 1 per second) would be rated −4; markedly accelerated rate would be rated +3, and so on. Similarly, mildly irregular AMRs would be rated 1, moderately irregular AMRs rated 2, and so on.

Range of movement of the jaw and lips during speech AMRs should be observed because range is reduced or variable in some dysarthrias. The

Table 3–3 AMR and SMR performance for normal adults across studies of young and elderly adults, summarized in Kent, Kent, and Rosenbek's (1987) review of maximum performance tests of speech production. Standard deviations are given in parentheses.

Motion rate task	Median*	Minimum[†]	Maximum[‡]
/pʌ/	6.3 (0.7)	5.0 (0.4)	7.1 (1.2)
/tʌ/	6.2 (0.8)	4.8 (0.4)	7.1 (1.1)
/kʌ/	5.8 (0.8)	4.4 (0.6)	6.4 (1.1)
/pʌtʌkʌ/	5.0 (0.7)	3.6 (0.3)	7.5 (1.3)

* Median value of the means and standard deviations reported across studies.
[†] Lowest mean and lowest standard deviation reported across studies.
[‡] Highest mean and highest standard deviation reported across studies.
Note: The median of the minimum values in the ranges reported for /pʌ/ = 4.8; for /tʌ/ = 4.4; for /kʌ/ = 4.4; for /pʌtʌkʌ/ = 4.3.

rhythmicity of jaw and lip movements should also be observed because evidence of incoordination can sometimes be seen. Finally, interruptions or extraneous movements of the jaw, lip, and tongue should be noted (for example, tongue protrusion, lip retraction or pursing, lip smacking) because they may represent an underlying movement disorder.

Speech AMRs are generally slow or normal in rate in patients with motor speech disorders, although accelerated rate can be pathologic. Irregular AMRs are encountered in some but not all dysarthrias. Abnormalities of rate and regularity of AMRs are very useful in the identification of several dysarthria types.

3. Sequential motion rate. Sequential motion rate (SMR) is a measure of ability to move quickly from one articulatory position to another. Relative to AMRs, sequencing demands for SMRs are heavy and, for this reason, they are especially useful when apraxia of speech is suspected.

The patient should be asked to *"take a breath and repeat 'puh-tuh-kuh' over and over again until I tell you to stop."* This should be followed by a 2 to 3 second example by the clinician. Some people need reinstruction in the sequence, and slow or unison practice is sometimes necessary for the task to be grasped. When the sequence cannot be learned, repetition of "buttercup, buttercup, buttercup . . ." is acceptable, but the meaningfulness of the word makes it a simpler task than /pʌ tʌ kʌ /.

4. Contextual speech. The most useful task for evaluating the integrated function of all components of speech, and each of the primary valves, is contextual speech. This includes conversational and narrative speech, as well as reading aloud a standard paragraph containing a representative phonetic sample. The well-known Grandfather Passage is often used for this purpose (see Appendix B on p. 95).

Conversational speech is elicited during history taking, but the clinician's formal identification of deviant speech characteristics may be deferred so the facts of the history can be attended to. Open-ended questions asking about the patient's family, work, or hobbies usually elicit a sample sufficient to judge speech characteristics, but sometimes personality traits, depression, anxiety, or cognitive deficits limit responsiveness. Some patients respond more readily with narratives about pictured scenes than they do to more open-ended requests for narratives.

Reading a standard passage can provide a good sample of connected speech and, when repeatedly used, the clinician develops a sense of what is normal for the standard content. However, the ability among people to read aloud varies widely. Less skilled readers may read slowly, hesitantly, and with pronunciation errors and prosodic features that are inconsistent with their conversational prosody. When such reading problems are pronounced, reading is of little value because they can mask or superficially resemble the speech characteristics present in some dysarthrias.

5. Stress testing. Patients with motor speech disorders are susceptible to the effects of fatigue. In fact, regardless of dysarthria type, they will often complain of speech deterioration with prolonged conversation or with general physical fatigue over the course of a day. Because fatiguing of speech is so common, it is usually unnecessary for diagnostic purposes to observe speech under conditions of fatigue. However, whenever LMN weakness of unknown cause is present, or when the patient complains of rapid or dramatic changes in speech with continued speaking or general physical effort, speech stress testing should be pursued.

The patient should be asked to *"count as precisely as possible"* at a rate of about two digits per second. This should be continued without rest for

TASKS FOR ASSESSING MOTOR SPEECH PROGRAMMING CAPACITY
(APRAXIA OF SPEECH)

The tasks below require imitation or speaking in response to simple requests. Other tasks that are useful and important for assessing motor programming ability include conversation, narrative picture description, and reading aloud.

Scoring: The following codes may be used to capture response characteristics that may reflect apraxic behaviors.

Distortion (D)

Groping (audible or visible) (G)

Substitution (S)

Attempt at articulatory self-correction (SC)

Delayed response initiation (DR)

Awareness of errors (AOE)

Sequencing errors (SE)

Slow rate (SR)

Syllable × syllable production of
multisyllabic words, phrases (S×S)

A numeric code, adapted from the *Porch Index of Communicative Ability* (Porch, 1967) may also be useful.

15 = correct in all respects

14 = distorted

13 = delayed

10 = self-corrected articulatory
error

9 = correct after a stimulus
repetition

7 = error clearly related to
target

6 = error unrelated to target

5 = rejection or stated inability
to respond

4 = unintelligible but
differentiated from other
responses

3 = unintelligible & relatively
undifferentiated from other
responses

Broad or narrow transcription of aberrant responses is very useful.

I. "Repeat these sounds after me"

1. /i/ _____
2. /a/ _____
3. /u/ _____
4. /ei/ _____
5. /ai/ _____
6. /au/ _____
7. /m/ _____
8. /b/ _____
9. /p/ _____
10. /t/ _____
11. /n/ _____
12. /k/ _____
13. /g/ _____
14. /ʃ/ _____
15. /s/ _____
16. /tʃ/ _____
17. /f/ _____
18. /Ɵ/ _____

II. "Repeat these words after me"

1. mom _____
2. Bob _____
3. peep _____
4. bib _____
5. tot _____
6. deed _____
7. kick _____
8. gay _____
9. fife _____
10. sis _____
11. zoos _____
12. church _____
13. shush _____
14. lull _____
15. roar _____

III. "Repeat these words"

1. cat _____
   catnip _____
   catapult _____
   catastrophe _____
2. please _____
   pleasing _____
   pleasingly _____
3. thick _____
   thicken _____
   thickening _____

IV. "Repeat these words three times"

1. animal _____ _____ _____
2. snowman _____ _____ _____
3. artillery _____ _____ _____
4. stethoscope _____ _____ _____
5. rhinocerous _____ _____ _____
6. volcano _____ _____ _____
7. harmonica _____ _____ _____
8. octopus _____ _____ _____
9. statistical analysis _____ _____ _____
10. Methodist Episcopal Church
    _____ _____ _____

V. "Repeat these sentences"

1. We saw several wild animals. _____
2. My physician wrote out a prescription. _____
3. The municipal judge sentenced the criminal. _____

TASKS FOR ASSESSING MOTOR SPEECH PROGRAMMING CAPACITY
(APRAXIA OF SPEECH)—cont'd

VI. "Repeat the following as fast and as steadily as possible"

1. /p∧p∧p∧p∧ . . ./ _____   3. /k∧k∧k∧k∧ . . ./ _____

2. /t∧t∧t∧t∧ . . ./ _____   4. /p∧t∧k∧p∧t∧k∧ . . ./ _____

VII. "Count from one to ten"   **VIII. "Say the days of the week"**

1. _____	6. _____	1. Sunday _____	5. Thursday _____
2. _____	7. _____	2. Monday _____	6. Friday _____
3. _____	8. _____	3. Tuesday _____	7. Saturday _____
4. _____	9. _____	4. Wednesday _____	
5. _____	10. _____		

IX. "Sing" ("Happy Birthday," "Jingle Bells," or another familiar tune)

1. How well is the tune carried? _____

2. How adequate is articulation? _____

X. Description of conversation and narrative speech. _____
_____
_____

XI. Description of reading aloud. _____
_____
_____

Adapted and modified from Wertz, LaPointe, and Rosenbek (1984) and unpublished Mayo Clinic tasks for assessing apraxia of speech.

2 to 4 minutes. Significant deterioration of voice quality, resonance, or articulation consistent with perceptual characteristics associated with weakness may reflect the presence of myasthenia gravis, especially if speech improves significantly after a minute or two of rest. Testing speech muscle strength before and after stress testing may provide confirmatory evidence of weakness.

6. Assessing motor speech programming capacity. Sometimes patients produce articulatory substitutions, omissions, repetitions or additions. They may block, hesitate, or engage in trial-and-error groping for correct articulatory postures during conversation or reading. When this occurs, or when dominant hemisphere pathology is suspected, further assessment of speech motor programming ability should be pursued. An apraxia of speech may be present.

If speech is moderately to mildly or equivocally impaired, the patient should be asked to perform speech SMRs and to repeat complex multisyllabic words and sentences. The box above provides a list of words, word series, and sentences that have proven useful for this purpose.

If the patient is mute or barely able to speak, tasks that facilitate speech or place minimal demands on novel motor programming should be attempted. These tasks include singing a familiar

tune, counting, saying the days of the week, completing redundant sentences, and imitating consonant-vowel-consonant (CVC) syllables with identical initial and final consonants. Sometimes, patients find it easier to imitate isolated sounds than syllables or words. Patients with apraxia of speech often will improve in response to these simple tasks. A mismatch between speech adequacy on complex voluntary tasks and simpler "automatic" tasks increases the likelihood that apraxia of speech and not dysarthria is the correct diagnosis.

Published tests for the diagnosis of dysarthria. Only one standardized published test quantifies dysarthria in a manner that distinguishes among dysarthria types. A few published measures are available for assessing intelligibility in dysarthric speakers.

The only standardized diagnostic test is the *Frenchay Dysarthria Assessment (FDA)* (Enderby, 1983). The FDA relies on a 9-point rating scale applied to patient-provided information, observations of oral structures and functions, and speech. Measures of intelligibility and speaking rate are also made, as well as judgments about hearing, vision, dentition, language, mood, posture, and sensation. The task-oriented portion of the test focuses on reflexes, speech and nonspeech activities of respiration, the lips, jaw, soft palate, tongue and laryngeal function, and the measurement of intelligibility (the intelligibiltiy portion of the test will be discussed in the section on intelligibility assessment). The FDA is brief and does not require extensive training to administer and score.

Interjudge reliability coefficients for the test are acceptably high after three hours of training. It appears that the test can distinguish among flaccid, spastic, ataxic, hypokinetic, and mixed flaccid-spastic dysarthria with a high degree of accuracy. For example, a discriminant analysis of FDA results for 85 patients with confirmed neurologic diagnoses consistent with sites of damage associated with each of the five dysarthria types correctly classified 91% of the patients. Correct classification across dysarthria types ranged from 83% to 100%. The test manual also indicates that an "independent diagnosis" based only on FDA profiles—not direct observation of patients—was in agreement with the patients' therapists for 91% of 112 dysarthric patients. Enderby (1986) concluded, "One may speculate that accurate information on dysarthria may assist neurologic diagnosis."

The test manual provides graphs of the means and standard deviations for each of the five dysarthria types examined (three of the five groups had fewer than 15 patients). Although the profile for each dysarthria type is discussed, it is clear that there is considerable overlap among the groups for many of the FDA subtests. Specific criteria for objectively determining dysarthria type are not provided, nor are the discriminant function formulas that would permit quantitated subject placement into a dysarthria category.

The FDA demonstrates that distinctions among patients with different dysarthria types can be quantified and that the distinctions correlate with neurologic diagnosis. The test relies heavily on patient report and ratings of nonspeech oral activities, and it does not yield a comprehensive description of specific deviant speech characteristics associated with each dysarthria type. For these reasons, it may more appropriately be viewed as a test that distinguishes among patients with different lesion loci on the basis of nonverbal oral findings and certain speech characteristics, rather than a differential diagnostic test of dysarthria per se. With the addition of data for other dysarthria types (for example, hyperkinetic dysarthria), an increase in the number of cases per dysarthria type to the data base and discriminant analyses, and provision of discriminant function formulas or other criteria for quantitatively determining dysarthria type for individual patients, the FDA would have increased value as a standardized measure for dysarthria diagnosis.

Published tests for assessing apraxia of speech. There are only two published measures for the assessment of apraxia of speech. Their development as psychometrically valid and reliable standardized tests is incomplete. They do, however, represent organized approaches to assessment that have good face validity. They can be useful in establishing the presence of the disorder. These measures are:

1. Apraxia Battery for Adults (ABA) (Dabul, 1979). The ABA was developed in response to the need for a systematic method for measuring the presence and severity of apraxia of speech, and for quantifying speech changes over time. It represents a revision of an earlier version administered to 40 patients, 17 of whom were apraxic and aphasic, the remainder being aphasic or dysarthric but not apraxic.

The ABA contains six subtests. Five assess aspects of speech that are usually deficient in apraxia of speech; the sixth assesses limb and oral apraxia, deficits that tend to co-occur with apraxia of speech. The speaking subtests include measures of: diadochokinetic rates (SMRs for two and three syllable sequences); articulatory adequacy for imitation of words of increasing length; latency between presentation of a pictured multisyllabic noun and intiation of a naming response, and the time required from initiation to completion of the naming response; adequacy of articulation across three repetitions of verbally presented multisyllabic words; and an inventory of 15 behaviors or observations that are often associated with apraxia of speech.

Although norms have not been published, general guidelines for interpretation based on the performance of 40 patients are provided. The guidelines relate to distinctions in performance on each subtest among apraxic-aphasic patients, aphasic patients, and dysarthric patients. Guidelines are provided for determining the severity of apraxia of speech and suggestions are made for treatment based on test performance.

The advantage of the ABA is that it represents a series of tasks with face validity that can be administered in a standard fashion to patients with diagnosed or suspected apraxia of speech. Scores can be used to describe patient performance, compare performance over time, and quantify the diagnosis and severity of the problem in research studies. Shortcomings include a lack of normative data and an absence of demonstrated interjudge, intrajudge, and test-retest reliability, and measures of validity other than face validity.

2. Comprehensive Apraxia Test (CAT) (Di Simoni, 1989). The CAT is similar to the ABA in organization and degree of development as a standardized test. It contains a group of nonverbal oral volitional tasks and speech tasks that tend to distinguish apraxia of speech from other speech disorders. Administration and scoring guidelines are presented but reliability data are not. Although subtests and items have high face validity, data on the test's validity are not available.

Similar to the ABA, the CAT contains six subtests, five of which assess speech and one which assesses nonverbal oral postures and movements. The nonverbal oral volitional subtest requires imitation of oral postures and movements; responses are scored for degree of accuracy or inaccuracy, speed, completeness, and awkwardness. The speech subtests include imitative measures of isolated phonemes; AMRs and SMRs; single syllable production (words and nonsense syllables); utterances of increasing length (for example, "cowboy," "tax simplification instructions"); and contextual interference. The contextual interference subtest examines the effect of phonetic environment on the production of particular sounds. Stimuli are bisyllabic CVC-CVC in form. For each stimulus, one consonant in the sequence is the target to be scored; remaining consonants are identical or differ to varying degrees from the target. For example, imitation of the initial /ʃ/ in "sheep-shug" can be compared to its imitation in "sheet-mush." Voicing, manner, and place of production errors are scored. Error analysis examines the degree to which errors follow lawful patterns and the effect of particular phonetic environments on response accuracy.

The advantages of the CAT are similar to those of the ABA: good face validity, standard stimuli and approach to administration and scoring. It also provides information about phonetic environment influences on error frequency and type. Its weaknesses are also similar to those of the ABA: lack of normative data, absence of data on interjudge reliability, intrajudge reliability and test-retest reliability, and absence of validity data other than face validity.

Intelligibility assessment

Dysarthria does not always affect intelligibility. Nevertheless, the degree to which speech is understandable should always be addressed because it has great face and ecologic validity as an index of severity. This can range from an estimate of intelligibility during interaction with the patient to formal standardized quantitative testing. The degree to which assessment of intelligibility is pursued depends on the purposes of examination.

If the primary purpose of examination is diagnosis or to decide about the necessity for treatment, a general rating of intelligibility may suffice. Such a rating may include judgments about intelligibility by the patient, their significant others, and the clinician. The patient (and significant others) can be asked if being understood is a problem, how frequently and under what circumstances, and what is generally done to ensure the message is understood (for example, repetition, yes-no questioning, writing, etc.). The clinician may estimate a percentage of intelligible speech based on observations during examination, noting the circumstances under which the judgment is based (in quiet, with visual contact, when the topic of conversation is known, etc.). A projected estimate of intelligibility in other (usually less ideal) situations may also be made. Table 3–4 contains a scale that may be of value for this purpose. It reflects judgments of intelligibility and communicative efficiency in different environments and for different degrees of message complexity or predictability.

A formal quantitated estimate of speech intelligibility is important as a baseline or measure of progress when the patient will be treated or is being treated to improve intelligibility; when an objective quantified estimate of disability or handicap must be made for medical-legal purposes; when treatment may not be pursued but the patient is to be followed over time to document improvement, stability, or deterioration as a function of medical or surgical intervention, disease progression, and so on; or for research purposes.

Only a few measures have been developed for assessing intelligibility in adult dysarthric speakers. Virtually none have been designed specifically for apraxia of speech (although some of those available for dysarthria can probably be adapted for patients with apraxia of speech if aphasia is not a significant problem).

Assessment of intelligibility in dysarthric speakers (AIDS). (Yorkston and Beukelman, 1981a). The AIDS is probably the most widely used standardized test for measuring intelligibility, speaking rate, and communicative efficiency in dysarthria. It quantifies intelligibility of single words and sentences and provides an estimate of communication efficiency by examining the rate of intelligible words per minute in sentences. A computerized version, the *Computerized Assessment of Intelligibility of Dysarthric Speech* (Yorkston, Beukelman, and Traynor, 1984) is also available.

The single word task requires the patient to read or imitate a series of 50 words. The word list is generated by randomly selecting one of twelve

Table 3–4 Intelligibility rating scale for motor speech disorders

Rating	Dimension	Intelligibility
10	Environment* Content[†] Efficiency[‡]	Normal in all environments without restrictions on content without need for repairs
9	Environment Content Efficiency	Sometimes[§] reduced under adverse conditions when content is unrestricted but adequate with repairs
8	Environment Content Efficiency	Sometimes reduced under ideal conditions when content is unrestricted but adequate with repairs
7	Environment Content Efficiency	Sometimes reduced under adverse conditions even when content is restricted but adequate with repairs
6	Environment Content Efficiency	Sometimes reduced under ideal conditions when content is unrestricted even when repairs are attempted
5	Environment Content Efficiency	Usually[‖] reduced under adverse conditions when content is unrestricted even when repairs are attempted
4	Environment Content Efficiency	Usually reduced under ideal conditions even when content is restricted but adequate with repairs
3	Environment Content Efficiency	Usually reduced under adverse conditions even when content is restricted even when repairs are attempted
2	Environment Content Efficiency	Usually reduced under ideal conditions even when content is restricted even when repairs are attempted
1	Speech is not a viable means of communication in any environment, regardless of restrictions in content or attempts at repair	

*Environment may be "ideal" (for example, face-to-face, without visual or auditory deficits in the listener, without competition from noise or visual distractions) or "adverse" (for example, at a distance, with visual or auditory deficits or distractions).

[†] Content may be "unrestricted" (include all pragmatically appropriate content, new topics, lengthy narratives, etc.) or "restricted" (for example, limited to brief responses to questions or statements by the listener that allow for some degree of prediction of response content).

[‡] Efficiency may be "normal" (rarely in need of repetition or clarification because of poor motor speech production) or "repairs" may be necessary (repetition, restatement, responses to clarifying questions, modified production such as oral spelling, word-by-word confirmation of listener's repetition, spelling, etc.)

[§] Intelligibility is reduced in 25% or less of the individual's utterances.

[‖] Intelligibility is reduced in 50% or more of the individual's utterances, but not for all utterances.

Note: Not all possible combinations of deviant dimensions can be captured by a 10-point scale, and there is an obvious "gray area" between the meaning of "sometimes" and "usually." The point on the scale that most closely approximates the clinician's judgment should be used. Many patients will fit into more than one point on the scale. It may be prudent to assign a range rather than a single point in such cases (for example, 5–6).

phonetically similar words for each of the 50 items. A judge listens to an audio recording of the responses and identifies the spoken words in a multiple choice format in which the 12 choices for each word are listed or in a transcription format in which the spoken word is transcribed. The intelligibility score is the percentage of words correctly identified.

In the sentence task, the patient reads or imitates two sentences each, of 5 to 15 words in length, for a total of 220 words. Sentences are selected randomly from a master pool of 100 sentences of each length. The judge transcribes the sentences word by word. The intelligibility score is the percentage of words correctly transcribed.

At least two people must be involved in assessment, one to select the sample for assessment and the other to listen and transcribe or respond in a multiple choice format to the recorded sample. Repeated assessments for a given patient over time must either use the same judge or groups of judges to control for interjudge variability.

A measure of speaking rate during the sentence task is derived by dividing the number of words (220) by the duration of the sentence sample. Rate of intelligible speech is the number of correctly transcribed words divided by the total duration; a similar measure for rate of unintelligible words can also be computed. The rate of intelligible speech per minute is then divided by 190 (the mean rate of intelligible speech produced by normal speakers, who are nearly 100% intelligible on the test); this yields a *communicative efficiency ratio*. This measure of communicative efficiency may be particularly useful for mildly impaired speakers whose rate may be slow in spite of good intelligibility (Yorkston and Beukelman, 1981b).

The AIDS provides an index of severity of impairment, an estimate of the patient's deviation from normal, and a standard for monitoring change over time. Test-retest variability for the word-list test, allowing for differences between stimuli and day-to-day variability, is under 5%. Variability between sentence lists for the sentence test, however, even within the same day, is higher (approximately 9% to 11%). This latter degree of variability led Yorkston and Beukelman to recommend establishment of stable baseline measures of intelligibility before starting intervention, if the test is to be used to help document efficacy of treatment.

Frenchay Dysarthria Assessment (Enderby, 1983). The FDA (already discussed) has a component that evaluates the intelligibility of words, sentences, and conversation. In the word task, 10 stimuli are drawn randomly from a set of 50 words. The 10 words, unknown to the examiner, are read by the patient. Performance on the task is rated on a 5-point scale, with points on the scale reflecting differences in the number of words correctly recognized or the ease with which they are recognized. Although some of the words on the 50-item list are distinguished by minimal contrasts (park, dark), the 50 stimuli are heterogenous in frequency of occurrence, number of phonemes and syllables, and stress pattern. Kent and others (1989) have pointed out that word heterogeneity causes problems in selecting equivalent lists, and that the intervals between points on the 5-point rating scale may not be equal.

The sentence task is administered and scored like the word task. The sentences actually consist of a standard carrier phrase "the man is ___" with the final word represented by one of 50 randomly selected words ending with "ing." Consequently, this task is more a measure of single word intelligibility than sentence intelligibility.

The conversation task is based on about 5 minutes of conversation that is graded on a 5-point severity scale ranging from "no abnormality" to "totally unintelligible" speech. Although the scale represents a ranking of impaired intelligibility, its quantiative value is limited.

A word intelligibility test. Kent and others (1989) have designed two word intelligibility tests for use with dysarthric speakers. Although not published as standardized tests, they deserve mention because their characteristics are different from published tests and may provide valuable clinical information beyond percentage scores for intelligibility and efficiency.

Both tests are single word measures. An intelligibility score representing percentage of intelligible words is generated by judgments of words read by a speaker. The word stimuli and the organization of response choices permit the examination of 19 phonetic contrasts that may be vulnerable in dysarthric speech (for example, front-back vowel contrasts, voicing contrasts for initial and final consonants, fricative-affricate contrasts). The phonetic contrasts have acoustic correlates (for example, voice onset time and preceding vowel duration for initial and final voicing contrasts, respectively) that permit a more in-depth exploration of features associated with decreased intelligibility.

In the multiple choice version, the speaker reads one of four words distinguished by minimal phonetic contrasts (for example, beat, boot, bit, meat). There are 70 minimal contrast items in the test and any of the four contrasting words for each item can be used (therefore, there are 280 test words). This allows random selection of one of the four words for each of the 70 items, so repeated assessments may be conducted with the same judges.

The paired-word test is designed for use with severely dysarthric patients who cannot reliably produce more complex CVC syllables. Its items consist almost entirely of minimal contrasts within CV or VC syllables (for example, shoe-chew, eat-it). Sixteen contrasts are tested in three-word pairs each.

Data for patients with amyotrophic lateral sclerosis (ALS) demonstrate the test's ability to detect varying degrees of intelligibility impairment. Phonetic analyses also demonstrate the test's capacity to identify the locus of phonetic difficulties that contribute most to reduced intelligibility. For example, for their ALS patients, velopharyngeal function and laryngeal contrasts were particularly impaired, consistent with findings of perceptual studies by Carrow and others (1974) and Darley, Aronson, and Brown (1969a & b). Kent and others (1989) point out that the phonetic feature analysis extends perceptual findings by identifying the effect on articulation/phonetic outcomes of laryngeal and velopharyngeal dysfunction.

The promise of this kind of assessment, at least for research purposes, is that it provides information about the phonetic contributors to reduced intelligibility. Such information could aid decisions about treatment focus and, possibly, diagnosis. Because the contrasts examined in the test have corresponding measurable acoustic contrasts, test results may also influence the choice of relevant acoustic analyses for individual speakers or specific dysarthria types. In sum, these attributes have the potential to refine perceptual analyses, direct acoustic and physiologic analyses, document severity, identify attributes of speech to receive emphasis in treatment, and perhaps to establish distinctive patterns of phonetic deficits associated with specific dysarthria types.

Acoustic and physiologic measures

There are a large and expanding number of instrumental analyses that can be used to study motor speech disorders. In the past, many of these have been inaccessible or seldom used by clinicians because of cost, the time-consuming requirements to develop competence for data acquisition and interpretation, and a relative lack of information about the practical contribution of such analyses to diagnosis and management. More recently, instrumentation has become more affordable and user-friendly.

The need to integrate traditional clinical auditory-perceptual and nonspeech task assessment with instrumental procedures has been recognized (Kent, 1990). Instrumentation for acoustic and physiologic analyses is being evaluated for its applicability to clinical questions that can be addressed within the clinical setting (for example, Read, Buder, and Kent, 1990). These efforts have been reflected since 1982 in the biennial Conference on Motor Speech Disorders (and its subsequent publications: Berry, 1983; Yorkston and Beukelman, 1989; Moore, Yorkston, and Beukelman, 1991; Till, Yorkston, and Beukelman, 1994), a conference that includes reports of efforts to translate clinical observations and questions into research investigation, and to translate research findings into clinical practice (Yorkston and Beukelman, 1989). Many of the papers involve instrumental analyses of motor speech disorders.

In spite of increasing accessibility, instrumental analyses are not widely used in the clinical evaluation and management of motor speech disorders. Gerratt and others (1991), in a survey of Department of Veterans Affairs Medical Center Speech Pathology Services, found limited use of acoustic,

kinematic, aerodynamic, and imaging measures for clinical evaluation purposes. Instrumental measures were rated as less frequently used and less valuable than published and unpublished auditory-perceptual and nonspeech assessment techniques. The relatively limited use of instrumentation was felt to reflect unavailability, inability to use instrumentation, and clinical preference. Another possible explanation is that the clinical value of instrumental analysis has not been established (McNeil, 1986). Gerratt and others concluded, " . . . clinicians' reluctance to use instrumentation may result from a lack of knowledge and a lack of evidence to support the contribution of instrumentation in dysarthria management. The former requires the attention of training programs; the latter demands the attention of clinical research" (pp. 86–87).

Instrumental analyses have contributed to the description and understanding of motor speech disorders. Some acoustic and physiologic measures have potential value for clinical diagnosis and some have demonstrated value in management. As Kent (1990) pointed out, however, the operative word for diagnosis is *potential*. The intelligibility test described by Kent and others (1989) and the manner in which it is being used (for example, Kent and others, 1989; Kent and others, 1990; Kent and others, 1991) may represent a prototype for the kind of research that may bridge the gap between clinical practice that uses auditory perceptual and nonspeech assessment and instrumental approaches that can quantify and help parse the components of the speech system that are disordered. That is, clinical perceptual assessment, the results of which can be quantified into patterns of phonetic breakdown and then further quantified acoustically and physiologically, may help identify the loci of speech deficits, the physiology and acoustic correlates of decreased intelligibility and deviant perceptual speech characteristics, and, perhaps, those aspects of deviant speech whose improvement would lead to the greatest gains with treatment. To the degree that acoustic and physiologic analyses yield patterns of impairment that can be associated with specific dysarthria types or lesion loci, they may also contribute to refinements in clinical differential diagnosis.

It is beyond the scope of this book to review in-depth acoustic and physiologic approaches to the dysarthrias. The current uncertainty regarding reliability, validity, and clinical applicability of acoustic and physiologic methods to clinical differential diagnosis and management justifies a peripheral role for instrumental analysis in the clinical examination and diagnosis of motor speech disorders at this time. In fact, perceptually based clinical assessment will always be the mainstay of clinical diagnosis. It should be recognized, however, that instrumental analyses help us understand the underpinnings of motor speech disorders, and that they may someday be widely applicable and important to clinical diagnostic and management efforts. Because they have contributed significantly to the description and understanding of motor speech disorders, frequent reference will be made to studies employing them in each of the following chapters on the dysarthrias and apraxia of speech.

SUMMARY

1. Diagnosis of motor speech disorders is dependent on adequate examination of speech and the speech mechanism. Examination goals and activities include description and problem detection, establishing diagnostic possibilities, establishing a speech diagnosis, establishing implications for localization and disease diagnosis, and specifying severity.
2. The essential components of the motor speech examination include the history, the examination of the oral mechanism, the assessment of salient features of speech, the estimation of intelligibility and severity, and the determination of appropriate acoustic and physiologic measures.
3. The history requires goal-setting with the patient and the acquisition of information about: relevant events prior to the development of speech deficits; the onset and course of the speech problem; the course and nature of associated deficits; the patient's perception of the speech problem and its consequences; current or prior management of the speech problem; the patient's awareness of the medical diagnosis and prognosis.
4. Speech assessment relies heavily on identification of deviant speech characteristics. Speech tasks include: vowel prolongation, AMRs, SMRs, contextual speech, stress testing, and tasks for stressing or facilitating motor speech programming. Accurate diagnosis ideally relies on a combination of an analytic approach in which deviant speech characteristics and clusters are identified and a synthetic appreciation of the "global" product of all speech characteristics interacting with one another.
5. Examination of the oral mechanism at rest and during nonspeech activities provides confirmatory evidence and information about the size, strength, symmetry, range, tone, steadiness, speed, and accuracy of orofacial structures and movements. Observations of the speech structures are made at rest, during sustained postures and movement, and in response to tests for normal and primitive reflexes. Assessing voluntary versus automatic nonspeech movements of the speech muscles is also important when nonverbal oral apraxia is suspected.
6. Judgments of speech intelligibility should always be made. Estimates of intelligibility can range from impressionistic estimates by the clinician and the patient and their significant others to formal assessment with standard intelligibility tests.
7. Many acoustic and physiologic measures are available to study motor speech disorders. Information derived from such measures has potential to quantify and explain clinical perceptual observations and to increase our understanding of the pathophysiologic underpinnings of deviant speech. The value of instrumental analysis for day-to-day clinical diagnosis and management has not yet been clearly established.

Appendix A

DEVIANT SPEECH DIMENSIONS ENCOUNTERED IN DYSARTHRIAS

Label	Description
Mayo Clinic Dysarthria Study Dimensions (Darley, Aronson, and Brown, 1975, used with permission)	
1. Pitch level	Pitch of voice sounds consistently too low or too high for age and sex
2. Pitch breaks	Pitch of voice shows sudden and uncontrolled variation (falsetto breaks)
3. Monopitch	Voice is characterized by a monopitch or monotone. Voice lacks normal pitch and inflectional changes. It tends to stay at one pitch level.
4. Voice tremor	Voice shows shakiness or tremulousness.
5. Monoloudness	Voice shows monotony of loudness. It lacks normal variations in loudness.
6. Excess loudness variation	Voice shows sudden, uncontrolled alterations in loudness, sometimes becoming too loud, sometimes too weak.
7. Loudness decay	There is progressive diminution or decay of loudness.
8. Alternating loudness	There are alternating changes in loudness.

Continued.

Label	Description
Mayo Clinic Dysarthria Study Dimensions (Darley, Aronson, and Brown, 1975, used with permission)—cont'd	
9. Loudness level (overall)	Voice is insufficiently or excessively loud.
10. Harsh voice	Voice is harsh, rough, and raspy.
11. Hoarse (wet) voice	There is wet, "liquid-sounding" hoarseness.
12. Breathy voice (continuous)	Voice is continuously breathy, weak, and thin.
13. Breathy voice (transient)	Breathiness is transient, periodic, and intermittent.
14. Strained-strangled voice	Voice (phonation) sounds strained or strangled (an apparently effortful squeezing of voice through glottis).
15. Voice stoppages	There are sudden stoppages of voice airstream (as if some obstacle along vocal tract momentarily impedes flow of air).
16. Hypernasality	Voice sounds excessively nasal. Excessive amount of air is resonated by nasal cavities.
17. Hyponasality	Voice is denasal.
18. Nasal emission	There is nasal emission of airstream.
19. Forced inspiration-expiration	Speech is interrupted by sudden, forced inspiration and expiration sighs.
20. Audible inspiration	There is audible, breathy inspiration.
21. Grunt at end of expiration	There is a grunt at the end of expiration.
22. Rate	Rate of actual speech is abnormally slow or rapid.
23. Short phrases	Phrases are short (possibly because inspirations occur more often than normal). Speaker may sound as if he has run out of air. He may produce a gasp at the end of a phrase.
24. Increase of rate in segments	Rate increases progressively within given segments of connected speech.
25. Increase of rate overall	Rate increases progressively from beginning to end of sample.
26. Reduced stress	Speech shows reduction of proper stress or emphasis patterns.
27. Variable rate	Rate alternates from slow to fast.
28. Prolonged intervals	There is prolongation of interword or intersyllable intervals.
29. Inappropriate silences	There are inappropriate silent intervals.
30. Short rushes of speech	There are short rushes of speech separated by pauses.
31. Excess and equal stress	There is excess stress on usually unstressed parts of speech (e.g., monosyllabic words and unstressed syllables of polysyllabic words).
32. Imprecise consonants	Consonant sounds lack precision. They show slurring, inadequate sharpness, distortions, and lack of crispness. There is clumsiness in going from one consonant sound to another.
33. Prolonged phonemes	There are prolongations of phonemes.
34. Repeated phonemes	There are repetitions of phonemes.
35. Irregular articulatory breakdowns	There is intermittent, nonsystematic breakdown in accuracy of articulation.
36. Distorted vowels	Vowel sounds are distorted throughout their total duration.
37. Intelligibility (overall)	This is a rating of overall intelligibility or understandability of speech.
38. Bizarreness (overall)	This is a rating of the degree to which overall speech calls attention to itself because of its unusual, peculiar, or bizarre characteristics.
Other relevant dimensions (not used in Mayo Clinic dysarthria studies)	
39. Diplophonia	Simultaneous perception of two different pitches.
40. Flutter	Rapid, relatively low amplitude voice tremor (perceived as in the 7 to 12 Hz range), usually most apparent during vowel prolongation.
41. Inhalatory stridor	Similar to audible inspiration (#20) but characterized by actual rough phonation due to vocal cord approximation and vibration during inhalation.
42. Myoclonus	1 to 4 Hz rhythmic "beats" in the voice, sometimes sufficient to cause brief voice arrests, usually heard only during vowel prolongation.
43. Weak pressure consonants	Pressure consonants lack acoustic distinctiveness or are weak because of excessive nasal airflow during their production.
44. Slow AMRs/Fast AMRs	Speech alternating motion rates are slow or fast.
45. Irregular AMRs	Speech alternating motion rates are irregular in duration, pitch, or loudness.

Label	Description
46. Simple vocal tics	Repetitive, rapid, apparently involuntary noises or sounds (e.g., throat clearing, grunting) produced in isolation or during voluntary speech.
47. Palilalia	Compulsive repetition of words or phrases, usually in a context of accelerating rate and decreasing loudness.
48. Coprolalia	Involuntary, compulsive, repetitive obscene language or swearing, often uttered loudly, softly, or incompletely.

Appendix B

GRANDFATHER PASSAGE

You wish to know all about my grandfather. Well, he is nearly 93 years old, yet he still thinks as swiftly as ever. He dresses himself in an old black frock coat, usually several buttons missing. A long beard clings to his chin, giving those who observe him a pronounced feeling of the utmost respect. Twice each day he plays skillfully and with zest upon a small organ. Except in the winter when the snow or ice prevents, he slowly takes a short walk in the open air each day. We have often urged him to walk more and smoke less, but he always answers, "Banana oil!" Grandfather likes to be modern in his language.

REFERENCES

Berry WR: Clinical dysarthria, San Diego, 1983, College-Hill.

Brazis P, Masdeu JC, and Biller J: Localization in clinical neurology, Boston, 1985, Little-Brown.

Carrow E et al: Deviant speech characteristics in motor neuron disease, Arch Otolaryngol 100:212, 1974.

Dabul B: Apraxia battery for adults, Tigard, Oregon, 1979, CC Publications.

Dalston R, Warren DW, and Dalston ET: The modified tongue-anchor technique as a screening test for velopharyngeal inadequacy: a reassessment, J Speech Hear Disord 55:510, 1990.

Darley FL, Aronson AE, and Brown JR: Clusters of deviant speech dimensions in the dysarthrias, J Speech Hear Res 12:462, 1969a.

Darley FL, Aronson AE, and Brown JR: Differential diagnostic patterns of dysarthria, J Speech Hear Res 12:246, 1969b.

Darley FL, Aronson AE, and Brown JR: Motor speech disorders, Philadelphia, 1975, WB Saunders.

DeSimoni FG: Comprehensive apraxia test (CAT), Dalton, Pennsylvania, 1989, Praxis House Publishers.

Enderby P: Frenchay dysarthria assessment, San Diego, 1983, College-Hill.

Enderby P: Relationships between dysarthric groups, Br J Disord Commun 21:189, 1986.

Fox DR and Johns DF: Predicting velopharyngeal closure with a modified tongue-anchor technique, J Speech Hear Disord 35:248, 1970.

Gerratt BR et al: Use and perceived value of perceptual and instrumental measures in dysarthria management. In Moore CA, Yorkston KM, and Beukelman DR, editors: Dysarthria and apraxia of speech: perspectives on management, Baltimore, 1991, Paul H. Brookes.

Gilroy J and Meyer JS: Medical neurology, New York, 1979, Macmillan.

Hager JC and Ekman P: The asymmetry of facial actions is inconsistent with models of hemispheric specialization, Psychophysiology 23:307, 1985.

Hixon TJ, Hawley JL, and Wilson KJ: An around-the-house device for the clinical determination of respiratory driving pressure: a note on making the simple even simpler, J Speech Hear Disord 47:413, 1982.

Jacobs L and Gossman MD: Three primitive reflexes in normal adults, Neurology 30:184, 1980.

Kearns KP and Simmons NN: Interobserver reliability and perceptual ratings: more than meets the ear, J Speech Hear Res 31:131, 1988.

Kent RD: The acoustic and physiologic characteristics of neurologically impaired speech movements. In Hardcastle WJ and Marchal A, editors: Speech production and speech modelling, The Netherlands, 1990, Kluwer Academic Publishers.

Kent RD, Kent JF, and Rosenbek JC: Maximum performance tests of speech production, J Speech Hear Disord 52:367, 1987.

Kent RD et al: Impairment of speech intelligibility in men with amyotrophic lateral sclerosis, J Speech Hear Disord 55:721, 1990.

Kent RD et al: Toward phonetic intelligibility testing in dysarthria, J Speech Hear Disord 54:482, 1989.

Kent RD et al: Speech deterioration in amyotrophic lateral sclerosis: a case study, J Speech Hear Res 34:1269, 1991.

McNeil MR: A critical appraisal of methods in the evaluation and management of dysarthria. Paper presented at the Clinical Dysarthria Conference, Tucson, Arizona, 1986.

Monrad-Krohn GH: On the dissociation of voluntary and emotional innervation in facial paresis of central origin, Brain 47:22, 1924.

Moore CA, Yorkston M, and Beukelman DR, editors: Dysarthria and apraxia of speech: perspective on management, Baltimore, 1991, Brooks Publishing.

Netsell R and Hixon TJ: Noninvasive method for clinically estimating subglottal air pressure, J Speech Hear Disord 43:326, 1978.

Porch BE: Porch index of communicative ability, Palo Alto, California, 1967, Consulting Psychologists Press.

Read C, Buder EH, and Kent RD: Speech analysis systems: an evaluation, J Speech Hear Res 35:314, 1992.

Rowland LP: Signs and symptoms in neurologic diagnosis. In Rowland LP, editor: Merritt's textbook of neurology, ed 8, Philadelphia, 1989, Lea and Febiger.

Spriestersbach DC, Morris HL, and Darley FL: Examination of the speech mechanism. In Darley FL and Spriestersbach D, editors: Diagnostic methods in speech pathology, ed 2, New York, 1978.

Thompson JK: Right brain, left brain: left face, right face: hemisphericity and the expression of facial emotion, Cortex 21:281, 1985.

Till JA, Yorkston KM, and Beukelman DR, editors: Motor speech disorders: advances in assessment and treatment, Baltimore, 1994, Brookes Publishing.

Walton J: Essentials of Neurology, London, 1982, Pitman.

Wertz RT, LaPointe LL, and Rosenbek JC: Apraxia of speech: the disorder and its treatment, New York, 1984, Grune and Stratton.

Yorkston KM, Beukelman DR, and Traynor CD: Computerized assessment of intelligibility of dysarthric speech, Tigard, Oregon, 1984, CC Publications.

Yorkston KM and Beukelman DR: Assessment of intelligibility of dysarthric speech, Tigard, Oregon, 1981a, CC Publications.

Yorkston KM and Beukelman DR: Communication efficiency of dysarthric speakers as measured by sentence intelligibility and speaking rate, J Speech Hear Disord 46:296, 1981b.

Yorkston KM and Beukelman DR: Recent advances in clinical dysarthria, Boston, 1989, College-Hill.

PART TWO

The Disorders and
Their Diagnoses

4 Flaccid Dysarthria

Flaccid dysarthria is a perceptually distinguishable motor speech disorder produced by injury or malfunction of one or more of the cranial or spinal nerves. *It reflects problems in the nuclei, axons, or neuromuscular junctions that make up the motor units of the final common pathway (FCP)*, and it may be manifest in any or all of the respiratory, phonatory, resonatory, and articulatory components of speech. Its primary deviant speech characteristics can be traced to muscular weakness and reduced muscle tone and their effects on the speed, range, and accuracy of speech movements. The primacy of weakness as an explanation for the speech characteristics of this disorder leads to its designation as *flaccid* dysarthria.

Flaccid dysarthria is encountered in a large medical practice at a frequency comparable to that of the other major single dysarthria types. From 1987 to 90 at the Mayo Clinic it accounted for 10.5% of all dysarthrias and 9.6% of all motor speech disorders seen in the Section of Speech Pathology (Figure 1–3).

Unlike most other dysarthria types, flaccid dysarthria sometimes results from damage confined to isolated muscle groups. As a result, it is justifiable to think of subtypes of the disorder, each characterized by speech abnormalities attributable to unilateral or bilateral damage to a specific cranial or spinal nerve or combination of cranial or spinal nerves. Accurate identification of the cranial or spinal nerve source for the deviant speech features can help localize the offending lesion that, in flaccid dysarthria, will always be somewhere between the brain stem or spinal cord and muscles of speech.

Close attention to the clinical features of flaccid dysarthria can help solidify the clinician's knowledge of peripheral nervous system (PNS) anatomy and physiology. More than any other dysarthria type, it can teach us about the course and muscular innervations of the cranial nerves, the roles of specific muscle groups in speech production, and some of the remarkable and often spontaneous ways in which people adapt and compensate for weakness in order to maintain intelligible speech.

CLINICAL CHARACTERISTICS OF FLACCID PARALYSIS

Because flaccid paralysis reflects FCP damage, reflexive, automatic, and voluntary movements all are affected. Recognition of this principle is important to distinguishing lower motor neuron (LMN) lesions from lesions to other parts of the motor system.

Weakness, hypotonia, and diminished reflexes are the primary characteristics of flaccid paralysis. Atrophy, fasciculations, and fibrillations commonly accompany them. Occasionally, rapid weakening with use and recovery with rest are distinguishing features. The presence or absence of these characteristics is dependent to some extent on the portion of the motor unit that has been damaged. These characteristics are discussed below and summarized in Table 4–1.

Table 4–1 Components of the motor unit associated with characteristics of flaccid paralysis (+ = present; − = absent; +/− = may or may not be present)

Feature	Damaged component			
	Cell body	Axon	Neuromuscular junction	Muscle
Weakness	+	+	+	+
Hypotonia	+	+	+	+
Diminished reflexes	+	+	+	+
Atrophy	+	+	−	+
Fasciculations	+	+/−	−	−
Fibrillations	+	+/−	−	−
Rapid weakening & recovery with rest	−	−	+	−

Weakness

Weakness in flaccid paralysis stems from damage to any portion of the motor unit, including cranial and spinal nerve cell bodies in the brain stem or spinal cord, the peripheral or cranial nerve leading to muscle, and the neuromuscular junction. It can also result from pathology of the muscle itself. When damaged, motor units are inactivated and the ability to contract is lost or diminished in the muscles. When motor unit disease inactivates all of the LMN input to a muscle, *paralysis*, the complete inability to contract muscle, is the result. If some input to muscle remains viable, *paresis*, or reduced contraction and weakness, is the result.

The effects of weakness on muscle can be observed during single (phasic) contractions, during repetitive contractions, and during sustained (tonic) contractions.

Hypotonia and reduced reflexes

Flaccid paralysis is also associated with *hypotonia* (reduced muscle tone) and reduced or absent normal reflexes. In flaccid paralysis, the ability of a muscle to contract in response to stretch is compromised because the motor component of the stretch reflex* operates through the FCP. This results in the flabbiness that can be seen or felt in muscles with reduced tone. Weakness and hypotonia, therefore, are roughly synonymous with the concept of flaccidity.

Atrophy

Muscle structure can be altered by FCP and muscle diseases. When cranial or spinal nerve nuclei (cell bodies), the peripheral nerve (axons), or muscle fibers are involved, muscles will eventually *atrophy* or lose bulk. Atrophy is almost always associated with significant weakness.

Fasciculations and fibrillations

When motor neuron cell bodies are damaged (and less prominently, when their axons are damaged),

*The stretch reflex was discussed in Chapter 2.

fasciculations and *fibrillations* may develop. Fasciculations are visible, arrhythmic, isolated twitches or dimplings in resting muscle that result from spontaneous motor unit discharges in response to nerve degeneration or irritation. Fibrillations are invisible, spontaneous, independent contractions of individual muscle fibers that reflect slow repetitive action potentials. They can be detected electromyographically (EMG) within about 1 to 3 weeks after a muscle is deprived of motor nerve supply. Fasciculations and fibrillations are generally not present in muscle disease.

Progressive weakness with use

When disease affects the neuromuscular junction, progressive and rapid weakening of muscle with use, and recovery with rest, can occur. Even though fatigue is common in people with flaccid paresis, *rapid* weakening and recovery with rest is prominent only in neuromuscular junction disease (for example, myasthenia gravis).

ETIOLOGIES

Flaccid dysarthria can be caused by any process that damages the motor unit. These include degenerative, inflammatory, toxic, metabolic, neoplastic, traumatic, and vascular diseases. FCP diseases are associated with these broad etiologic categories with varying frequency, however, and this is also true for flaccid dysarthria. The exact distribution of causes of flaccid dysarthria is unknown and, in fact, probably varies as a function of the particular cranial or spinal nerves involved, the involvement of multiple versus single nerves, and the location of the pathology within the motor unit.

Some common terminology

A number of terms are used to describe pathologies of the FCP and muscle. The following definitions may facilitate comprehension of information presented in the remainder of this chapter:

Neuropathy—A general term that refers to any disease of nerve, regardless of cause, although usually of noninflammatory etiology.

Neuritis—An inflammatory disorder of nerve.

Peripheral neuropathy—Any disorder of nerve in the PNS. Peripheral neuropathies can affect motor, sensory, or autonomic fibers. They may be axonal, demyelinating, or mixed in their effects.

Cranial neuropathies—Peripheral neuropathies involving the cranial nerves.

Mononeuropathy—Neuropathy of a single nerve.

Polyneuropathy—A generalized process producing widespread bilateral and often symmetric effects on the PNS.

Radiculopathy—A PNS disorder involving the root of a spinal nerve, often just proximal to the intervertebral foramen.

Plexopathy—PNS involvement at the point where spinal nerves intermingle (in plexuses) before forming nerves that go to the extremities.

Myelitis—A nonspecific term that indicates inflammation of the spinal cord.

Myelopathy—Any pathologic condition of the spinal cord, but most often refers to those that result from compression, or toxic or altered metabolic states (Kincaid and Dyken, 1987).

Myopathy—Muscle disease. Myopathies are not associated with sensory disturbances or CNS pathology. The most common types of myopathy affect proximal rather than distal muscles.

Myositis—Inflammatory muscle disease.

Some associated diseases and conditions

At this point, it may be useful to review some conditions that are relatively unique to FCP or muscle diseases whose presence have a strong association with flaccid but not other forms of dysarthria. The conditions discussed here represent only a few of the potential etiologies of flaccid dysarthria.

Neuromuscular junction disease. Some diseases affect only the neuromuscular junction. *Myasthenia gravis* (MG) is the most common of these. MG is a chronic autoimmune disease characterized by abnormally rapid weakening of voluntary muscles with use and improvement with rest. It appears that antibodies destroy acetylcholine (ACh) receptors on muscle, in effect making muscle less responsive to the ACh that triggers muscle contraction. As a consequence, muscle contractions become progressively reduced with repeated use. Strength may improve with rest as nerves are able to replenish the supply of ACh. In men, MG occurs most often after age 50; women are affected most often between the ages of 20 and 40.

Ptosis (drooping of the eyelid), weakness of facial muscles, flaccid dysarthria, and dysphagia are very frequent presenting signs of MG (Penn and Rowland, 1989). Beyond clinical neurologic examination, MG is commonly diagnosed by EMG, pulmonary function tests, ACh receptor antibody blood tests, and a Tensilon (edrophonium chloride) test. Injection of Tensilon produces temporary recovery from weakness brought on by prolonged muscular effort. Sometimes speech stress testing is the task used for the Tensilon test. Patients with MG will show rapid development or worsening of flaccid dysarthria during stress testing, but rapid improvement after Tensilon injection, even as they continue to speak. Occasionally, a placebo (saline) will be used instead of Tensilon when there is suspicion that a patient's symptoms are psychogenic in origin. Such patients may improve with the placebo, ruling out MG and increasing suspicions about a psychological disorder.

Eaton-Lambert syndrome is a disorder of neuromuscular transmission in which there is inadequate release of ACh from nerve terminals. It is characterized by an incremental (improved) response to repetitive nerve stimulation, a pattern opposite of MG. That is, weakness is greatest at the initiation of muscle use or with slow rates of stimulation; strength increases with repetitive rapid stimulation, apparently because high rates of activation facilitate release of ACh. The syndrome occurs mostly in men with oat cell carcinoma of the lung, less frequently in the absence of neoplasm but with evidence of immune system abnormality (Penn, 1989).

Botulism is a deadly disease in which botulinum toxin acts on presynaptic membranes for the release of ACh, thus blocking neuromuscular transmission. Contaminated food is the most common cause. Facial, oropharyngeal, and respiratory paralysis can be among presenting signs (Penn, 1989). Botulism toxin in very small doses is an effective treatment for a number of movement disorders, including certain forms of spasmodic dysphonia. Its therapeutic use will be discussed in Chapter 17.

Vascular disorders. Brainstem stroke affecting cranial nerve nuclei can lead to flaccid dysarthria. A number of specific vascular syndromes are associated with flaccid dysarthria. *Wallenberg's lateral medullary syndrome* is among the more common of these. It is usually caused by ischemia in the territory of the posterior inferior cerebellar artery and affects the posterolateral portion of the medulla. It leads to ipsilateral facial sensory loss, contralateral trunk and extremity sensory loss, ipsilateral cerebellar signs, ipsilateral neurophthalmologic abnormalities, and ipsilateral nucleus ambiguus involvement with subsequent palatal, pharyngeal, and laryngeal weakness and associated dysarthria and dysphagia (Brazis, 1992).

Collet-Sicord syndrome is characterized by unilateral involvement of cranial nerves IX–XII. It can be caused by vascular lesions of the jugular vein and carotid artery below the skull base (and also by carotid artery dissection, skull base fractures, inflammatory lesions, and various tumors such as neurinomas, metastases, and jugular glomus tumors) (Waespe and others, 1988).

Infectious processes. *Polio (poliomyelitis)* is a viral disease with an affinity for LMN cell bodies, most often in the lumbar and cervical regions of the spinal cord. Bulbar involvement occurs in 10 to 15% of cases, with the IXth and Xth cranial nerves being affected most often, but involvement of the Vth and VIIth nerves not uncommon. The dorsal area of the medulla is generally involved in the bulbar form of the disease; respiratory and circulatory centers in the medulla can also be affected (Adams and Victor, 1991). Survivors often recover function of muscles that were not completely paralyzed, usually within six months. Occasionally, polio victims will develop the insidious onset of progressive weakness long after the acute attack (*"post-polio syndrome"*); this may occur by chance alone, but it may be that previously involved nerves are more susceptible to the effects of aging (Kincaid and Dyken, 1987).

Herpes zoster is a viral infection that may affect the Vth and VIIth nerve ganglia. It most often produces pain. When it causes facial paresis, it is known as the *Ramsay-Hunt syndrome*. The herpes virus may also cause superior laryngeal nerve paralysis and dysphonia (Andour, Schneider, and Hilsinger 1980; Hartman, Daily, and Morin, 1989).

Sarcoidosis is a nonviral, chronic granulomatous infection that can occur in all organs and tissues. It occasionally affects the PNS or central nervous system (CNS), most often single or multiple cranial nerves, especially the VIIth nerve. Sometimes, cranial neuropathies associated with sarcoidosis result from basilar meningitis (Pleasure and Schotland, 1989).

Individuals infected with HIV who develop AIDS may develop neurologic complications as the result of opportunistic infections. *Cryptococcal meningitis* is the most common fungal infection in AIDS. The resulting meningeal inflammation can affect posterior fossa structures, leading to multiple cranial nerve palsies. Other neurologic complications of AIDS that can lead to cranial nerve involvement include *CNS lymphoma* (the most common CNS tumor in AIDS) and *neurosyphilis* (Singer, 1991). The involvement of cranial nerves for speech may lead to flaccid dysarthria in such cases.

Demyelinating disease. *Guillain-Barré* syndrome is a disorder of unknown cause but is frequently preceded by viral infection. It is characterized by the acute or subacute onset of PNS dysfunction. Histologically, focal demyelinization occurs in peripheral and cranial nerves. When severe, axonal degeneration may occur. Proximal muscles are affected more severely than distal muscles. Facial, oropharyngeal, and ocular muscles are occasionally affected first, and more than half of affected individuals have facial weakness, dysphagia, and flaccid dysarthria. Recovery is sometimes rapid and complete but may take several months in others. Some individuals are left with permanent weakness (Griffin, 1983).

Chronic demyelinating polyneuritis is similar to Guillain-Barré syndrome but less acute in onset and more prolonged in course. Affected individuals may suffer frequent, recurrent attacks (Pleasure and Schotland, 1989). Weakness may be asymmetric.

Muscle disease. *Muscular dystrophy* is a genetic degenerative disease. There are several types, including Duchenne, fascioscapulohumeral, and limb girdle. They are associated with degeneration of muscle fibers and proliferation of connective tissue. The effects are usually diffuse, chronic, and progressive. The fascioscapulohumeral form may affect bulbar muscles; facial weakness may be prominent.

Myotonic muscular dystrophy is an inherited autosomal dominant disease that can affect several organ systems. A characteristic diagnostic sign is failure of muscle to relax promptly after forcible contraction. *Percussion myotonia* is a persistent myotonic contraction that follows strong percussion. It may be observed in the tongue, after pressure is exerted on it, as an obvious depression that persists for several seconds (Roses, 1989). Muscle atrophy gives the face a characteristic long, lean, and expressionless appearance, with weak voluntary and emotional facial movements. Articulation, phonation, and resonance may be affected. Velopharyngeal incompetence has been reported as the presenting symptom in one case (Salomonson, Kawamoto, and Wilson, 1988).

Polymyositis is a disease of striated muscle that can be idiopathic or associated with a number of infectious processes. The tongue, jaw, pharyngeal, and laryngeal muscles may be affected, causing dysarthria and dysphagia (Adams and Victor, 1991).

Degenerative disease. *Motor neuron diseases* are a group of disorders that involve degeneration of motor neurons. *Progressive bulbar palsy* is a motor neuron disease that primarily affects LMNs supplied by cranial nerves. Although it may also include upper motor neurons (UMNs) that supply the bulbar muscles, it can be limited to LMNs. *Amyotrophic lateral sclerosis (ALS)*, the most common motor neuron disease, affects the bulbar, limb, and respiratory muscles. By definition, ALS is a disease of both UMNs and LMNs; its initial manifestations may be confined to the LMNs of bulbar muscles, however. Therefore, progressive bulbar palsy and ALS may produce flaccid dysarthria associated with multiple cranial nerve involvement. These conditions will be discussed in more detail in Chapter 10 which discusses mixed dysarthrias.

Anatomic anomalies. *Arnold-Chiari malformation* is a congenital anomaly of undetermined etiology characterized by downward elongation of the brain stem and cerebellum into the cervical spinal cord. Signs and symptoms reflect injury to the cerebellum, medulla, and lower cranial nerves. Onset of symptoms is infrequently delayed until adulthood. The damage to the brain stem may lead to flaccid dysarthria.

Syringomyelia (syrinx = a tube) is a developmental abnormality characterized by elongated cavities lined by glia close to the central canal of the spinal cord. Cavity expansion and compression of the anterior horns of the gray matter cause atrophy of the anterior horn cells and axonal degeneration in the spinal cord. The condition may extend upward into the fourth ventricle, where it is called *syringobulbia*. When the brain stem is involved, Vth nerve sensory loss, vertigo, and cranial nerve weakness can occur (Bannister, 1985). Flaccid dysarthria may be associated with the condition.

Other. Radiation therapy for the treatment of carcinoma can cause neuropathy, including cranial neuropathies and, possibly, associated flaccid dysarthria. Pathology usually involves axonal degeneration and fibrosis (Pleasure and Schotland, 1989).

Cranial mononeuropathies, particularly facial and vocal cord paralyses, are frequently idiopathic (of unknown origin). Recovery from such conditions is often quite good.

SPEECH PATHOLOGY
Distribution of etiologies in clinical practice

The box on page 104 summarizes the etiologies for 108 quasirandomly selected cases seen at the Mayo Clinic with a primary speech pathology diagnosis of flaccid dysarthria. The reader is cautioned that these data may not represent the distribution of etiologies of flaccid dysarthria in the general population or its distribution in many speech pathology practices. They probably approximate the most frequent etiologies encountered in speech pathology practices within large multidisciplinary primary and tertiary medical settings where patients are referred for diagnosis as well as management of communication disorders.

The data establish that flaccid dysarthria can result from a wide variety of medical conditions. Surgical trauma, most often but not always limited to the laryngeal branches of the vagus nerve, was a frequent cause. Trauma to the laryngeal branches of the vagus occurred in cervical disk, thyroid, cardiac, and upper lung surgeries because of the proximity of the vagus nerve to the surgical field. Carotid endarterectomy—to remove occlusive or ulcerative plaque from the carotid artery in the neck—reportedly damages the VIIth, Xth, or XIIth cranial nerves in about 15% of cases (Massey and others, 1984); such injuries are usually transient and probably the result of retraction or clamping of nerves rather than nerve division. Neurosurgical trauma was more likely to result in multiple cranial nerve lesions than was otorhinolaryngologic, plastic, dental, or chest surgery. Neck surgery, most often thyroid surgery, was the most frequent cause of isolated laryngeal nerve lesions.

It is noteworthy that a substantial proportion of flaccid dysarthrias were due to cranial neuropathies of undetermined origin, and that the Xth nerve was most often implicated when the lesion was confined to a single nerve (note that even though facial palsy occurs relatively frequently in the general population (Katusic and others, 1986), it apparently either did not often result in dysarthria or did not lead to referral for speech pathology assessment or management). The remaining etiologies were associated with muscle disease, tumor, myasthenia gravis, ALS, stroke, infectious processes, anatomic malformations, demyelinating disease, or the effects of radiation therapy.

Patient perceptions and complaints

People with flaccid dysarthria may offer complaints that differ from those of people with other dysarthria types; these complaints may provide clues to speech diagnosis and its localization, especially when they can be attributed to muscles supplied by a single cranial nerve. Such complaints will be noted in the review of deficits associated with each of the cranial nerves because they provide clues about some of the questions that should be asked when weakness is suspected as the primary cause of speech difficulty.

The next several sections will address the cranial and spinal nerves that may be involved in flaccid dysarthria. The anatomic course and function of each nerve will be reviewed briefly (greater detail was provided in Chapter 2), as will some of the conditions that can damage each nerve. Nonspeech findings that may be encountered will also be discussed. Finally, the salient features of the motor speech examination will be discussed, including the primary auditory perceptual character-

ETIOLOGIES OF FLACCID DYSARTHRIA FOR 108 QUASIRANDOMLY SELECTED CASES WITH A PRIMARY SPEECH DIAGNOSIS OF FLACCID DYSARTHRIA AT THE MAYO CLINIC FROM 1969–90. PERCENTAGE OF CASES UNDER EACH BROAD ETIOLOGIC HEADING IS GIVEN IN PARENTHESES. SPECIFIC ETIOLOGIES UNDER EACH HEADING ARE ORDERED FROM MOST TO LEAST FREQUENT.

Traumatic (33%)
Surgical (28%)
1. Neurosurgical (14%)
   Cervical disk
   Carotid endarterectomy
   Carotid artery tumor, posterior fossa tumor, pontine tumor
   Carotid aneurysm, brainstem vascular
   Jugular and acoustic tumors
2. Otorhinolaryngologic/plastic and dental surgery (8%)
   Thyroid
   Parathyroid, maxillectomy for carcinoma, dental surgery, facelift with liposuction
3. Chest/cardiac surgery (7%)
   Left upper lobectomy for lung carcinoma
   Cardiac

Nonsurgical (6%)
Closed-head injury, skull fracture
Neck injury

Neuropathies of undertermined origin (27%)
Xth nerve, superior and/or recurrent laryngeal branches
X (all branches) + XII
X, all branches
(VII), (XII), (VII + X), (IX + X + XI, jugular foramen syndrome)

Muscle disease (8%)
Muscular dystrophy, myotonic dystrophy, myopathy

Tumor (6%)
Posterior fossa (foramen magnum, jugular foramen)
Tongue/neck
Nasopharynx, widespread metastases

Myasthenia gravis (6%)

Degenerative (6%)
ALS

Vascular (5%)
Brainstem stroke (pons, medulla)

Infectious (3%)
Polio
Meningitis

Anatomic malformation (3%)
Arnold-Chiari malformation, syringobulbia, syringomyelia

Demyelinating (1%)
Guillain-Barré

Other (1%)
Radiation therapy (palate, nasopharynx)

ALS, amyotropic lateral sclerosis.

istics, accompanying visible deficits, some of the compensatory behaviors that may develop in response to the neuromuscular deficit, and some of the evidence from instrumental studies that further delineate the characteristics and neurologic bases of the speech deficits. The neuromuscular deficits associated with flaccid dysarthria are summarized in Table 4–2.

Trigeminal (Vth) nerve lesions

Course and function. The three main branches of the Vth nerve arise in the trigeminal ganglion in the petrous bone of the middle cranial fossa. Central connections from the trigeminal ganglion enter the lateral aspect of the pons and are distributed to various nuclei in the brain stem.

The peripheral distribution of the Vth nerve through its three branches includes (1) the sensory ophthalmic branch, which exits the skull through the superior orbital fissure to innervate the upper face; (2) the sensory maxillary branch, which exits the skull through the foramen rotundum to supply the midface; and (3) the motor and sensory mandibular branch, which exits the skull through the foramen ovale to supply the jaw muscles, tensor tympani, and tensor veli palatini.

Trigeminal functions for speech are mediated through its maxillary and mandibular branches. Sensory roles are to provide tactile and proprioceptive information about jaw, face, lip, and tongue movements and their relationship to stationary articulatory structures within the mouth (teeth, alveolus, palate). Motor functions are associated with jaw movements during speech.

Etiologies and localization of lesions. Damage to the Vth nerve is usually associated with involvement of other cranial nerves. *It is rarely the only cranial nerve involved in flaccid dysarthria* (see Table 4–5). Any pathology that can affect the middle cranial fossa can produce weakness or sensory loss in its distribution. Etiologies most often include stroke, infection, arteriovenous malformation (AVM), tumors in the middle fossa or cerebellopontine angle, and trauma to the skull or anywhere along its course to muscle. Peripheral branches are most often damaged in isolation by tumors or fractures of the facial bones or skull.

Disease of the neuromuscular junction can cause jaw weakness, as can disease affecting the jaw muscles themselves (myopathies).

Pain of trigeminal origin can indirectly affect speech. *Trigeminal neuralgia* (tic douloureux) is characterized by sudden brief periods of pain in one or more of the sensory divisions of the trigeminal nerve. It is often idiopathic but many cases may be due to compression or irritation of the trigeminal sensory roots (Brazis, Masdeu, and Biller, 1985). Pain can be triggered by sensory input from facial or jaw movements, sometimes leading to restricted lip, face, or jaw movements during speech to avoid triggering pain.

Nonspeech oral mechanism. In patients with unilateral mandibular branch lesions, the jaw may deviate to the weak side when opened, and the partly opened jaw may be pushed easily to the weak side by the examiner. The degree of masseter or temporalis contraction felt on palpation when the patient bites down may be decreased on the weak side.

With bilateral weakness, the jaw may hang open at rest. The patient may be unable to close it or may move it slowly or with reduced range. The patient may be unable to resist the examiner's attempts to open or close the jaw and may be unable to clench the teeth strongly enough for normal masseter or temporalis contraction to be felt (Figure 3–2). Patient complaints that may relate to jaw weakness include chewing difficulty, drooling, and overt recognition that the jaw is difficult to close or move.

If sensory branches to speech structures are affected, the patient may complain of decreased face, cheek, tongue, teeth, or palate sensation. This can be assessed while the patients' eyes are closed by asking them to indicate when they detect touch or pressure applied to the affected areas. Decreased sensation of undetermined origin in one or more of the peripheral branches of the Vth nerve is often referred to as *trigeminal sensory neuropathy*. Viral etiology is common, but association with diabetes, sarcoidosis, and connective tissue disease has also been noted. Facial numbness is occasionally a presenting symptom in multiple sclerosis (Regli, 1981).

Table 4–2 Neuromuscular deficits associated with flaccid dysarthria.

Direction	Rhythm	Rate		Range		Force	Tone
Individual movements	Repetitive movements	Individual movements	Repetitive movements	Individual movements	Repetitive movements	Individual movements	Muscle tone
Normal	Regular	Normal	Normal	Reduced	Reduced	Weak	Reduced

Adapted from Darley FL, Aronson AE, and Brown JR: Differential diagnostic patterns of dysarthria, J Speech Hear Res 12:246, 1969a.

Speech. Effects of Vth nerve lesions on speech are most apparent during reading and conversation and during AMRs. During AMRs, imprecision or slowness for "puh" should be greater than that for "tuh" or "kuh." Vowel prolongation may be normal. In myasthenia gravis, progressive weakening of jaw movements during speech may be observed.

Unilateral damage to the motor division of the Vth nerve generally does not perceptibly affect speech. In contrast, bilateral lesions can have a devastating impact on articulation. The inability to elevate the bilaterally weak jaw can *reduce precision or make impossible bilabial, labiodental, linguadental, and linguaalveolar articulation, as well as lip and tongue adjustments for many vowels, glides, and liquids.* Speech rate may be slowed; this may be either a direct effect of weakness or reflect compensation for weakness. The effects of Vth nerve motor weakness on speech are summarized in Table 4–3.

Lesions to the sensory portion of the mandibular branch, especially if bilateral, can cause loss of face, lip, lingual, and palatal sensation sufficient to result in imprecise articulation of bilabial, labiodental, linguaalveolar, and linguapalatal sounds. This can occur without weakness and is presumably due to reduced sensory information about articulatory movements or contacts. Technically, the articulatory distortions resulting from decreased sensation should not be classified as a dysarthria because the source of the speech deficit is not neuromotor. However, because the source is neurologic and does affect the precision of motor activity, it could be viewed as a "sensory dysarthria." Nonetheless, it is probably best simply to describe these difficulties as deficits resulting from decreased oral sensation, rather than using the term dysarthria or sensory dysarthria for them.

Individuals with relatively isolated severe jaw weakness will sometimes manually hold the jaw closed to facilitate articulation. Patients with mandibular branch sensory loss sometimes produce exaggerated movements of the jaw, lips, and face during speech, presumably in an attempt to increase sensory feedback. These movements can sometimes be mistaken for, or difficult to distinguish from, hyperkinetic movement disorders. However, sensory loss is usually detectable on touch or pressure sensation testing in patients with trigeminal sensory loss and not in patients with true hyperkinesias.

Finally, as noted previously, patients with trigeminal neuralgia may restrict jaw movement during speech to reduce sensation that might trigger pain. Although apparent visually, this compensatory restriction of movement may not be apparent auditorily. Mild articulatory distortions and decreased loudness or altered resonance, however, could result from such a strategy.

Facial (VIIth) nerve lesions

Course and function. The VIIth nerve is motor and sensory in function, but only its motor component has a clear role in speech. Motor fibers originate in the facial nucleus in the lower third of the pons and exit the cranial cavity, along with fibers of the VIIIth nerve, through the internal auditory meatus. They pass through the facial canal, exit at the stylomastoid foramen below the ear, pass through the parotid gland, and innervate the muscles of facial expression. The facial muscles crucial for speech are those that move the lips and firm the cheeks to permit impounding of intraoral air pressure and bilabial and labiodental articulation.

Etiologies and localization of lesions. The VIIth nerve can be damaged in isolation or along with other cranial nerves. Pathology in the brain stem and posterior fossa can cause VIIth nerve damage, but a lesion anywhere along the nerve may affect its functions for speech.

Because the VIIth and VIth (abducens) nerves are in close proximity within the pons, especially in the floor of the fourth ventricle, lesions of both the VIth and VIIth nerves implicate that part of the brain stem. If the VIIth and VIIIth nerves are involved, as they frequently are with acoustic neuromas, a lesion is suspected in the area of the internal auditory meatus where both nerves exit the brain stem.

Known causes of facial paralysis include but are not limited to infection by herpes zoster, mononucleosis, otitis media, meningitis, Lyme disease, syphilis, sarcoidosis, and inflammatory polyradiculoneuropathy. Common neoplastic causes include acoustic neuroma, cerebellopontine angle meningioma, neurofibroma of the facial nerve, and leptomeningeal carcinomatosis (*Clinical Examinations in Neurology,* 1991; Brazis, Masdeu, and Biller, 1985). Vascular lesions and trauma can also cause VIIth nerve lesions.

Bell's palsy is a relatively common condition of undetermined etiology characterized by isolated unilateral VIIth nerve weakness. Upper and lower facial muscles are affected and the ability to close the eye on the affected side may be limited. Depending on the exact site of lesion, the patient may also have decreased lacrimation, salivation, and taste sensation, as well as hyperacusis (possibly due to involvement of the portion of the nerve that innervates the stapedius). Most cases of isolated facial paralysis have no apparent cause and 86% have been reported to make full recovery (Katusic and others, 1986). Proposed causes include an autoimmune-mediated inflammatory fo-

Table 4–3 Effects on speech of unilateral and bilateral cranial nerve and spinal respiratory nerve lesions. The IXth and XIth nerves are not included because of the negligible or unclear effects of lesions of them on speech.

[handwritten annotations: "S. Accessory" pointing to XIth; "Glossopharyngeal" pointing to IXth]

Cranial nerves	Respiratory-phonatory		Resonance		Articulation		Prosody	
	Unilateral	Bilateral	Unilateral	Bilateral	Unilateral	Bilateral	Unilateral	Bilateral
V	None	None	None	None	None	Imprecise consonants Bilabial Labiodental Linguadental Lingual-alveolar Distorted vowels, glides, liquids	None	Slow rate (compensatory or primary)
VII	None	None	None	None	Mild distortion of bilabial & labiodentals Distortion of anterior lingual fricatives & affricates	Distortion or inability to produce bilabials & labiodentals ? Vowel distortions ? Anterior lingual fricative & affricate distortions	None	Slow rate (compensatory or primary)
X Above pharyngeal branch	Breathiness Reduced loudness Reduced pitch Short phrases Hoarseness Diplophonia	Breathiness Aphonia Short phrases Inhalatory stridor	Mild hypernasality Nasal emission	Moderate + hypernasality Nasal emission	None (? mildly weak pressure consonants)	Weak pressure consonants	Short phrases	Short phrases

Continued.

Table 4–3 Effects on speech of unilateral and bilateral cranial nerve and spinal respiratory nerve lesions. The IXth and XIth nerves are not included because of the negligible or unclear effects of lesions of them on speech—cont'd

Cranial nerves	Respiratory-phonatory		Resonance		Articulation		Prosody	
	Unilateral	Bilateral	Unilateral	Bilateral	Unilateral	Bilateral	Unilateral	Bilateral
X Below pharyngeal branch	Same as above	Same as above	None	None	None	None	Short phrases	Short phrases
X Superior branch only	Breathy hoarseness	Breathy, hoarse Reduced loudness Reduced pitch range	None	None	None	None	Short phrases	Short phrases
	Respiratory-phonatory		Resonance		Articulation		Prosody	
X	Breathy, hoarse	Breathy, hoarse	None	None	None	None	Short phrases	Short phrases
Recurrent branch only	Reduced loudness Diplophonia	Reduced loudness	None	None	None	None		
XII	None	None	None	? altered	Mildly imprecise lingual consonants	Mild-severe imprecise lingual consonants Vowel distortions	None	Slow rate (compensatory or primary)
Spinal Respiratory Nerves	None	Reduced loudness Reduced pitch variability Strained voice (compensatory)	None	None	None	None	None	Short phrases Reduced pitch & loudness variability

cal neuropathy, herpes simplex viral infection of the nerve, and swelling of the nerve induced by exposure to cold or allergic factors leading to compression by the bony facial canal (*Clinical Examinations in Neurology*, 1991).

Nonspeech oral mechanism. The visible effects of unilateral VIIth nerve lesions can be striking. At rest, the affected side sags and is hypotonic. The forehead may be unwrinkled, the eyebrow drooped, and the eye open and unblinking. The tip of the nose and corner of the mouth may be drawn toward the unaffected side. Drooling on the affected side may occur. The nasolabial fold is often flattened and the nasal ala may be immobile during respiration. During smiling the face will retract more toward the intact side (see Figure 4–1). Food may squirrel between the teeth and cheek on the weak side because of buccinator weakness. The patient may complain of biting the cheek or lip when chewing or speaking and have difficulty keeping food in the mouth. With milder weakness, asymmetry may be apparent only with use, as in voluntary retraction, pursing, and cheek puffing, with or without resistance from the examiner. Reduced or absent movement will be observable during voluntary, emotional, and reflexive activities. Fasciculations and atrophy may be apparent on the affected side.

Bilateral VIIth nerve lesions are less common than unilateral lesions. With bilateral lesions, the effects of weakness are on both sides, but may be less striking visually because of the symmetric appearance. At rest, the mouth may be lax and the space between the upper and lower lips wider than normal. During reflexive smiling the mouth may not pull upward, giving the smile a "transverse" appearance. The patient may be unable to retract, purse, or puff the cheeks, or the seal on puffing may be overcome easily by the examiner. Fasciculations in the perioral area and chin may be present; patients are usually unaware of them. Patients may complain that their face or the lips do not move well during speech and that they lose food or liquid out of their mouth when eating. Drooling during speech, when concentrating on another activity, during eating, or during sleep may be reported or observed.

Abnormal movements of the face sometimes occur with VIIth nerve lesions. They are worthy of mention because they are unexpected in the context of FCP disease and may be confused with hyperkinesias of CNS origin. *Synkinesis* (see Figure 4–1) is the abnormal contraction of muscle adjacent to muscle that is contracting normally (for example, a normal reflexive or voluntary eye blink may cause a simultaneous movement of lower facial muscles). It reflects aberrant branching or misdirection of regenerating axons of the facial nerve, or abnormal activity of residual motor units, and is most commonly seen after recovery from Bell's palsy (Brazis, Masdeu, and Biller, 1985; *Clinical Examinations in Neurology*, 1991). *Hemifacial spasm* is characterized by paroxysmal, rapid, irregular, usually unilateral tonic twitching of facial muscle. It may be due to irritation of the nerve by a pulsating blood vessel in the area of the cerebellopontine angle or facial canal, but it may also be due to tumor, aneurysm, or AVM (*Clinical Examinations in Neurology*, 1991; Levin and Lee, 1987; Nishi and others, 1987). *Facial myokymia* is characterized by rhythmic, undulating movements on an area of the face in which the surface of the skin moves like a "bag of worms." These are more prolonged than fasciculations and reflect alternating brief contractions of adjacent motor units. They are often benign but, if widespread, may be associated with multiple sclerosis, brainstem tumors, or demyelinating cranial neuropathies (*Clinical Examinations in Neurology*, 1991; Nudelman and Starr, 1983).

Speech. The speech tasks that are most revealing of VIIth nerve lesions are conversational speech and reading, speech AMRs, and stress testing.

A *flutter of the cheeks* may be present during conversation because hypotonicity results in less resistance to intraoral air pressure peaks during pressure sound production. Poor bilabial closure on one or both sides may be apparent. There may be a noticeable mismatch between speech AMRs for "puh" versus those for "tuh" and "kuh," with reduced precision and perhaps slowness of "puh" because of lip weakness. In general, precision is reduced more than speed, unless weakness is bilateral and severe. If myasthenia gravis is present, stress testing may generate visible and auditory perceptual deficits attributable to lower-face weakness.

The effect of unilateral facial nerve lesions on speech may be more visible than audible. There may be mild perceptible distortion of bilabial and labiodental consonants and, less frequently, anterior lingual fricatives and affricates. There is usually no perceptible effect on vowels.

Bilateral facial weakness, depending on its degree, can result in distortions or complete inability to produce /p/, /m/, /w/, /hw/, /f/, and /v/. The distortion of bilabial stops is often in the direction of frication or spirantization. If lip rounding and spreading are markedly reduced, vowels may be distorted. The effects of VIIth nerve lesions on speech are summarized in Table 4–3.

Patients with unilateral and bilateral facial weakness will sometimes spontaneously compensate in an effort to improve speech and physical

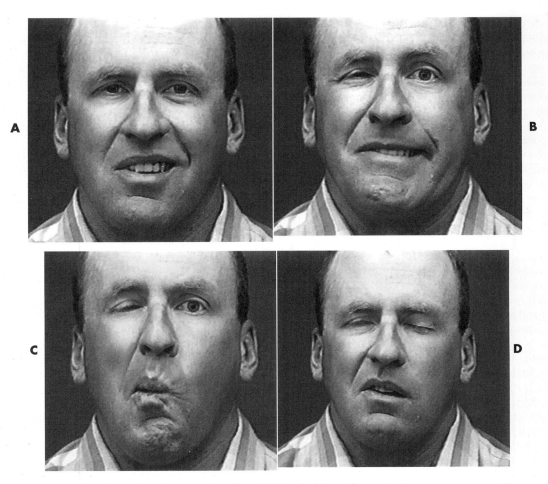

Figure 4–1 A, partially recovered unilateral right facial weakness during spontaneous smile; **B,** voluntary lip retraction; and **C,** lip pursing, with **D,** paradoxical, involuntary right-lip retraction (synkinesis) when voluntarily closing the eyes. Synkinetic eye closing is also apparent during voluntary lip retraction (**B**) and pursing (**C**).

appearance. In unilateral weakness, they may use a finger to prop up the sagging weak side at rest and during speech or, rarely, actually assist the movement of their lower lip in producing bilabial and labiodental sounds. Some patients will exaggerate jaw closure in an effort to approximate the lips. If weakness is bilateral, severe, isolated to the face, and chronic (as may occur in some cases of myopathy), substitution of lingual alveolar consonants for bilabial consonants (for example, t/p) may occur.

Glossopharyngeal (IXth) nerve lesions

Course and function. Motor fibers of the IXth nerve that are relevant to speech originate in the nucleus ambiguus within the reticular formation of the lateral medulla. The rootlets of the IXth nerve emerge from the medulla, pass through the jugular foramen in the posterior fossa, and eventually into

the pharynx to innervate the stylopharyngeus muscle that elevates the pharynx during swallowing and speech. Afferent fibers originate in the inferior ganglion in the jugular foramen and terminate in the nucleus of the tractus solitarius in the medulla; they carry sensation from the pharynx and posterior tongue and are important to the sensory component of the gag reflex.

Etiologies and localization of lesions. The IXth nerve is rarely damaged in isolation (at the least, the Xth nerve is also typically involved). It is susceptible to the same pathologic influences that affect the other cranial nerves in the lower brain stem. Intramedullary and extramedullary lesion localization is usually tied to localization of Xth and XIth nerve lesions.

Nonspeech oral mechanism. The IXth nerve is assessed clinically by examining the gag reflex, particularly asymmetry in the ease with which the reflex is elicited. A reduced gag may implicate the sensory or motor components of the reflex, the sensory component if the patient reports decreased sensation in the area. However, a normal gag can be present after intracranial section of the IXth nerve, suggesting that the Xth nerve is also involved in pharyngeal function. Therefore, the gag reflex may not be a reliable test for IXth nerve function (*Clinical Examinations in Neurology*, 1991). It is clear, however, that the IXth nerve may be implicated in patients with dysphagia, with lesions to the nerve presumably affecting pharyngeal elevation during the pharyngeal phase of swallowing.

Some individuals with IXth nerve lesions develop brief attacks of severe pain that begin in the throat and radiate down the neck to the back of the lower jaw. Pain can be triggered by swallowing or tongue protrusion. This condition is known as *glossopharyngeal neuralgia.*

Speech. The IXth nerve's role in speech cannot be assessed directly. It probably has some influence on resonance and perhaps phonatory functions because of the effects of lesions on pharyngeal elevation. Because IXth nerve lesions are usually associated with Xth nerve lesions, and because the Xth nerve has a crucial and relatively clearly defined role in speech, the IXth nerve's importance in the assessment of dysarthria can be considered indeterminate for practical purposes.

Vagus (Xth) nerve lesions

Course and function. Cell bodies of the Xth nerve that are relevant to speech originate in the nucleus ambiguus. Cell bodies of relevant sensory fibers originate in the inferior ganglion located in or near the jugular foramen; central processes of the sensory fibers terminate in the nucleus of the tractus solitarius in the brain stem.

The Xth nerve exits the skull through the jugular foramen, along with the IXth and XIth nerves. From there it divides into the pharyngeal branch, which enters the pharynx; the superior laryngeal branch, which enters the pharynx and larynx; and the recurrent laryngeal branch, which passes down to the upper chest where it loops around the subclavian artery on the right, and around the aorta on the left, before traveling back up the neck to enter the larynx.

The pharyngeal branch supplies the muscles of the pharynx, except the stylopharyngeus (IXth nerve), the muscles of the soft palate, except the tensor veli palatini (mandibular branch of the Vth nerve), and the palatoglossus muscle. It is responsible for pharyngeal constriction and palatal elevation and retraction during speech and swallowing.

The internal laryngeal nerve, a component of the superior laryngeal nerve, transmits sensation from mucus membranes of portions of the larynx, epiglottis, base of the tongue, and aryepiglottic folds, and from stretch receptors in the larynx. The external laryngeal nerve, the motor component of the superior laryngeal nerve, supplies the inferior pharyngeal constrictors and the cricothyroid muscles. Its innervation of the cricothyroid muscle is important because cricothyroid contraction lengthens the vocal cords for pitch adjustments.

The recurrent laryngeal branch of the Xth nerve innervates all of the intrinsic laryngeal muscles except the cricothyroid. Its sensory fibers carry general sensation from the vocal cords and larynx below them.

Etiologies and localization of lesions. The localization of Xth nerve lesions is more complicated than that for other cranial nerves, owing to its long course and its three major branches. The degree of weakness, positioning of paralyzed vocal cords, and degree and type of voice or resonance abnormality depend on the localization of the lesion along the course of the nerve and on whether the lesion is unilateral or bilateral. Careful consideration of signs and symptoms stemming from Xth nerve lesions can often distinguish among lesions that are intramedullary, extramedullary, or above the pharyngeal branch; below the pharyngeal branch but above the superior and recurrent laryngeal branches; or below the superior laryngeal branch.

Vagus nerve lesions can be intramedullary, extramedullary, or extracranial. *Intramedullary lesions* damage the nerve in the brain stem. *Extramedullary lesions* damage the trunk of the nerve as it leaves the body of the brain stem but while it is still within the cranial cavity (that is, before it exits from the jugular foramen). *Extracranial lesions* damage the nerve after it exits the skull. It is generally the case that as the distance of a lesion from the brain stem increases, the number of muscles, structures, and functions affected by the lesion decreases. Therefore, intracranial lesions are more likely than extramedullary and extracranial lesions to be bilateral or associated with multiple cranial nerve involvement. Extramedullary lesions are more likely to be unilateral but may still affect several cranial nerves (for example, the IXth, Xth, and XIth nerves all exit through the jugular foramen on each side of the posterior fossa). Extracranial lesions are more likely to be isolated to the Xth nerve and perhaps only one of its branches.

The relationships between Xth nerve lesion loci and impairment of muscle function are summarized in Table 4–4. The most important relationships include the following.

1. Intramedullary, extramedullary, and extracranial lesions above the separation of the pharyngeal, superior laryngeal, and recurrent laryngeal branches will affect all muscles supplied by the nerve below the level of the lesion. Therefore, pharyngeal and palatal muscles supplied by the pharyngeal branch, the cricothyroid muscle supplied by the superior laryngeal branch, and the remaining intrinsic laryngeal musculature supplied by the recurrent laryngeal branch will be weak or paralyzed on the side of the lesion (see Figure 4–2).

2. Lesions below the pharyngeal branch, but still high enough in the neck to affect the superior and recurrent branches, will spare the upper pharynx and velopharyngeal mechanism, but will cause paralysis or weakness of the cricothyroid and remaining intrinsic muscles on the side of the lesion.

3. Lesions of the superior laryngeal branch but not the recurrent laryngeal or pharyngeal branches will affect the cricothyroid but not the velopharyngeal mechanism or the remaining intrinsic laryngeal musculature.

4. Lesions affecting only the recurrent laryngeal nerve will cause weakness or paralysis of the intrinsic laryngeal musculature on the side of the lesion, except the cricothyroid.

Intramedullary and extramedullary lesions affecting the Xth nerve can be caused by primary and metastatic tumor, infection, stroke, syringobulbia, Arnold-Chiari malformation, Guillian-Barré syndrome, polio, motor neuron disease, and other inflammatory or demyelinating diseases (Aronson, 1990). Not infrequently, lesions in the posterior fossa affect cranial nerves IX, X, and XI in combination. When this occurs in the area of the jugular foramen it is called the *jugular foramen syndrome.*

Extracranial Xth nerve disorders can be caused by myasthenia gravis; tumors in the neck or thorax; aneurysms in the aortic arch, internal carotid, or subclavian artery; and surgery (Aronson, 1990; Brazis, Masdeu, and Biller, 1986). Thyroidectomy is a common cause of vocal cord paralysis, and Xth (and VIIth and XIIth) nerve damage can occur during carotid endarterectomy (Massey and others, 1984). Vagus nerve degeneration and dysphonia have been reported in individuals with severe alcoholic neuropathies (Guo, McLeod, and Baverstock, 1987).

Nonspeech oral mechanism. Unilateral pharyngeal branch lesions are manifest by the following:

1. The soft palate hangs lower on the side of the lesion.

2. It pulls toward the nonparalyzed side on phonation (Figures 4–2 and 4–3). A palate that hangs low at rest but elevates symmetrically may not be weak. It may be asymmetric as a normal variant or the result of scarring from tonsillectomy. If palatal asymmetry on phonation is ambiguous, the clinician should look for a levator "dimple" representing the point of

Table 4–4 Effects on the vocal cords and soft palate of Xth nerve lesions. Note that many lesions do not cause complete paralysis, so the vocal cords and soft palate may be weak but capable of some movement.

Level of lesion	Vocal cords		Soft palate	
	Unilateral	**Bilateral**	**Unilateral**	**Bilateral**
I. Pharyngeal, superior, & recurrent laryngeal branches	One cord fixed in abducted position	Both cords fixed in abducted position	One side low, immobile	Both sides low, immobile
II. Superior & recurrent laryngeal branches	One cord fixed in abducted position	Both cords fixed in abducted position	Normal	Normal
III. Superior laryngeal nerve	Both cords can adduct Affected cord shorter Epiglottis & anterior larynx shifted toward intact side on phonation	Absent tilt of thyroid on cricoid cartilage Inability to see full cord length because of epiglottis overhang Bowed cords	Normal	Normal
IV. Recurrent laryngeal nerve	One cord fixed in paramedian position	Both cords fixed in paramedial position	Normal	Normal

Adapted from Aronson AE: Clinical voice disorders, New York, 1990, Thieme.

maximum contraction of the levator veli palatini muscle. If it is centered, the palate may not be weak; if it is displaced to one side, the palate is probably weak on the opposite side.

3. The gag reflex may be diminished on the weak side.

In bilateral lesions the palate will hang low in the pharynx at rest and move minimally or not at all during phonation. The gag reflex may be difficult to elicit or absent (recall that this may be normal in some individuals), and nasal regurgitation may occur during swallowing.

Unilateral and bilateral superior laryngeal branch lesions that spare the recurrent laryngeal branch are frequently missed because the vocal cords can look normal. However, in unilateral lesions, even though both cords adduct, the affected vocal cord will appear shorter than normal and the epiglottis and anterior larynx will be shifted toward the intact side. In bilateral cricothyroid paralysis, both cords appear short and will be bowed, and the epiglottis will overhang and obscure the anterior portion of the vocal cords (Aronson, 1990).

Unilateral lesions of the recurrent laryngeal nerve but not the pharyngeal or superior laryngeal nerve will leave the affected vocal cord fixed in the paramedian position. When bilateral, both

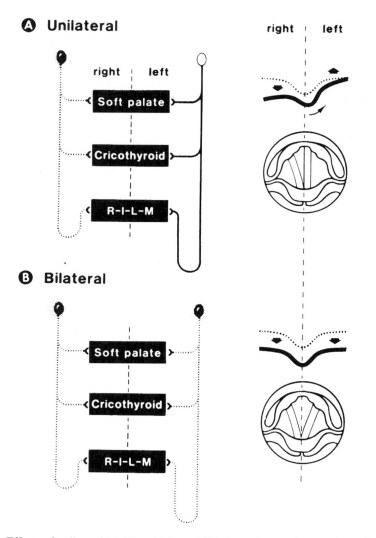

Figure 4–2 Effects of unilateral (right) and bilateral Xth (vagus) nerve lesions above the origin of the pharyngeal, superior laryngeal, and recurrent laryngeal branches of the nerve. When unilateral, the soft palate hangs lower on the right and pulls toward the left on phonation. The right vocal fold is fixed in an abducted position, while the left fold adducts to the midline on phonation. When bilateral, the palate rests low bilaterally and does not move on phonation. Both vocal folds remains in the abducted position on phonation. (From Aronson AE: Clinical voice disorders, New York, 1990, Thieme.)

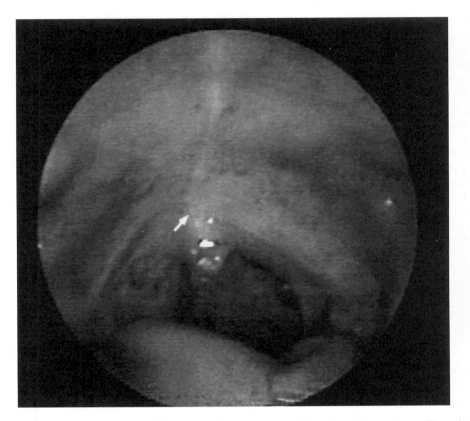

Figure 4–3 Palatal movement during phonation in a patient with left palatal weakness. The palate pulls to the right. The arrow identifies the levator eminence (dimple), which is also displaced to the right. This patient also has left lingual weakness secondary to a left XIIth (hypoglossal) nerve lesion; note the smaller left than right side of the tongue because of atrophy on the left.

cords will be in the paramedian position. The cords are not completely abducted because the intact cricothyroid maintains its adductor function and pulls the cord closer to the midline. In unilateral paralysis, dysphagia may be present, and the cough and glottal coup will be weak. There may be airway compromise. In bilateral paralysis, airway compromise and inhalatory stridor often occur because abductor paralysis prevents widening of the glottis during inhalation. The resulting respiratory distress may require tracheostomy.

Lesions affecting both the recurrent and superior laryngeal branches of the vagus will leave the affected vocal cords paralyzed in the abducted position because all laryngeal adductors are affected. The cough and glottal coup are weak and dysphagia is common. Signs of weakness are worse with bilateral than unilateral vocal cord lesions.

Speech. Table 4–3 summarizes the effects of unilateral and bilateral Xth nerve lesions on speech. The effects cross several aspects of speech production, including phonation, resonance, articulation, and prosody, but the effects on resonance and phonation are generally most pronounced. When the pharyngeal branch is affected unilaterally, there may be little or no perceptible effect or mild-to-moderate hypernasality and nasal emission during pressure-consonant production. If weakness is bilateral, *hypernasality* can be marked to severe, *audible nasal emission* may be very apparent, and *pressure consonants may be noticeably imprecise* because of inability to impound intraoral pressure. *Loudness may be mildly reduced* because of the damping effects of the nasal cavity on the emitted sound, and *phrase length may be reduced* because of nasal air wastage. Facial grimacing may develop in an effort to valve the air stream at the nares. The imprecision of pressure consonants sometimes generates suspicions about tongue, face, or jaw weakness. If consonant imprecision is solely due to velopharyngeal incompetence, occluding the nares during speech will facilitate intraoral pressure for articulation and aid assessment of the adequacy of the other articulators.

Unilateral lesions of the Xth nerve below the pharyngeal branch but including the superior and recurrent laryngeal branches can result in *breathiness* or *aphonia, reduced loudness, diplophonia, reduced pitch*, and *pitch breaks. Phrases may be short* because of air wastage through the incompletely adducted glottis during phonation. A *rapid vocal flutter* may be present during vowel prolongation. In bilateral paralysis these characteristics are exaggerated.

Lesions of the superior laryngeal nerve that spare the pharyngeal and recurrent laryngeal nerves cause subtle changes in voice. When unilateral, mild *breathiness* or *hoarseness* and mild *inability to alter pitch* may be present. Loudness may be normal or mildly reduced. The inability to alter pitch may generate complaints about decreased ability to sing. Bilateral cricothyroid paralysis can cause mild to moderate breathiness and hoarseness, *decreased loudness*, and markedly reduced ability to alter pitch.

Unilateral recurrent laryngeal nerve lesions that spare the superior laryngeal nerve and pharyngeal branch will cause *breathy-hoarse voice quality, decreased loudness*, and sometimes *diplophonia* and *pitch breaks*. Bilateral weakness or paralysis will cause *inhalatory stridor*, but the voice may be relatively unaffected because the cords are adducted close to the midline. *Airway compromise*, however, is a serious problem.

Acoustic and physiologic studies. Videofluoroscopy or nasendoscopy are useful for documenting weakness of the velopharyngeal valve during speech. Bilateral velopharyngeal weakness can be demonstrated by nasendoscopy and videofluoroscopy in lateral, frontal, and base views. Laryngoscopic examination is essential in cases with suspected vocal cord weakness, not only for diagnostic purposes but also for management considerations.

The visible characteristics of weak vocal cord activity have been described beyond simple observations of paralysis. Videostroboscopy and high-speed laryngeal photography in patients with unilateral vocal cord paralysis have documented: a lack of firm glottal closure during phonation; "light touch" glottic closure, reflecting either less than complete paralysis or assistance to medial cord approximation by the Bernoulli effect; irregular vocal cord vibration; exaggeration in the affected vocal cord of the mucosal wave during phonation; and abnormal frequency and amplitude perturbations in vocal cord activity (Hirano, Koike, and von Leden, 1968; Wattersen, McFarlane, and Menicucci, 1990). Greater vibratory amplitude and exaggerated mucosal waves are consistent with what might be expected with hypotonicity. These observations are consistent with the perception of breathiness (lack of firm glottal closure), hoarseness, and perhaps diplophonia (irregular and asymmetric vibratory characteristics) in patients with vocal cord weakness.

Aerodynamic studies of people with unilateral or bilateral vocal cord weakness have identified increased airflow rates during speech. These findings are consistent with neuromuscular weakness of the vocal cords, with subsequent incomplete vocal cord adduction and excessive air escape through the glottis during phonation (Hirano, Koike, and von Leden, 1968; Iwata, von Leden, and Williams, 1972; Till and Alp, 1991; von Leden, 1968). Relatedly, Till and Alp (1991) have established that dysarthric speakers with laryngeal "hypovalving" had increased mean air flow during connected speech and inspired twice the volume of air per minute than normals, mostly through increased breaths per minute. In contrast, their mean speech duration per breath group was only half of normal. They also expired more air than normal during pauses but tended to have reduced pause frequency and duration, possibly secondary to poor vocal cord valving or a compensatory effort to increase speaking time. These findings are consistent with the perception of breathiness and short phrases in people with laryngeal weakness. They define some of the efforts that individuals may make to compensate for vocal cord weakness, such as increased breaths per minute, increased inspiratory volume, and a tendency to reduce pause frequency and duration.

Acoustic studies of people with unilateral vocal cord paralysis or weakness have documented the following characteristics: a breakdown of formant structure, reflected in a long-term average acoustic spectrum characterized by high fundamental frequency amplitude with a marked dropoff of harmonics above the first formant; random noise in spectrograms and increased spectral energy levels in high frequency regions, possibly reflecting turbulent air flow through a partially open glottis; restricted standard deviation and range of fundamental frequency, suggesting reduced ability to reach upper pitch ranges (Hammarberg, Fritzell, and Schiratzki, 1984; Murry, 1978; Rontal, Rontal, and Rolnick, 1975). These studies have noted a relationship between some of these characteristics and perceptual judgments of breathiness and hypofunctional voice (Hammarberg, Fritzell, and Schiratzki, 1984; Reich and Lerman, 1978). Findings of restricted fundamental frequency range and variability (Murry, 1978) are consistent with Darley, Aronson, and Brown's (1975) finding that monopitch is frequently perceived in flaccid dysarthria.

Aerodynamic, acoustic, videofluoroscopic, and nasendoscopic studies have repeatedly shown a relationship between velopharyngeal inadequacy (VPI) and hypernasality, nasal emission, and weak pressure consonants. Although most studies have examined people with palatal clefts or undefined or mixed dysarthrias, their general findings can probably be generalized to those with velopharyngeal weakness associated with Xth nerve lesions. In addition to increased nasal air flow with VPI, there are a number of acoustic correlates of listeners' perception of hypernasality. These include: decreased energy and higher frequency of the first formant; change or shift in center frequencies of formants; increased formant bandwidth; reduced vowel intensity and dynamic intensity range; reduced vocal pitch range; and extra resonances (Curtis, 1968; Johns, 1985). Reduced formant and overall intensity probably reflect the damping characteristics of the nasal cavity. Finally, the connection of the pharyngeal tube to a side branching tube (nasal cavity) leads to the development of antiresonances in the spectrum (that is, a sharp drop in intensity in a portion of the spectrum where energy is expected). Because these acoustic attributes are correlated with VPI and perceptions stemming from it, they represent quantifiable indices of velopharyngeal weakness that may be useful for documentation of deficits, comparisons over time, and the effects of management.

Accessory (XIth) nerve lesions

Course and function. The cranial portion of the XIth nerve arises from the nucleus ambiguus, emerges from the side of the medulla, and exits the skull through the jugular foramen along with the IXth and Xth nerves. It intermingles with fibers of the Xth nerve to help innervate the uvula, levator veli palatini, and intrinsic laryngeal muscles. The spinal portion arises from the first 5 to 6 cervical segments of the spinal cord, ascends and enters the posterior fossa through the foramen magnum, and then leaves the skull with fibers of the IXth, Xth, and cranial portion of the XIth nerve, where it innervates the sternocleidomastoid and trapezius muscles.

Etiologies and localization of lesions. Etiologies of lesions to the cranial portion of the XIth nerve are similar to those described for the Xth nerve. The spinal portion can be damaged by lesions in the cervical spinal cord, and by compression from lesions in the area of the foramen magnum. Radical neck surgery is another source of XIth nerve lesions.

Nonspeech oral mechanism. Lesions of the spinal portion of the XIth nerve reduce shoulder elevation on the side of the lesion and weaken head-turning to the side opposite the lesion. Such lesions do not generally affect speech. If bilateral weakness causes significant shoulder weakness and head drooping, then respiration, phonation, and resonance may be indirectly and mildly affected by the postural deficit.

Because it is impossible clinically to separate the effects of Xth nerve lesions from those of lesions to the cranial portion of the XIth nerve, and because some argue that the cranial portion of the XIth nerve is more appropriately considered part of the Xth nerve, it is unnecessary to treat the XIth nerve as distinctly important to motor speech function.

Hypoglossal (XIIth) nerve lesions

Course and function. The XIIth nerve originates in the medulla. Its fibers exit the brain stem as a number of rootlets that converge and pass through the hypoglossal foramen just lateral to the foramen magnum. The nerve travels medial to the IXth, Xth, and XIth nerves in the vicinity of the common carotid artery and internal jugular vein, and passes above the hyoid bone to reach the intrinsic and extrinsic muscles of the tongue.

The XIIth nerve innervates all of the intrinsic and extrinsic muscles of the tongue, except the palatoglossus (Xth nerve). It is crucial for lingual articulatory movements as well as chewing and swallowing.

Etiologies and localization of lesions. Hypoglossal nerve lesions can be intramedullary, extramedullary, and extracranial. They can be caused by any etiologic factor that can affect the lower cranial nerves. Lesions to it often damage other cranial nerves, especially IX, X, and XI, but, for example, intracranial metastasis (Keane, 1984) or basilar skull lesions from tumor or trauma may affect only the XIIth nerve. It can also be damaged by lesions in the neck, including surgery (for example, carotid endarterectomy) or by accidental trauma, carotid and vertebral artery aneurysms, local infection, infectious mononucleosis, common cold, and tumors (for example, in the neck, salivary glands, base of tongue) (Affi, Ziyad, and Faris, 1984; Brazis, Masdeu, and Biller, 1985).

Nonspeech oral mechanism. In unilateral hypoglossal lesions the tongue may be atrophic and shrunken on the weak side (see Figure 4–3). Fasciculations may be apparent. The tongue will deviate to the weak side on protrusion because the action of the unaffected genioglossus muscle is unopposed (Figure 4–4). The ability to curl the tip

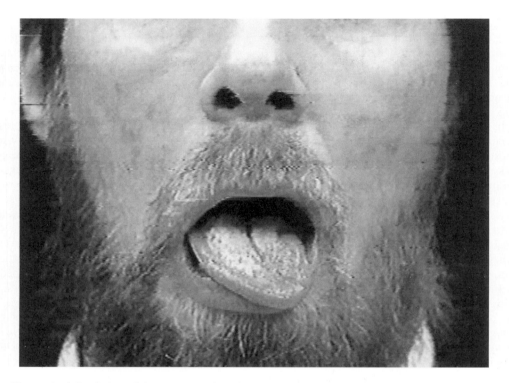

Figure 4–4 Deviation of the tongue to the left on protrusion, reflecting a left XIIth (hypoglossal) nerve lesion.

of the tongue to the weak side inside the mouth will be diminished as will the ability to push the tongue into the cheek against resistance. Voluntary tongue lateralization within the mouth occasionally yields paradoxic results, with ability to push the tongue into the cheek on the weak side sometimes appearing normal. It may be that some people push the tongue to the weak side with the unaffected side instead of attempting to use the longitudinal fibers on the weak side to turn the tongue to the weak side.

With bilateral lesions the tongue may be atrophic bilaterally, with bilateral fasciculations. It may protrude symmetrically but with limited range, or not at all. Lateralization and elevation may be impossible. Saliva may accumulate in the mouth and food may squirrel in the cheeks. Patients may note an inability to move food around in the mouth and may alter their diet to accommodate to this problem. They may complain that the tongue feels "heavy" or "thick," or that it doesn't move well for eating and speaking. Drooling complaints may be related to lingual weakness.

Speech. The overriding speech characteristic in unilateral and bilateral XIIth nerve lesions is *imprecise articulation* that can be isolated to lingual phonemes. Table 4–3 summarizes the effects of unilateral and bilateral XIIth nerve lesions on speech.

Isolated unilateral XIIth nerve lesions are often compensated for to a degree that allows perceptually normal speech. Articulatory distortions are generally mild and do not affect intelligibility.

Bilateral lingual weakness produces difficulty with sounds requiring elevation of the tip or back of the tongue. When weakness is mild, anterior lingual consonant distortion is often detected more readily than velar distortions because of their greater number and frequency of occurrence in the language. The movements for the traditionally difficult-to-produce linguals, /s/, /ʃ/, /tʃ/ and their voiced cognates, as well as /r/ and /l/, are most susceptible to lingual weakness and may be the "first to go" when weakness develops. When weakness is pronounced, however, velars may be particularly devastated, perhaps because a greater mass must be moved to produce them relative to that for anterior lingual consonants.

Resonance differences are occasionally noted in people with bilateral tongue weakness. The resonance abnormality is sometimes labeled hypernasality or hyponasality, but this is probably inaccurate. Although the reason for resonance alterations is unclear, it may be that the weak tongue tends to fall back into the pharynx, altering the shape of the pharyngeal tube and, hence, resonance characteristics; reduced tongue movement reduces variability of oral cavity shapes during speech, thereby reducing normal resonance variability, leading to a perception of abnormal resonance; or atrophy alters the size of the oral and pharyngeal cavities, leading to resonance changes.

The most useful tasks for assessing lingual movement are connected speech (including stress testing, if myasthenia gravis is suspected) and speech AMRs. Connected speech places heavy demands on rapid, variable movements and may be most useful for identifying lingual distortions. AMRs are useful because, if weakness is limited to the tongue, AMRs for "puh" should be normal, whereas those for "tuh" and "kuh" may be imprecise or slow. A noticeable mismatch in precision or rate between bilabial and lingual AMRs usually suggests isolated or relatively greater lingual weakness or, if the difference is in favor of lingual AMRs, isolated or relatively greater bilabial weakness. Imprecision and slowness for "kuh" generally exceeds that for "tuh" when the tongue is weak, possibly because elevation of the back of the tongue, with its greater mass, places increased demands on strength (note, however, that AMRs for "kuh" are also somewhat slower than "tuh" in normal speakers).

Speakers with bilateral tongue weakness will often compensate well if other muscles are intact. For example, they may exaggerate jaw movement to facilitate lingual articulation, or they may restrict jaw movement to keep the tongue closer to articulatory targets in the maxilla. Compensatory exaggerated movements occasionally are mistaken for hyperkinetic movement disorders, although the physical mechanism examination usually clarifies the issue.

Acoustic and physiologic studies. Studies of strength have demonstrated lingual weakness in individuals with flaccid dysarthria. Dworkin and Aronson (1986) compared tongue strength in normal and dysarthric adults using a strain gauge force transducer to measure maximal sustained lingual force. Two of their 18 subjects had flaccid dysarthria with XIIth nerve lesions. They were weaker than controls on anterior and lateral strength measures, and their AMRs were slower than normal. However, for the entire dysarthric group there was no relationship between tongue strength and ratings of speech intelligibility. It therefore appears that tongue strength measures may be useful in quantifying lingual weakness but may not have any predictive relationship with speech rate or intelligibility. The lack of relationship between tongue strength and speech rate is consistent with the general perceptual impression that speech rate is noticeably reduced in flaccid dysarthria only when weakness is quite severe.

Spinal nerve lesions

Course, function, and localization of lesions. Upper cervical spinal nerves supplying the neck are indirectly implicated in voice, resonance, and articulation (see discussion of the spinal component of the XIth cranial nerve). These effects are indirect and poorly understood.

Spinal nerves involved in respiration are spread from the cervical through the thoracic divisions of the spinal cord. Those supplying the diaphragm arise from the 3rd to 5th cervical segments. They combine to form the phrenic nerves, each of which innervates half of the diaphragm, the most important inspiratory respiratory muscle. Remaining inhalatory muscles are supplied by branches of the lower cervical nerves, intercostal nerves, and phrenic nerves. Muscles of forced exhalation, important for control of exhalation during speech, are innervated by motor fibers of the thoracic and intercostal nerves.

Diffuse impairment of spinal nerves supplying respiratory muscles is required to interfere significantly with respiration. The exception is damage to the 3rd to 5th segments of the cervical spinal cord, which can paralyze the diaphragm bilaterally and severely compromise breathing.

Etiologies. Spinal cord injuries above C3 can isolate the respiratory muscles from the brain stem respiratory control centers and cause respiratory paralysis. Diseases such as myasthenia gravis, amyotrophic lateral sclerosis, Guillain-Barré syndrome, and spinal cord injuries affect respiration by weakening muscles or interfering with their innervation.

Nonspeech oral and respiratory mechanisms. Compromised respiratory nerve function can result in rapid, shallow breathing. Flaring of the nasal alae and use of upper chest and shoulder neck muscles to elevate and enlarge the rib cage suggest respiratory compromise. Thoracic expansion may be visibly restricted during inhalation and patients may be unable to hold their breath for more than a few seconds. They may be unable to generate or sustain subglottal air pressure sufficient to support speech as measured by a U-*tube or waterglass manometer.*

Speech. Flaccid dysarthria due to isolated respiratory disturbance is rare in most speech pathology practices. It is not clear if this is because the incidence of such disturbances is low, if such patients rarely complain of the effects of such disturbances on speech or spontaneously compensate for them, or if the respiratory compromise for basic life support is so overriding that its effect on speech is of low priority to the patient and their medical caregivers. Such speech problems certainly exist, as exemplified in a case history report by Hixon, Putnam, and Sharp (1983) and in the majority of the individuals with cervical spinal cord injuries studied by Hoit and others (1990). Patients with respiratory weakness sufficient to affect speech usually also have weakness that interferes with quiet breathing or breathing during other physical activities. These deficits have usually been identified prior to speech examination. Table 4–3 summarizes the effects of respiratory weakness on speech.

Respiratory weakness reduces the amount and force of expelled air. Reduced vital capacity and control of expiration can result in *short phrases* and *reduced loudness*. Prosodic abnormalities secondary to *altered phrasing* may result, as may *decreased pitch and loudness variability*. Such problems are not universally present, but are not uncommon. For example, in Hoit and others' (1990) study of 10 adults with cervical spinal cord injury, three were perceived as normal speakers, three had reduced loudness, two were breathy, two had short phrases, and one had prolonged inspiration that presumably affected prosody.

Patients with respiratory weakness may inhale with obvious effort, sometimes raising their shoulders and extending their neck in compensation for diaphragmatic weakness. They may attempt to speak on residual air and the voice may actually sound *strained*, perhaps secondary to efforts to achieve vocal cord adduction with limited subglottic pressure or to maximize efficient use of the restricted respiratory supply (Hixon, Putnam, and Sharp, 1983). Many of these characteristics are present in patients with severe asthma, chronic obstructive pulmonary disease, and other respiratory disturbances of a nonneurologic nature. Finally, inability to extend the duration of exhalation for normal phrase length in speech leads some patients to *speak on inhalation.*

Respiratory weakness in combination with cranial nerve weakness in flaccid dysarthria is not unusual, and distinguishing between phonatory and prosodic abnormalities due to respiratory versus laryngeal weakness can be difficult. Some clues that may help to identify which level is more involved include:

1. Gasping for air, nares flaring, shoulder elevation, and neck retraction on inhalation during speech are rare in isolated laryngeal weakness but not uncommon in respiratory weakness.
2. Patients with isolated laryngeal adductor weakness do not complain of shortness of breath at times other than during speech. Those with respiratory weakness do.

3. Patients with isolated respiratory weakness may have reduced loudness and breathy or strained voice quality, but they are generally not hoarse or harsh, and never diplophonic. Those with laryngeal weakness are frequently hoarse or harsh, and sometimes diplophonic.
4. Patients with greater laryngeal than respiratory weakness may have a glottal coup that is less adequate than their cough (good respiratory force during coughing may overcome vocal cord weakness). The opposite can occur when respiratory weakness exceeds laryngeal weakness (less respiratory force is required for a glottal coup than cough).

Physiologic studies. Acoustic and physiologic studies of speech in people with isolated respiratory weakness are few. Hixon, Putnam, and Sharp (1983) conducted a detailed kinematic analysis of respiratory movements in a person with flaccid paralysis of respiratory muscles. The patient demonstrated considerable capacity for compensatory speech respiratory activities in the form of "neck breathing" and "glossopharyngeal breathing" (these will be discussed in Chapter 17 on the treatment of dysarthria). The data support contentions that reduced vital capacity need not result in speech difficulty if valving of the airstream can be made more efficient.

Hoit and others' (1990) study of individuals with cervical spinal injury documented abnormal chest wall movement consistent with loss of abdominal muscle function. They also found speech breathing patterns that reflected compensations for expiratory muscle weakness. Speakers inspired to larger lung and rib cage volumes (they inhaled more deeply) and terminated speech at larger volumes than nonimpaired speakers, presumably to take advantage of higher elastic recoil pressure at those volumes that could drive the upper airway and larynx during phonation. Speakers also used larger lung volumes when asked to increase loudness. These compensatory strategies were developed spontaneously in most cases.

Multiple cranial nerve lesions

When several cranial nerves are damaged, the condition is often referred to as *bulbar palsy.* Damage to more than a single cranial nerve is not unusual. The jaw, face, lips, tongue, palate, pharynx, and larynx can be affected in varying combinations and to varying degrees depending on the particular cranial nerves involved and whether damage is unilateral or bilateral.

Conditions that affect multiple cranial nerves tend to be associated with intracranial pathology. This is because the smallest lesion that can do the most damage is in the brain stem where the cranial nerves are closer together than anywhere else along their course. This is not always the case, however, because multiple cranial nerves may be involved in neuromuscular junction diseases (myasthenia gravis), and myopathies can affect muscles in the distribution of more than one cranial nerve.

Etiologies. Multiple cranial nerve involvement can be caused by many of the same conditions that affect single cranial nerves. Multiple rather than single cranial nerve involvement is more common in certain diseases, however, including ALS, myasthenia gravis, and brainstem tumors or vascular disturbances.

Nonspeech oral mechanism. Clinical examination findings in patients with multiple cranial nerve involvement are no different than those with damage to single cranial nerves. The cumulative effects on function, however, can be much more devastating than the effects of single cranial nerve lesions.

Speech. Deviant speech characteristics associated with multiple cranial nerve lesions are similar to those associated with isolated cranial nerve damage, but the effects are heard in combination. Consequently, they may be more difficult to isolate. In general, the dysarthria will be perceived as more severe than in single cranial nerve lesions, but this is not always the case, especially if the measure of severity is intelligibility. For example, a bilateral lesion of the hypoglossal nerve could have a greater impact on intelligibility than combined unilateral lesions of the Vth, VIIth, and Xth nerves.

Distribution of cranial nerve involvement in flaccid dysarthria

The distribution of cranial nerve involvement in the population of people with flaccid dysarthria is unknown, but a retrospective review of cases seen in a large medical setting provides some clues about the distribution encountered in some practices.

Table 4–5 summarizes the distribution of involvement of cranial nerves V, VII, X, and XII in 107 out of 108 of the cases whose etiologies are summarized in the box on page 104 (the missing case was insufficiently documented to specify cranial nerves). Cautious interpretation should be exercised regarding the representativeness of these data for the general population or for all speech pathology practices. In addition, these data represent speech pathologists' judgment about the contribution of cranial nerve weakness to the dysarthria and not necessarily all of the cranial nerves that might have been involved (for example, unilateral Vth nerve weakness was not included if it did not appear relevant to the speech deficit).

Several characteristics of the distribution are of interest. First, Vth nerve and respiratory contributions to flaccid dysarthria were infrequent; this probably means that they are usually not affected in flaccid dysarthria or, if they are, are not often judged to contribute to the speech characteristics that represent the dysarthria. The VIIth and XIIth nerves were involved much more frequently, and the Xth nerve more often than any other speech cranial nerve. Among the branches of the Xth nerve, the pharyngeal branch was only infre-

Table 4–5 Distribution of involvement of the Vth, VIIth, Xth, and XIIth cranial nerves, and spinal respiratory nerves, in 106 quasirandomly selected cases with a primary speech diagnosis of flaccid dysarthria at the Mayo Clinic from 1969–90. Number of instances in which each nerve was the only speech nerve involved and the number of instances in which each nerve was involved along with other speech nerves are given. *Sixty-eight percent of the cases had isolated unilateral or bilateral involvement of a single cranial nerve. Thirty-two percent had more than one cranial nerve involved.* As a result, the total number of different nerves reported is 144.

Nerve	Isolated unilateral	Isolated bilateral	Multiple unilateral	Multiple bilateral	% of total
V	—	—	2	1	2
VII	—	3	5	8	11
X - Pharyngeal branch only	—	2	—	2	3
Laryngeal branch(es) only	41	2	—	2	31
All branches	9	11	5	19	31
XII	1	4	8	17	21
Respiratory	—	—	—	2	1
% of Total	35	15	14	35	100

quently implicated without involvement of the superior or recurrent laryngeal branches. In contrast, the laryngeal branches were frequently implicated without pharyngeal branch involvement; this reflects the high frequency of surgery-related or idiopathic vocal cord paralyses below the pharyngeal branch of the Xth nerve. Finally, about two-thirds of the sample had unilateral or bilateral involvement of a single cranial nerve (most often the Xth nerve). The remaining one-third of the sample had involvement of more than one cranial nerve.

Clusters of deviant speech dimensions

Darley, Aronson, and Brown (1969b) found three clusters of deviant dimensions in their group of 30 patients with bulbar palsy. These clusters are useful in understanding the presumed neuromuscular deficits, the components of the speech system that are most prominently involved, and features of flaccid dysarthria that distinguish it from other dysarthria types (see Table 4–6).

The first cluster was *phonatory incompetence*. It included *breathy voice*, *audible inspiration*, and *short phrases*. The cluster represents incompetence at the laryngeal valve, including inadequate vocal cord adduction (breathiness due to inadequate vocal cord adduction, and short phrases due to air wastage through the glottis) and abduction (audible inspiration due to inadequate vocal fold abduction during inspiration).

The second cluster was *resonatory incompetence*. It included *hypernasality*, *nasal emission*, *imprecise consonants*, and *short phrases*. The relationship among these features reflect weakness of the velopharyngeal valve leading to excessive nasal resonance (hypernasality) and nasal air flow during attempts to produce consonants requiring

intraoral pressure (nasal emission). Imprecise consonants in this cluster reflect the secondary effect of nasal emission on pressure consonant precision. Short phrases reflect the effect of air wastage through the velopharyngeal port during speech.

The final cluster was *phonatory-prosodic insufficiency*. It consisted of *harsh voice, monopitch*, and *monoloudness*. Darley, Aronson, and Brown felt these characteristics reflected hypotonia in laryngeal muscles. This hypothesis has received support from acoustic and physiological studies and from direct observation of weak or paralyzed vocal cords (already discussed).

The phonatory and resonatory incompetence clusters are especially important for differential diagnosis because they were not found in other dysarthria types. Therefore, the presence of phonatory or resonatory incompetence is suggestive of flaccid dysarthria and implicates LMN weakness at the laryngeal and velopharyngeal valves (Xth cranial nerve). The third cluster, phonatory-prosodic insufficiency, was not isolated to flaccid dysarthria (it also occurred in ataxic dysarthria). Its recognition is important for the description and diagnosis of dysarthria, but it may not contribute as much to differential diagnosis among dysarthria types as the first two clusters.*

Table 4–7 summarizes the most deviant speech characteristics that were found by Darley, Aron-

Table 4–6 Deviant clusters of abnormal speech characteristics in flaccid dysarthria.

Cluster name	Speech characteristics
Phonatory incompetence	Breathiness, short phrases, audible inspiration
Resonatory incompetence	Hypernasality, imprecise consonants, nasal emission, short phrases
Phonatory-prosodic insufficiency	Harsh voice, monoloudness, monopitch

Based on Darley FL, Aronson AE, and Brown JR: Differential diagnostic patterns of dysarthria, J Speech Hear Res 12:246, 1969b.

*The reader may be struck by the restriction of these clusters to Xth nerve abnormalities. This does not mean that speech abnormalities attributable to weakness of other cranial nerves do not occur in flaccid dysarthria, nor does it imply that recognition of other abnormalities is not helpful to diagnosis. The absence of obvious influences of other cranial nerves in the cluster analysis of Darley, Aronson, and Brown probably reflects several influences, the most clinically relevant of which may be: the distribution of cranial nerve involvement in their sample (and those with flaccid dysarthria in general, as suggested by the findings summarized in Table 4–5) may have been biased toward Xth nerve lesions; the grouping of all articulatory deficits under the global designation of imprecise consonants and vowel distortions may have "washed out" the unique specific effects of Vth, VIIth, and XIIth nerve lesions on speech; imprecise consonants can occur in all dysarthria types, so their presence is not likely to be distinctive within clusters that distinguish among types of dysarthria; and the primary purpose of the studies was to distinguish among dysarthria types rather than the differential effects on speech of damage to specific cranial nerves within a specific dysarthria type (that is, flaccid dysarthria).

The important point here is that investigating the functions of each cranial nerve and the loci of specific speech characteristics is important to examination, description, and diagnosis, regardless of Darley, Aronson, and Brown's cluster analysis results. Also, because flaccid dysarthria can be manifest by damage to only a single cranial nerve, and because other dysarthrias are rarely manifest through a single cranial nerve, identification of the offending muscle group is important to differential diagnosis and treatment decisions.

Table 4–7 The most deviant speech characteristics encountered in flaccid dysarthria by Darley, Aronson, and Brown (1969a), listed in order from most to least severe. Also listed are the cranial nerves and muscle groups most likely associated with the deviant speech characteristics.

Dimension	Primary cranial nerve	Level
Hypernasality*	X	Velopharyngeal
Imprecise consonants	V	Articulatory
		Jaw
	VII	Face
	X	Valopharyngeal
	XII	Tongue
Breathiness* (continuous)	X	Laryngeal
Monopitch	X	Laryngeal
Nasal emission*	X	Velopharyngeal
Audible inspiration*	X	Laryngeal
Harsh voice quality	X	Laryngeal
Short phrases*	X	Laryngeal and/or
	Spinal respiratory	Respiratory
Monoloudness	X	Laryngeal and/or
	Spinal respiratory	Respiratory

*Tend to be distinctive or more severely impaired in flaccid dysarthria than any other single dysarthria type.

son, and Brown in their patients with bulbar palsy. The cranial or spinal nerve and the component of the speech mechanism that is most likely implicated in the production of each of the characteristics are also given. Table 4–8 summarizes the acoustic and physiologic correlates of flaccid dysarthria that were reviewed within the discussion of deficits associated with each of the speech cranial nerves.

CASES

The following cases review the histories, examination findings, and neurologic findings and diagnoses for several patients with flaccid dysarthria. As a group, they illustrate some of the commonalities and differences that exist among people with this type of dysarthria. Several cases illustrate the prominence of speech deficits in neurologic disease and the importance of speech diagnosis to medical/neurologic diagnosis.

Case 4.1

A 44-year-old woman presented to neurology with an eight-month history of speech difficulty, which she thought was caused by ongoing stress. Neurologic exam was normal. The neurologist was uncertain, but wondered if her complaint was stress-related. Speech pathology consultation was requested.

During speech consultation the patient revealed that her speech deteriorated when she was tired or under stress. She described it as "slurred, almost like my mouth freezes–.–.–.almost sounds like it goes nasal." She vaguely described an alteration of chewing and swallowing ability at such times, but denied choking or drooling. The speech problem would persist until she rested. The primary sources of stress were a busy

schedule caring for her three school-age children and coaching a high school volleyball team daily. She noted that her speech frequently changed while she was coaching. She described her family life and work as stable and happy, but very busy.

Speech was initially normal. After six minutes of continuous reading aloud, mild sibilant distortions became apparent, along with equivocal hoarseness and intermittent vocal flutter. Speech AMRs were normal and the patient did not become hypernasal; however, inconsistent nasal air flow was detected on a mirror held at the nares during repetition of nonnasal sounds and phrases. After another 4.5 minutes of reading, she began to interdentalize /s/ and /z/, distort affricates, and mildly distort /r/. AMRs remained normal and hypernasality was not perceived. Oral mechanism exam immediately following stress testing demonstrated only equivocal lingual weakness. The patient was upset and cried during this period of speech deterioration, making it difficult to separate the probable effects of weakness from her emotional response. Speech returned to normal after 30 seconds of rest.

She was asked to return the following day at 5 P.M., after volleyball practice. Speech was initially normal but deteriorated quickly and significantly, and its character was the same as that noted the day before. In addition, pitch breaks and some fluttering of the cheeks during speech were apparent.

The speech diagnosis was "flaccid dysarthria characterized by weakness of, at the least, cranial nerves VII, X, and XII, bilaterally, with rapid deterioration with stress testing, consistent with the pattern of breakdown seen in myasthenia gravis." Subsequent EMG and improvement of her symptoms with Mestinon treatment confirmed the diagnosis of myasthenia gravis. She subsequently did well with Mestinon treatment.

Commentary. *(1) Speech difficulty can be the first sign of neurologic disease. (2) The presence of*

Table 4–8 Summary of direct observations and acoustic and physiologic findings in flaccid dysarthria (based on literature summarized in text). Some findings may reflect efforts to compensate for weakness and not just the primary effects of weakness.

Level	Direct, acoustic, & physiologic observations
Respiratory	Reduced vital capacity
	Termination of speech at larger than normal lung volumes*
	Larger than normal inspiratory & rib cage volumes*
	Abnormal chest wall movements*
	Neck and glossopharyngeal breathing*
Laryngeal/respiratory	Vocal cord immobility/sluggishness
	Incomplete glottal closure
	Abnormal vocal cord frequency & amplitude perturbations
	Increased amplitude of vocal cord mucosal wave
	Increased airflow rate
	Increased inspiratory volume*
	Increased breaths per minute*
	Reduced pause frequency & duration*
	Reduced speech duration/syllables per breath group*
	Reduced range & variability of f_o
	High amplitude of f_o with reduced energy of harmonics
	Reduced formant intensity & definition
	Increased high-frequency spectral energy (noise)
Velopharyngeal	(including findings from studies of velopharyngeal incompetence associated with cleft palate)
	Reduced/absent palatal movement
	Reduced/absent pharyngeal-wall movement
	Increased nasal air flow
	Decreased energy in f_o
	Increased frequency of f_o
	Reduced pitch range
	Increased formant bandwidth
	Reduced overall intensity & intensity range
	Extra resonances
	Antiresonances
Lingual	Reduced sustained lingual force

*Compensatory or possibly compensatory.

psychological/emotional stress at the onset of speech difficulty is insufficient proof of psychogenic etiology. Patients often attribute their physical problem to stress when neurologic disease presents insidiously. In such cases, neurologic and psychologic factors deserve equal attention until a clear cause emerges. (3) Speech diagnosis can localize disease in the motor system. In some cases, speech diagnosis provides strong evidence for a specific neurologic diagnosis.

Case 4.2

A 37-year-old man presented with a complaint of speech difficulty, problems with "tongue control," and headache and neck pain of two months' duration. He described his speech as "slurred" and complained of excess saliva accumulation and difficulty moving food with his tongue.

Oral mechanism exam identified a bilaterally atrophic tongue, but no fasciculations. He was barely able to move his tongue in any direction and tongue strength

was rated −4 bilaterally. Saliva pooled in the mouth. Phonation and resonance were normal, as were AMRs for "puh" and "tuh," but those for "kuh" were equivocally slowed and reduced in precision. Lingual sounds were distorted during connected speech. Nonlingual sounds, rate, and prosody were normal. Jaw and facial movements during speech were exaggerated in apparent compensation for his lingual weakness. Intelligibility was remarkably good.

Neurologic exam was otherwise normal except for mild weakness of neck flexor muscles. Skull radiographs showed destruction of the interior portion of the clivus (the bony part of the posterior fossa anterior to the foramen magnum) and an associated nasopharyngeal soft tissue mass. Magnetic resonance imaging (MRI) and computed tomography scans identified a destructive tumor mass in the anterior rim of the foramen magnum bilaterally. The patient underwent neurosurgery for radical subtotal removal of a chordoma tumor of the clivus. Postoperatively, articulatory imprecision was mildly worse but no other speech deficits developed. The patient underwent radiation therapy and his speech gradually improved, but not to normal. Lingual atrophy and weakness persisted. He did well but two years later developed headache, nausea, vomiting, and double vision. There was evidence of tumor recurrence, but further radiation therapy or surgery were not advised because of risks and unlikely benefit. The patient lived outside of the geographic area and was not seen for further follow-up.

Commentary. (1) Flaccid dysarthria can be caused by damage to a single cranial nerve, unilaterally or bilaterally. (2) Speech difficulty can be the first sign of neurologic disease. (3) Speech intelligibility can be remarkably preserved in isolated bilateral tongue weakness.

Case 4.3

A 51-year-old woman presented with a one-year history of left facial numbness, achiness of the left eye, and mild headache. Neurologic exam was normal with the exception of decreased facial sensation. MRI demonstrated an abnormality in the left middle cerebellar peduncle, left side of the pons, and left cerebellopontine angle cistern. She underwent a left suboccipital craniectomy and resection of a cerebellopontine angle cavernous hemangioma. She did very well postoperatively but had decreased sensation of the left face, a decreased left corneal reflex, and equivocal weakness of the left jaw. She complained that it was difficult to know if she had swallowed all of her food and that food would remain on the left side of her mouth after swallowing. She also felt her left face drooped and that her speech was distorted.

Speech examination failed to identify weakness of the face, tongue, or palate. There was equivocal weakness of the left masseter muscle but it did not appear significant enough to impact on speech (that is, range and rate of jaw movement was good). Her connected speech was normal with the exception of mild, inconsistent lingual articulatory imprecision. Speech AMRs and vowel prolongation were normal. Face, lip, and jaw movements were exaggerated during speech and the patient said that she was trying to articulate carefully to compensate for her speech problem. Tactile and pressure sensation of the face, perioral area, and tongue were reduced on the left and were normal on the right. Her articulatory precision actually improved after she was instructed to reduce exaggerated face, lip, and jaw movements. She felt reassured by this observation and was pleased to hear that her distortions were only barely detectable.

It was concluded that her speech deficit was secondary to decreased face and tongue sensation and perhaps to her exaggerated efforts to increase sensory feedback during speech.

Commentary. (1) Speech deficits can result from sensory loss, but tend to be mild. (2) Efforts at compensation for speech deficits are not always productive. (3) Management of speech deficits is sometimes accomplished by counseling, some simple suggestions, and reassurance.

Case 4.4

A 40-year-old millwright presented with an eight-month history of voice difficulty. His dysphonia began after anterior-approach cervical disk surgery. He had been unable to return to work as a millwright because coworkers were unable to hear his directions and responses in the noisy work environment. He occasionally coughed and choked after swallowing and had to clear his throat frequently.

Speech and oral mechanism exam were normal except for a markedly breathy-hoarse voice quality, moderately decreased loudness, and short phrases secondary to presumed air wastage through the glottis. He could sustain "ah" and "z" for only 2 seconds but sustained "s" for 12 seconds. His cough and glottal coup were markedly weak. There was no evidence of palatal asymmetry, the palate was mobile, and the gag reflex was normal.

The speech pathologist's impression was "suspect vocal cord paralysis secondary to recurrent laryngeal nerve damage caused by surgical trauma." Subsequent laryngeal examination identified a right vocal cord paralysis (paramedian position) and agreed it was probably secondary to surgical trauma. Teflon injection of the right vocal cord resulted in normal conversational loudness, ability to sustain "ah" for 14 seconds, /s/ for 12 seconds, and /z/ for 10 seconds. The patient remained unable to produce a loud, shouting voice. He was, however, pleased with his voice improvement and was able to return to work as a millwright, although with some fatigue in his voice by the end of the work day.

Commentary. (1) Flaccid dysarthria can result from damage to a single cranial nerve. (2) The degree of deficit perceptually does not always predict the impact of the problem on a person's day-to-day functioning (this patient could not work). (3) Some speech deficits can be managed very effectively with medical intervention.

Case 4.5

A 76-year-old mildly retarded man presented to Ear, Nose, and Throat (ENT) with a 10 to 11 week history of speech and swallowing difficulty. A swallowing study conducted elsewhere was normal. Except for the patient's obvious speech difficulty and suspected tongue fasciculations, ENT examination was normal. The physician thought the patient might have ALS. He was referred for speech and neurologic examinations.

Speech examination the following day was difficult because of the patient's immature affect, anxiety, and difficulty following directions. He did report that his swallowing problem was present upon awakening one morning and that his speech difficulty followed 1 to 2 days later. He reported greater difficulty swallowing food than liquids but had had nasal regurgitation when swallowing water. He believed all of his problems had worsened since onset.

Oral mechanism examination revealed left ptosis and difficulty closing both eyes completely. His face was moderately weak bilaterally. The tongue was tremulous on protrusion but there were no fasciculations or atrophy; it was −2,3 weak bilaterally. Palatal movement gradually decreased over repeated repetitions of "ah ah ah−.−.−." There was consistent nasal air escape during speech. There was some reduction in speed and range of movement during alternating retraction and pursing of the lips. Cough and glottal coup were weak. Gag reflex was normal. Sucking reflex was positive, but not necessarily abnormal for an adult of his age.

Speech examination was difficult because of his anxiety and difficulty following directions. However, the following characteristics were apparent: hypernasality (3); weak pressure consonants (3,4); imprecise articulation (2); reduced rate (0,1). Prolonged "ah" was breathy (0,1) and inhalatory stridor was apparent after maximum vowel prolongation. The patient prolonged "ah" for 20 seconds initially, but over multiple trials this decreased to 12 seconds. It was difficult to get him to persist in speaking for stress testing but hypernasality and weak pressure consonants appeared to increase over time.

The speech pathologist's impression was "flaccid dysarthria implicating, at the least, cranial nerves X, XII, and VII, bilaterally. There is no evidence of a spastic dysarthria or other CNS-based dysarthria. There is some deterioration of speech during stress testing, raising suspicions about neuromuscular junction disease (does this patient have myasthenia gravis?)."

Subsequent clinical neurologic exam, EMG, and an ACh receptor antibody test confirmed a diagnosis of myasthenia gravis. The patient improved rapidly when treated with Mestinon, but within three months his bulbar symptoms worsened and he developed respiratory compromise. The patient underwent plasmaphoresis and was placed on high-dose steroids, but died one month later.

Commentary. (1) Speech can be among the first signs of neurologic disease. (2) Careful speech examination sometimes is more enlightening than anatomic examination of speech structures. (3) The presence of cognitive deficits can make examination difficult. (4) The value of accurate localization and disease diagnosis by speech examination, unfortunately, is not always matched by long-term benefit to the patient.

Case 4.6

A 45-year-old man presented to Neurology with a three-month history of swallowing difficulty that began with a choking episode, followed by continuing difficulty swallowing solid foods, but not liquids. Speech difficulty began about one month later, which the patient described as "slurring" and "difficulty with pronunciation." The neurologic examination was normal with the exception of possible palatal or tongue weakness. EMG failed to find evidence of neuromuscular junction disease but did find an abnormality of the hypoglossal nerve or its nuclei. MRI scan failed to find evidence of abnormality in the brainstem or posterior fossa. A video swallow study was normal. ENT examination was normal.

During speech evaluation, the patient complained of some dull, aching pain in his ears, tongue, jaw, and gums, which he attributed to increased effort to chew food completely before swallowing. He noted mild difficulty with chewing and a tendency to put food to the left in his mouth. He felt he was able to initiate a swallow but often gagged and had to bring food back up and reinitiate a swallow. He was not aware of drooling during the day but noted that his pillow was frequently wet upon awakening in the morning.

During the examination, the patient cleared his throat frequently. Jaw strength was normal. There was equivocal weakness of lip rounding. The tongue was moderately weak bilaterally. Tongue protrusion and lateralization were limited (2,3), and there were equivocal fasciculations on the right side of the tongue. The palate elevated more extensively toward the right. There was a trace of nasal emission during pressure-sound production. Cough and glottal coup were normal. Speech was characterized by imprecise articulation, primarily on lingual consonants (0,1) and by hypernasality with occasional audible nasal emission (1). Voice quality was hoarse-breathy (0,1). He was able to sustain a vowel for 25 seconds. Speech AMRs for "puh" and "tuh" were normal but "kuh" was slow (−1). There was no significant deterioration of speech during stress testing.

The clinician's impression was "flaccid dysarthria associated with, at the least, weakness of cranial nerves XII and X, most likely bilateral. There was no significant deterioration of speech during stress testing, as might be encountered in myasthenia gravis. Finally, I hear no evidence to suggest the presence of a spastic component to his dysarthria."

All other laboratory and imaging tests, including tests for myasthenia gravis, were normal. The patient received counseling for management of his dysphagia and was discharged. He returned three months later complaining of increased dysphagia and tongue pain. ENT examination revealed a tender swollen tongue. Computed tomography scan of the head and neck identified a mass extending posteriorly from the posterior aspect of the left superior tongue. Subsequent surgery identified extensive squamous cell carcinoma of the tongue with neck metastases. Right and left neck dissection and total glossectomy and laryngectomy were carried out. To the present, three years post surgery, there has been no tumor recurrence.

Commentary. (1) Speech difficulty can be among the first signs of neurologic or other organic disease. (2) The apparent involvement of more than one cranial nerve does not always place the lesion inside the skull, even when muscle disease and neuromuscular junction disease are not present. (3) Neurologic signs and symptoms do not always mean the patient has primary nervous system disease. Although cranial nerves were affected, the neoplasm in this case was nonneurologic.

SUMMARY

1. Flaccid dysarthria results from damage to the motor units of cranial or spinal nerves that serve the speech muscles. It occurs at a frequency comparable to that of other single dysarthria types. It sometimes reflects weakness in only a small number of muscles and can be isolated to lesions of single cranial or spinal nerves. Weakness and hypotonia are the underlying neuromuscular deficits that explain most of the speech characteristics associated with flaccid dysarthria.

2. Lesions anywhere within the motor unit can cause flaccid dysarthria, and a variety of etiologies can produce such lesions. Surgery and trauma from accidents are common causes. Neuropathies leading to flaccid dysarthria are often of undetermined etiology. Muscle disease, tumor, myasthenia gravis, stroke, infections, degenerative and demyelinating diseases, and anatomic malformations are among the remaining commonly encountered causes.

3. The speech characteristics and nonspeech examination findings differ among lesions of the Vth, VIIth, Xth, and XIIth cranial nerves and spinal respiratory nerves. Examination can localize the effects of disease to one or a combination of these nerves.

4. Lesions of the mandibular branch of the Vth (trigeminal) cranial nerve lead to weakness of jaw muscles. When bilateral, jaw weakness can have significant effects on articulation. Lesions of the Vth nerve that affect sensation from the jaw, face, lip, and tongue and stationary points of articulatory contact may also affect speech, primarily articulatory precision.

5. Lesions of the VIIth (facial) cranial nerve can lead to facial weakness and flaccid dysarthria. Unilateral weakness of the face can be associated with mild articulatory distortions. Bilateral lesions may lead to significant distortion of all consonants and vowels requiring facial movement.

6. Lesions of the Xth (vagus) cranial nerve can lead to weakness of velopharyngeal and laryngeal muscles and to some of the most prominent and frequently encountered manifestations of flaccid dysarthria. Lesions of the pharyngeal branch of the nerve can lead to resonatory incompetence, with hypernasality, nasal emission, and weakening of pressure consonant sounds. Lesions of the superior laryngeal and recurrent laryngeal branches can lead to a variety of dysphonias, the perceptual attributes of which are consistent with weakness and hypotonia of laryngeal muscles. Lesions above the pharyngeal branch of the vagus nerve can lead to both resonatory and laryngeal incompetence, whereas lesions below the pharyngeal branch are associated with laryngeal manifestations only.

7. Lesions of the XIIth (hypoglossal) cranial nerve cause tongue weakness. The resulting flaccid dysarthria is reflected in imprecision of lingual articulation, with severity dependent upon degree of weakness and whether the lesion is unilateral or bilateral.

8. Lesions affecting spinal respiratory nerves can reduce respiratory support for speech. Weakness at this level can lead to reduced loudness and pitch variability, as well as a shortening of phrase length.

9. Phonatory and resonatory incompetence are commonly encountered distinguishing features of flaccid dysarthria. Although they are tied to involvement of the Xth cranial nerve, it is nonetheless important to attend to speech movements generated through the Vth, VIIth, and XIIth cranial nerves. This is important both for a complete description of the speech disorder, and because speech deficits isolated to any of the cranial or spinal nerves are possible in flaccid dysarthria and unusual in other dysarthria types.

10. Flaccid dysarthria can be the only, the first, or among the first and most prominent manifestations of neurologic disease. Its recognition as a motor speech disorder and its localization to motor units subserving speech may aid the localization and diagnosis of neurologic disease. Its diagnosis and description are important to decision-making regarding medical and behavioral management of the individual and the speech disorder.

REFERENCES

Adams RD and Victor M: Principles of neurology, New York, 1991, McGraw-Hill.

Affi AK, Ziyad HR, and Faris KB: Isolated, reversible hypoglossal nerve palsy, Arch Neurol 41:1218, 1984.

Andour KK, Schneider G, and Hilsinger RL: Acute superior laryngeal nerve palsy: analysis of 78 cases, Otolaryngol Head Neck Surg 88:418, 1980.

Aronson AE: Clinical voice disorders, New York, 1990, Thieme.

Bannister R: Brain's clinical neurology, London, 1985, Oxford University Press.

Brazis PW: Ocular motor abnormalities in Wallenberg's lateral medullary syndrome, Mayo Clin Proc 67:365, 1992.

Brazis PW, Masdeu JC, and Biller J: Localization in clinical neurology, Boston, 1985, Little, Brown.

Clinical examinations in neurology, ed 3, Philadelphia, 1971, WB Saunders.

Curtis JF: Acoustics of speech production and nasalization. In Spriestersbach DC and Lerman DS, editors: Cleft palate and communication, New York, 1968, Academic Press.

Darley FL, Aronson AE, and Brown JR: Clusters of deviant speech dimensions in the dysarthrias, J Speech Hear Res 12:462-496 1969a.

Darley FL, Aronson AE, and Brown JR: Differential diagnostic patterns of dysarthria, J Speech Hear Res 12:246, 1969b.

Darley FL, Aronson AE, and Brown JR: Motor speech disorders, Philadelphia, 1975, WB Saunders.

Dworkin JP and Aronson AE: Tongue strength and alternate motion rates in normal and dysarthric subjects, J Commun Disord 19:115, 1986.

Griffin JW: Diseases of the peripheral nervous system. In Rosenberg RN, editor: The clinical neurosciences, New York, 1983, Churchill Livingstone.

Guo YP, McLeod JG, and Baverstock J: Pathologic changes in the vagus nerve in diabetes and chronic alcoholism, J Neurol Neurosurg Psychiatry 50:1449, 1987.

Hammarberg B, Fritzell B, and Schiratzki H: Teflon injection in 16 patients with paralytic dysphonia: perceptual and acoutic evaluations, J Speech Hear Disord 49:72, 1984.

Hartman DE, Daily WW, and Morin KN: A case of superior laryngeal nerve paresis and psychogenic dysphonia, J Speech Hear Disord 54:526, 1989.

Hirano M, Koike Y, and von Leden H: Maximum phonation time and air wastage during phonation, Folia Phoniatr 20:185, 1968.

Hixon TJ, Putnam AHB, and Sharp JT: Speech production with flaccid paralysis of the rib cage, diaphragm, and abdomen, J Speech Hear Disord 48:315, 1983.

Hoit JD and others: Speech breathing in individuals with cervical spinal cord injury, J Speech Hear Res 33:798, 1990.

Iwata S, von Leden H, and Williams D: Air flow measurements during phonation, J Commun Disord 5:67, 1972.

Johns DF: Surgical and prosthetic management of neurogenic velopharyngeal incompetency in dysarthria. In Clinical management of neurogenic communication disorders, New York, 1985, Little, Brown.

Katusic SK and others: Incidence, clinical features, and prognosis in Bell's palsy, Rochester, MI, 1968–1982, Ann Neurol 20:622, 1986.

Keane JR: Tongue atrophy from brainstem metastases, Arch Neurol 41:1219, 1984.

Kincaid JC and Dyken ML: Myelitis and myelopathy. In Baker AB and Joynt RJ, editors: Clinical neurology, vol 3, Philadelphia, 1987, Harper & Row.

Levin JM and Lee JE: Hemifacial spasms due to cerebellopontine angle lipoma: case report, Neurology 37:337, 1987.

Massey WE and others: Cranial nerve paralysis following carotid endarterectomy, Stroke 15:157, 1984.

Murry T: Speaking fundamental frequency characteristics associated with voice pathologies, J Speech Hear Disord 43:374, 1978.

Nishi T and others: Hemifacial spasm due to contralateral acoustic neuroma, Neurology 37:339, 1987.

Nudelman KL and Starr A: Focal facial spasm, Neurology 33:1092, 1983.

Penn AS and Rowland LP: Myasthenia gravis. In Rowland LP, editor: Merritt's textbook of neurology, Philadelphia, 1989, Lea & Febiger.

Penn AS: Other disorders of neuromuscular transmission. In Rowland LP editor: Merritt's textbook of neurology, Philadelphia, 1989, Lea & Febiger.

Pleasure DE and Schotland DL: Acquired neuropathies. In Rowland LP, editor: Merritt's textbook of neurology, Philadelphia, 1989, Lea & Febiger.

Regli F: Symptomatic trigeminal neuralgia. In Samii M and Janetta PJ, editors: The cranial nerves, New York, 1981, Springer-Verlag.

Reich AR and Lerman JW: Teflon laryngoplasty: an acoustical and perceptual study, J Speech Hear Disord 43:496, 1978.

Rontal E, Rontal M, and Rolnick M: The use of spectrograms in the evaluation of voice cord injection, Laryngoscope, 85:47, 1975.

Roses AD: Progressive muscular dystrophies. In Rowland LP, editor: Merritt's textbook of neurology, Philadelphia, 1899, Lea & Febiger.

Salomonson J, Kawamoto H, and Wilson L: Velopharyngeal incompetence as the presenting symptoms in myotonic dystrophy, Cleft Palate J 25:296, 1988.

Singer EJ: Central nervous system (CNS) complications of HIV disease. Special interest divisions, Division 2, Neurophysiology and neurogenic speech and language disorders, Rockville, MD, November, 1991, American Speech-Language-Hearing Association.

Till JA and Alp LA: Aerodynamic and temporal measures of continuous speech in dysarthric speakers. In Moore CA, Yorkson KM, and Beukelman DR, editors: Dysarthria and apraxia of speech: perspectives on management, Baltimore, 1991, Brooks Publishing.

von Leden H: Objective measures of laryngeal function and phonation, Ann N Y Acad Sci, 155:56, 1968.

Waespe W and others: Lower cranial nerve palsies due to internal carotid dissection, Stroke 19:1561, 1988.

Watterson T, McFarlane SC, and Menicucci AL: Vibratory characteristics of teflon-injected and noninjected paralyzed vocal folds, J Speech Hear Disord 55:61, 1990.

5 Spastic Dysarthria

Spastic dysarthria is a perceptually distinguishable motor speech disorder produced by damage to the direct and indirect activation pathways of the central nervous system (CNS), bilaterally. It may be manifest in any or all of the respiratory, phonatory, resonatory, and articulatory components of speech, but it is generally not confined to a single component. Its characteristics reflect the combined effects of weakness and spasticity in a manner that slows movement and reduces its range and force. Excessive muscle tone (spasticity) seems to be an important contributor to the distinguishing features of the disorder, hence its designation as *spastic* dysarthria. The correct identification of spastic dysarthria can aid the diagnosis of neurologic disease and may help localize the sites of lesions to the CNS motor pathways.

Spastic dysarthria is encountered as the primary speech pathology in a large medical practice at a rate comparable to that of the other major single dysarthria types. From 1987 to 90 at the Mayo Clinic, spastic dysarthria accounted for 10.3% of all dysarthrias and 9.4% of all motor speech disorders seen in the Section of Speech Pathology (Figure 1–3).

The clinical features of spastic dysarthria reflect the effects of excessive muscle tone and weakness on speech. They illustrate very well the distinction between speech deficits attributable to weakness alone (as in flaccid dysarthria) from those in which the barriers to normal speech also include neuromuscular resistance to movement.

ANATOMY AND BASIC FUNCTIONS OF THE DIRECT AND INDIRECT ACTIVATION PATHWAYS

The direct activation pathway, also known as the *pyramidal tract* or *direct motor system*, forms part of the upper motor neuron (UMN) system, the activities of which direct movements through the final common pathway (lower motor neurons). The direct activation pathway includes the *corticobulbar tracts*, which influence the activities of cranial nerves, and the *corticospinal tracts*, which influence the activities of spinal nerves.

The course of the direct activation pathway within the CNS was reviewed in Chapter 2. The important features of this system for speech can be summarized as follows: the pathway is bilateral, one originating in the cortex of the right cerebral hemisphere, the other in the cortex of the left cerebral hemisphere; its course leads rather directly to the cranial and spinal nerve nuclei in the brain stem and spinal cord that innervate the speech muscles; its fibers primarily innervate muscles on the side of the body opposite the cerebral cortex of origin but, for the speech muscles, this applies only to the muscles of the lower face, and, to a lesser extent, the tongue. The remaining cranial nerves subserving speech receive bilateral input from the direct (and indirect) activation pathway. This bilateral innervation serves a protective function in the sense that unilateral UMN lesions generally do not have a pronounced effect on jaw, velopharyngeal, laryngeal, or (usually) tongue movements for speech. This neural redundancy may exist to ensure survival by minimizing the effects of unilateral UMN lesions on chewing, swallowing, and airway protection functions.

The direct activation pathway is predominantly *facilitatory*. That is, impulses through it tend to lead to movement, particularly *skilled discrete movements.*

The indirect activation pathway, also known as the *extrapyramidal* or *indirect motor system,* is also part of the UMN system. It originates in the cortex of each cerebral hemisphere, but its course is more complicated than the direct activation pathway's because synapses occur along its course from the cortex to the brain stem and spinal cord. Crucial interneuronal connections include those with the basal ganglia, cerebellum, reticular formation, vestibular nuclei, and red nucleus. The indirect activation pathway is crucial for *regulating reflexes and maintaining posture, tone,* and *associated activities that provide a framework for skilled movements.* Many of its activities are *inhibitory.*

CLINICAL CHARACTERISTICS OF UMN LESIONS AND SPASTIC PARALYSIS

Damage to the direct activation pathway leads to a loss or reduction in its ability to facilitate fine, discrete movements. Hence, fine, skilled movements are lost or reduced. Initially, lesions lead to reduced muscle tone and weakness but they generally evolve to increased tone and spasticity. Weakness is usually more pronounced in distal than proximal muscles (the distal and speech muscles are those most involved in finely controlled skilled movement). Reflexes tend to be diminished initially but become more pronounced over time.

Direct activation pathway lesions are also associated with a *positive Babinski sign,* a pathologic reflex elicited by applying pressure with a relatively sharp point from the sole of the foot on the side of the heel forward to the little toe and across to the great toe. The normal response is a planting of the toes. The Babinski response is an extension of the great toe and fanning of the other toes. When present in adults, a Babinski sign is associated with CNS disease, reflecting a release of a primitive reflex from CNS inhibition (a Babinski reflex is normal in infants). *Pathologic oral reflexes* are also common in bilateral UMN disease, including suck, snout, and jaw jerk reflexes (defined in Chapter 3).

Damage to the indirect activation pathway affects its predominantly inhibitory role in motor control. As a result, lesions tend to lead to "positive signs" or overactivity such as increased muscle tone, spasticity, and hyperactive reflexes. These signs are interrelated. Spasticity, for example, is the result of hyperactivity of stretch reflexes and it goes hand-in-hand with increased muscle tone. It results in resistance to movement that is generally more pronounced at the beginning of movement or in response to quick movements. In the limbs, spasticity tends to be "biased" toward lower extremity extension (that is, the legs resist bending) and upper extremity flexion (that is, the arms resist straightening). The extension

bias in the lower extremity often leads physical therapists to hope for spasticity to develop in the legs of patients with UMN lesions because it facilitates standing.

Patients with UMN lesions and hyperactive reflexes will sometimes exhibit *clonus,* a kind of repetitive reflex contraction response that occurs when a muscle is kept under tension (stretch) by the examiner; for example, when the foot is continuously dorsiflexed by the examiner, the reflex response may look like a rhythmic tremor (*Clinical Examinations in Neurology,* 1991).

Selective damage to only the direct or only the indirect activation pathway is uncommon because both pathways arise in adjacent and overlapping areas of the cortex and travel in close proximity through much of their course to lower motor neurons (LMNs). As a result, people with spastic paralysis commonly exhibit decreased skilled movement and weakness from direct activation pathway damage as well as increased muscle tone and spasticity from indirect activation pathway damage.

Direct and indirect activation pathway signs of UMN lesions are summarized in Table 5–1. The major abnormalities that affect movement in spastic paralysis include *spasticity, weakness, reduced range of movement,* and *slowness of movement.* These abnormalities also appear to represent the most salient features of disordered movement in patients with spastic dysarthria.

THE RELATIONSHIP OF SPASTIC DYSARTHRIA TO SPASTIC PARALYSIS

The neuropathophysiologic underpinnings of spastic dysarthria are more complex and less well understood than those of flaccid dysarthria. This is partly a product of the complexity of the CNS motor pathways and the fact that spastic dysarthria is usually associated with damage to two components of the motor system, the direct and indirect activation pathways. In addition, the degree to which the concept of spasticity can be applied to the cranial nerve innervated portion of the speech system has been questioned (Abbs, Hunker, and Barlow, 1983; Abbs and Kennedy, 1982; Barlow and Abbs, 1984), as has the ability of spasticity in general to explain impaired motor performance (Landau, 1974).

Most of what we know about the clinical manifestations of spastic paralysis is based on studies of limb movement, which require the movement of joints in agonist and antagonistic relationships with each other. Many speech movements do not involve the movement of joints, and different speech structures have varying numbers of muscle spindles that are important in the mediation of stretch reflexes. For example, the jaw is well

Table 5–1 Direct and indirect activation pathway signs of UMN lesions.

Damage to	
Direct activation pathway (pyramidal tracts)	**Indirect activation pathway (extrapyramidal tracts)**
Loss of fine, → Increased muscle tone skilled movement	
Hypotonia → Clonus	
Weakness → Spasticity (distal > proximal)	
Absent abdominal reflexes	Decorticate or decerebrate posture
Babinski sign → Hyperactive stretch reflexes	
Hyporeflexia → Hyperactive gag reflex	

UMN, upper motor neuron.

endowed with spindles, the intrinsic muscles of the tongue have some, and the face has none (Barlow and Abbs, 1984). Furthermore, lip movements do not require the movement of bone, and the tongue is a muscular hydrostat the movements of which do not involve joints. Relatedly, it is likely that the different speech structures are affected in somewhat different ways by UMN lesions (Abbs, Hunker, and Barlow, 1983). Finally, unlike the limbs, speech requires symmetric movements of bilaterally innervated structures. That is, jaw, face, tongue, palate, and laryngeal movements require the synchronous movement of each of their halves so that the structures move as a single unit.

In spite of the differences between bulbar and limb movements, and uncertainty about the degree to which understanding spastic paralysis in the limbs can explain what occurs in the bulbar muscles during speech, it appears that, for practical clinical purposes at least, several of the *general* principles and observations about spastic paralysis discussed in the previous section can be usefully applied to our clinical conceptions of spastic dysarthria.

ETIOLOGIES

Spastic dysarthria can be caused by any process that damages the direct and indirect activation pathways of the CNS bilaterally. These include degenerative, inflammatory, toxic, metabolic, traumatic, and vascular diseases. These etiologic categories produce bilateral CNS motor system damage and spastic dysarthria with varying frequency,

although the exact distribution of causes of spastic dysarthria is unknown.

Although no general etiologic category is uniquely associated with spastic dysarthria, vascular disorders are more frequently associated with spastic dysarthria than with most other dysarthria types. A few of these disorders are discussed below. Other diseases that can produce spastic dysarthria but are more frequently associated with other dysarthria types (especially mixed dysarthrias) will be discussed in the chapters that deal with those specific dysarthrias.

Vascular disorders

Infarcts in the distribution of the internal carotid and middle and posterior cerebral arteries, and less frequently the anterior cerebral artery, can produce spastic dysarthria. However, because these arteries mostly supply structures within the cortex and subcortical structures of the cerebral hemispheres—where the UMN pathways on the left and right are not in close proximity to one another—lesions in both the left and right hemisphere are required to produce the bilateral UMN damage associated with spastic dysarthria. In the brain stem, where the right and left UMN pathways are in close proximity to one another, a single infarct in the vertebrobasilar arterial distribution may be sufficient to produce the bilateral UMN damage required for spastic dysarthria. In general, therefore, *a single brainstem stroke can produce a spastic dysarthria, whereas a single cerebral hemisphere stroke cannot.*

Some patients with spastic dysarthria have had multiple *lacunes* or *lacunar infarcts,* small deep infarcts in the small penetrating arteries of the basal ganglia, thalamus, brain stem, and deep cerebral white matter.* They are nearly always associated with hypertension. *Lacunar state* is a term applied to patients with numerous lacunar infarcts who frequently have dementia, dysarthria (frequently spastic), pseudobulbar affect, dysphagia, hyperreflexia, and incontinence (Bayles and Kaszniak, 1987).

Relatedly, *Binswanger's subcortical encephalopathy* is a term sometimes applied to patients with multiinfarct dementia. It occurs in individuals who have had multiple infarcts over months or years, and is often associated with hypertension or diabetes. The major lesions are in the subcortical white matter with relative sparing of cortex and basal ganglia. The bilateral lesions can affect UMN pathways and lead to spastic dysarthria. The

---

*Lacunar stroke syndromes are discussed in more detail in Chapter 9, Unilateral Upper Motor Neuron Dysarthria.

association of spastic dysarthria with dementia is an important diagnostic observation because dysarthria is not commonly associated with degenerative cortical dementias such as Alzheimer's and Pick's disease.

Inflammatory disease

Leukoencephalitis is characterized by inflammation of the white matter of the brain or spinal cord. In acute *hemorrhagic leukoencephalitis* the white matter of both hemispheres is destroyed, with similar changes in the brainstem and cerebellar peduncles. This destruction is associated with necrosis of small blood vessels and surrounding brain tissue, with inflammatory reactions in the meninges. There is a tendency for large focal lesions to form in the cerebral hemispheres (Adams and Victor, 1991). The bilateral and multifocal effects of this white matter disease can affect UMN pathways and cause spastic dysarthria (or mixed dysarthrias).

Degenerative disease

Primary lateral sclerosis (PLS) is a rarely occurring subcategory of motor neuron disease (of which amyotropic lateral sclerosis [ALS] is a major subcategory). It is manifest by corticospinal and corticobulbar tract signs alone, with no evidence of LMN involvement (Rowland, 1980). It usually begins in the fifth decade or later. It seems that dysarthria is very frequently present in PLS, and sometimes is the presenting problem (Pringle and others, 1992). Because clinical findings are limited to descending UMN tracts, it is presumed that the type of dysarthria is spastic. The distinction between PLS and ALS is of more than academic interest because the median disease duration until death for PLS (19 years, as reported by Pringle and others, 1992) is much longer than for ALS (only a few years). Because the dysarthria of PLS is presumably spastic only, the correct distinction between spastic and the mixed spastic-flaccid dysarthria often associated with ALS can be of some assistance to neurologic differential diagnosis.

SPEECH PATHOLOGY
Distribution of etiologies, lesions, and severity in clinical practice

The box on page 132 summarizes the etiologies for 107 quasirandomly selected cases seen at the Mayo Clinic with a primary speech pathology diagnosis of spastic dysarthria. The cautions expressed in Chapter 4 about generalizing these observations to the general population or all speech pathology practices apply here as well.

The data establish that spastic dysarthria can result from a number of medical conditions, the distribution of which are quite different from that associated with flaccid dysarthria. Over 90% of the cases were accounted for by vascular, degenerative, traumatic, demyelinating, and undetermined etiologies. Over 60% were accounted for by vascular and degenerative etiologies.

Nonhemorrhagic strokes accounted for most of the vascular causes. This is not surprising because nonhemorrhagic strokes account for the highest proportion of neurovascular disturbances in general. Many patients in this group had multiple strokes and most with only a single stroke had a brainstem lesion. Those with only a single confirmed (by computed tomography [CT] or magnetic resonance imaging [MRI]) stroke in one of the cerebral hemispheres had nonspeech clinical signs and symptoms of bilateral involvement, suggesting the presence of "silent" or undetected infarcts or other neuropathology in the "intact" hemisphere or brain stem.

A few patients with a neurologic diagnosis of stroke had no identifiable lesion on CT or MRI, and a few had neuroimaging data and nonspeech clinical findings of only unilateral UMN involvement. This suggests that *spastic dysarthria may be the only evidence of bilateral pathology in some individuals,* or that characteristics of spastic dysarthria can sometimes be encountered with unilateral UMN lesions.*

The localization of infarcts associated with spastic dysarthria was widespread within the UMN system, and included the cortex (usually posterior frontal lobe), the centrum semiovale, internal capsule, basal ganglia, pons, and medulla, bilaterally. Degenerative diseases associated with spastic dysarthria were usually unspecified. It is not unusual for neurodegenerative disease to defy a more specific diagnosis, especially early in the course of the disease; this sometimes remains the case until autopsy. ALS and progressive supranuclear palsy (PSP) were the most commonly diagnosed neurodegenerative diseases. It should be noted, however, that ALS and PSP can be associated with other dysarthria types and very frequently with mixed dysarthrias. (PSP and ALS will be discussed further in Chapter 10). PLS was the clinical neurologic diagnosis for a few patients in the sample.

Traumatic brain injury (TBI) was a fairly frequent cause of spastic dysarthria. Yorkston, Beukelman, and Bell (1988) indicate that ataxic, flaccid, and mixed flaccid-spastic and spastic-ataxic

---

*In the author's experience, apparent spastic dysarthria in cases of presumed unilateral stroke, with no other clinical evidence of bilateral pathology, is encountered most frequently early postonset of a single unilateral stroke. If true, the reasons for this occurrence are unclear.

ETIOLOGIES OF SPASTIC DYSARTHRIA FOR 107 QUASIRANDOMLY SELECTED CASES WITH A PRIMARY SPEECH PATHOLOGY DIAGNOSIS OF SPASTIC DYSARTHRIA AT THE MAYO CLINIC FROM 1969–90. PERCENTAGE OF CASES UNDER EACH BROAD ETIOLOGIC HEADING IS GIVEN IN PARENTHESES.

Vascular (31%)
Nonhemorrhagic stroke (single or multiple) (27%)
Ruptured aneurysm (2%)
Hemorrhagic stroke (1%)
Hypoxic encephalopathy (1%)

Degenerative (30%)
Unspecified degenerative CNS disease (14%)
Amyotrophic lateral sclerosis (9%)
Progressive supranuclear palsy (5%)
Primary lateral sclerosis (2%)

Traumatic (12%)
Traumatic brain injury (10%)
Neurosurgical (for example, tumor resection) (2%)

Undetermined (12%)
Undetermined CNS disease (7%)
Stroke vs ALS (2%)
Indeterminate pontine lesion; leukoencephalopathy; pseudobulbar palsy (3%)

Demyelinating (6%)
Multiple sclerosis

Tumor (4%)
CNS tumor (3%)
Paraneoplastic syndrome (1%)

Multiple causes (3%)
Stroke + dementia; tumor + radiation therapy; TBI + alcoholism + PSP

Inflammatory (2%)
Inflammatory brainstem disorder; postencephalitic

Infectious (1%)
Infectious encephalopathy

CNS, central nervous system.
ALS, amyotropic lateral sclerosis.
TBI, traumatic brain injury.
PSP, progressive supranuclear palsy.

---

dysarthria have been reported in patients with TBI. However, the occurrence of isolated spastic dysarthria in TBI in the sample reviewed here is not surprising given the frequent occurrence of bilateral, multifocal, and diffuse brain injury in TBI. Trauma from intracranial surgery is another possible traumatic cause of spastic dysarthria.

A number of patients had spastic dysarthria of indeterminate etiology. Some of them had several possible diagnoses (for example, stroke versus ALS) or diagnoses compatible with bilateral UMN involvement. Two patients had only dysarthria and dysphagia; they received a diagnosis of pseudobulbar palsy, a descriptive but not an etiologic diagnosis.

Several patients had multiple sclerosis (MS) (to be discussed in Chapter 10). A few had tumors. CNS tumors, particularly if localized in the brain stem, can cause spastic dysarthria, as can unilateral hemispheric tumors if they exert mass effects on the brain stem or opposite hemisphere. Only a few patients had inflammatory or infectious disorders.

The data also illustrate that spastic dysarthria can arise from multiple causes or events in the same patient (for example, stroke plus atrophy associated with dementing illness; TBI plus alcoholism plus PSP). This observation is important because some patients being evaluated for a condition that ordinarily might not be associated with spastic dysarthria might develop it because their current illness is added to the effects of a prior or concurrent condition. It is not unusual, for example, to discover in a patient who has developed signs of unilateral stroke and spastic dysarthria that there is a history of prior stroke on the opposite side of the brain (with or without speech disturbance).

The distribution of lesions for the cases summarized in the box on page 132 was widespread through the UMN system, including the *cortex, corona radiata, basal ganglia, internal capsule, pons,* and *medulla.* Focal lesions were most obvious when the etiology was vascular. Generalized or diffuse atrophy was frequently the only evidence of CNS damage in TBI, degenerative disease, and undetermined etiologies. About one-fourth of the patients had no evidence of cerebral pathology on neuroimaging studies. It is important to note that the only clinical sign of bilateral pathology in some patients was their spastic dysarthria and frequently accompanying dysphagia and pathologic oral reflexes. Many of these patients, however, did have neuroimaging evidence of bilateral or diffuse pathology.

This retrospective review did not permit a precise delineation of dysarthria severity. However, in the sample of 107 patients reviewed in the box on page 132 intelligibility was specifically commented upon in 77%; in those cases, *54% were judged to have reduced intelligibility.* The degree to which this figure accurately estimates intelligibility impairments in the population with spastic dysarthria is unclear. It is likely that many patients for whom an observation of intelligibility was not made had normal intelligibility; however, the sample probably contains a larger number of mildly impaired patients than is encountered in a typical rehabilitation setting.

Finally, because of its association with bilateral, multifocal or diffuse CNS disease, it is not usual for spastic dysarthria to be accompanied by cognitive disturbances that may include dementia or cognitive-communication deficits associated with right hemisphere impairment, TBI, and aphasia. For the patients in this sample whose cognitive abilities were explicitly judged or formally assessed (72% of the sample), *43% had some impairment of cognitive ability.*

Patient perceptions and complaints

Patients with spastic dysarthria often offer complaints or descriptions that provide clues or confirmatory evidence for the speech diagnosis and its localization. Some of these are only infrequently associated with other dysarthria types.

A frequent complaint is that speech is *slow* or *effortful.* When asked, patients will often confirm that it feels as if they are speaking against resistance. The descriptors, "slow" and "effortful," are not often heard from patients with other dysarthria types (with the exception of several forms of hyperkinetic dysarthria). They often will complain of *fatigue* with speaking, sometimes with accompanying deterioration of speech. With the exception of myasthenia gravis, the complaint of fatigue occurs more frequently in spastic than flaccid dysarthria, even though deterioration of speech in spastic dysarthria is not usually dramatic and almost never rapid.* Patients also often note that they must speak more slowly to be understood, but may admit that they really are unable to speak any faster. Finally, they often complain of *"nasal"* speech; this complaint is heard more frequently in patients with flaccid dysarthria.

Swallowing complaints are common and often can be associated with both oral and pharyngeal phases of swallowing.† In some patients, a precursor to dysphagia and evidence of a lowered gag reflex threshold is increased susceptibility to gagging when brushing teeth. Patients will also complain of *drooling,* moreso than for most other single dysarthria types. Finally, many patients with spastic dysarthria will complain of *difficulty controlling their expression of emotion,* especially laughter and crying. This "pseudobulbar effect" is rarely encountered in other single dysarthria types. It will be discussed in more detail in the next section.

Clinical findings

Spastic dysarthria is often associated with bilateral motor signs and symptoms in the arms and legs

---

*Fatigue is a common complaint in patients with spastic paresis of the limbs and is usually assumed to be of CNS origin, secondary to impaired recruitment of alpha motoneurons. However, there is also some evidence that biochemical changes in muscles of patients with UMN lesions may contribute to excessive fatigability (Miller and others, 1990). The etiology of the muscle changes may be due to partial immobilization and disuse. That there is reduced muscle volume and weight following a period of disuse has been demonstrated by Duchateau and Hainaut (1987).

†In degenerative or gradually developing neurologic disease, speech and swallowing problems very often emerge concurrently. In the author's experience, which may be subject to referral bias, when one preceds the other, speech difficulty tends to develop first.

that make the presence of bilateral CNS involvement obvious.* However, it can occur in the absence of bilateral or even unilateral limb findings and may, sometimes along with dysphagia and pathologic oral reflexes, be the only sign of neurologic disease. This is not unusual in certain degenerative nervous system diseases.

Bilateral spastic paralysis affecting the bulbar muscles traditionally has been called *pseudobular palsy*. Many neurologists use the term to describe the speech of spastic dysarthria. Pseudobulbar palsy is a clinical syndrome that derives its name from its superficial resemblance to bulbar palsy (associated with LMN lesions and flaccid dysarthria). It reflects bilateral lesions of corticobulbar fibers and is most commonly associated with multiple or bilateral stokes, CNS trauma, degenerative CNS disease, encephalopathies, and CNS tumors. Its clinical features include dysarthria, dysphagia, and other oral mechanism abnormalities that will be discussed below.

Nonspeech oral mechanism. Several oral mechanism findings are frequently associated with spastic dysarthria. *Dysphagia* is common and may be severe. Although some patients will deny chewing or swallowing difficulties, on questioning they may admit that they must be careful when swallowing, that chewing meat has become more difficult, or that they chew more slowly or more carefully than before. Nasal regurgitation is unusual in pure spastic dysarthria.

Drooling is common, and patients often attribute it to excessive saliva production; it is more likely due to decreased frequency of swallowing or poor control of secretions. It may occur when the patient concentrates on some nonspeech activity, particularly if the neck is flexed (for example, during writing). Patients with or without daytime drooling will sometimes note that their pillow is wet upon awakening in the morning or that saliva has dried around the mouth during the night. Reflexive swallowing of secretions may be characterized by obviously slowed jaw, lip, and facial movement, sometimes to a degree that appears effortful; occasionally it is audible.

At rest, the nasolabial folds may be smoothed or flattened or the face may be held in a somewhat fixed, subtle smiling or pouting posture. Reflexive or emotional facial responses are frequently slowly emergent but may then overflow and be excessive.

Patients with spastic dysarthria frequently exhibit lability of affect, often called *pseudobulbar affect* or *pathological laughing and crying*. When subtle, the patient may have an "on the verge of tears" facial expression. When more obvious, they may cry or laugh in a stereotypic manner for no apparent reason, may fluctuate between laughing and crying, and may have difficulty inhibiting laughter and crying once they begin. The ease with which the response is elicited tends to be related to the emotional loading of the interaction, but the emotional response may occur spontaneously or simply when the patients are asked if they have difficulty controlling emotional expression. Patients often report that their inner emotional state does not match their physical expression of emotion. The behaviors can occur during speech, sometimes with significant effects on intelligibility or efficiency of communication. Pseudobulbar affect can convey an impression of emotional instability or dementia, but may occur without any clear evidence of those disorders, and sometimes without other evidence of pseudobular palsy (Asfora and others, 1989), including dysarthria. These uncontrollable emotional responses are often extremely upsetting to patients. Aronson (1990) points out that "the reduced threshold for crying and laughter has clinical diagnostic importance and needs to be recognized as one of the great social and psychological burdens borne by patients with pseudobulbar palsy" (p. 92).

Examination of nonspeech oromotor functions usually demonstrates normal jaw strength. The face may be weak bilaterally and range of lip retraction and pursing may be decreased; however, lower facial weakness is usually not as pronounced as with LMN lesions. The tongue is usually full and symmetric but range of movement may be reduced and weakness apparent on strength testing. Nonspeech alternating motion rates (AMRs) for jaw, lip retraction and pursing, and lateral or anterior tongue movements are often slow and reduced in range of movement, but are generally regular in rhythm.

The palate is usually symmetric but may move slowly or minimally on phonation. The gag reflex is often hyperactive. The cough and glottal coup may be normal in sharpness if respiratory and laryngeal movements are not too slowed, but they may be weak if slowness is prominent.

Pathologic oral reflexes are common. *Positive sucking, snout, and jaw jerk reflexes* are frequently present and are suggestive of bilateral UMN involvement.

Speech. Conversational speech and reading, speech AMRs, and vowel prolongation are the most useful tasks for eliciting the salient and

---

*Unilateral UMN lesions produce a syndrome of signs and symptoms that affect movements on the contralateral side of the body. This syndrome sometimes includes unilateral UMN dysarthria, a dysarthria that is distinguishable from spastic dysarthria. Unilateral UMN dysarthria is discussed in Chapter 9.

Table 5–2 Neuromuscular deficits associated with spastic dysarthria.

Direction	Rhythm	Rate		Range		Force	Tone
Individual movements	**Repetitive movements**	**Individual movements**	**Repetitive movements**	**Individual movements**	**Repetitive movements**	**Individual movements**	**Muscle tone**
Normal	Regular	Slow	Slow	Reduced (weak)	Reduced biased	Reduced	Excessive

Adapted from Darley FL, Aronson AE, and Brown JR: Clusters of deviant speech dimensions in the dysarthrias, J Speech Hearing Res 12:462, 1969b.

distinguishing characteristics of spastic dysarthria. Speech stress testing and sequential motion rates (SMRs) are not particularly revealing.

The deviant speech characteristics associated with spastic dysarthria are not easily described by listing each cranial nerve and the speech characteristics associated with its abnormal function. This is because spastic dysarthria is associated with *impaired movement patterns rather than weakness of individual muscles.* This reflects the organization of CNS motor pathways for the control of movement patterns rather than isolated muscle movements, and it represents an important distinction between LMN and UMN lesions. Therefore, spastic dysarthria is usually associated with deficits at all of the speech valves and for all components of the speech system, although not always equally. The involvement of multiple speech valves may explain why intelligibility is so frequently affected.

Table 5–2 summarizes the neuromuscular deficits assumed by Darley, Aronson, and Brown (1969a and b, 1975) to underlie spastic dysarthria. In general, direction and rhythm or timing of movement are unaffected. The chief disturbances are *slowness and reduced range of individual and repetitive movements, reduced force of movement, and excessive or biased muscle tone or spasticity.* The bias of muscle tone is most apparent at the laryngeal valve, in which the bias is toward hyperadduction during phonation, and the velopharyngeal valve, in which bias is toward reduced velopharyngeal closure. The relationship between these neuromuscular deficits and the prominent deviant clusters and speech characteristics of spastic dysarthria will become apparent in subsequent description of those characteristics. Experimental support for the presumed underlying neuromuscular deficits, especially slowness and reduced range of movement, will be reviewed in the section on acoustic and physiologic studies.

Clusters of deviant dimensions and prominent deviant speech characteristics. Darley, Aronson, and Brown (1969b) found four clusters of deviant dimensions in their group of 30 patients

Table 5–3 Deviant clusters of abnormal speech characteristics in spastic dysarthria.

Cluster	Speech characteristics
Prosodic excess	Excess & equal stress Slow rate
Articulatory-resonatory incompetence	Imprecise consonants Distorted vowels Hypernasality
Prosodic insufficiency	Monopitch Monoloudness Reduced stress Short phrases
Phonatory stenosis	Low pitch Harshness Strained-strangled voice Pitch breaks Short phrases Slow rate

Based on Darley FL, Aronson AE, and Brown JR: Clusters of deviant speech dimensions in the dysarthrias, J Speech Hearing Res 12:462, 1969b.

with pseudobulbar palsy. These clusters are useful to understanding the neuromuscular deficits that seem to underlie spastic dysarthria, the components of the speech system that are most prominently involved, and the features of spastic dysarthria that distinguish it from other dysarthria types (see Table 5–3).

The first cluster is *prosodic excess,* represented by *excess and equal stress* and *slow rate* of speech. These characteristics are probably related to slowness of individual and repetitive movements. Slowness of movement logically reduces speech rate. It probably also contributes to excess and equal stress by reducing the speed of the muscular adjustments necessary for the rapid pitch, loudness, and durational adjustments associated with normal speech stress patterns. Slow overall speech rate may also lead to a perception of excess and equalized stress because longer syllable duration is associated with stressed syllables.

The second cluster is *articulatory-resonatory incompetence,* represented by *imprecise consonants, distorted vowels,* and *hypernasality.* This cluster represents the probable effects of reduced range and force of articulatory movements (presumably including the lips, tongue, jaw, and face) and velopharyngeal movements. The strong interrelationships among velopharyngeal and articulatory features in this cluster implicate the velopharyngeal mechanism's articulatory role, not its resonatory role (that is, inadequate velopharyngeal closure results in weak, imprecise pressure consonants).

The third cluster is *prosodic insufficiency,* consisting of *monopitch, monoloudness, reduced stress,* and *short phrases.* For the most part, these characteristics are attributable to reduced vocal variability, with stressed syllables left unstressed or insufficiently different from unstressed syllables, and reduced pitch and loudness variability. Darley, Aronson, and Brown felt decreased range of movement was the most likely explanation for this cluster.

The fourth cluster is *phonatory stenosis,* characterized by *low pitch, harshness, strained-strangled voice, pitch breaks, short phrases,* and *slow rate.* These phonatory characteristics seem to reflect efforts to produce voice through a narrowed glottis with secondary reduction of phrase length and speech rate. The assumption is that laryngeal hypotonus is present with a bias toward excessive adduction or resistance to abduction. The features of slow rate and short phrases may also be related to slowness of movement and inefficient valving at the velopharyngeal and articulatory valves.

Darley, Aronson, and Brown also noted the presence of *breathiness* in patients with spastic dysarthria, a characteristic that was uncorrelated with any of the clusters found for the disorder. This breathiness could reflect a degree of vocal-cord weakness, but could also represent a compensatory response rather than a primary problem. For example, some patients may actively maintain incomplete adduction to prevent laryngeal stenosis, or, alternatively, may intermittently actively abduct the cords to facilitate exhalation or provide relief from the effort induced by laryngeal stenosis.

Table 5–4 summarizes the most deviant speech dimensions found by Darley, Aronson, and Brown (1969a). It should be noted that the rankings in Table 5–4 represent the order of prominence (severity) of the speech characteristics, and not the features that are most distinctive of spastic dysarthria. For example, imprecise consonants, although rated as the most severely impaired characteristic in spastic dysarthria, is found in all major dysarthria types and, therefore, is not a *distinguishing* characteristic of spastic dysarthria.

A number of studies support Darley, Aronson, and Brown's identification of slow rate as a pervasive and perceptually salient feature of spastic dysarthria. For example, Kammermeier (1969, as summarized by Darley, Aronson, and Brown, 1975), found a mean reading rate of 104 words per minute in patients with spastic dysarthria, slower than those with bulbar palsy, Parkinson's disease, cerebellar disease, and dystonia. Slow speech

Table 5–4 The most deviant speech dimensions encountered in spastic dysarthria by Darley, Aronson, and Brown (1969a), listed in order from most to least severe. Also listed is the component of the speech system associated with the deviant speech characteristics. The component "prosodic" is listed when several components of the speech system may contribute to the dimension.

Dimension	Speech component
Imprecise consonants*	Articulatory
Monopitch	Laryngeal
Reduced stress	Prosodic
Harshness*	Laryngeal
Monoloudness	Laryngeal-respiratory
Low pitch*	Laryngeal
Slow rate*	Articulatory-prosodic
Hypernasality	Velopharyngeal
Strained-strangled quality*	Laryngeal
Short phrases*	Laryngeal-respiratory-velopharyngeal or articulatory
Distorted vowels	Articulatory
Pitch breaks*	Laryngeal
Breathy voice (continuous)	Laryngeal
Excess and equal stress	Prosodic

*Tend to be distinctive or more severely impaired in spastic dysarthria than any other single dysarthria type.

AMRs have been documented in several studies (Dworkin and Aronson, 1986; Hirose, 1986; Portnoy and Aronson, 1982). In studies in which comparisons have been made to other dysarthria types, patients with spastic dysarthria have had the slowest AMRs. Linebaugh and Wolfe (1984) documented slow rate of syllable production in spastic dysarthria, as well as a moderate relationship between rate and intelligibility and speech naturalness ratings.

What features of spastic dysarthria help distinguish it from other types of motor speech disorders? Among all of the characteristics that may be detected in spastic dysarthria, *strained-strangled voice quality, slow speech rate, and slow and regular speech AMRs are the most distinctive clues to the presence of spastic dysarthria.*

Table 5–5 summarizes the primary distinguishing speech characteristics and common oral mechanism exam and patient complaints encountered in spastic dysarthria.

Acoustic and physiologic findings

Acoustic and physiologic studies of acquired spastic dysarthria have been limited, with relatively greater attention having been paid to children and adults with cerebral palsy. This brief summary will focus primarily on acoustic and physiologic studies of acquired spastic dysarthria. The results of these studies are summarized in Table 5–6. Figure 5–1 illustrates some acoustic correlates of perceived slow and regular AMRs and Figure 5–2 illustrates some acoustic correlates of perceived slow connected speech rate and prosodic abnormalities commonly associated with spastic dysarthria.

Respiration. Little is known about speech-related respiratory characteristics of acquired spastic dysarthria. It is quite possible, however, that they bear a resemblance to some of the documented respiratory difficulties of children and adults with spastic cerebral palsy. These abnormalities include reduced inhalatory and exhalatory respiratory volumes leading to shallow breathing; paradoxical breathing, in which abdominal muscles fail to relax during inhalation, with resultant opposition to abdominal lowering and restriction of respiratory intake; and reduced vital capacity (Aronson, 1990; Darley, Aronson, and Brown, 1975).

The degree to which respiratory anomalies affect speech in spastic dysarthria is unclear. Complicating its understanding is the fact that laryngeal valve hyperadduction is nearly always present, so even normal expiratory capacity must work against laryngeal resistance to air flow. In some cases, efforts to overcome severe glottic constriction during speech are so great that the speaker will seek momentary relief by suddenly releasing a considerable quantity of air. The result is intermittent breathiness and air wastage that sometimes leads to reduced utterance length per breath group (Aronson, 1990). Therefore, deviations of respiratory activity in spastic dysarthria may reflect the primary effects of underlying respiratory deficits but also secondary effects from abnormal laryngeal (and possibly resonatory and articulatory) activities as well.

Laryngeal function. Laryngeal examination may reveal normal-appearing vocal cords at rest, although Ziegler and von Cramon (1986) have reported incomplete abduction during respiration. Bilateral hyperadduction of the true and false vocal cords during speech may be apparent (Aronson, 1990; Ziegler and von Cramon, 1986).

Kammermeier (1969, as reported by Darley, Aronson, and Brown, 1975) reported decreased pitch variability in a group of males with pseudobulbar palsy. Fundamental frequency was lower in comparison to other dysarthria groups, but was still within the normal range for males. These findings lend support to the perception of monopitch by Darley, Aronson, and Brown, but not to their finding of low pitch. Fortunately, the presence of monopitch seems more salient than low pitch to the differential diagnosis of spastic dysarthria.

Velopharyngeal function. On oral inspection, the palate may appear to move sluggishly or not at all during vowel prolongation. Palatal immobility, slow movement, and incomplete velopharyngeal closure may be apparent on videofluoroscopy and

Table 5–5 Primary distinguishing speech and speech-related findings in spastic dysarthria.

Perceptual
Phonation
Strained-strangled voice quality

Articulation-Prosody
Slow rate
Slow & regular AMRs

Physical
Dysphagia, drooling
Weak face & tongue
Pathological reflexes (suck, snout, jaw jerk)
Pseudobulbar affect

Patient complaints
Slow speech rate
Increased effort to speak
Fatigue when speaking
Swallowing-chewing difficulty
Poor control of emotional expression

Table 5–6 Summary of acoustic and physiologic findings in studies of spastic dysarthria.*

Speech component	Acoustic or physiologic observation

Respiratory (or respiratory/laryngeal) (based on studies of spastic cerebral palsy)	Reduced:
	    Inhalatory & exhalatory volumes (shallow breathing)
	    Respiratory intake
	    Vital capacity
	    Rate of amplitude variations
	Poor visuomotor tracking with respiratory movements

Laryngeal	Decreased:
	    Vocal cord abduction during respiration
	    Fundamental frequency variability
	    Hyperadduction of true & false cords during speech
	    Poor visuomotor tracking with pitch variations

Velopharyngeal	Increased pharyngeal constriction Slow, sluggish velopharyngeal movement Incomplete velopharyngeal closure

Articulatory/rate/prosody	Reduced:
	    Completeness of articulatory contacts
	    Completeness of consonant clusters
	    Speed and range of tongue movement
	    Range of jaw movement
	    Acceleration & deceleration of articulators
	    Tongue strength
	    Articulatory effort for final word stress
	    Frequency & intensity increases for initial word stress
	    SPL contrasts in consonants
	    Voice-onset-time for stops
	    Amplitude of release bursts for stops
	    Overall speech rate
	Increased:
	    Syllable & word durations
	    Duration of nonphonated intervals
	    Spirantization during stops
	    Prolonged phonemes
	    Slow phoneme-to-phoneme transitions
	    Centralization of vowel formants
	    Voicing of voiceless stops

*Note that many of these observations are based on studies of only one or a few speakers and that not all speakers with spastic dysarthria will exhibit these features. Note also that these characteristics may not be unique to spastic dysarthria; some may also be found in other motor speech disorders or nonneurologic conditions.

nasendoscopy studies. Ziegler and von Cramon (1986) noted the tendency of some of their spastic subjects to voice voiceless stops. They speculated that such distortions may be facilitated by incomplete velopharyngeal and oral cavity contacts that prevent interruption of phonation, even if vocal cord capacity is normal. This explanation was supported by one of their subject's ability to produce voiceless stops when air wastage through the velopharyngeal port was decreased with a nose clamp. This observation illustrates the interactions at different levels of the speech system that may affect articulatory outcomes (note that the rapid laryngeal adjustments necessary for producing

voiceless consonants may represent another source of voicing errors).

Articulation, rate, and prosody. Several studies have documented slowness and reduced range of movement of the tongue, (Hirose, Kiritani, and Sawashima, 1982a & b; Kent, Netsell, and Bauer, 1975). A study by Kent, Netsell, and Bauer (1975) illustrates the physiologic approaches and results of such studies. They studied tongue, lip, jaw, and velar movement in normal and dysarthric speakers using cineradiography, with small radiopaque markers placed on the tongue and lip. Although not described by dysarthria type, it is likely that two of their subjects had spastic dysar-

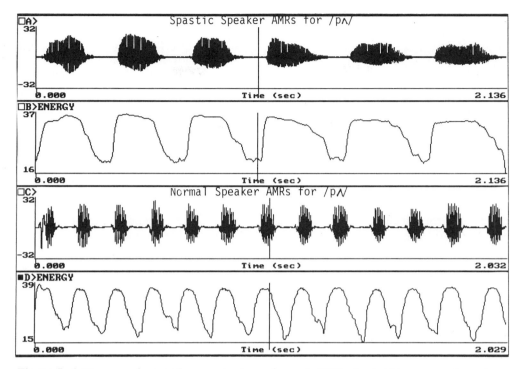

Figure 5–1 Raw waveform and energy tracings of speech AMRs for /pʌ/ by a normal speaker (bottom two panels) and a speaker with spastic dysarthria. The Normal Speaker's AMRs are normal in rate (∼ 6.5 Hz) and relatively regular in duration and amplitude. In contrast, the Spastic Speaker's are very slow (∼ 3.0 Hz) and regular. These attributes represent the acoustic correlates of perceived slow and regular AMRs that are common in spastic dysarthria.

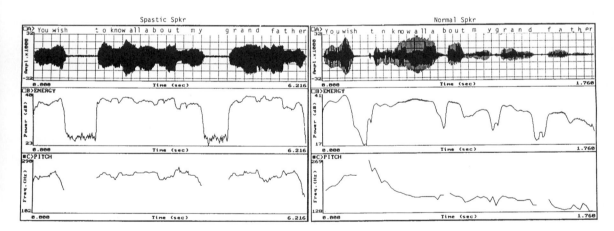

Figure 5–2 Raw waveform and energy and pitch (f$_o$) tracings for the sentence "You wish to know all about my grandfather" by a normal female speaker (tracings on right) and a female speaker with spastic dysarthria (tracings on left).

The Normal Speaker completes the sentence in < 2 secs with normal variability in syllable duration and amplitude (energy tracing), and normal variability and declination in f$_o$ across the sentence (picth tracing).

In contrast, the Spastic Speaker is very slow (∼ 6.2 secs for the utterance). The silent breaks evident in all tracings between "wish" and "to" and between "my" and "grandfather" are considerably lengthened and reflect slowness in achieving and releasing stop closure for 't' and 'g', respectively. Other portions of the utterance in the energy and pitch tracings show little syllable distinctiveness, reflecting continuous voicing and restricted loudness and pitch variability. These acoustic attributes reflect the perceptible slow rate and monopitch and monoloudness that are characteristic of many speakers with spastic dysarthria.

thria. Results documented slowness and decreased range of movement for the tongue and palate. One of the two subjects had adequate range of jaw movement whereas the other had limited jaw movement. Hirose (1986) has also documented slowed jaw and tongue movements and reduced range of tongue movements in a patient with spastic dysarthria.

Acoustic studies have found evidence for prolongation of phonemes, slow transitions from one phoneme to another, increased syllable and word durations, slow speech AMRs, centralization of vowel formants (indicating restricted range of movement), reduced rate of amplitude variations, increased duration of nonphonated intervals, and reduced overall speech rate (Dworkin and Aronson, 1986; Hirose, 1986; Kammermeier, 1969 (as summarized by Darley, Aronson, and Brown, 1975); Linebaugh and Wolfe, 1984; Portnoy and Aronson, 1982; Ziegler and von Cramon, 1986). All of these findings provide evidence of slowness of movement or reduced range of movement during speech.

Several other acoustic attributes provide evidence of imprecise articulation that may be related to slowness, reduced range of movement, or weakness at the articulatory, velopharyngeal, or laryngeal valves. These attributes include reduced sharpness of voiceless stops with a tendency toward voicing and reduced sound pressure level (SPL) contrasts in consonants (Alajouanine, Sabouraud, and Gremy, 1959, as summarized by Darley, Aronson, and Brown, 1975; Ziegler and von Cramon, 1986). Ziegler and von Cramon (1986) attributed reduced SPL differences to inadequate voicing and hypernasality, as well as to the presence of friction noise (spirantization) with decreased amplitude of release bursts during production of stops. They also noted that adequate production of stops and vowels was usually accomplished at the expense of articulatory rate.

Physiologic studies also provide evidence for imprecision and reduced fine motor control. Hardcastle, Barry, and Clark (1985) used electropalatography and pneumotachography to examine tongue-palate contacts and voice onset time (VOT) in one subject with spastic dysarthria. Patterns of articulatory contact were generally incomplete, sequences of consonant clusters were often reduced or incomplete, and VOT for voiceless stops were shorter than normal or characterized by spirantization. Dworkin and Aronson (1986) found reduced tongue strength in speakers with spastic dysarthria, although not disproportionately in comparison to individuals with other dysarthria types.

In a nonspeech visuomotor tracking study, McClean, Beukelman, and Yorkston (1987) required subjects to track a sinusoidal wave with lower-lip and jaw movement (using strain gauge tranducers), respiratory activity (by transducing air pressure changes in a face mask), and laryngeal activity (by altering fundamental frequency). Their one subject with spastic dysarthria had subnormal levels of respiratory tracking and greatly reduced tracking with the larynx, but normal control of the jaw and lip. These observations suggest that spastic dysarthria may be associated with fine motor control difficulties that may vary across levels of the speech system.

A few additional studies have found differential effects among speech structures. For example, Ziegler and von Cramon (1986), in an acoustic analysis of consonant-vowel-consonant (CVC) sequences, found disproportionate impairment of tongue-back movements relative to tongue-blade movements. Several studies have found relative preservation of range and control of jaw movement (Hirose, 1986; McClean, Beukelman, and Yorkston 1987). Hirose (1986) speculated that the relative preservation of jaw movement may permit it to compensate to some degree for inadequate tongue and lip articulatory movements.

Slow speech rate helps explain the presence of prosodic abnormalities in spastic dysarthria, but few investigations have examined vocal-stress patterns. Murry (1983) tested the ability of five individuals with spastic dysarthria to vary stress during multiple productions of three-word sentences in which stress was to be placed on varying words. Peak intraoral pressure, integrated pressure time (duration of the pressure pulse), fundamental frequency, vowel duration, and vowel intensity were measured. Normal subjects showed expected stress patterns on all measures. In contrast, the spastic speakers conveyed phrase final word stress only with fundamental frequency and intensity changes and they generally imparted stress less adequately than normal. Stress appeared to be conveyed by compensation; for example, subjects seemed to use increased articulatory effort for phrase initial word stress. For final word stress, fundamental frequency and intensity increased but articulatory effort was compromised. Murry concluded that when spastic dysarthric subjects use consonant-related cues to stress a word, vowel-related cues are decreased relative to baseline (for initial word stress). For final word stress, they switch to a vowel strategy and reduce articulatory effort. They did not generally use vowel duration cues to vary stress in any position.

CASES

Case 5.1

A 65-year-old woman presented to neurology with a six-month history of "slurred speech" and dysphagia. Prior history was unremarkable, except for hypertension that did not require medication. Her initial difficulty with swallowing was greater for liquids than solids, and had progressed to a point where she had extreme difficulty with liquids. However, she had not lost weight nor had she had difficulty with aspiration or nasal regurgitation. A short time after her dysphagia developed, she noted speech difficulty, which also had gradually progressed. She had been placed on Mestinon for myasthenia gravis by a neurologist at another institution, without benefit.

The neurologic exam, beyond her speech difficulty and dysphagia, revealed mild bilateral facial weakness and bilaterally increased deep tendon and Babinski reflexes. AMRs of arms and legs were diminished slightly on the left. Laboratory tests were essentially normal, as were screenings for hereditary demyelinating syndromes. Nerve conduction studies and EMG were normal, including EMG examination of the tongue. MRI of the head was normal.

During speech examination, the patient said she initially attributed her swallowing difficulty to her dentures. At onset, her tongue felt "thick" and she was aware of a "nasal tone" to her voice. Psychologic stress and prolonged speaking made speech worse. She admitted to occasionally biting her cheek when chewing; food sometimes squirreled in her cheeks. She had compensated by chewing more slowly and eating smaller amounts to prevent choking. She admitted to difficulty controlling emotional expression.

She frequently had an "on the verge of crying" facial expression. Jaw strength was normal. The lower face was weak (−1) on voluntary lip retraction. The tongue was full and symmetric but lateral tongue movements were slow (−2,3). The tongue was moderately weak bilaterally, slightly more so on the left. The palate was symmetric and mobile. Gag reflex, cough, and glottal coup were normal. A sucking reflex was equivocally present.

Conversational speech and reading were characterized by: reduced rate (−2); monopitch and monoloudness (2); strained-harsh-groaning voice quality (1,2); occasional pitch breaks; hypernasality (0,1); and imprecise articulation (1,2). Prolonged "ah" was sustained for 11 seconds and was equivocally strained. Her speech AMRs were slow (−2,3) but regular. Intelligibility was judged normal in the quiet one-to-one setting but probably mildly compromised in noise.

Acoustic analysis showed fundamental frequency (242 Hz) and measures of jitter and shimmer to be grossly normal. Speech AMRs for /pʌ/, /tʌ/, and /kʌ/ were 2.8, 2.8, and 2.5 Hz, respectively. The clinician concluded: "Spastic dysarthria, suggestive of bilateral UMN involvement affecting the bulbar muscles. There are no clear-cut features of flaccid dysarthria, nor do I note characteristics that could be interpreted as ataxic." Speech therapy and management of her dysphagia were recommended.

The neurologist concluded that the patient had progressive UMN dysfunction of undetermined etiology, but wondered about primary lateral sclerosis. Reevaluation in 3 to 6 months was recommended. She has not yet been seen for follow-up.

Commentary. (1) Degenerative neurologic disease can present as dysarthria or dysphagia. (2) Diagnosis of spastic dysarthria places the lesion in the CNS, bilaterally, and can help to rule out disease isolated to LMNs (for example, myasthenia gravis). (3) It is not unusual for degenerative diseases in which spastic dysarthria and dysphagia are the primary signs to defy more specific neurologic diagnosis, and for neuroimaging studies to be normal.

Case 5.2

A 41-year-old right-handed man from Saudi Arabia was hospitalized for management of hypertension, and speech and swallowing difficulties. According to his family, he had fairly adequate English language skills.

The patient had a two-year history of hypertension for which he had refused to take medication. Eleven months ago, over the course of an evening, he developed left hemiplegia. Ten days later he lost consciousness and upon awakening 17 days later was unable to speak or swallow. His left hemiplegia persisted, but he had no motor signs on the right side of the body. With therapy his left-sided weakness improved, but swallowing and speech remained significantly impaired. He had been fed through a nasogastric tube, but more recently he had been eating blenderized foods while lying supine.

Neurologic exam revealed a left hemiparesis. Upper limb reflexes were hyperactive bilaterally, left greater than right. He was unable to speak. Questions were raised about whether the patient had an "expressive aphasia," or if a component of his speech difficulty was psychogenic. It was assumed that his lesion was unilateral (right).

On speech examination, he was nearly anarthric (without speech). He could produce a low volume, nasally emitted and resonated, strained-strangled undifferentiated vowel with great effort, but little else. With his lips closed he produced a prolonged and strained /m/. Lip and jaw movements were very slow and limited in range, but were more extensive during reflexive swallowing; the jaw opened widely during a reflexive yawn. Suck, snout, and jaw jerk reflexes were present. At rest, the tongue sat in a relatively retracted position. Tongue movement was minimal and slow; he was unable to extend it beyond the edge of the lower teeth and unable to elevate or move it laterally. The palate hung so low in the pharynx that the uvula could not be seen; a gag reflex could not be elicited. Surprisingly, his cough was sharp.

There was no evidence of language difficulty. He followed two-step commands and communicated effectively through writing, although with occasional spelling errors.

It was concluded that he had a "severe spastic dysarthria without any evidence of aphasia or apraxia of speech, and no clear evidence of a psychogenic contribution to his speechlessness. To produce a dysarthria like this, the lesion should be bilateral."

Subsequent CT scan revealed old infarcts in the centrum semiovale of both hemispheres, as well as an infarction in the right posterior parietal cortex (see Figure 5–3).

A brief period of speech therapy was undertaken but it was rapidly apparent that intelligible speech would not be achieved. It was noted that vocal loudness increased and hypernasality decreased when the palate was elevated from the surface of the tongue with a tongue depressor. A palatal lift prosthesis was made in the hope that it would make swallowing easier, but the weight of the velum on the device made it impossible to keep the prosthesis securely fastened. The patient underwent pharyngeal flap surgery and was then able to eat pureed food while sitting in an upright position, although it took two hours for him to complete a meal. He also was able to breathe orally. Writing was an effective, portable, but somewhat inefficient means of communication for him. He returned to his homeland before other means of augmentative communication could be thoroughly investigated.

Commentary. *(1) The presence of significant spastic dysarthria should raise questions about bilateral UMN involvement, even when limb findings suggest that the lesion is only unilateral. (2) Lesions do not have to be large to produce devastating consequences for speech. The patient's centrum semiovale lesions were small but their locus was sufficient to interrupt UMN pathways to the bulbar speech muscles bilaterally. (3) Severe spastic dysarthria is almost always accompanied by significant dysphagia. (4) Accurate diagnosis of the speech deficit helped to rule out aphasia as well as significant psychogenic influences. This information was useful in counseling the patient and family, particularly their understanding of the nature of the problem and*

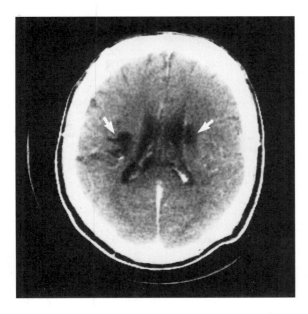

Figure 5–3 CT scan for Case 5.2. Relatively small infarcts in the centrum semiovale of both hemispheres (*arrows*) produced a severe spastic dysarthria.

their acceptance about limitations on future recovery of speech.

Case 5.3

A 71-year-old woman presented to Ear, Nose, and Throat (ENT) with a three-month history of "lost voice." Prior medical history was unremarkable. The only abnormality on ENT exam was decreased tongue mobility. "Neurologic dysphonia" and possible "lower motor neuron disease" was suspected. Speech pathology and neurology consultations were arranged.

During speech evaluation, the patient recalled that her progressing speech difficulty had been present for about 15 months. She complained that her voice was strained, that speech was slow, and that speaking was effortful. She had difficulty swallowing liquids, with occasional choking and very infrequent nasal regurgitation. She had not had to modify her diet nor had she lost weight. She denied change or difficulty controlling emotional expression, drooling, and difficulty with memory or other cognitive skills.

Speech AMRs of the jaw, lower face, and tongue were slow (−2) but regular. Jaw and lower face strength were normal; there was equivocal weakness of the left tongue. There was a very slight droop at the right corner of the mouth and a subtle "snarl" of the left upper lip at rest. The palate was symmetric and relatively immobile during vowel prolongation, but moved normally during gagging. Nasal emission was apparent during pressure sound production. Her cough was normal. Suck, snout, and jaw jerk reflexes were not detected.

Connected speech was characterized by a strained-harsh-groaning voice quality (2), reduced rate (−1,2), hypernasality (1,2), imprecise articulation (1), and monopitch and monoloudness (1,2). Lip and jaw movements were slightly exaggerated during speech, possibly reflecting compensatory efforts to maintain intelligibility. Speech AMRs were slow (−2,3). "Ah" was sustained for only 6 seconds and was strained (3).

The clinician concluded, "Spastic dysarthria, moderately severe. No clear evidence of a flaccid (LMN) component. Speech characteristics are strongly suggestive of bilateral UMN dysfunction affecting the bulbar musculature." She was referred for speech therapy and management of her dysphagia, which she pursued closer to home.

Neurologic examination noted brisk muscle stretch reflexes, but there were no other pathologic reflexes. No fasciculations were detected. Subsequent EMG failed to identify fibrillations or fasciculation potentials. MRI of the head, with special attention to the brain stem, was normal. The neurologist concluded that the patient had a pseudobulbar palsy with spastic dysarthria plus very minimal findings in the upper limbs. ALS was suspected, but a diagnosis could not be confirmed. She was not seen for subsequent follow-up.

Commentary. *(1) Speech difficulty can be the presenting complaint in neurologic disease. (2) Spastic dysarthria can occur in the absence of other significant neurologic deficits and can progress without significant clinical findings in the limbs. (3) Spastic dysarthria is frequently accompanied by dysphagia. (4) Dysarthria* *affecting the bulbar musculature, in the absence of limb findings, is sometimes misinterpreted as LMN disease (frequently myasthenia gravis). Careful speech examination can help establish the presence of bilateral UMN involvement in such cases.*

Case 5.4

An 80-year-old woman was admitted to the hospital neurology service with the sudden onset of speech difficulty. She had a 10-year history of hypertension. About a year prior to the current admission she had the sudden onset of dysarthria, dysphagia, and right-hand clumsiness, all of which resolved within 10 days.

Neurologic examination identified significant dysarthria, dysphagia, and left-hand weakness, as well as hyperactive reflexes on the left. A diagnosis of a right internal capsule or pontine infarct was made. Subsequent MRI and CT scans identified moderate generalized atrophy and multiple focal areas of abnormality in the hemispheric white matter bilaterally, consistent with subcortical ischemic disease.

Speech examination revealed both left and right lower facial weakness with reduced range of movement on smiling, lip rounding, and lip puffing. Tongue protrusion and lateralization were limited in range. Gag reflex was hypoactive. A sucking reflex was not present. Contextual speech was characterized by a hoarse, strained voice quality, reduced loudness, imprecise articulation, hypernasality, and monopitch and monoloudness. Speech AMRs were slow (2) but regular. Speech intelligibility was reduced. There was no evidence of aphasic language impairment or apraxia of speech.

The clinician concluded that the patient had a "marked spastic dysarthria with significantly reduced speech intelligibility. The tongue is markedly weak, but this is probably on a bilateral UMN basis."

Speech therapy was recommended, which she pursued closer to home. Neuropsychologic assessment identified moderate generalized cognitive dysfunction, most evident in areas of attention and concentration, new learning and memory, and reasoning and problem solving.

Commentary. *(1) Although full recovery from unilateral UMN lesions causing dysarthria is possible, additional lesions on the other side of the brain can result in spastic dysarthria with significant reduction of speech intelligibility. (2) When spastic dysarthria is present following an apparent unilateral cerebral event, suspicions should be raised about bilateral lesions. In this case, the history and current event helped establish the presence of more than one lesion.*

SUMMARY

1. Spastic dysarthria results from damage to the direct and indirect activation pathways (upper motor neurons) bilaterally. It occurs at a frequency comparable to that of other single dysarthria types. It generally is associated with deficits in many of the components of speech production. The combined effects of spasticity and weakness on the speed, range, and force of movement seem to account for most of the deviant speech characteristics associated with spastic dysarthria.

2. Clinical signs that accompany spastic dysarthria usually reflect the combined effects of direct and indirect activation pathways damage and, therefore, include weakness, loss of skilled movement, spasticity, hyperactive reflexes, and pathological reflexes. The salient effects of UMN lesions on speech movements include spasticity, weakness, reduced range of movement, and slowness of movement.

3. Vascular and degenerative etiologies may account for a majority of cases of spastic dysarthria, but traumatic, demyelinating, and undetermined etiologies are probably not uncommon. Most patients with spastic dysarthria have other clinical signs or neuroimaging evidence of bilateral UMN dysfunction, but spastic dysarthria can be the only neurologic sign in some cases. The distribution of offending lesions can be widespread in the UMN system, including pathways ranging from the cortex to brain stem.

4. Dysphagia and pseudobulbar affect are common in patients with spastic dysarthria. Complaints that speech is slow and effortful and deteriorates with fatigue are also common.

5. The deviant speech characteristics in spastic dysarthria reflect impaired movements and movement patterns. Deficits in all components of speech are common.

6. The major clusters of deviant speech characteristics in spastic dysarthria include prosodic excess, articulatory-resonatory incompetence, prosodic insufficiency, and phonatory stenosis. Although many deviant speech characteristics can be detected in spastic dysarthria, strained-strangled voice quality, slow speech rate, and slow and regular speech AMRs are the most distinctive clues to the presence of spastic dysarthria. In general, acoustic and physiologic studies of individuals with spastic dysarthria have provided quantitative support for its clinical perceptual characteristics. They have helped to specify more completely the location and dynamics of abnormal movement that lead to the perceived speech disturbance.

7. Spastic dysarthria can be the only, the first, or among the first or most prominent manifestations of neurologic disease. Its recognition and correlation with bilateral UMN dysfunction can aid the localization and diagnosis of neurologic disease and may contribute to the medical and behavioral management of individuals and their speech disorders.

REFERENCES

Abbs JH and Kennedy JG: Neurophysiological processes of speech movement control. In Lass NJ, McReynolds LV, Northern JL, and Yoder DE, editors: Speech, language, and hearing, vol 1, normal processes, Philadelphia, 1982, WB Saunders.

Abbs JH, Hunker CJ, and Barlow SM: Differential speech motor subsystem impairments with suprabulbar lesions: neurophysiological framework and supporting data. In Berry WR, editor: Clinical dysarthria, San Diego, 1983, College-Hill.

Adams RD and Victor M: Principles of neurology, New York, 1991, McGraw-Hill.

Aronson AE: Clinical voice disorders, New York, 1990, Thieme.

Asfora WT, DeSalles AAF, Abe M, and Kjellberg RN: Is the syndrome of pathological laughing and crying a manifestation of pseudobulbar palsy? J Neurol Neurosurg Psychiat 52:523, 1989.

Barlow SM and Abbs JH: Orofacial fine motor control impairments in congenital spasticity: evidence against hypertonus-related performance deficits, Neurology 34:145, 1984.

Bayles KA and Kaszniak AW: Communication and cognition in normal aging and dementia, Boston, 1987, College-Hill.

Clinical examinations in neurology, ed 6, members of the Department of Neurology, Mayo Clinic, Mayo Foundation for Medical Education and Research, St Louis, 1991 Mosby–Year Book.

Darley FL, Aronson AE, and Brown JR: Differential diagnostic patterns of dysarthria, J Speech Hear Res 12:246, 1969a.

Darley FL, Aronson AE, and Brown JR: Clusters of deviant speech dimensions in the dysarthrias, J Speech Hear Res 12:462, 1969b.

Darley FL, Aronson AE, and Brown JR: Motor speech disorders, Philadelphia, 1975, WB Saunders.

Duchateau J and Hainaut K: Electrical and mechanical change in immobilized human muscle, J Appl Psychol 62:2168, 1987.

Dworkin JP and Aronson AE: Tongue strength and alternate motion rates in normal and dysarthria subjects, J Commun Disord 19:115, 1986.

Hardcastle WJ, Barry RA, and Clark CJ: Articulatory and voicing characteristics of adult dysarthric and verbal dyspraxia speakers: an instrumental study, Brit J Commun Disord 20:249, 1985.

Hirose H: Pathophysiology of motor speech disorders (dysarthria), Folia Phoniatr 38:61, 1986.

Hirose H, Kiritani, S, and Sawashima J: Patterns of dysarthric movement in patients with amyotrophic lateral sclerosis and pseudobulbar palsy, Folia Phoniatr 34:106, 1982a.

Hirose H, Kiritani S, and Sawashima J: Velocity of articulatory movements in normal and dysarthric subjects, Folia Phoniatr 34:210, 1982b.

Kammermeier MA: A comparison of phonatory phenomena among groups of neurologically impaired speakers: PhD dissertation, University of Minnesota, 1969.

Kent R, Netsell R, and Bauer LL: Cineradiographic assessment of articulatory mobility in the dysarthrias, J Speech Hear Disord 40:467, 1975.

Landau WM: Spasticity: the fable of a neurological demon and the emperor's new therapy, Arch Neurol 31:217, 1974.

Linebaugh CW and Wolfe VE: Relationships between articulation rate, intelligibility, and naturalness in spastic and ataxic speakers. In McNeal M, Rosenbek J, and Aronson A, editors: The dysarthrias: physiology acoustics perception management, Austin, TX, 1984, Pro-Ed.

McClean MD, Beukelman DR, and Yorkston KM: Speech-muscle visuomotor tracking in dysarthric and nonimpaired speakers, J Speech Hear Res 30:276, 1987.

Miller RG and others: Excessive muscular fatigue in patients with spastic paraparesis, Neurology 40:1271, 1990.

Murry T: The production of stress in three types of dysarthric speech. In Berry W, editor: Clinical dysarthria, Boston, 1983, College-Hill.

Portnoy RA and Aronson AE: Diadochokinetic syllable rate and regularity in normal and in spastic ataxic dysarthric subjects, J Speech Hear Disord 47:324, 1982.

Pringle CE and others: Primary lateral sclerosis, Brain 115:495, 1992.

Rowland LP: Motor neuron diseases: the clinical syndromes. In Mulder DW, editor: The diagnosis and treatment of amyotrophic lateral sclerosis, Boston, 1980, Houghton Mifflin.

Yorkston KM, Beukelman D, and Bell K: Clinical management of dysarthric speakers, San Diego, 1988, College-Hill.

Ziegler W and von Cramon D: Spastic dysarthria after acquired brain injury: an acoustic study, Brit J Commun Disord, 21:173, 1986.

6 Ataxic Dysarthria

Ataxic dysarthria is a perceptually distinguishable motor speech disorder associated with damage to the cerebellar control circuit. It may be manifest in any or all of the respiratory, phonatory, resonatory, and articulatory levels of speech, but its characteristics are most evident in articulation and prosody. Its speech characteristics reflect the effects of incoordination and reduced muscle tone on speech, the products of which are slowness and inaccuracy in the force, range, timing, and direction of speech movements. Ataxia is an important contributor to the speech deficits of patients with cerebellar disease, hence the disorder's designation as *ataxic* dysarthria. The identification of ataxic dysarthria can aid the diagnosis of neurologic disease and may assist lesion localization because its presence is so strongly associated with cerebellar dysfunction.

Ataxic dysarthria is encountered as the primary speech pathology in a large medical practice at a rate slightly higher than that for the other major single dysarthria types. From 1987 to 1990 at the Mayo Clinic, ataxic dysarthria accounted for 14.6% of all dysarthrias and 13.3% of all motor speech disorders seen in the Section of Speech Pathology (Figure 1–3).

The clinical features of ataxic dysarthria help to illustrate the important role of the cerebellum in speech motor control. Of all of the individual dysarthria types, it most clearly reflects a breakdown in motor organization and control, rather than in neuromuscular execution that characterizes most other dysarthria types. When one listens to the speech of a person with ataxic dysarthria, the impression is not one of underlying weakness, resistance to movement, or restriction of move-

ment, but rather one of an activity that is being poorly controlled or coordinated.

ANATOMY AND BASIC FUNCTIONS OF THE CEREBELLAR CONTROL CIRCUIT

The cerebellar control circuit consists of the cerebellum and its connections. The components of the circuit were described in some detail in Chapter 2. Here we will briefly summarize structures and pathways of the cerebellar control circuit that are most relevant to speech.

The *vermis* forms the midportion of the anterior and posterior lobes of the cerebellum. To the sides of the vermis are the right and left *cerebellar hemispheres*, each of which is connected to the opposite thalamus and cerebral hemisphere. Each cerebellar hemisphere is involved in controlling movement on the ipsilateral side of the body. Therefore, the left cerebral and right cerebellar hemispheres cooperate in controlling movement on the right side of the body, and the right cerebral and left cerebellar hemispheres cooperate in controlling movement on the left side of the body. The lateral cerebellar hemispheres of the posterior cerebellar lobe are particularly important to the *coordination of skilled voluntary muscle activity and tone.*

Purkinje cells, the functions of which are inhibitory, are the sole output neurons of the cerebellar cortex. They synapse with deep cerebellar nuclei and their output exits the cerebellum through the *superior* or *inferior cerebellar peduncles.*

The cerebellum influences, and is informed about, activities at several levels of the motor system. The primary and essential connections for its role in speech control include: reciprocal con-

145

nections with the cerebral cortex; auditory and proprioceptive feedback from speech muscles, tendons, and joints; reciprocal connections with brainstem components of the indirect activation pathway; and cooperation with the basal ganglia control circuit through loops among the thalamus, cereberal cortex, and components of the indirect motor system.

From a functional standpoint, the cerebellum presumably receives notice of intended movements from the cerebral cortex and monitors the adequacy of movement outcomes based on feedback from muscles, tendons, and joints. It can influence subsequent cortical motor output based on that feedback and on ongoing information from the cortex about upcoming movement goals. This permits it to make modifications that smooth the coordination of movement.

LOCALIZATION OF SPEECH WITHIN THE CEREBELLUM

The localization of speech within the cerebellum is uncertain. Brown, Darley, and Aronson (1970), examining disparities in gait, limb, and speech disturbances in people with cerebellar disease, concluded that areas other than the anterior portion of the vermis were probably important or sufficient for motor speech control. Similarly, Victor, Adams, and Mancal (1959) noted that dysarthria is unusual in chronic alcoholic patients, who tend to have extensive degeneration in the anterior lobe of the cerebellum, including the superior vermis, suggesting that the superior vermis and anterior portion of the anterior lobes are not crucial for speech. Brown, Darley, and Aronson (1970) concluded that *ataxic dysarthria usually results from bilateral or generalized cerebellar disease,* even though it may sometimes be due to a more focal lesion.

Where are such focal lesions? Several studies of people with cerebellar tumors or small cerebellar infarcts implicate the paravermal (posteromedial) areas and lateral hemispheres of the cerebellum (Ackerman and others, 1992; Amarenco and others, 1991; Amici, Avanzini, and Pacini, 1976; Lechtenberg and Gilman, 1978). Clinical evidence also indicates that ataxic dysarthria can result from lesions to the superior cerebellar peduncle, the major cerebellar-cortical pathway for fiber tracts involved in voluntary movement control (von Cramon, 1981). In general, therefore, ataxic dysarthria is probably most commonly associated with bilateral or generalized cerebellar disease. *When lesions are focal, the lateral hemispheres and posteromedial or paravermal regions of the cerebellum or the area of the superior cerebellar peduncle are implicated.*

Might speech functions be lateralized within the cerebellum, similar to the lateralization of speech and language within the cerebral hemispheres? Holmes (1922) observed that disease limited to one lateral cerebellar hemisphere could affect speech, but he also noted that speech usually improves rapidly when lesions are unilateral.

Lechtenberg and Gilman (1978), in a review of 122 patients with nondegenerative cerebellar disease, identified 31 with dysarthria. Seventy-one percent of those with dysarthria had exclusive or predominantly left cerebellar disease; 23% had right cerebellar hemisphere disease (two patients had lesions of the vermis). Fifty-four percent of those with exclusively or predominantly left cerebellar hemisphere lesions had disordered speech before surgical intervention, compared to only 15% of patients with right hemisphere lesions and 6% of patients with vermal lesions. The authors concluded that speech was most frequently disordered with lesions to the superior portion of the left cerebellar hemisphere* and that speech was more strongly represented in the cerebellar hemispheres than in the vermis. Because prosodic disturbances are prominent in ataxic dysarthria, they felt that the "dominance" of the left cerebellar hemisphere is logically related to its strong cerebellar-cortical ties to the right cerebral hemisphere and its apparently important role in prosodic functions. Kent and Rosenbek (1982) have discussed the relationship of cerebellar functions to speech prosody and the relationship of prosodic disturbances in cerebellar disease to the aprosody and dysprosody that may occur with right and left hemisphere lesions, respectively. They point out that "We should not conclude that the cerebellum is normally a generator of prosody. It may instead be part of a larger neuronal circuit that regulates the prosodic base of speech" (p. 286).

The notion of lateralized cerebellar dominance for speech is very interesting and relevant to our understanding of speech motor control. That there may be an asymmetric distribution of cerebellar lesions that lead to ataxic dysarthria also raises the possibility of different "types" of ataxic dysarthria dependent upon the lateralization of cerebellar lesions. It should be noted, however, that ataxic dysarthria is not just a prosodic disturbance (articulation, at the least, is also affected) and that left cerebral hemisphere lesions that produce apraxia of speech also typically affect prosody (although in a manner very different from that resulting from

---

*In contrast, Ackerman and others (1992) reported that three of their four patients with dysarthria resulting from unilateral cerebellar infarcts had *right*-sided lesions.

right cerebral hemisphere lesions). As Gilman, Bloedel, and Lechtenberg (1981) state, "... it is unlikely that only one cerebellar locus could be responsible for all of the facets of speech disorder occurring with cerebellar disease" (p. 229). Therefore, at this point in time, caution should be exercised in drawing conclusions about the lateralization of speech functions within the cerebellum.

CLINICAL CHARACTERISTICS OF CEREBELLAR LESIONS AND ATAXIA

The distinctive effects of cerebellar lesions are summarized in Table 6–1. They are grouped according to their association with lesions to the gross anatomic divisions of the cerebellum. Localizing signs of cerebellar disease to the midline versus lateral areas should be viewed cautiously because "each of the signs classically attributed to midline cerebellar disease can occur with disease in the lateral zones of the cerebellum" (Gilman, Bloedel, and Lechtenberg, 1981, p. 195). Difficulties with standing and walking are the most common signs of cerebellar disease, and gait is often referred to as ataxic. *Stance and gait are usually broad-based* and *truncal instability* may lead to falls. Steps may be irregularly placed and the legs lifted too high and slapped to the ground. There may be no difference in steadiness when standing with the feet together with the eyes open versus closed (the Romberg test). In contrast, patients with hysteria, vestibular dysfunction, or a loss of proprioception in the lower extremities are less steady with the eyes closed than open (a

positive Romberg finding) (Daube and others, 1986).

Titubation is a rhythmic tremor of the body or head that can occur with cerebellar disease. It is usually manifest as rocking of the trunk or head forward or back, side to side, or in a rotary motion, several times per second. Tremor of the head and neck can also occur as a benign condition in the elderly (essential tremor) without other evidence of cerebellar dysfunction.

Abnormal eye movements can occur in cerebellar disease. The most common of these is *nystagmus* (the rapid oscillation or jerkiness back and forth of the eyes at rest or with lateral or upward gaze). Patients may also exhibit *oculodysmetria* in which small rapid eye movements develop as the patient attempts to fix on a visual target and attempts to correct for inaccurate fixation (Gilman, Bloedel, and Lechtenberg, 1981).

Hypotonia, a decrease in resistance to passive movement and common in lower motor neuron (LMN) weakness, can occur in cerebellar disease. It may be associated with excessive *pendulousness,* in which an extremity, allowed to swing freely in a pendular manner, will exhibit a greater than average number of oscillations before coming to rest; this is a function of decreased muscle tone or decreased resistance to movement. A related phenomenon, known as *impaired check and excessive rebound* may also occur. For example, when asked to maintain the arm in an outstretched position with the eyes shut, a light tap on the wrist usually results in a large displacement of the limb followed by overshoot beyond the original position when it returns; return may be associated with oscillation of the arm about the initial position. The wide excursion reflects impaired check whereas overshoot reflects excessive rebound.

Dysmetria, a common sign of cerebellar disease, is a disturbance in the trajectory of a body part during movements or the inability to appropriately control range of movement. It is often characterized by overshooting or undershooting of targets and by abnormalities in speed, giving movements an irregular appearance. It is frequently detected when the patient is asked to repetitively touch the tip of the index finger to the nose and then to fully extend the arm to touch the examiner's finger (nose-finger-nose test) (*Clinical Examinations in Neurology,* 1991).

Dysdiadochokinesis is a manifestation of *decomposition of movement* that occurs in cerebellar disease. Decomposition of movement refers to errors in the sequence and speed of component parts of a movement, with a resultant lack of coordination. *Dysynergia* is another term often applied to the inability to perform components of

Table 6–1 Common clinical signs of cerebellar disease.

Midline zone (vermis, flocculonodular lobe, fastigial nuclei)
  Disordered stance and gait
  Truncal titubation
  Rotated or tilted head postures
  Ocular motor abnormalities
  Dysarthria

Lateral hemispheric zone (hemispheres, dentate, and interposed nuclei)
  Hypotonia
  Dysmetria
  Dysdiadochokinesis
  Ataxia
  Tremor
  Ocular motor abnormalities
  Dysarthria

Based on Gilman S, Bloedel JR, and Lechtenberg R: Disorders of the cerebellum, Philadelphia, 1981, FA Davis.

movements at the right time and place. These difficulties are elicited by testing alternating or fine repetitive movements. A common task is the knee-pat test in which the patient pats the knee alternately with the palm and dorsum of the hand, gradually increasing to a maximum rate. Poor performance is characterized by abnormalities in rate, rhythm, amplitude, and precision. This task falls under the category of alternating motion rates (AMR) tasks, in which irregularities of repetitive movements often reflect cerebellar disease. Other AMR tasks used to elicit dysdiadochokinesis include side-to-side tongue wiggling, up and down finger wiggling, and patting the floor with the ball of the foot. Speech AMRs are analogous to these tests of coordination and speed.

Ataxia is the product of dysmetria, dysdiadochokinesis, and decomposition of movement. Ataxic voluntary movements are halting, imprecise, jerky, poorly coordinated, and lacking in speed and fluidity or smoothness. Ataxia is generally associated with disease of the cerebellar hemispheres.

Cerebellar disease is sometimes associated with *intention* or *kinetic tremor* that is apparent during movement or sustained postures; it is usually most pronounced as a target is approximated (*terminal tremor*). This cerebellar tremor usually occurs with disorders of the lateral cerebellar hemispheres.

Some signs may occur in conjunction with cerebellar disease but do not reflect cerebellar dysfunction per se. For example, patients with cerebellar tumors, hemorrhage, or infarct that produce increased intracranial pressure may have *papilledema* or swelling of the optic discs. Gilman, Bloedel, and Lechtenberg (1981) note that mild facial weakness, often limited to the lower face, occurs frequently with focal cerebellar lesions, more often with cerebellar hemisphere than midline lesions. Although pressure effects on the VIIth nerve are a possible explanation, they note that there may be other, as yet undetermined, explanations. Other cranial nerve abnormalities may also be encountered in individuals with cerebellar lesions, including Vth, VIth, and VIIIth nerve lesions. Finally, disturbances of cognition and consciousness may be present, presumably in association with effects on cerebral function by degeneration, hydrocephalus, or brainstem compression (Gilman, Bloedel, and Lechtenberg, 1981).

ETIOLOGIES

Ataxic dysarthria can be caused by any process that damages the cerebellum or cerebellar control circuit pathways. These processes include degenerative, inflammatory, neoplastic, toxic, metabolic, traumatic, and vascular diseases (defined in Chapter 2). These etiologic categories are associated with cerebellar disease and ataxic dysarthria with varying frequency. The exact distribution of causes of ataxic dysarthria is unknown.

Several diseases are associated with ataxic dysarthria more frequently than with other dysarthria types. In addition, some diseases specifically affect the cerebellum and, therefore, are uniquely associated with ataxic dysarthria. In general, however, the presence of ataxic dysarthria by itself is not diagnostic of any specific neurologic disease. Some of the more common neurologic conditions that are associated with ataxic dysarthria more frequently than with other dysarthria types are discussed below. Other diseases that can produce ataxic dysarthria but are more frequently associated with other dysarthria types (especially mixed dysarthria) are discussed in the chapters dealing with those specific dysarthrias.

Degenerative diseases

Degenerative diseases that prominently affect the cerebellum are not uncommon, but their mechanisms are generally unknown. They are usually nonfatal, begin in adulthood, and evolve over several decades. Those in which degeneration is largely confined to the cerebellum are often referred to as *cerebelloparenchymal*. Those that also affect the spinal cord tracts are *spinocerebellar,* and those that also affect the inferior olive and pontine nuclei are called *olivopontocerebellar* (Gilman, Bloedel, and Lechtenberg, 1981).

Hereditary ataxias may be dominant or recessive. Many of the recessively inherited progressive ataxias manifest initial symptoms in childhood. *Friedreich's ataxia* is among the most common of these and is considered due to an inborn error of metabolism that is inherited in an autosomal recessive pattern. It usually begins before adolescence and evolves to incapacitation and death over a course of about 20 years. It is predominantly spinocerebellar in character. In addition to ataxia, there may be other signs of cerebellar involvement, sensory disturbances, spasticity, LMN weakness, and extrapyramidal features that can include dystonia, chorea, and other movement disorders. Dysarthria is common in Friedreich's ataxia, although it is not usually a presenting sign. Several studies have examined the dysarthria associated with the disorder (Gentil, 1990; Gilman and Kluin, 1984; Joanette and Dudley, 1980; Murry, 1983). They all describe speech characteristics associated with ataxic dysarthria. Some imply that the dysarthria may be mixed in character, most often with features suggestive of an accompanying spastic component (Joanette and Dudley, 1980; Murry, 1983). Because the disease is known to affect portions of the motor system beyond the cerebellum, it is not surprising that its associated dysarthria is not always only ataxic in character.

Dominantly inherited hereditary ataxias tend to begin between 20 and 40 years of age. *Olivopontocerebellar atrophy (OPCA)* is an example of such a disease. It is a heterogeneous condition associated with neurologic diseases that are broadly grouped under the heading of *multiple systems atrophy (MSA)* (Quinn, 1989). OPCA is associated with degeneration of the pontine, arcuate and olivary nuclei, the middle cerebellar peduncles, and the cerebellum, but not infrequently also associated with degenerative changes in the basal ganglia, cerebral cortex, spinal cord, and even peripheral nerves. The clinical features are variable, but cerebellar findings are the most common; parkinsonism, movement disorders, pyramidal and ophthalmologic signs, bulbar and pseudobulbar palsy, and dementia may also occur (Harding, 1987).

Multiple sclerosis (MS) may be associated with cerebellar lesions and ataxic dysarthria. Discussion of MS will be deferred to Chapter 10, Mixed Dysarthrias, because MS lesions often are not confined to the cerebellum. However, a condition associated with MS, known as *paroxysmal ataxic dysarthria (PAD),* deserves mention here because its occurrence is strongly suggestive of MS or familial cerebellar ataxia (Espir and Walker, 1969). In PAD, brief episodes of ataxic dysarthria occur in an individual whose speech may be otherwise normal; it may be accompanied by limb ataxia and visual symptoms. The mechanism is unclear but it is speculated that during active stages of MS, neurons are especially sensitive to changes in oxygen supply, and that the paroxysms are triggered by such changes.

Netsell and Kent (1976) reviewed 10 cases in the literature and three cases of their own with PAD and an established or provisional diagnosis of MS. The group's distinctive characteristics included: a few to several hundred episodes per day, each lasting for 5 to 30 seconds; speech characteristics consistent with those of ataxic dysarthria; the possibility of remission and reappearance at a later time, with or without new symptoms; no evidence of associated seizures; overbreathing sometimes evoking the paroxysms; and remittance of paroxysms in each case with administration of carbamazepine (Tegretol).

Vascular disorders

Vascular lesions can affect cerebellar function and lead to ataxic dysarthria. Lesions are most commonly caused by aneurysms, arteriovenous malformations (AVMs), cerebellar hemorrhage, or occlusion in the vertebrobasilar system. The lateral regions of the vertebrobasilar system, including the posterior inferior cerebellar artery at the level of the medulla, the anterior inferior cerebellar artery at the level of the pons, and the superior cerebellar artery at the level of the midbrain, are most often implicated in cerebellar and cerebellar pathway (that is, superior cerebellar peduncle) vascular lesions that may lead to ataxic dysarthria (Brown, 1949).

Neoplastic disorders

Tumors within or exerting mass effects on the cerebellum can lead to cerebellar signs, including ataxic dysarthria. Cerebellopontine angle tumors, which often arise from the meninges (meningiomas) or supporting cells of cranial nerves, may lead to early cerebellar signs because of pressure on the middle cerebellar peduncle, dentate nucleus, and posterior cerebellar lobes. There also may be involvement of multiple cranial nerves, including V, VI, VII, VIII, and X, plus other signs of brainstem dysfunction (Brown, 1949). Such tumors can lead to ataxic dysarthria, as well as to flaccid and spastic dysarthria. Most tumors of the cerebellopontine angle are acoustic neuromas (Gilman, Bloedel, and Lechtenberg, 1981).

Some posterior fossa tumors are more common in children and young adults. Ependymomas and medulloblastomas frequently arise around the fourth ventricle and can produce cerebellar signs. Astrocytomas of the cerebellar hemispheres are relatively common in children (Daube and others, 1986).

Twenty-five percent of metastatic brain tumors develop in the cerebellum (Gilman, Bloedel, and Lechtenberg, 1981). Signs and symptoms of cerebellar disease may be the first evidence that the patient has a tumor, the primary tumor remaining occult. *Paraneoplastic disorders* may affect the central nervous system (CNS), particularly the cerebellum. They tend to occur in patients with carcinoma outside of the CNS and, although they affect neurologic function, do not reflect actual invasion by tumor. Paraneoplastic syndromes affecting the cerebellum are often associated with lung and ovarian cancer. Purkinje cells are predominantly affected and diffuse degenerative changes in the cerebellar cortex and deep cerebellar nuclei occur. Antibodies to Purkinje cells may be present in patients with paraneoplastic cerebellar disease and may precede clinical symptoms. Along with nystagmus and ataxia of gait and limbs, dysarthria is a common clinical manifestation of paraneoplastic cerebellar disease (Anderson, Rosenblum, and Posner, 1988). Neoplasm outside of the CNS is frequently suspected in patients with signs of nonfamilial cerebellar degeneration of late onset (Adams and Victor, 1991).

Trauma

Traumatic brain injury (TBI) is often associated with limb ataxia and dysarthria (Brink, Imbus, and

Woo-Sam, 1980; Chester and Reznick, 1987; Gilchrist and Wilkinson, 1979; Roberts, 1976). Anoxia secondary to TBI is often invoked as the cause of cerebellar deficits, but damage to the superior cerebellar peduncles, which are vulnerable to the rotational injuries associated with TBI, has also been associated with cerebellar signs, including dysarthria (Chester and Reznick, 1987).

"Punch-drunk" encephalopathy or *dementia pugilistica* is often encountered in boxers who have sustained repeated cerebral injuries. These individuals may be ataxic. The cerebellum is among the areas of the CNS that undergo pathologic changes (Adams and Victor, 1991). Ataxic dysarthria may occur in this condition.

Toxic/metabolic conditions

Acute and chronic alcohol abuse can produce cerebellar signs and symptoms, the most common of which are abnormal stance and gait. True alcoholic cerebellar degeneration is probably the result of nutritional deficiency rather than the direct effect of alcohol. Although ataxic speech frequently occurs with acute alcohol intoxication (Victor, 1986), permanent dysarthria in chronic alcoholism is not common (Gilman, Bloedel, and Lechtenberg, 1981). Signs of cerebellar dysfunction can also develop with severe malnutrition and associated vitamin deficiencies (the cerebellum and brain stem are particularly vulnerable to thiamin deficiency).

Neurotoxic levels of several drugs may produce cerebellar signs and symptoms. These drugs frequently include anticonvulsants, such as phenytoin (Dilantin), carbamazepine (Tegretol), valproic acid (Depakote), and primidone (Mysoline). Lithium, used to treat manic depressive illness, can produce neurotoxic effects that include postural or intention tremor, ataxia, hyperkinesia, and dysarthria (Judd, 1991), which can be ataxic in character (and sometimes spastic and hyperkinetic, in the author's experience). Valium, an antianxiety drug, has also been associated with ataxic dysarthria (Miller and Groher, 1990).

Other

Hypothyroidism is an endocrine disturbance that, when severe, can lead to ataxic dysarthria (Jordan, 1985). It is caused by insufficient secretion of thyroxin by the thyroid glands. When severe, the condition is known as *myxedema*. The ataxic dysarthria of hypothyroidism may be accompanied by a hoarse, gravelly, and excessively low-pitched dysphonia caused by mass loading of the vocal cords with myxomatous material (Aronson, 1990).

Normal pressure hydrocephalus (NPH) is a condition in which the ventricles may be enlarged while normal cerebrospinal fluid (CSF) pressure is maintained; it has been associated with subarachnoid hemorrhage or inflammatory conditions, but etiology is often unclear. It is recognized by a triad of symptoms that include progressive gait disorder, impaired mental function, and urinary incontinence (Adams and Victor, 1991). Dysarthria may occur in NPH and it may be ataxic in character.

SPEECH PATHOLOGY
Distribution of etiologies, lesions, and severity in clinical practice

The box on page 151 summarizes the etiologies for 107 quasirandomly selected cases seen at the Mayo Clinic with a speech pathology diagnosis of ataxic dysarthria. The cautions expressed in Chapter 4 about generalizing these data to the general population or all speech pathology practices also apply here.

The data establish that ataxic dysarthria can result from a number of medical conditions. Over 90% of the cases are accounted for by degenerative, vascular, demyelinating, undetermined, toxic/metabolic, and traumatic etiologies. Degenerative, vascular, and demyelinating diseases account for over 60% of the etiologies.

Degenerative diseases were the most frequent cause (34%), with nearly half of the degenerative conditions accounted for by relatively isolated cerebellar degenerative disease of undetermined etiology. The remainder of the degenerative etiologies included more specific entities such as OPCA, Shy-Drager syndrome, multiple systems atrophy, progressive supranuclear palsy (PSP), and cerebellar and brainstem degeneration. Most of these latter conditions are typically associated with CNS degeneration that affects more than the cerebellum; consequently, they are often associated with other dysarthria types, most often mixed dysarthria. They will be described more completely in Chapter 10. The remaining etiologies (Friedreich's ataxia, spinocerebellar degeneration, hereditary cerebellar atrophy) have already been defined.

Nonhemorrhagic stroke accounted for most of the vascular causes. About three-quarters of the vascular cases had a single event, with the remainder having had multiple strokes. Nearly half of the vascular cases had an identifiable lesion in the cerebellum; most of the remaining cases had lesions in the brain stem or midbrain. Two cases had supratentorial lesions (one in the posterior right frontal lobe, the other with multiple lesions in the periventricular white matter). Whether the lesions in these latter cases were responsible for the ataxic dysarthria is a matter of conjecture. If they were responsible, it suggests either an incorrect speech diagnosis or the possibility that the speech charac-

ETIOLOGIES OF ATAXIC DYSARTHRIA FOR 107 QUASIRANDOMLY SELECTED CASES WITH A PRIMARY DIAGNOSIS OF ATAXIC DYSARTHRIA AT THE MAYO CLINIC FROM 1969–1990. PERCENTAGE OF CASES UNDER EACH BROAD ETIOLOGIC HEADING IS GIVEN IN PARENTHESES.

Degenerative (34%)

Cerebellar degeneration, unspecified etiology (15%)
OPCA (7%)
Shy-Drager (3%)
Multiple systems atrophy (2%)
Cerebellar atrophy, hereditary (2%)
Other degenerative conditions (6%)
Cerebellar and brainstem degeneration; PSP; Friedreich's ataxia; spinocerebellar degeneration; hereditary degenerative CNS disease; hereditary cerebral calcinosis

Vascular (16%)

Nonhemorrhagic stroke (single or multiple) (10%)
Hemorrhagic stroke (3%)
Ruptured aneurysm (2%)
Lupus, intracranial arteritis (1%)

Demyelinating (15%)

Multiple sclerosis (14%)
Unspecified demyelinating disease (1%)

Undetermined (14%)

Undetermined cerebellar ataxia (4%)
Undetermined cerebellar atrophy (2%)
Other (8%)
Dysarthria only; paroxysmal periodic ataxia; corticobulbar and extrapyramidal abnormality; undetermined cerebellar and brainstem disease; Wilson's disease vs. liver disease; encephalitis vs. undetermined brainstem disease; tumor vs. AVM; undetermined neurologic problem.

Toxic/metabolic (7%)

Prescribed medication (usually anticonvulsant) (4%)
Other (alcohol/drug abuse; anoxic encephalopathy associated with intentional drug overdose) (3%)

Traumatic (6%)

Closed head injury (5%)
Penetrating head injury (1%)

Inflammatory (5%)

Meningitis (2%)
Encephalitis (2%)
Multifocal leukoencephalopathy (1%)

Tumor (3%)

Brainstem tumor; cerebellopontine angle tumor; paraneoplastic syndrome

Multiple (1%)

Stroke + ? CNS degenerative disease

Other (1%)

Depression/personality disorder

OPCA, olivopontocerebellar atrophy; *PSP,* progressive supranuclear palsy; *CNS,* central nervous system; *AVM,* arteriovenous malformation.

teristics associated with ataxic dysarthria can be associated with supratentorial lesions (cerebellar symptoms have been reported in supratentorial lesions; see Chapter 9 for further discussion of this possibility).

The association of ataxic dysarthria with brainstem and midbrain lesions deserves comment. It is likely that the dysarthria in such cases is due to lesions affecting major cerebellar pathways in the brain stem or midbrain. For example, lesions of the superior cerebellar peduncles can lead to the same abnormalities that occur with cerebellar hemispheric lesions (von Cramon, 1981).

Multiple sclerosis accounted for nearly all of the demyelinating etiologies. Its representation of 14% of the sample suggests that ataxic dysarthria is not uncommon in MS and that it may occur as the only dysarthria type in MS more frequently than does spastic dysarthria (MS accounted for 6% of the cases of spastic dysarthria that were reviewed in Chapter 5). However, because lesions may be disseminated in many locations of the nervous system in MS, mixed dysarthria or other dysarthria types are common. Multiple sclerosis will be discussed in more detail in Chapter 10.

A substantial number of patients did not receive a definitive etiologic diagnosis. Within this group were patients with several possible diagnoses (for example, tumor versus arteriovenous malformation) and a number whose symptoms and course were too subtle or short-lived to be understood. It is likely that at least several of these cases had degenerative cerebellar diseases and probable that a clearer diagnostic picture emerged as the disease progressed or as more sophisticated diagnostic tests (for example, magnetic resonance imaging [MRI]) became available.

Toxic/metabolic causes for ataxic dysarthria are noteworthy because they were not evident in the samples of flaccid or spastic dysarthria (although this does not eliminate toxic/metabolic etiologies for those dysarthrias). Most often, ataxic dysarthria was secondary to anticonvulsant medications prescribed for epilepsy. Medication effects should always be suspected as a possible cause of ataxic dysarthria in individuals with seizure disorders who are on anticonvulsant medications.

The association of ataxic dysarthria with TBI in this sample is in agreement with the discussion by Yorkston, Beukelman, and Bell (1988). TBI accounted for a somewhat smaller proportion of cases of ataxic dysarthria reviewed here than cases of spastic dysarthria reviewed in Chapter 5. This does not necessarily mean that isolated spastic dysarthria occurs more frequently than isolated ataxic dysarthria in the TBI population because

these cases were selected on the basis of dysarthria diagnosis and not on the basis of etiology.

The data also establish that ataxic dysarthria may occur in association with inflammatory disease such as encephalitis and meningitis. This demonstrates that focal deficits can occur in conditions that are often diffuse in nature. Tumors associated with ataxic dysarthria were relatively uncommon, but were consistently located in the brain stem, were adjacent to the cerebellum (cerebellopontine angle) or affected cerebellar function indirectly (paraneoplastic syndrome).

The distribution of lesions for the cases summarized in the box on page 151 was usually in the *cerebellum or posterior fossa*. Because so many of the causes of ataxic dysarthria in the sample defied detection by neuroimaging (for example, degenerative, toxic, undetermined etiologies), clinical findings must be relied on for localization. In this regard, nearly 90% of the sample had nonspeech clinical signs of cerebellar involvement. Nearly 40% either did not have neuroimaging studies or had negative neuroimaging studies. Of those patients who had abnormalities detected by neuroimaging, about 55% had lesions or atrophy that were confined to or included the cerebellum, with about an additional 15% having lesions more generally localized to the brain stem or posterior fossa. Nearly 25% had evidence of generalized, diffuse, or multifocal abnormalities. Less than 10% had evidence of cerebral hemisphere lesions without evidence of cerebellar or posterior fossa abnormalities. This latter finding obviously does not rule out cerebellar or brainstem lesions in such patients (for example, many posterior fossa lesions went undetected before the advent of MRI) but, as already discussed, it raises the possibility that ataxic speech characteristics may occur in individuals with supratentorial lesions. In general, however, the clinical neurologic findings and neuroimaging data indicate that most patients with ataxic dysarthria have lesions or clinical signs that are localizable to the cerebellum or to the cerebellar pathways in the brain stem. This is reassuring because the sample was selected on the basis of speech diagnosis and not localization of disease; therefore, it helps confirm the localizing value of a diagnosis of ataxic dysarthria.

This retrospective review did not permit a clear delineation of dysarthria severity. However, in those patients for whom a judgment of intelligibility was explicitly stated (64% of the sample), *41% had reduced intelligibility*. The degree to which this figure accurately estimates the frequency of intelligibility impairments in the population with ataxic dysarthria is unclear. It is likely that many patients for whom an observation of intelligibility was not made had normal intelligibility; however, the sample probably contains a larger number of mildly impaired patients than is encountered in a typical rehabilitation setting.

Finally, cognitive deficits may be present in some people with ataxic dysarthria. Of the patients in this retrospective sample whose cognitive abilities were explicitly commented on or formally assessed (79% of the sample), *33% had some impairment of cognitive ability.* The reasons for such deficits are not entirely clear, but it is presumed that such patients had disorders that affected functions in noncerebellar structures.

Patient perceptions and complaints

People with ataxic dysarthria may describe their speech in ways that provide clues to their speech diagnosis and its localization. Similar to people with other dysarthria types, they often complain that their speech is *slurred.* Unlike patients with other dysarthria types, however, they also often refer to the *"drunken" quality* of their speech, either as they perceive it ("I sound like I'm drunk") or as others have commented upon it ("People ask me if I've been drinking"). They may also report dramatic deterioration in their speech with limited alcohol intake. Patients will occasionally complain that they are unable to coordinate their breathing with speaking, and sometimes note that they bite their cheeks or tongue while talking. When their dysarthria is mild, they may observe that speech proceeds normally until they suddenly *"stumble over" words.*

Patients may complain about the negative effects of fatigue on their speech, but perhaps less so than those with flaccid or spastic dysarthria. They do not often complain of increased physical effort in speaking. They often report that slowing speech rate generally improves intelligibility. Drooling is infrequently a complaint, but patients may comment that they bite their cheek or tongue when eating. Swallowing complaints are much less frequent than encountered in patients with flaccid or spastic dysarthria; this is consistent with observations that the cerebellum does not play an important role in swallowing (Logemann, 1983).

Clinical findings

Ataxic dysarthria usually occurs with other signs of cerebellar disease. In some cases it is the initial or only sign of cerebellar dysfunction. For example, Brown, Darley, and Aronson (1968) noted that ataxic dysarthria was the initial symptom in 7 of their 30 patients with cerebellar disease. In such cases, recognition of the dysarthria as ataxic can be valuable to neurologic localization, especially because there may be no other oromotor evidence of neurologic disease.

Nonspeech oral mechanism. The oral mechanism examination is often normal. That is, the size, strength and symmetry of the jaw, face, tongue, and palate may be normal at rest, during emotional expression, and during sustained postures. The gag reflex is usually normal and pathologic oral reflexes are generally absent. Drooling is uncommon and the reflexive swallow is usually normal on casual observation.

Nonspeech AMRs of the jaw, lips, and tongue may be irregular. This is usually most apparent on lateral wiggling of the tongue or retraction and pursing of the lips; judgments that nonspeech AMRs are irregular should be interpreted cautiously and only after observing many normal individuals, because normal performance is frequently somewhat irregular on these tasks. It is more relevant and valuable to observe the direction and smoothness of jaw and lip movements during connected speech and speech AMRs for evidence of dysmetria; irregular movements during speech are often observable, are not frequently observed in normal speakers, and are more relevant to the speech diagnosis than nonspeech AMRs.

Speech. Conversational speech or reading and speech AMRs are the most useful tasks for observing the salient and distinguishing characteristics of ataxic dysarthria. Repetition of sentences containing multisyllabic words (for example, "We saw several wild animals"; "My physician wrote out a prescription"; "The municipal judge sentenced the criminal") may promote distinctive irregular articulatory breakdowns and prosodic abnormalities. Speech AMRs can be particularly revealing; *irregular speech AMRs are a distinguishing characteristic of ataxic dysarthria* (Figure 6-1).

Similar to spastic dysarthria, the deviant speech characteristics of ataxic dysarthria are not easily described by listing each cranial nerve and the speech characteristics associated with its abnormal function. Ataxic dysarthria is associated with *impaired coordination of movement patterns rather than with deficits in individual muscles,* and it is the breakdown in coordination among simultaneous and sequenced movements that give it its distinctive character. It is *predominantly an articulatory and prosodic disorder.*

Table 6-2 summarizes the neuromuscular deficits presumed by Darley, Aronson, and Brown (1969a and b, 1975) to underlie ataxic dysarthria. In general, it is characterized by inaccurate movements, slow movements, and hypotonia of affected

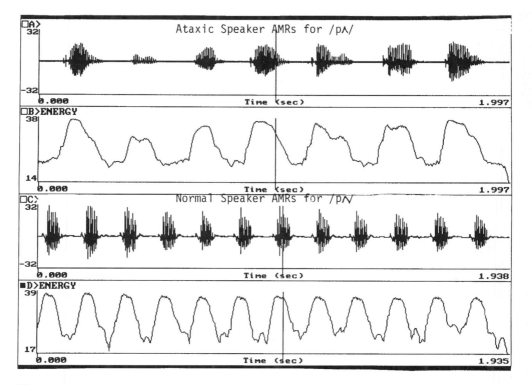

Figure 6–1 Raw waveform and energy tracings of speech AMRs for /pʌ/ by a normal speaker (*bottom two panels*) and a speaker with ataxic dysarthria. The normal speaker's AMRs are normal in rate (~ 6.5 Hz) and are relatively regular in duration and amplitude. In contrast, the ataxic speaker's are slow (~ 3.5 Hz) and irregular in amplitude, syllable duration, and intersyllable interval; these latter attributes represent the acoustic correlates of perceived irregular alternating motion rates.

Table 6–2 Neuromuscular deficits associated with ataxic dysarthria.

Direction	Rhythm	Rate		Range		Force	Tone
Individual movements	**Repetitive movements**	**Individual movements**	**Repetitive movements**	**Individual movements**	**Repetitive movements**	**Individual movements**	**Muscle tone**
Inaccurate	Irregular	Slow	Slow	Excessive to normal	Excessive to normal	Normal to excessive	Reduced

Adapted from Darley FL, Aronson AE, and Brown JR: Differential diagnostic patterns of dysarthria, J Speech Hear Res 12:246, 1969b.

muscles. As a result, individual and repetitive movements contain errors in timing, force, range, and direction, and tend to be slow with an unpredictable character. The relationships among these characteristics and the specific deviant characteristics associated with ataxic dysarthria are discussed below. Experimental support for the presumed underlying neuromuscular deficits, especially those that reflect the global impression of incoordination, will be reviewed in the section on acoustic and physiologic findings.

Clusters of deviant dimensions and prominent deviant speech characteristics. Darley, Aronson, and Brown (1969b) found three distinct clusters of deviant speech dimensions in their group of 30 patients with cerebellar disorders. These clusters are useful to understanding the neuromuscular deficits that underlie ataxic dysarthria, the components of the speech system that are most prominently involved, and the features that distinguish ataxic dysarthria from other dysarthria types. These clusters are summarized in Table 6–3.

Table 6–3 Deviant clusters of abnormal speech characteristics in ataxic dysarthria.

Cluster	Speech characteristics
Articulatory inaccuracy	Imprecise consonants Irregular articulatory breakdowns Distorted vowels
Prosodic excess	Excess and equal stress Prolonged phonemes Prolonged intervals Slow rate
Phonatory-prosodic insufficiency	Harshness Monopitch Monoloudness

Based on Darley FL, Aronson AE, and Brown JR: Differential diagnostic patterns of dysarthria, J Speech Hear Res 12:246, 1969b.

The first cluster is *articulatory inaccuracy,* comprised of *imprecise consonants, irregular articulatory breakdowns,* and *vowel distortions.* These features reflect inaccuracy in the direction of articulatory movements and dysrhythmia of repetitive movements. They implicate movements of the jaw, face, and tongue primarily, but do not exclude inaccurate movements at the velopharyngeal valve.

The second cluster is *prosodic excess,* composed of *excess and equal stress, prolonged phonemes, prolonged intervals,* and *slow speech rate.* This cluster seems related to the slowness of individual and repetitive movements that are prominent in ataxia in general. Darley, Aronson, and Brown (1975) noted that the slowing of repetitive movements seems to include "slowness, even metering of patterns, and excessive vocal emphasis on usually unemphasized words and syllable . . ." (pp. 167-168). This cluster is probably related to descriptions of speech in individuals with cerebellar disease as "scanning" in character, a term defined in slightly different ways by various authors (for example, Walshe, 1973; DeJong, 1967; Scripture, 1916). It refers to slowness, a word-by-word or "sing-song" cadence, and equal and obvious emphasis on each syllable or word whether normally stressed or unstressed.

The third cluster is *phonatory-prosodic insufficiency,* composed of *harshness, monopitch,* and *monoloudness.* Darley, Aronson, and Brown attributed this cluster to insufficient excursion of muscles (presumably laryngeal and, possibly, respiratory) as a result of hypotonia.

Table 6–4 summarizes the most deviant speech dimensions found by Darley, Aronson, and Brown (1969a). The component of the speech system most prominently associated with each characteristic is also included. The rankings in the table represent the order of prominence (severity) of the speech characteristics and not necessarily the features that best distinguish ataxic dysarthria from other dysarthria types.

A few additional comments are warranted about some of the clusters and prominent speech characteristics because they bear on clinical diagnosis. These are based on some data embedded within those presented by Darley, Aronson, and Brown (1969a & b) or reflect clinical impressions from assessments of many patients with cerebellar disease.

1. The cluster of prosodic excess, particularly the deviant dimensions of excess and equal stress and prolonged phonemes and intervals, although quite distinctive of ataxic dysarthria, is not prominent in all patients. For example, only 20 to 24 of Darley, Aronson, and Brown's 30 subjects with cerebellar disease exhibited the speech features of this cluster. This lack of pervasiveness is not simply a function of severity because some patients with marked ataxic dysarthria and decreased intelligibility do not have prominent prosodic excess. In such cases, it may be the cluster of articulatory inaccuracy that predominates with irregular articulatory breakdowns giving speech an "intoxicated," irregular character rather than a measured quality.

2. Relatedly, not all patients with ataxic dysarthria have irregular speech AMRs, even though irregular AMRs are a distinctive and fairly pervasive marker of the disorder. It is the author's impression that irregular AMRs occur less frequently in patients with prominent prosodic excess (whose AMRs may be quite slow) and are more prominent in those with significant articulatory inaccuracy. Of course, many patients with ataxic dysarthria have both prosodic excess and articulatory inaccuracy.

3. Irregular articulatory breakdowns are sometimes associated with "*telescoping,*" an occurrence that refers to an inconsistent breakdown of articulation in which a syllable or series of syllables are suddenly or unpredictably run together, giving speech a transient accelerated character.

4. Some ataxic speakers exhibit "*explosive loudness*" and poorly modulated pitch and loudness variations. These characteristics do not appear within the most deviant characteristics or clusters of ataxic dysarthria but are striking when present. Darley, Aronson, and Brown observed excess loudness variability in one third of their

Table 6–4 The most deviant speech dimensions encountered in ataxic dysarthria by Darley, Aronson, and Brown (1969a), listed in order from most to least severe. Also listed is the component of the speech system associated with each characteristic. The component "prosodic" is listed when several components of the speech system may contribute to the dimension. Characteristics listed under "other" include features not among the most deviant but which were judged deviant in a number of subjects and are not typical of most other dysarthria types.

Dimension	Speech component
Imprecise consonants	Articulatory
Excess and equal stress*	Prosodic
Irregular articulatory breakdowns*	Articulatory
Distorted vowels*	Articulatory-prosodic
Harsh voice quality	Phonatory
Prolonged phonemes*	Articulatory-prosodic
Prolonged intervals	Prosodic
Monopitch	Phonatory-prosodic
Monoloudness	Phonatory-prosodic
Slow rate	Prosodic
Other	
Excess loudness variations*	Respiratory-phonatory-prosodic
Voice tremor	Phonatory

*Tend to be distinctive or more severely impaired than in any other single dysarthria type.

subjects and noted that this feature is probably a component of what some have described as *"explosive speech."* Although it may not occur frequently, explosive loudness has traditionally been associated with cerebellar dysfunction (Mavlov and Kehaiov, 1969; Grewel, 1957; Kammermeier, 1969).

5. *Voice tremor* is not frequently encountered in ataxic dysarthria and does not emerge among the clusters of deviant speech characteristics or among its most deviant speech characteristics (Darley, Aronson, and Brown, 1969a, b). However, cerebellar disease can be associated with tremor of the laryngeal and respiratory muscles that results in a slow voice tremor of approximately 3 Hz (Ackerman and Ziegler, 1991; Aronson, 1990).

6. Abnormal resonance is rare in ataxic dysarthria. However, intermittent *hyponasality* may be perceived in some ataxic speakers. These infrequent occurrences presumably reflect improper timing of velar and articulatory gestures for nasal consonants.

7. If some patients with ataxic dysarthria have predominant prosodic excess whereas others have predominant articulatory inaccuracy, if the two clusters can occur relatively independently, and if some patients with ataxic dysarthria truly have predominant explosive loudness, then there may be subtypes of ataxic dysarthria. If true, subtypes might be tied to differences in lesion location within the cerebellar control circuit. The hypothesis of Gilman, Bloedel, and Lechtenberg (1981) about differences in the

incidence of ataxic dysarthria between right and left cerebellar hemisphere lesions may also be relevant to the possible existence of subtypes of ataxic dysarthria.

What features of ataxic dysarthria help distinguish it from other motor speech disorders? Among all of the characteristics that may be detected, *irregular articulatory breakdowns, irregular speech AMRs, excess and equal stress, distorted vowels,* and *prolonged phonemes* are the most distinctive clues to its presence. Table 6–5 summarizes the primary distinguishing speech characteristics, common oral mechanism findings, and patient complaints associated with ataxic dysarthria.

Acoustic and physiologic findings

Respiratory and laryngeal function. Darley, Aronson, and Brown's (1969a) ataxic patients had excess loudness variations that they felt might have been due to altered respiratory patterning. They noted, however, that the hypothesis requires confirmation by direct observations of respiratory function during speech.

There have been only a few physiologic studies of respiratory function in ataxic dysarthria, but it is clear that respiratory speech functions can be disturbed. Brown, Darley, and Aronson (1970) studied respiratory function in four patients. Although respiratory rate was unremarkable, vital capacity was reduced in two patients and ability to sustain "ah" was limited in three. They also observed "a breakdown in the timing of onset of respiration and phonation leading to air wastage" (p. 309).

Table 6-5 Primary distinguishing speech and speech-related findings in ataxic dysarthria.

Perceptual

    Phonation-respiration
        Excessive loudness variations
    Articulation-prosody
        Irregular articulatory breakdowns
        Irregular AMRs
        Distorted vowels
        Excess and equal stress
        Prolonged phonemes

Physical

    Dysmetric jaw, face, and tongue AMRs

Patient complaints

    "Drunk"/intoxicated speech
    Stumble over words
    Bites tongue/cheek when speaking or
        eating
    Speech deteriorates with alcohol
    Poor coordination of breathing with
        speech

Abbs, Hunker, and Barlow (1983) studied rib cage and abdominal movements during speech in one patient with ataxic dysarthria. They found evidence of incoordination between chest wall components but did not find incoordination between labial and mandibular movements. They suggested that the findings were indicative of differential impairments between and among portions of the cranial and spinal motor systems.*

In a comprehensive study employing spirometric and kinematic techniques, Murdoch and others (1991) examined respiratory function during speech and nonspeech tasks in 12 people with cerebellar disease and ataxic dysarthria. A number of differences were found between normal controls and a significant proportion of ataxic speakers during vowel prolongation, syllable repetition, and reading and conversational tasks. The most salient findings for ataxic speakers included: (1) reduced vital capacity, (2) paradoxical movements or abrupt changes in movements of the rib cage and abdomen, and (3) a tendency to initiate utterances at lower than normal lung volume levels. These abnormalities were interpreted as reflecting poor coordination of the chest wall components of respira-

---

*The validity of Abbs, Hunker, and Barlow's (1983) findings and interpretations, however, were questioned on a number of grounds by Hixon and Hoit (1984), and Putnam (1988) has suggested that the study and subsequent criticisms of it is "an instructive tutorial on the dubious value of macrosomic inferences from microsomic perspectives on a single subject" (1988, p. 147).

tion during speech. The authors noted that such aberrations could contribute to some of the prosodic abnormalities perceived in ataxic dysarthria.

McClean, Beukelman, and Yorkston (1987) examined the ability of one ataxic subject to track a visually presented sinusoidal target by controlling respiratory movements or by varying voice fundamental frequency. The subject's control of respiratory movements bore only a limited relationship to target movements and there was marked variability in performance. The subject was also unable to vary fundamental frequency to perform the tracking task (nondysarthric and some individuals with other dysarthria types could), suggesting that the task's demands far exceeded the subject's motor control ability.

Darley, Aronson, and Brown (1975) summarized a number of acoustic studies that bear on the issue of laryngeal speech control. The subjects in a number of these studies had multiple sclerosis and may, therefore, have had mixed dysarthrias or dysarthrias other than ataxic, so their conclusions should be viewed cautiously; the speech disorder was attributed to cerebellar dysfunction in many cases, however (Haggard, 1969; Janvrin and Worster-Drought, 1932; Kammermeier, 1969; Lehiste, 1965; Mavlov and Kehaiov, 1969; Scripture, 1916; and Zemlin, 1962). In general, these studies suggest that patients with cerebellar involvement may display "somewhat elevated vocal pitch level, restricted pitch and intensity variability, and individual patterns of aberrant vocal fold vibration that may be related to perceived voice quality deviations or may precede the development of audible changes in voice" (Darley, Aronson, and Brown, 1975, p. 162). Darley, Aronson, and Brown pointed out that what may be perceived as phonatory abnormalities could also be the result of dysfunction at another level of speech production, such as respiration.

More recently, Gentil (1990), in an acoustic study of 14 patients with Friedreich's disease who apparently had ataxic dysarthria, found abnormal variability in fundamental frequency and intensity during vowel prolongation and a speech AMR task. This supports the frequent clinical perception of irregular speech AMRs and unsteadiness of vowel prolongation in ataxic dysarthria.

Finally, Ackerman and Ziegler (1991) acoustically analyzed the voice of a woman with chronic cerebellar atrophy who had ataxic dysarthria and a voice tremor. The voice tremor was measured at about 3 Hz, a rate consistent with other forms of cerebellar postural tremor. The voice tremor was interpreted as laryngeal in origin because rhythmic oscillations were not present during sustained voiceless fricatives, an occurrence that would have suggested the presence of respiratory or articulatory tremor.

Articulation, rate, and prosody. Several studies have documented rate abnormalities. Acoustic measures of speech AMRs and word and sentence production have generally confirmed the presence of reduced rate and, interestingly, *excessive* or *reduced* variability of speech segment durations.

Gentil (1990) found that some subjects with Friedreich's disease could not produce a fast rate, that speech AMRs were always slow, and that the group had larger than normal standard deviations and coefficients of variation (standard deviation divided by the mean) for one-, two-, and three-syllable utterances. There was also evidence of relatively sudden abnormal variations in fundamental frequency and intensity, characteristics that may alter prosody. Slowness was attributed to hypotonia. Irregularity of segment durations was attributed to ataxia or timing errors among lip, jaw, tongue, velopharyngeal, laryngeal, and respiratory subsystems.

In a spectrographic study of a speaker with Friedreich's ataxia, Lehiste (1965) documented alterations in articulatory manner that included frication of plosives, substitution of affricates for fricatives, substitution of stops for fricatives, and occasional glottal stop substitutions. Omissions of nasals with compensatory nasalization were also noted.

Tatsumi and others (1979) acoustically analyzed the rate, regularity, and intensity of speech AMRs in a group of ataxic speakers. Most had slow AMRs and considerable irregularity in AMR rate or intensity. Dworkin and Aronson (1986) and Portnoy and Aronson (1982) have also documented the slowness of speech AMRs in ataxic speakers. Portnoy and Aronson also found AMRs of ataxic speakers to be more variable than those of normal speakers and those with spastic dysarthria.

Linebaugh and Wolfe's (1984) acoustic analysis of syllable duration documented greater than normal durations in 14 ataxic speakers (mean syllable duration in ataxic speakers of 249 msec versus 198 msec in normal speakers). There was no relationship between duration and measures of intelligibility or speech naturalness in the ataxic speakers, suggesting that factors other than slow rate may be responsible for deficits in those dimensions. In contrast to Darley, Aronson, and Brown (1969a), Linebaugh and Wolfe did not find syllable duration differences between their groups of ataxic and spastic speakers. They noted that Darley, Aronson, and Brown's perceptual ratings were based on total utterance duration, which included interword pauses plus speech segments, instead of their method that measured only the audible portions of speech samples. This implies that spastic speakers

may be slower than ataxic speakers because of longer interword pauses rather than longer speech segment durations.

Kent, Netsell, and Abbs (1979) examined the acoustic characteristics of speech in five ataxic speakers. They (and Kent, 1979) found evidence of reduced rate, including longer syllable durations and formant transitions, and occasionally longer voice onset time. Consonant clusters and vowel nuclei of words were usually lengthened, and in some instances were three times longer than normal. Voice onset time was sometimes shorter than normal and segment durations were often more variable than normal, suggesting abnormal variability in movements beyond general slowness. The normal tendency to reduce base word duration as the number of syllables in words increases was inconsistent (for example, the duration of the syllable "please" in the sequence "please, pleasing, pleasingly" showed inconsistent reductions, small reductions, and occasional lengthening of the base word as the number of syllables increased). Although lengthened segments seemed characteristic of the ataxic speakers, inconsistent degrees of lengthening altered speech stress and timing patterns. Lax and unstressed vowels were more likely to be disproportionately lengthened, a finding that fits well with the perception of excess and equal stress or "scanning" in some ataxic speakers. Simmons (1983) also spectrographically documented equalized syllable durations in an ataxic speaker.

Kent, Netsell, and Abbs (1979) concluded that general timing control is a major problem in ataxic dysarthria. They speculated that ataxic speakers do not decrease syllable duration when it is appropriate because such reductions require flexibility in sequencing complex motor instructions. The lack of flexibility may lead to a syllable-by-syllable motor control strategy with subsequent abnormal stress patterns. The authors also speculated that if a damaged cerebellum is unable to revise basic cortical motor programs, it may be necessary to rely more heavily on cortical control of speech. Because cortical revisions of a motor program presumably take longer than cerebellar revisions, speech segment durations might be increased to allow time for the longer and slower cortical loops to operate. This explanation is intriguing, and it raises questions about whether imposition of cortical control in response to cerebellar damage occurs "automatically," is dependent on the specific nature of the cerebellar deficit, reflects an intentional compensatory response by the speaker, or represents a combination of these possibilities.

In a spectrographic analysis of one ataxic speaker, Kent and Netsell (1975) documented slow rate, but not within all speech intervals. They did find evidence of prolonged vowels and marked and inappropriate changes in fundamental frequency, which may have contributed to the perception of inappropriate stress patterns. Many of their acoustic (and physiologic) observations were consistent with Darley, Aronson, and Brown's (1969a and b) perceptual analyses. However, they questioned whether Darley, Aronson, and Brown's clusters of prosodic excess and phonatory-prosodic insufficiency have independent physiologic-acoustic bases, because monopitch and monoloudness and stress abnormalities might be explained by common factors. They also felt that excess and equal stress may not be independent of slow rate and prolonged intervals and phonemes, as implied by Darley, Aronson, and Brown. Finally, Kent and Netsell suggested that hypotonia may not, as suggested by Darley, Aronson, and Brown, just be related to laryngeal/phonatory function but may also explain some articulatory and prosodic abnormalities. That is, ataxic dysarthria may be characterized by "a generalized hypotonia, which results in a delay in the generation of muscular forces (hence producing the speech abnormality of prolongation), a reduced rate of muscular contraction (hence producing slowness of movement), and reduced range of movement (hence producing the phenomenon of telescoping)" (p. 129–130). Netsell and Kent (1976) have also reported a cinefluorographic and spectographic analysis of a subject with paroxysmal ataxic dysarthria with characteristics very similar to the subject presented in their 1975 study.*

Kent and Rosenbek (1982) summarized the spectrographic analysis of an ataxic speaker with "scanning" speech. The speaker had limited variation in syllable duration, fairly regular spacing between syllabic nuclei, and a generally flat fundamental frequency contour. In general, these features were consistent with "an equalization across syllables with respect to their prosodic content" (p. 262). Therefore, in the scanning speech of ataxic dysarthria, variability of segment durations and fundamental frequency may actually be less than normal.

Yorkston and others (1984) examined three ataxic speakers' ability to control fundamental frequency, duration, and intensity in order to stress targeted words in short sentences. They all showed some abnormalities compared to normal speakers,

even though they often varied speed adequately enough to accurately signal stress. Some of the abnormalities included exaggerations in fundamental frequency, duration and intensity changes, restriction of fundamental frequency variation, excessive interword pauses, and poor use of durational shifts.

Murry (1983) also found a lack of homogeneity among acoustic correlates of stress among five ataxic speakers, including differences in "strategies" used to signal stress on initial as opposed to final words in sentences. For example, ataxic speakers tended to use increased articulatory effort (for example, as reflected in peak intraoral air pressure) but not vowel duration increases to stress initial words; in the final position they used changes in fundamental frequency and intensity, but tended not to increase articulatory effort. The use of a "consonant strategy" for initial stress and a "vowel strategy" for final word stress was in contrast to normal speakers who used both consonant and vowel strategies for initial and final words. Murry noted that the acoustic correlates of stress in his subjects were in general agreement with the results of perceptual studies of ataxic dysarthria.

A few physiologic studies have shed further light on the underlying dynamics of ataxic dysarthria. Hirose and others (1978) used an x-ray microbeam system and electromyography (EMG) to examine articulatory movements, range, velocity, and consistency of articulatory movements. Their one ataxic speaker had difficulty initiating movement and inconsistency in the range and velocity of repetitive articulatory movements (as in speech AMRs). EMG showed a breakdown of rhythmic patterns in articulatory muscles during syllable repetition, but jaw and lip movements were generally synchronous with each other. In general, the data were consistent with perceptions of ataxic speech as containing irregular articulatory breakdowns.

McNeil and others (1990) studied isometric force and static position control of the upper and lower lip, tongue, and jaw during nonspeech tasks in four ataxic speakers. They had greater force and position instability than normal speakers, although impairment on one task did not necessarily predict impairment on other tasks. McClean, Beukelman, and Yorkston's (1987) ataxic speaker performed poorly on a nonspeech visuomotor tracking task involving the lower lip and jaw. Both of these studies support a conclusion that ataxic speakers are impaired in motor control.

Using cineradiography, Kent and Netsell (1975, 1976) analyzed articulatory positions and movements in ataxic speech. They observed abnormally small adjustments of anterior-posterior tongue

---

*This work of Kent and Netsell is an excellent example of how inferences derived from acoustic and physiologic studies can lead to refinements or modifications of hypotheses generated by perceptual analyses of the dysarthrias.

Table 6–6 Summary of acoustic and physiologic findings in studies of ataxic dysarthria. Note that many of these observations are based on studies of only one or a few speakers, and that not all speakers with ataxic dysarthria will exhibit these features. Note also that these characteristics are not necessarily unique to ataxic dysarthria; some may also be characteristic of other motor speech disorders, or non-neurologic conditions.

Speech component	Acoustic or physiologic observation
Respiratory/laryngeal	Abnormal and paradoxical rib cage and abdominal movements Reduced vital capacity (probably secondary to incoordination) Poor visuomotor tracking with respiratory movements Poor visuomotor tracking with f_o Increased variability of f_o and intensity during vowel prolongation and AMRS

Articulation, rate, & prosody	Reduced rate:
	    Increased syllable duration
	    Increased duration of formant transitions
	    Longer voice onset time (but sometimes shorter)
	    Lengthened consonant clusters & vowel nuclei
	    Slow AMRs
	    Disproportionate lengthening of lax/unstressed vowels
	    Difficulty initiating purposeful movement
	    Slow lip, tongue, & jaw movements
	Increased variability, inconsistency, or instability of:
	    Segment durations
	    Rate
	    Intensity
	    AMR rate & intensity
	    f_o
	    Range & velocity of articulatory movements, especially AMRS
	    Increased instability of force & static position control in lip, tongue, & jaw on nonspeech tasks
	    Inconsistent reduction of base word (first syllable) duration with increases in number of syllables in words
	    Inconsistent velopharyngeal closure
	Reduced variability or restriction of:
	    Anterior-posterior tongue movements during vowel production
	    Syllable duration
	    Spacing between syllabic nuclei
	    f_o contour in connected speech
	Other
	    Breakdown in rhythmic EMG patterns in articulatory muscles during syllable repetition
	Poor visuomotor tracking with lower lip & jaw movements on nonspeech tasks
	Occasional failure of articulatory contact for consonants.

AMR, alternating motion rate; *EMG,* electromyography; f_o, fundamental frequency.

movements during vowel production and felt that such restrictions may help explain the perception of vowel distortions. Individual movements of the lips, tongue, and jaw were often slow but movements among those structures were generally coordinated. They also observed occasional incomplete velopharyngeal closure and failure of articulatory contact for consonants.

The general observations derived from acoustic and physiologic studies reviewed in this section are summarized in Table 6–6. Figure 6–2 illustrates some of the typical acoustically measurable rate and prosodic abnormalities that may be present in ataxic dysarthria.

CASES

Case 6.1

A 53-year-old woman presented with a 2 to 3 year history of intermittent "jumping" of her vision. For nine months she had double vision, imbalance when walking, and "mild slurring of speech," all of which had gradually worsened.

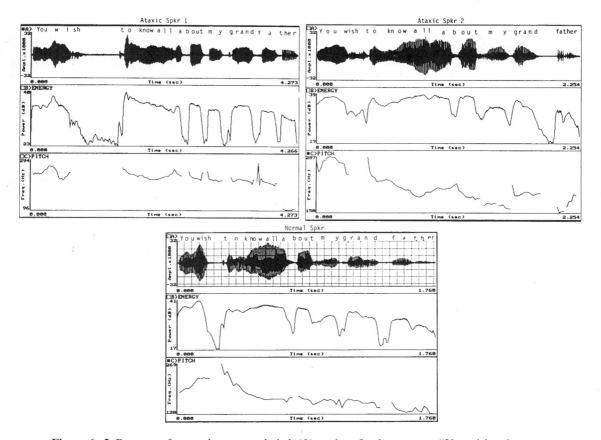

Figure 6–2 Raw waveform and energy and pitch (f_o) tracings for the sentence "You wish to know all about my grandfather" by a normal female speaker (*bottom tracings*) and two females with ataxic dysarthria (*upper tracings*). The normal speaker completes the sentence in < 2 secs with normal variability in syllable duration and amplitude (*energy tracing*), and normal variability and declination in f_o across the sentence (*pitch tracing*). Ataxic Speaker 1 is very slow (~ 4.3 secs for the utterance). Note also the relatively equal amplitude and duration of syllables for ". . . about my grandfather" in the energy tracing, and the relative absence of f_o variability and declination in the pitch tracing. These represent acoustic correlates of the slow rate, excess and equal stress, and monoloudness and monopitch that is often apparent in ataxic dysarthria. Ataxic Speaker 2 is not dramatically slow and the energy and pitch tracings are grossly similar to the Normal Speaker's. Note, however, that the word "grandfather" is produced more rapidly, particularly the syllables for "father;" the stressed syllable "fa" is shorter than the unstressed "ther" (*energy tracing*). These alterations are associated with perceivable breakdowns in articulation, as well as dysprosody characterized by abnormal stress and syllable durations.

Neurologic exam revealed abnormal extraocular movements, nystagmus, mild proximal weakness in all limbs, severe gait ataxia, and moderate limb ataxia. A Babinski sign was present bilaterally. Magnetic resonance imaging scan revealed several areas of abnormality in the white matter of both hemispheres, suggestive of demyelinating disease. Multiple sclerosis was suspected but she had a very high cereberospinal fluid white blood cell count. A serum Purkinje cell antibody test was ordered.

The patient reported that her speech initially was "slightly slurred." It had worsened over the last five months and was suceptible to fatigue. She sometimes bit her tongue when eating and occasionally drooled when laughing or crying. The speech mechanism was normal in size, strength, and symmetry. Jaw and lateral tongue movements were dysmetric. Voluntary cough and glottal coup seemed poorly coordinated.

Conversational speech was characterized by: irregular articulatory breakdowns (3); dysprosody (3); excess and equal stress (scanning) (2,3); inappropriate loudness variability (1). Overall speech rate was slow (−2). Speech AMRs were irregular (3) and slow (−2). Vowel prolongation was breathy and unsteady (1,2).

The clinician concluded, "Unambiguous, moderately severe ataxic dysarthria suggestive of cerebellar dysfunction. Unless she is emotionally upset while talking, speech intelligibility is good. In fact, the scanning quality to her speech works to her advantage in terms of intelligibility." Speech therapy was not recommended.

Subsequently, her serum Purkinje cell antibody test was positive, strongly suggestive of paraneoplastic cerebellar degeneration associated with underlying malignancy. She was unable to remain at the clinic for full work-up for malignancy, but this was pursued at home. Initial work-ups there were negative, but an ovarian malignancy was discovered about five months later.

Commentary. *(1) Ataxic dysarthria is not uncommon in cerebellar disease and frequently occurs in paraneoplastic syndromes that affect the cerebellum. In such cases, the dysarthria (and other neurologic signs) may be apparent prior to detection of the primary malignancy. (2) The presence of ataxic dysarthria (and other dysarthrias) does not dictate that therapy should be undertaken. The patient's intelligibility was normal and there was nothing obvious about her speech that suggested that therapy would alter speech in a direction of greater normalcy. (She was advised to pursue therapy if her dysarthria worsened, however).*

Case 6.2

A 41-year-old woman presented for speech evaluation prior to neurologic assessment. She had been aware of a change in her speech for about a year and people frequently asked if she was "on drugs or drinking." Speech deteriorated under conditions of stress or fatigue, but she felt intelligibility remained normal. She denied chewing-swallowing difficulty. She mentioned that her 49-year-old brother also had gait, balance, and speech difficulties.

Oral mechanism exam was normal in size, strength, and symmetry. Gag reflex was hypoactive. Cough and glottal coup were normal. Snout, sucking, and jaw jerk reflexes were absent.

Conversational speech was characterized by: irregular articulatory breakdowns (1,2); reduced rate (1,2); dysprosody (1); occasional excess and equal stress (0,1); reduced pitch (0,1); and nonspecific subtle hoarseness (0,1). Speech AMRs were slow and irregular (1,2). Prolonged "ah" was unsteady (1). Speech intelligibility was normal.

The clinician concluded, "ataxic dysarthria, relatively mild." Both the patient and clinician felt therapy was unnecessary, but she was advised to pursue reassessment and possibly therapy if her speech difficulties progressed.

Neurologic evaluation identified multiple signs of cerebellar involvement, particularly pronounced gait and balance difficulties. Computed tomography (CT) scan and MRI identified marked cerebellar atrophy involving both cerebellar hemispheres and the vermis, most marked in the inferior cerebellar vermis. Family history established that her brother and father probably had the same condition. It was suspected that the patient had an autosomal dominant, primary cerebellar degenerative disease. Genetic counseling was provided; the patient's three children were felt to have a one-in-two risk of inheriting cerebellar degenerative disease.

Commentary. *(1) Ataxic dysarthria is a common and sometimes presenting sign of degnerative cerebellar disease, including inherited conditions. Its accurate diagnosis helps confirm disease localization. (2) Diagnosis of dysarthria and its specific type can be made when the problem is mild and intelligibility is unaffected.*

Case 6.3

A 27-year-old woman presented to neurology with a 10-year history of progressive gait imbalance, incoordination of the hands, and "slurred speech." Her symptoms worsened around her menstrual periods and when she was nervous or fatigued; they had worsened slightly during a pregnancy. Neurologic exam confirmed the presence of ataxic gait, upper limb ataxia, and nystagmus.

During speech examination, she admitted to an approximately 10-year history of "slurred speech," which did not seem to have progressed recently. Conversational speech was characterized by occasional irregular articulatory breakdowns (0,1) that were most apparent during consonant clusters and affricates. Infrequently, rate was mildly slowed and multisyllabic words were produced with excess and equal stress. Prolonged "ah" was unsteady (1). Speech AMRs were slow (−1) but not noticeably irregular.

The clinician concluded that the patient had a "mild ataxic dysarthria" that was not pervasively apparent and did not affect intelligibility. Therapy was not recommended.

Electromyography revealed a severe disorder of primary sensory neurons and other findings that were consistent with the diagnosis of spinocerebellar degeneration. Her neurologist concluded that she had a form of spinocerebellar degeneration but that the course of disease was more slowly progressive and milder than commonly encountered in Friedreich's ataxia. The diagnosis and hereditary implications were discussed with the patient.

She was seen for follow-up six years later. There was some worsening of her gait disturbance, but no worsening of her other deficits, including speech.

Commentary. *(1) Ataxic dysarthria can be among the presenting signs of cerebellar degenerative disease. Its characteristics can be quite subtle but its recognition can help confirm cerebellar dysfunction. (2) Some degenerative CNS diseases that affect speech may be so slowly progressive that intelligibility is preserved over many years and perhaps never significantly affected.*

Case 6.4

A 56-year-old woman presented for neurologic assessment with a primary complaint of speech difficulty. This had developed gradually, with some progression, over the previous eight months. It was accompanied by general "awkwardness" when sewing or running and some memory problems. Neurologic examination was normal with the exception of her speech deficit, although questions were raised about depression and possible cognitive decline. Subsequent psychometric assessment was normal. Computed tomography scan and MRI scans were negative. A complete general medical work-up was normal. Psychiatric consultation confirmed the presence of depression, but felt that it had developed in response to her neurologic/speech difficulties.

Speech examination was notable for the presence of irregular articulatory breakdowns during connected speech (2), irregular speech AMRs (2), and unsteadiness of vowel prolongation (1,2). Intelligibility was mild-moderately reduced. There was no evidence of aphasia.

The clinician concluded "dysarthria, ataxic (cerebellar), moderate-marked."

The neurologist concluded that the patient had a cerebellar dysarthria of undetermined etiology and stated that the underlying disease might "declare itself more clearly with time." She was seen about 18 months later for reassessment. Her dysarthria had worsened and she had a clear-cut gait ataxia. Magnetic resonance imaging scan was again normal. Repeat psychometric assessment was unchanged and no other abnormalities were identified during a complete medical work-up. Again, the diagnosis was "cerebellar syndrome of unknown origin."

The patient experienced progression of her deficits over the next 18 months but her only new symptom was a mild and vaguely described swallowing problem. These were reported through correspondence and not observed during formal reassessment. She was not seen for further follow-up.

Commentary. (1) Ataxic dysarthria can be the first and most prominent finding in degenerative neurologic disease. (2) It may precede the development of other signs of cerebellar degeneration and may be present in the absence of neuroimaging evidence of cerebellar degeneration or lesions.

Case 6.5

A 63-year-old woman was hospitalized for evaluation and treatment of cardiovascular problems. She had a history of myocardial infarction and had had coronary bypass surgery six months ago. Three weeks prior to admission she developed the sudden onset of speech difficulty and problems with gait. She had no difficulties with language, chewing, or swallowing.

Oral mechanism examination was normal. Speech was characterized by irregular articulatory breakdowns (1,2); irregular speech AMRs (1); and unsteady vowel prolongation (2). Intelligibility was normal.

The clinician concluded that the patient had a "mild ataxic dysarthria." Because intelligibility was essentially normal, and because the patient was compensating well for her deficit and was generally unconcerned about it, therapy was not recommended.

Subsequent CT scan identified a 2 cm area of low attenuation in the right cerebellar hemisphere consistent with a diagnosis of infarct.

Commentary. (1) Ataxic dysarthria can result from cerebellar stroke and may be among the most prominent signs of such an event. (2) Ataxic dysarthria can result from a unilateral lesion affecting the cerebellar hemispheres. (3) Although some studies suggest that ataxic dysarthria resulting from unilateral cerebellar lesions occurs more frequently with lesions of the left cerebellar hemisphere, it can occur with lesions to the right cerebellar hemisphere. (4) The presence of dysarthria does not lead automatically to a recommendation for treatment. Such a recommendation is based on the degree of disability and the patient's judgment about and compensations for the problem, among other things.

SUMMARY

1. Ataxic dysarthria results from damage to the cerebellar control circuit, most frequently damage to the lateral hemispheres or vermis of the cerebellum. It may occur at a frequency slightly higher than that for other major single dysarthria types. Although it may reflect deficits at all levels of speech production, it is most evident in articulation and prosody. Incoordination and reduced muscle tone appear responsible for the slowness of movement and inaccuracy in the force, range, timing, and direction of speech movements in ataxic dysarthria.

2. Degenerative disease may account for the largest proportion of cases of ataxic dysarthria; vascular, demyelinating, and undetermined etiologies are also common. Most patients have clinical evidence of cerebellar involvement other than ataxic dysarthria. When positive, neuroimaging studies frequently identify cerebellar lesions or abnormalities in the brain stem or posterior fossa.

3. People with ataxic dysarthria frequently complain of slurred speech and a "drunken" quality to their speech. Complaints of dysphagia and difficulty with drooling are infrequent.

4. The major clusters of deviant speech characteristics in ataxic dysarthria include articulatory inaccuracy, prosodic excess, and phonatory-prosodic insufficiency. Although many abnormal speech characteristics can be detected in ataxic dysarthria, irregular articulatory breakdowns, irregular speech AMRs, excess and equal stress, distorted vowels, and prolonged phonemes are the most distinctive clues to the presence of ataxic dysarthria.

5. In general, acoustic and physiologic studies of ataxic dysarthria have provided quantitative supportive evidence for the clinical perceptual characteristics of the disorder. They have helped to specify more completely the locus and dynamics of abnormal movements underlying the perceived speech disturbance.

6. Ataxic dysarthria can be the only, the first, or among the first or most prominent manifestations of neurologic disease. Its correlation with cerebellar abnormalities can aid the localization and diagnosis of neurologic disease and may contribute to the medical and behavioral management of the individual and the speech disorder.

REFERENCES

Abbs JH, Hunker CJ, and Barlow SM: Differential speech motor subsystem impairments with suprabulbar lesions:

neurophysiological framework and supporting data. In Berry WR, editor: Clinical dysarthria, San Diego, 1983, College-Hill.

Ackerman H and Ziegler W: Cerebellar voice tremor: an acoustic analysis, J Neurol Neurosurg Psychiatry 54:74, 1991.

Ackerman H and others: Speech deficits in ischemic cerebellar lesions, J Neurol 239:223, 1992.

Adams RD and Victor M: Principles of neurology, New York, 1991, McGraw-Hill.

Amarenco P and others: Paravermal infarct and isolated cerebellar dysarthria, Ann Neurol, 30:211, 1991.

Amici R, Avanzini G, and Pacini L: Cerebellar tumors. In Monographs in neural sciences, vol 4, Basel, Switzerland, 1976, Karger.

Anderson NE, Rosenblum MK, and Posner JB: Paraneoplastic cerebellar degeneration: clinical-immunological correlations, Ann Neurol 24:559, 1988.

Aronson AE: Clinical voice disorders, New York, 1990, Thieme.

Brink JD, Imbus C, and Woo-Sam J: Physical recovery after severe closed head trauma in children and adolescents, J Pediatr, 97:721, 1980.

Brown JR: Localizing cerebellar syndromes, J Amer Med Assoc 141:518, 1949.

Brown JR, Darley FL, and Aronson AE: Deviant dimensions of motor speech in cerebellar ataxia. In Transactions of the American Neurological Association, 93:193, 1968.

Brown JR, Darley FL, and Aronson AE: Ataxic dysarthria, Int J Neurol 7:302, 1970.

Chester CS and Reznick BR: Ataxia after severe head injury, Ann Neurol 22:77, 1987.

Clinical examinations in neurology, ed 6, members of the Department of Neurology, Mayo Clinic, Mayo Foundation for Medical Education and Research, St Louis, 1991, Mosby–Year Book.

Darley FL, Aronson AE, and Brown JR: Clusters of deviant speech dimensions in the dysarthrias, J Speech Hear Res 12:462, 1969a.

Darley FL, Aronson AE, and Brown JR: Differential diagnostic patterns of dysarthria, J Speech Hear Res 12:246, 1969b.

Darley FL, Aronson AE, and Brown JR: Motor speech disorders, Philadelphia, 1975, WB Saunders.

Daube JR and others, Medical neurosciences, Boston, 1986, Little, Brown.

DeJong RN: The neurological examination, ed 3, New York, 1967, Hoeber.

Dworkin JP and Aronson AE: Tongue strength and alternate motion rates in normal and dysarthric subjects, J Commun Disord 19:115, 1986.

Espir MLE and Walker ME: Carbamazepine in multiple sclerosis, Lancet 1:280, 1969.

Gentil M: Dysarthria in Friedreich's disease, Brain Lang 38:438, 1990.

Gilchrist E and Wilkinson M: Some factors determining prognosis in young people with severe head injuries, Arch Neurol 36:355, 1979.

Gilman S and Kluin D: Perceptual analysis of speech disorders in Friedreich disease and olivopontocerebellar atrophy. In Bloedel JR and others, editors: Cerebellar functions, Berlin, 1984, Springer-Verlag.

Gilman S, Bloedel JR, and Lechtenberg R: Disorders of the cerebellum, Philadelphia, 1981, FA Davis.

Grewel F: Classification of dysarthrias, Acta Psychiatr Scand 32:325, 1957.

Haggard MP: Speech waveform measurements in multiple sclerosis, Folia Phoniatr Logop 21:307, 1969.

Harding AE: Commentary: olivopontocerebellar atrophy is not a useful concept. In Marsden CN and Fahn S, editors: Movement disorders 2, New York, 1987, Butterworth.

Hirose H and others: Analysis of abnormal articulatory dynamics in two dysarthric patients, J Speech Hear Disord 4:96, 1978.

Hixon TJ and Hoit J: Differential subsystem impairment, differential subsystem impairments and decomposition of respiratory movement in ataxic dysarthria: a spurious trilogy, J Speech Hearing Disord 49:436, 1984.

Holmes G: Clinical symptoms of cerebellar disease, Lancet 59, 1922.

Janvrin F and Worster-Drought C: Diagnosis of disseminated sclerosis by graphic registration and film tracks, Lancet 2:1348, 1932.

Joanette Y and Dudley JG: Dysarthric symptomatology of Friedreich's ataxia, Brain Lang 10:39, 1980.

Jordan JE: Thyroid disorder, Semin Neurol 5:304, 1985.

Judd LL: The therapeutic use of psychotropic medications. In Wilson and others, editors: Harrison's principles of internal medicine, New York, 1991, McGraw-Hill.

Kammermeier MA: A comparison of phonatory phenomena among groups of neurologically impaired speakers, Ph.D. dissertation, University of Minnesota, 1969.

Kent R and Netsell R: A case study of an ataxic dysarthric: cineradiographic and spectrographic, J Speech Hear Disord 40:115, 1975.

Kent RD and Rosenbek JC: Prosodic disturbance and neurologic lesion, Brain Lang 15:259, 1982.

Kent R: Isovowel lines for the evaluation of vowel formant structure in speech disorders, J Speech Hear Disord 44:513, 1979.

Kent R, Netsell R, and Abbs JH: Acoustic characteristics of dysarthria associated with cerebellar disease, J Speech Hear Disord 22:627, 1979.

Lechtenberg R and Gilman S: Speech disorders in cerebellar disease, Ann Neurol 3:285, 1978.

Lehiste I: Some acoustic characteristics of dysarthric speech, Bibliotheca Phonetica, Fasc 2, Basel, 1965, S Karger.

Linebaugh CW and Wolfe VE: Relationships between articulation rate, intelligibility, and naturalness in spastic and ataxic speakers. In McNeil MR, Rosenbek JC, and Aronson AE, editors: The dysarthrias: physiology, acoustics, perception, management, San Diego, 1984, College-Hill.

Logemann J: Evaluation and treatment of swallowing disorders, San Diego, California, 1983, College-Hill.

Mavlov L and Kehaiov A: Le rôle des cordes vocales dans la parole scandée et explosive lors de lésions cérébelleuses, Rev Laryngol Otol Rhino (Bord) 90:320, 1969.

McClean MD, Beukelman DR, and Yorkston KM: Speech-muscle visuomotor tracking in dysarthric and nonimpaired speakers, J Speech Hear Res 30:276, 1987.

McNeil MR and others: Oral structure nonspeech motor control in normal, dysarthric, aphasic, and apraxic speakers: isometric force and static position, J Speech Hear Res 33:255, 1990.

Miller RM and Groher ME: Medical speech pathology, Rockville, MD, 1990, Aspen.

Murdoch BE and others: Respiratory kineumatics in speakers with cerebellar disease, J Speech Hear Res 34:768, 1991.

Murry T: The production of stress in three types of dysarthric speech. In Berry W, editor: Clinical dysarthria, Boston, 1983, College-Hill.

Netsell R and Kent R: Paroxysmal ataxic dysarthria, J Speech Hear Disord 41:93, 1976.

Portnoy RA and Aronson AE: Diadochokinetic syllable rate and regularity in normal and in spastic ataxic dysarthria subjects, J Speech Hear Disord 47:324, 1982.

Putnam AHB: Review of research in dysarthria. In Winitz H, editor: Human communication and its disorders, a review 1988, Norwood, NJ, 1988, Ablex Publishing.

Quinn N: Multiple system atrophy—the nature of the beast, J Neurol Neurosurg Psychiatry (special supplement):78, 1989.

Roberts AH: Long-term prognosis of severe accidental head injury, Proc R Soc Med 69:137, 1976.

Scripture EW: Records of speech in disseminated sclerosis, Brain 39:455, 1916.

Simmons N: Acoustic analysis of ataxic dysarthria: an approach to monitoring treatment. In Berry W, editor: Clinical dysarthria, Boston, 1983, College-Hill.

Tatsumi IF and others: Acoustic properties of ataxic and parkinsonian speech, in syllable repetition tasks. Annual bulletin, research institute of logopedics and phoniatrics 13:99, 1979.

Victor M: Neurologic disorders due to alcoholism and malnutrition. In Baker AB and Joynt RJ, editors: Clinical neurology, vol 4, Philadelphia, 1986, Harper and Row.

Victor M, Adams RD, and Mancal EL: Restricted form of cerebellar cortical degeneration occurring in alcoholic patients, Arch Neurol 1:579, 1959.

von Cramon D: Bilateral cerebellar dysfunctions in a unilateral mesodiencephalic lesion. J Neurol Neurosurg Psychiatry 44:361, 1981.

Walshe F: Diseases of the nervous system, ed 11, New York, 1973, Longman.

Yorkston KM and others: Assessment of stress patterning. In McNeil M, Rosenbek J, and Aronson A, editors: The dysarthrias: physiology, acoustics, perception, management, Austin, TX, 1984, Pro-Ed.

Yorkston KM, Beukelman D, and Bell K: Clinical management of dysarthric speakers, San Diego, 1988, College-Hill.

Zemlin WR: A comparison of the periodic function of vocal fold vibration in a multiple sclerosis and a normal population, PhD dissertation, University of Minnesota, 1962.

7 Hypokinetic Dysarthria

Hypokinetic dysarthria is a perceptually distinguishable motor speech disorder associated with
basal ganglia control circuit pathology. It may be
manifest in any or all of the respiratory, phonatory,
resonatory, and articulatory levels of speech, but
its characteristics are most evident in voice, articulation, and prosody. Its deviant speech characteristics reflect the effects of rigidity, reduced force and
range of movement, and slow individual but sometimes fast repetitive movements on speech. Decreased mobility or range of movement is a significant contributor to the disorder, hence its designation
as *hypokinetic* dysarthria.

Hypokinetic dysarthria is encountered as the
primary speech pathology in a large medical practice at a rate that approximates that for the other
major single dysarthria types. From 1987 to 1990
at the Mayo Clinic, it accounted for 9.1% of
all dysarthrias and 8.3% of all motor speech
disorders seen in the Section of Speech Pathology
(Figure 1–3).

Hypokinetic dysarthria is the only dysarthria in
which a prominent perceptual characteristic may
be *rapid* speech rate. Its identification can aid
neurologic diagnosis and localization. Its presence
is strongly associated with basal ganglia pathology
and is often tied to a depletion of, or functional
reduction in, the effect of the neurotransmitter,
dopamine, on the activities of the basal ganglia.
Parkinson's disease is the prototypic disease associated with hypokinetic dysarthria.

The clinical features of hypokinetic dysarthria
reflect the effects on speech of aberrations in the
maintenance of proper background tone and supportive neuromuscular activity on which the quick,
discrete, phasic movements of speech are superim-

posed. The disorder helps to illustrate the role of
the basal ganglia control circuit in providing an
adequate neuromuscular environment for voluntary motor activity. Hypokinetic speech may give
the impression that the movements and resultant
sounds are "all there" but have been attenuated in
their range or amplitude as well as their ability to
vary with normal flexibility and speed.

ANATOMY AND BASIC FUNCTIONS OF
THE BASAL GANGLIA CONTROL CIRCUIT

The basal ganglia control circuit consists of the
basal ganglia and their connections. Its components were described in some detail in Chapter 2.
Its structures and pathways that are most relevant
to speech are briefly summarized here.

The basal ganglia are located deep within the
cerebral hemispheres. They include the *striatum,*
comprised of the *caudate nucleus and putamen,*
and the *lentiform nucleus,* comprised of the *putamen* and *globus pallidus.* The *substantia nigra* and
subthalamic nuclei are anatomically and functionally related to the basal ganglia. Basal ganglia
activities are strongly associated with the actions
of the indirect activation pathways or extrapyramidal system.

The interconnections that make up the basal
ganglia control circuit are complex. The basic
components include: cortical, thalamic, and substantia nigra input to the striatum, with crucial
cortical input coming from the frontal lobe premotor cortex; striatum input to the substantia nigra
and globus pallidus; and globus pallidus input to
the thalamus, subthalamic nucleus, red nucleus,
and reticular formation in the brain stem. These
connections form loops in which information is

returned to its origin. For example, basal ganglia input to the thalamus is relayed to the cortex and returned to its origin in the basal ganglia; striatum input to the substantia nigra returns to the striatum; globus pallidus input to the subthalamic nucleus is returned to the globus pallidus. The major efferent pathways of the basal ganglia originate in the globus pallidus.

The functions of the circuit are to *regulate muscle tone, regulate movements that support goal-directed movements* (for example, the arm-swing during walking), *control postural adjustments during skilled movements* (for example, stabilize the shoulder during writing), *adjust movements to the environment* (for example, speaking with restricted jaw movement), and *assist in the learning of new movements.* Damage to the circuit either reduces movement or results in a failure to inhibit involuntary movement. In hypokinetic dysarthria, speech deficits are mostly associated with reductions of movement.

The primary influence of the basal ganglia control circuit on speech is through its connections with motor areas of the cerebral cortex. Its influence on the cortex appears inhibitory; that is, it damps or modulates cortical output that would otherwise be in excess of that required to accomplish movement goals. The circuit helps to maintain a stable musculoskeletal environment in which discrete movements can occur. Excessive or insufficient damping of cortical output results in disorders of motor control.

Imbalances among neurotransmitters are responsible for many of the motor problems associated with basal ganglia control circuit malfunction. The actions of *dopamine* are of particular importance to understanding Parkinson's disease and its associated hypokinetic dysarthria. Dopamine is normally produced in sufficient quantity in the substantia nigra and transmitted to the striatum where it probably acts as an inhibitory neurotransmitter. When substantia nigra neurons are destroyed, the dopamine supply to the striatum is reduced and its role in the circuit is diminished. The functional results of this are discussed in the next section.

CLINICAL CHARACTERISTICS OF BASAL GANGLIA CONTROL CIRCUIT DISORDERS ASSOCIATED WITH HYPOKINETIC DYSARTHRIA

Parkinsonism will serve as a model for discussing the clinical characteristics of basal ganglia control circuit disorders that result in hypokinesia. It is the most common cause of hypokinetic dysarthria, and it is generally accepted that dysarthria occurs in half of all cases with Parkinson's disease (Mlcoch,

1992), the percentage increasing with disease progression. Berry (1983) states that Parkinson's disease accounts for 98% of cases with hypokinetic dysarthria seen in speech pathology practices. The pathophysiology of Parkinson's disease and parkinsonism will be discussed in the next section. At this point, only nonoromotor characteristics of parkinsonism will be addressed.

The motor characteristics of parkinsonism are summarized in Table 7–1. The classic signs are *tremor at rest, rigidity, bradykinesia,* and *a loss of postural reflexes.*

The tremor in parkinsonism is a *static* or *resting tremor* that occurs at a rate of about 4 to 7 Hz (Darley, Aronson, and Brown, 1975). It is most apparent when the body part is relaxed, and it tends to decrease during voluntary movement. It is often apparent in the limbs and head, but may also be evident in the jaw, lips, and tongue. A *pill-*

Table 7–1 Common nonspeech clinical signs of parkinsonism.

Primary deficits	Examples
Resting tremor	Head Limb Pill-rolling Jaw, lip, tongue
Rigidity	Resistance to passive stretch in all directions through full range of movement Paucity of movement
Bradykinesia/ hypokinesia	Slow initiation & speed of movements "Freezing"
Akinesia	Festinating gait Reduced: Armswing during walking Limb gestures during speech Eye blinking Head movement accompanying vertical & horizontal eye movement Frequency of swallowing Micrographia Masked facies
Postural abnormalities	Stooped posture (flexed head & trunk) Poor adjustment to tilting or falling Difficulty turning in bed Difficulty going from sitting to standing

rolling movement between the thumb and forefinger may be present.

Rigidity is characterized by slowness of movement and a feeling of stiffness or tightness. It is apparent during passive stretch on muscles and probably contributes to the characteristic paucity of movement in parkinsonism. It may be the result of excessive central nervous system (CNS) influence on alpha motoneurons, which occurs because excessive cortical motor output is not properly inhibited by the basal ganglia (Adams and Victor, 1991). Unlike spasticity, in which resistance to movement is usually greatest at the beginning of stretch and is biased in one direction, rigidity is associated with resistance in all directions and through the full range of movement. *Cogwheel rigidity,* in which resistance of the limbs to passive stretch has a jerky or "off and on" character, is common.

Bradykinesia is characterized by delays or false starts at the beginning of movement and slowness of movement once begun. Movement may also be difficult to stop and repetitive movements may be decreased in amplitude and speed. In spite of a will to move, there may be intermittent *"freezing"* or immobility.

The terms *hypokinesia* (reduced movement) and *akinesia* (absence of movement) are often used interchangeably with bradykinesia (Jankovic, 1992). In addition to slowness, however, they also refer to underactivity or reduced range of movement, reduced use of an affected body part, and a reduction of the automatic, habitual movements that accompany natural movement. This cannot be attributed entirely to weakness, because strength is not notably affected in parkinsonism.

The underactivity of hypokinesia is reflected in a masked or expressionless and unblinking facial expression (*masked facies*), a classic feature of parkinsonism (Figure 7–1). Similarly, the normal armswing during walking and the limb gestures that automatically accompany speech may be reduced. Writing may be *micrographic* (small). Walking may be slowly initiated and then characterized by short, rapid shuffling steps, a phenomenon known as *festination.*

Posture tends to be characterized by involuntary flexion of the head, trunk, and arms. Because postural reflexes are impaired, the patient may be unable to make adjustments to tilting or falling and have difficulty turning in bed or moving from a sitting to standing position.

ETIOLOGIES

Hypokinetic dysarthria can be caused by any process that can damage the basal ganglia control circuit. These include degenerative, vascular, trau-

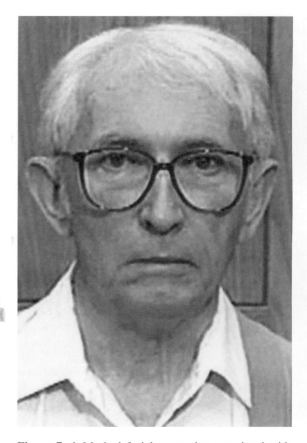

Figure 7–1 Masked facial expression associated with Parkinson's disease and hypokinetic dysarthria.

matic, inflammatory, neoplastic, toxic, and metabolic diseases (defined in Chapter 2). These broad etiologic categories are associated with hypokinetic dysarthria with varying frequency, but the exact distribution of causes is unknown.

Parkinson's disease and other related CNS degenerative diseases are almost certainly the most frequent cause of hypokinetic dysarthria. And, if other influences are not active (for example, medication effects), hypokinetic dysarthria is *the* dysarthria of Parkinson's disease. This sometimes leads to the interchangeable use of the terms hypokinetic dysarthria and "the dysarthria of Parkinson's disease" or "parkinsonian dysarthria." The term hypokinetic dysarthria is preferable, however, because conditions other than Parkinson's disease can be associated with it. In addition, patients with Parkinson's disease may have more than hypokinetic dysarthria. For example, medication used to treat Parkinson's disease can cause involuntary movements that result in hyperkinetic dysarthria. And, some patients with a diagnosis of Parkinson's disease ultimately receive a different diagnosis, one indicating the presence of more than basal ganglia dysfunction (for example, progressive supranuclear palsy).

Some of the common neurologic conditions associated with hypokinetic dysarthria with noticeably greater frequency than other dysarthria types are discussed in the following sections. Diseases that can produce the disorder but are more frequently associated with other dysarthria types (especially mixed dysarthria) are discussed in chapters dealing with those dysarthrias.

Degenerative diseases

Parkinson's disease (PD) is a common, slowly progressive idiopathic neurologic disease. It usually begins in mid-to-later life, sometimes with unilateral symptoms at the outset (Koller, 1992). Its occurrence is sporadic, although it is familial in 1% to 2% of cases (Beal, Richardson, and Martin, 1991). Many cases developed in the aftermath of an encephalitis epidemic after World War I; cases due to encephalitis are referred to as *postencephalitic parkinsonism.*

Parkinson's disease may affect more than motor function. One third to one half of PD patients have signs of dementia (Beal, Richardson, and Martin, 1991). Depression may also occur, either as part of the disease process or in response to its motor or cognitive disabilities. Sometimes akinesia and bradykinesia are mistaken for depression and the diagnosis of PD is missed.

The pathologic changes of PD most often involve nerve cell loss in the substantia nigra and locus ceruleus and decreased dopamine content in the striatum. The imbalance between dopamine and acetylcholine caused by the depletion of dopamine in the striatum is felt to be responsible for the clinical signs of the disease.

Parkinson's disease tends to be responsive to *dopaminergic drugs* (known as *dopamine agonists*), which restore the balance between dopamine and acetylcholine. Unfortunately, these agents do not affect the underlying disease process. *Levodopa* is the cornerstone of treatment of akinesia and postural problems; it works by increasing dopamine levels in the striatum. It is sometimes given in combination with *carbidopa* (this combination drug is *Sinemet*), which prevents destruction of levodopa in the bloodstream and minimizes side effects. *Bromocriptine,* also a dopamine agonist, acts directly on dopamine receptors and is often used in combination with Sinemet. *Anticholinergic drugs* may be used for resting tremor.

Unfortunately, the medications used to treat PD have side effects that include dystonia and dyskinesias, confusion, and *on-off effects.* On-off effects are symptom fluctuations that occur during a dosage cycle; they may include shifts from worsening of parkinsonian symptoms to the development of dystonia or dyskinesias at the beginning, peak, or end of a dosage cycle. Worsening of hypokinetic dysarthria or the emergence of hyperkinetic dysarthria may occur as reflections of on-off effects. Therefore, the dysarthria encountered in people with PD may represent the effects of the disease itself as well as the effects of medications used to treat it. The design of clinical and laboratory investigations of hypokinetic dysarthria in PD must take into account medication effects, and they need to control for the time at which observations are made during the dosage cycle, especially in longitudinal investigations.

The term Parkinson's disease is usually reserved for parkinsonism of unknown cause. The term *parkinsonism,* often used synonymously with PD, is usually used in a more general sense to refer to the clinical signs of the disease without regard to etiology. *Parkinson's syndrome* is sometimes used to refer to conditions with etiologies and pathophysiology that are different from PD (for example, vascular, Alzheimer's disease, drug-induced) (Olson and others, 1989), or when symptoms are not responsive to medications that are effective in managing PD.

Nigrostriatal degeneration is a rare condition that resembles PD, but its pathology is different and it is not responsive to dopaminergic drugs. In addition to parkinsonian signs, affected patients may have progressive ataxia or autonomic nervous system involvement (Adams and Victor, 1991). It is an example of diseases that fall under the broad heading of *multiple systems atrophy (MSA).* Other diseases captured under the MSA heading that can be associated with hypokinetic dysarthria include *olivopontocerebellar atrophy (OPCA)* (defined in Chapter 6), *progressive supranuclear palsy (PSP),* and *Shy-Drager syndrome.* Progressive supranuclear palsy and Shy-Drager syndrome will be described in Chapter 10 because they are frequently associated with mixed dysarthrias.

Alzheimer's disease (AD) is marked clinically by its progressive effects on memory, cognition, language, and personality, and histopathologically by neurofibrillary tangles, neuritic plaques, and granulovacuolar degeneration. Extrapyramidal signs are not uncommon and parkinsonian-like signs have been noted in 35% to 50% of patients with AD (Leverenz and Sumi, 1984; Mayeux, Stern, and Stanton, 1985). *Pick's disease,* another dementing illness with primary effects on the frontal and temporal lobes, is not usually associated with motor or sensory deficits; however, in its advanced stages parkinsonian-like symptoms may develop (Murdoch, 1990). Therefore, the development of hypokinetic dysarthria is possible in some degenerative diseases whose primary manifestations are in the cognitive domain.

Vascular conditions

Multiple or bilateral strokes affecting the basal ganglia can cause rigidity and akinesia, a condition sometimes referred to as "vascular parkinsonism" or "arteriosclerotic parkinsonism" (Critchley, 1929; Tolosa and Santamaria, 1984). *Cerebral hypoxia*, including that induced by carbon monoxide poisoning, can also produce extrapyramidal parkinsonian syndromes.

Toxic-metabolic conditions

Antipsychotic (neuroleptic) medications can have prominent blocking effects on dopamine receptors, leading to a variety of extrapyramidal symptoms (Judd, 1991). *Reserpine* and *phenothiazine drugs* can cause parkinsonian signs, including hypokinetic dysarthria, because they block dopaminergic transmission. *Bupropion* (*Wellbutrin*), an antidepressant, has infrequently been associated with bradykinesia, pseudoparkinsonism, and dysarthria (Smith and Faber, 1992); the dysarthria has not been described, but it is probably hypokinetic. Drug-induced parkinsonism usually develops within the first two months of treatment (Arana and Hyman, 1991). Parkinsonian symptoms may subside after drug withdrawal (Adams and Victor, 1991) or they may respond to drugs used to treat PD.

The illicit drug *MPTP* selectively destroys dopaminergic neurons of the substantia nigra and leads to a syndrome closely resembling PD. Parkinsonian symptoms persist after the drug is discontinued because substantia nigra neurons have been destroyed.

Chronic exposure to *heavy metals* (for example, manganese, lead, mercury) or to *chemicals* such as carbon disulphide, cyanide, and methyl chloride can create a parkinsonian syndrome. *Wilson's disease*, which involves increased copper depositions in the liver and brain, can produce parkinsonian signs, including hypokinetic dysarthria. It may also involve structures outside the basal ganglia, however, and is frequently associated with mixed dysarthria; it will be discussed further in Chapter 10.

Trauma

Repeated head trauma, as can occur in boxers with "punch drunk" encephalopathy, can damage the substantia nigra. This can lead to parkinsonian-like motor abnormalities, including hypokinetic dysarthria. A single-event *traumatic brain injury (TBI)* can also produce these abnormalities.

Parkinsonian patients with severe tremor that is unresponsive to drug treatment sometimes undergo *stereotactic ventrolateral thalamotomy* to relieve the tremor; the surgical placement of a lesion in the thalamus interrupts the circuit through which the tremor emerges. This often successfully abolishes the tremor but cognitive deficits, aphasia, and dysarthria (or worsening of dysarthria) are possible side effects. Therefore, in parkinsonian patients, hypokinetic dysarthria may be worsened, or a unilateral upper motor neuron dysarthria may be superimposed upon it (Andrianopoulos, Duffy, and Kelly, unpublished).

Infectious

Viral encephalitis has already been mentioned as a cause of PD. Infectious diseases that can lead to encephalitis include measles, mumps, mononucelosis, and rabies (Brown, 1980).

Other

Normal pressure hydrocephalus (NPH) (see Chapter 6 for definition) can be associated with parkinsonian symptoms, including hypokinetic dysarthria.

SPEECH PATHOLOGY
Distribution of etiologies, lesions, and severity in clinical practice

The box on page 171 summarizes the etiologies for 107 quasirandomly selected cases seen at the Mayo Clinic with a speech pathology diagnosis of hypokinetic dysarthria. The cautions expressed in Chapter 4 about generalizing these data to the general population or to all speech pathology practices also apply here.

The data establish that hypokinetic dysarthria can have a number of etiologies, the distribution of which are different from that associated with several other dysarthria types. Degenerative diseases accounted for 75% of the cases, of which three quarters had diagnoses of PD or parkinsonism. Unspecified "CNS degenerative disease" was the diagnosis for several cases; parkinsonism was suspected in some of these, but others had signs of more than basal ganglia degeneration (for example, dementia or cerebellar findings). The remaining degenerative diseases included conditions associated with multiple systems atrophy, such as PSP and Shy-Drager syndrome.

Nonhemorrhagic stroke accounted for the largest proportion of the relatively small number of vascular etiologies; this small number is consistent with clinical impressions that hypokinetic dysarthria is an uncommon result of stroke. The remaining vascular etiologies included hemorrhagic events and anoxia resulting from cardiac arrest.

Cases with undetermined etiology nonetheless

ETIOLOGIES OF HYPOKINETIC DYSARTHRIA FOR 107 QUASIRANDOMLY SELECTED CASES WITH A PRIMARY SPEECH PATHOLOGY DIAGNOSIS OF HYPOKINETIC DYSARTHRIA AT THE MAYO CLINIC FROM 1969 TO 1990. PERCENTAGE OF CASES UNDER EACH BROAD ETIOLOGIC HEADING IS GIVEN IN PARENTHESES.

Degenerative (75%)

Parkinson's disease (31%)

Parkinsonism (26%)

Progressive supranuclear palsy (7%)

Degenerative CNS disease (sometimes including suspicion of parkinsonism or Alzheimer's disease (5%)

Shy-Drager syndrome (3%)

Multiple systems atrophy, unspecified (2%)

Unspecified extrapyramidal and cerebellar degeneration (1%)

Vascular (10%)

Nonhemorrhagic stroke (5%)

Nonparenchymal bleeds (subarachnoid hemorrhage, subdural hematoma) (2%)

Ruptured aneurysm (1%)

Small vessel disease (1%)

Anoxia (cardiac arrest) (1%)

Undetermined (6%)

Extrapyramidal disorder (2%)

Parkinson's disease vs PSP (3%)

PSP vs stroke (1%)

Toxic/metabolic (3%)

Drug related (phenothiazines, unspecified) (2%)

Carbon monoxide (1%)

Traumatic (2%)

Closed head injury

Multiple (2%)

Parkinsonism + multiple sclerosis (1%)

Parkinsonism + stroke (1%)

Infectious (1%)

Postencephalitic parkinsonism

Other (1%)

Radiation necrosis

CNS, central nervous system; *PSP,* progressive supranuclear palsy.

had signs of basal ganglia involvement. The listed diagnostic possibilities usually included PD, PSP, or unspecified extrapyramidal disorder; in several cases, signs and symptoms were of recent onset or were very subtle; it is likely that a more definitive diagnosis emerged with passage of time.

The small number of cases with toxic or metabolic etiology generally were consistent with predictions from the literature (for example, one case with carbon monoxide poisoning, one associated with phenothiazine use).

Two cases had closed head injury, illustrating that its frequent significant effect on subcortical structures can produce hypokinetic dysarthria. A few cases had more than one disease, either or both of which may have caused the dysarthria (that is, parkinsonism, stroke, multiple sclerosis). The remaining causes included postencephalitic parkinsonism and an unusual case with parkinsonian signs following radiation therapy.

These cases support the status of PD and parkinsonism as prototypes of diseases associated with hypokinetic dysarthria. They also establish that vascular, toxic-metabolic, traumatic, and infectious conditions can produce the disorder.

As might be expected, 99% of the cases had nonspeech deficits that were clinically localized to the basal ganglia control circuit (but not necessarily limited to it). Neuroimaging (for example, computed tomography [CT], magnetic resonance imaging [MRI]) in most cases, however, was either negative or revealed only mild cerebral atrophy or enlarged ventricles; in some cases, cerebellar atrophy was also apparent. This is common in idiopathic PD and other related degenerative diseases that include, but are not necessarily limited to, the basal ganglia. Most of the vascular and traumatic cases had neuroimaging evidence of lesions in or near the basal ganglia, but not always bilaterally; however, patients with only unilateral lesions on neuroimaging nonetheless usually had bilateral clinical signs, indicating the presence of bilateral pathology.

This retrospective review did not permit a clear delineation of dysarthria severity. However, in those patients for whom a judgment of intellgibility was explicitly stated (69% of the sample), *78% had reduced intelligibility.* The degree to which this figure accurately estimates the frequency of intelligibility impairments in the population with hypokinetic dysarthria is unclear. It is likely that many patients for whom an observation of intelligibility was not made had normal intelligibility; however, the sample probably contains a larger number of mildly impaired patients than is encountered in a typical rehabilitation setting. It is reasonable to conclude, however, that intelligibility is frequently reduced by hypokinetic dysarthria.

Finally, cognitive impairment was common in this sample. For patients whose cognitive abilities were explicitly commented on or formally assessed (75% of the sample), *81% had some degree of cognitive impairment.*

Patient perceptions and complaints

Affected people may describe their speech in ways that provide clues to speech diagnosis and its localization. Complaints that the voice is *quieter, or weak, or cannot be heard in noise* are common. Many will complain that rate is *too fast* or that words are *indistinct,* and some note that their speech *lacks emotional tone.* Some complain that it is "difficult to get speech started" and others use the word "*stutter*" to describe difficulties with initiation of speech or repetitions of sounds, syllables, and even words. It is rare that complaints about dysfluencies are felt by the patient to be triggered by anxiety, anticipation of speech difficulty, specific word or sound fears, or circumlocution.

Complaints about negative effects of *fatigue* on speech are not uncommon. Those with drug responsive parkinsonism often note *variations in speech as a function of their medication cycle,* frequently characterized by deterioration just prior to their next dose. *Drooling* and *swallowing complaints* are not uncommon. Some patients complain that their upper lip feels stiff, perhaps reflecting the perception of reduced flexibility of movement.

Clinical findings

Hypokinetic dysarthria usually occurs with other signs of basal ganglia disease. It occurs frequently enough in parkinsonism for its recognition to serve as confirmatory evidence for the neurologic diagnosis. Even more important, it sometimes is the presenting complaint or first and only sign of parkinsonism. In such cases, recognition of the dysarthria as hypokinetic can be essential to localization and diagnosis.

Nonspeech oral mechanism. The oral mechanism examination can be very revealing and often confirmatory of the diagnosis of hypokinetic dysarthria. The face may be *unblinking* and *unsmiling, masked* or *expressionless at rest* (Figure 7–1) and *lack animation* during nonverbal social interaction. Movements of the eyes and face, hands, arms, and trunk that normally accompany speech and complement the emotions and indirect meanings conveyed through prosody may be attenuated. Chest and abdominal movements during quiet breathing may appear reduced or nonexistent, and they may remain reduced in excursion when the patient attempts to breathe deeply.

As the eyes may blink infrequently, so may the patient *swallow infrequently,* perhaps another reflection of rigidity or reduced automatic movements. This may lead to excessive saliva accumulation and *drooling.* When moving the eyes to look to the side or up or down, the normal tendency for head turning to accompany the gaze may be absent.

A tremor or *tremulousness* of the jaw and lips may be apparent at rest or during sustained mouth opening or lip retraction. Similarly, the tongue is often strikingly tremulous on protrusion or at rest within the mouth. The lips (particularly upper) may appear tight or immobile at rest and during movement, including speech.

The size, strength, and symmetry of the jaw, face, and tongue may be normal, often surprisingly so given their limited movement during speech. Nonspeech alternating motion rates (AMRs) of the jaw, lips, and tongue may be slowly initiated and completed, or rapid and markedly restricted in range. In contrast, range of motion for single movements (for example, lip retraction) may be distinctly greater than that observed during speech or expected emotional responses.

The overall impression derived during casual observation and formal oral mechanism examination is one of a lack of vigor or animation in the absence of a degree of weakness that might explain it. At rest, as well as during social interaction and speech, the patient's facial affect appears restricted, "flat," unemotional, and sometimes depressed. These impressions may not accurately reflect the patient's inner emotional state. Unfortunately, but predictably, their speech usually faithfully mirrors their nonverbal behaviors.

Speech. Conversational speech or reading, speech AMRs, and vowel prolongation all provide useful information about salient and distinguishing speech characteristics. Conversational speech and reading are essential for identifying the prosodic abnormalities that can be so prominent in the disorder. Speech AMRs are particularly useful for observing reductions in range of movement and rate abnormalities; rapid, accelerated, and sometimes "blurred" speech AMRs are distinguishing perceptual characteristics of hypokinetic dysarthria (see Figure 7–2). Vowel prolongation is useful for isolating some of the disorder's phonatory characteristics, especially those associated with loudness and quality.

Hypokinetic dysarthria usually reflects neuromuscular abnormalities in much of the speech musculature, usually related to restriction in the range or speed of movement patterns. The effects of these abnormalities give hypokinetic dysarthria its distinctive characteristics, most of which are associated with phonatory and articulatory activities, and the effects of those abnormalities on prosody.

Table 7–2 summarizes the neuromuscular deficits presumed by Darley, Aronson, and Brown (1969a & b, 1975) to underlie hypokinetic dysarthria. Speech movements and their timing are

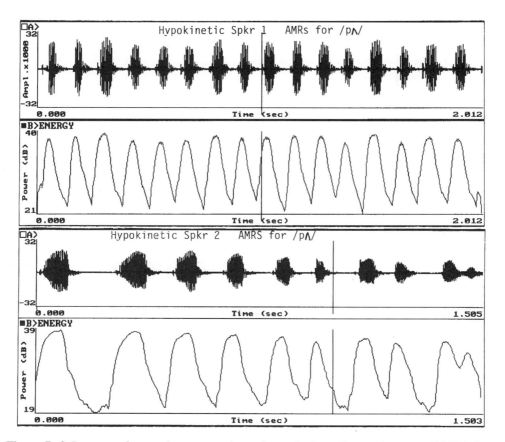

Figure 7–2 Raw waveform and energy tracings of speech alternating motion rates (AMRs) for /pʌ/ by two speakers with hypokinetic dysarthria. Speaker 1's AMRs (2 secs) are regular but rapid (~8 Hz). Speaker 2's productions (1.5 secs) are normal in rate (~6 Hz in the first sec), but show a trend toward increased overall rate and reduced amplitude and duration of each pulse, the acoustic correlate of perceived accelerated rate.

Table 7–2 Neuromuscular deficits associated with hypokinetic dysarthria.

Direction	Rhythm	Rate		Range		Force	Tone
Individual movements	Repetitive movements	Individual movements	Repetitive movements	Individual movements	Repetitive movements	Individual movements	Muscle tone
Normal	Regular	Slow	Fast	Reduced	Very Reduced	Reduced (paretic)	Excessive (balanced)

Adapted from Darley FL, Aronson AE, and Brown JR: Clusters of deviant speech dimensions in the dysarthrias, J Speech Hear Res 12:462, 1969b.

generally accurate. Individual movements are slowed but, especially when range of movement is limited, repetitive movements may be fast. The range and force of individual and repetitive movements are reduced. Muscle tone is excessive (that is, rigid) with resistance to movement in all directions, a condition that contributes to decreased range of movement. Limited range of movement may be the most significant underlying neuromuscular deficit in hypokinesia as it affects speech. The relationships among these characteristics and the specific deviant characteristics associated with hypokinetic dysarthria are discussed in the next section. Experimental support for the presumed underlying neuromuscular deficits will be reviewed in the section on acoustic and physiologic findings.

Prominent deviant speech characteristics and clusters of deviant dimensions. A general profile of the speech characteristics of hypokinetic dysarthria has been established by Logemann and others (1978). They determined the frequency of deviant voice and speech characteristics in a group of 200 people with PD. Only 11% had no speech deficit, attesting to the high incidence of dysarthria in the disease. Eighty-nine percent had voice disorders that were characterized by *hoarseness, roughness, tremulousness,* and *breathiness.* Forty-five percent had articulation problems (these will be described in the next section). Twenty percent had rate abnormalities that were characterized by *syllable repetitions, shortened syllables, lengthened syllables,* and *excessive pauses.* Ten percent were *hypernasal.* Of interest, 45% had voice abnormalities only and all patients with articulation problems had voice problems; the authors noted that this may reflect the existence of subgroups of dysarthrias in PD or the tendency for dysarthria to begin with laryngeal manifestations and eventually include articulation and other abnormalities. The higher frequency of laryngeal than articulatory impairment in PD has also been noted by Zwirner and Barnes (1992).

Darley, Aronson, and Brown (1969b) found only one cluster of deviant speech dimensions in

Table 7–3 The deviant cluster of abnormal speech characteristics found in hypokinetic dysarthria.

Cluster	Speech characteristics
Prosodic insufficiency	Monopitch Monoloudness Reduced stress Short phrases Variable rate* Short rushes of speech* Imprecise consonants*

*Considered a component of prosodic insufficiency in hypokinetic dysarthria but not in other dysarthria types with prosodic insufficiency.
Based on Darley FL, Aronson AE, and Brown JR: Clusters of deviant speech dimensions in the dysarthrias, J Speech Hear Res 12:462, 1969b.

their group of parkinsonian patients. They labeled it *prosodic insufficiency* to represent the attenuated patterns of vocal emphasis that result from the combined effects of the speech characteristics that make up the cluster. The characteristics of prosodic insufficiency are *monopitch, monoloudness, reduced stress, short phrases, variable rate, short rushes of speech,* and *imprecise consonants* (summarized in Table 7–3). Together, these features give hypokinetic dysarthria its distinctive *gestalt of a flat, attenuated, abbreviated, and sometimes accelerated quality.* The neuromuscular basis for the cluster was attributed to reduced range of movement and to the fast repetitive movements that are unique to parkinsonism.

Table 7–4 summarizes the most deviant speech dimensions encountered in hypokinetic dysarthria (Darley, Aronson, and Brown, 1969a). The component of the speech system most prominently associated with each speech characteristic is also included. The rankings in the table represent the order of prominence (severity) of the speech characteristics and not necessarily the features that best distinguish hypokinetic dysarthria from other dysarthria types.

Table 7–4 The most deviant speech dimensions encountered in hypokinetic dysarthria by Darley, Aronson, and Brown (1969a), listed in order from most to least severe. Also listed is the component of the speech system associated with each speech characteristic. The component "prosodic" is listed when several components of the speech system may contribute to the dimension.

Dimension	Speech component
Monopitch*	Phonatory-prosodic
Reduced stress*	Prosodic
Monoloudness*	Phonatory-respiratory-prosodic
Imprecise consonants	Articulatory
Inappropriate silences*	Prosodic
Short rushes of speech*	Articulatory-prosodic
Harsh voice quality	Phonatory
Breathy voice (continuous)	Phonatory
Low pitch	Phonatory
Variable rate*	Articulatory-prosodic
Other	
Increased rate in segments*	Prosodic
Increase of rate overall*	Prosodic
Repeated phonemes*	Articulatory

*Tend to be distinctive or more severely impaired than in any other single dysarthria type.

A few additional observations may help to complete the picture of the disorder.

1. The nature of imprecise consonants was not specifically rated by Darley, Aronson, and Brown (1969a). However, Logemann and Fisher (1981) did describe them in their narrow phonetic transcriptions of 90 patients with PD (Logemann and others, 1978). They found a predominance of highly consistent manner errors that occurred most frequently for stops, fricatives, and affricates. Stops, especially velars, were most frequently in error and were perceived as fricatives, presumably because of incomplete articulatory contact and continual emission of air during what should have been a stop period; this was also perceived for the stop portion of affricates. Fricatives were perceived as reduced in sharpness, presumably due to a reduced degree of air stream constriction. These features are related to the acoustic feature of *spirantization* and may be the result of *articulatory undershooting* resulting from accelerated rate or reduced range of movement, or both.

2. Some prominent features of hypokinetic dysarthria are not captured in the cluster of prosodic insufficiency (compare the speech characteristics in Tables 7–3 and 7–4). For example, frequently occurring *inappropriate silences* are not logically related to the neuromuscular deficits presumed to underlie prosodic insufficiency; they more likely reflect difficulty in initiating movements.

3. Breathiness, harshness, and reduced loudness can be particularly striking in some patients. When marked, they can extend to a *mildly strained, aphonic or whispered quality.* Even when not pervasively present, a strained-whispered aphonia will sometimes emerge from a breathy-harsh quality and persist for several seconds toward the end of a vowel prolongation task; in the author's experience, this rarely occurs in other dysarthria types. *Reduced loudness* and *breathy voice quality* can be an early sign of hypokinetic dysarthria and the presenting feature of parkinsonism (Aronson, 1991). In general, *dysphonia can be the presenting, most prominent and debilitating speech feature in people with hypokinetic dysarthria.*

4. Speech rate abnormalities can be a striking and highly distinctive feature of hypokinetic dysarthria. These often are apparent during AMRs, in which rate may be very *rapid or accelerated;* combined with reduced range of articulatory excursions, they may have a "blurred" quality, as if all syllables are run together. In conversation or reading, patients may demonstrate *short rushes of speech* in which several words are uttered together, sometimes rapidly, and are separated from the remainder of the utterance by pauses that may occur at inappropriate intervals. Some patients demonstrate an apparent *increased speech rate within segments,* a characteristic that appears analogous to the festinating gait so often present in parkinsonism. Finally, some patients' *overall speech rate is rapid.* Although not always present, features that lead to a perception of rapid rate are unique among the dysarthrias to hypokinetic dysarthria.*

*Note, however, that rapid speech rate can be idiosyncratically normal or associated with some nondysarthric neurologic and psychiatric conditions.

5. Dysfluencies, in the form of *repeated pho-nemes,* are not uncommon (about half of Dar-ley, Aronson, and Brown's patients exhibited them, and they were frequently present in the Logemann and others (1978) study). They tend to occur at the beginning of utterances or following pauses and are usually rapid and sometimes blurred and restricted in range of movement; when vowels and some consonants are "repeated," they may sound more like a prolonged vowel with a tremulous character. They may be analogous to the parkinsonian patient's difficulty in initiating walking, and the rapid, short shuffling steps that may occur as walking begins. Although dysfluencies or stut-teringlike behavior can occur in several neuro-logic conditions (see Chapter 13), the character of the repeated phonemes that occur in hypoki-netic dysarthria tend to be distinctive.

6. A speech disorder that may be strongly related to the repetition of phonemes in hypokinetic dysarthria is *palilalia.* Palilalia is characterized by "compulsive reiteration of utterances in a context of increasing rate and decreasing loud-ness" (LaPointe and Horner, 1981, p. 34). The repetitions usually involve words and phrases; phoneme repetitions are generally not sub-sumed in the disorder's definition. Palilalia is usually associated with bilateral subcortical pa-thology, especially involving the basal ganglia, but has also been noted in bilateral frontal lobe pathology (Brown, 1972). Palilalia will be dis-cussed further in Chapter 13.

7. True voice tremor is uncommon in hypokinetic dysarthria. However, the voice may be un-steady and tremorlike in character secondary to the prominent head and upper limb tremor that are present in some patients. In addition, the voice during vowel prolongation is sometimes characterized by a rapid, low-amplitude *tremu-lousness*; Logemann and others (1978) found vocal tremulousness in 14% of their 200 par-kinsonian patients.

8. Abnormal resonance is not prominent in hypo-kinetic dysarthria, but mild hypernasality was detected in about 25% of Darley, Aronson's, and Brown's, and 10% percent of Logemann and others' (1978) patients. Therefore, mild hypernasality, and even mild weakening of pressure consonants by nasal airflow, is an "acceptable" abnormality in the disorder; they need not raise strong suspicions about another dysarthria type in individuals whose other de-viant speech characteristics are consistent with hypokinetic dysarthria.

What features of hypokinetic dysarthria help distinguish it from other motor speech disorders?

Among the characteristics of the disorder, *mono-pitch, monoloudness, decreased loudness, reduced stress, variable rate, short rushes of speech, over-all increases in rate, increased rate within seg-ments, rapid speech AMRs, repeated phonemes,* and *inappropriate silences* are the most distinctive clues to the presence of hypokinetic dysarthria.

Table 7–5 summarizes the primary distinguish-ing distinctive speech characteristics and common oral mechanism findings and patient complaints encountered in hypokinetic dysarthria.

Acoustic and physiologic findings

Respiration. Abnormal respiratory functions could contribute to the reduced loudness, short phrases, short rushes of speech, and interruptions or pauses that may characterize hypokinetic dysar-thria (Aronson, 1991; Darley, Aronson, and Brown, 1975). Reduced vital capacity, reduced amplitude of chest wall movements during breath-ing, irregularities in breathing patterns, and in-creased respiratory rates have been documented (for example, Ewanowski, 1964; Kim, 1968; Laszewski, 1956; Solomon and Hixon, 1993). Many of these abnormalities have been attributed to alterations in the normal agonist-antagonist relationships of respiratory muscles during breath-ing (that is, rigidity).

Table 7–5 Primary distinguishing speech and speech-related findings in hypokinetic dysarthria.

Perceptual	
Phonatory-respiratory	Reduced loudness
Articulatory	Repeated phonemes, palilalia, rapid or "blurred" AMRs
Prosodic	Reduced stress, monopitch, monoloudness, inappropriate silences Short rushes of speech, variable rate, increased rate in segments, increased overall rate
Physical	Masked facial expression Tremulous jaw, lip, tongue Reduced range of motion on AMR tasks Head tremor
Patient complaints	Reduced loudness, rapid rate, "mumbling," "stuttering," difficulty initiating speech Stiff lips

The contribution of these abnormal respiratory functions to speech is not entirely clear. To the extent that maximum vowel prolongation reflects vital capacity and respiratory control, results have been contradictory. For example, Canter (1965a) and Boshes (1966) found reduced maximum vowel duration in patients with parkinsonism, but Ewanowski (1964) and Kreul (1972) did not. Mueller (1971) found shorter mean maximum phonation time and reduced airflow volume during vowel prolongation, and fewer syllables per breath group and reduced intraoral pressure during speech AMRs. Mueller noted that these deficiencies could reflect reduced respiratory efficiency or reduced glottal valving, either of which could result in insufficient generation of airflow necessary to normal speech. More recently, Solomon and Hixon (1993) found abnormally small rib cage volumes and abnormally large abdominal volumes at the initiation of speech breath groups in PD speakers. Although not clearly attributable to respiratory abnormalities, their PD speakers produced fewer words per breath group and spoke for less time per breath group than normal speakers.

Ewanowski (1964) documented the presence of longer latencies prior to beginning exhalation following forceful inhalation, as well as delayed initiation of phonation once exhalation had begun. Relatedly, Kim (1968) noted difficulty altering automatic respiratory rhythms for speech and documented the presence of more breath groups during reading. McClean, Beukelman, and Yorkston (1987) documented poor tracking of a sinusoidal target with respiratory movements in two of their three PD subjects.

Finally, in about half of their 19 subjects with PD and hypokinetic dysarthria, Murdoch and others (1989) found irregularities in chest wall movements during vowel prolongation and syllable repetition tasks, but not during reading or conversation. The abnormalities were characterized by abrupt movements of chest-wall parts and paradoxical movements of the rib cage and abdomen. There was no readily apparent explanation for the abnormalities, but the authors speculated that rigidity of respiratory muscles might have been responsible.

Reduced respiratory excursions, paradoxical respiratory movements, rapid breathing cycles, and difficulty altering vegetative breathing patterns for voluntary activities seem consistent with patterns of rigidity, hypokinesia, and difficulty initiating movements that occur in other muscle groups in parkinsonism. Such difficulties could contribute importantly to reduced physiologic support for speech and a number of the phonatory and prosodic abnormalities encountered in hypokinetic dysarthria.

Phonation. A number of acoustic and physiologic studies have examined laryngeal function in hypokinetic dysarthria. In general, they confirm hypotheses generated by perceptual analyses, and provide additional insights into the mechanisms underlying abnormal speech characteristics.

1. Fundamental frequency and intensity. Acoustic analyses have frequently found evidence of elevated fundamental frequency (f_o) (Canter, 1963, 1965; Illes and others, 1989; Kammermeier, 1969; Ludlow and Bassich, 1983, 1984) and sometimes of decreased intensity (Illes and others, 1988). For example, the median f_o for Canter's (1963) 17 male parkinsonian subjects was 129 Hz, compared to 106 Hz for age-matched male controls. In contrast, Metter and Hanson (1986) found f_o to fall mostly within the normal range in their PD patients, although they noted a tendency for f_o to increase with increased disease severity.

The tendency for f_o to be increased stands in contrast to the perceptual findings of Darley, Aronson, and Brown (1969a) who found a tendency for pitch to be perceived as low in parkinsonism. The reasons for this discrepancy are not clear. It may be that there is considerable intersubject variability in f_o/pitch or that factors other than f_o lead to a perception of low pitch (that is, monopitch, monoloudness, and reduced loudness could lead to perceptions of lower pitch). The mismatch between acoustic and perceptual studies on this dimension and the fact that ratings of low pitch and findings of elevated f_o are generally not extremely abnormal, suggest that pitch level and f_o alone are not likely to be highly sensitive distinguishing features of hypokinetic dysarthria.

Measures of f_o and intensity *variability* are much more revealing. Pitch and intensity variability have been examined in a wide variety of tasks, including vowel prolongation, spontaneous speech, reading, word and sentence imitation tasks, the expression of emotion, pitch glide tasks, and tasks requiring a range of loud and soft or high or low pitch productions. Findings consistently demonstrate a reduction of pitch and loudness variability in dysarthric parkinsonian patients (Caekebeke and others, 1991; Canter, 1963, 1965a; Darkins, Fromkin, and Benson, 1988; Ludlow and Bassich, 1983, 1984; Metter and Hanson, 1986; Kammermeier, 1969; Robin, Jordan, and Rodnitzky, 1986). This is dramatically illustrated by Canter's (1965b) observation that he was unable to measure speech AMR rate in some of his patients because of "flattened intensity peaks." In several studies, the acoustic findings correlated well with perceptual ratings of monopitch and monoloudness (Figure 7–3). In general, these results provide strong acoustic support for the clinical perception of monopitch and monoloudness.

2. Quality. There have been few acoustic investigations of voice quality. Lehiste (1965) found spectrographic evidence of laryngealization (slow or irregular vocal fold activity or biphasic phonation) and breathiness in parkinsonian speakers. Ludlow and Bassich (1984) found abnormal average amplitude perturbations (shimmer) that were correlated with perceptual measures of breathiness; they noted that this abnormality could be related to vocal cord bowing, with subsequent increased airflow turbulence and intensity variations.

3. Motor control. Several acoustic studies suggest that laryngeal control is reduced in hypokinetic dysarthria. There is evidence that some patients are slow to initiate phonation and that such events correlate with perceived inappropriate silences (Ludlow and Bassich, 1984). Relatedly, Lehiste (1965) found evidence of voiceless transitions from vowels to following consonants within syllables, possibly attributable to incoordination of articulation and voicing. Canter (1965b) noted that perceived omission of final consonants in parkinsonian patients could be due to poor phonatory control. Other studies have found evidence of continuous voicing (Figure 7–3) within sentences or on AMR tasks containing voiceless consonants (Kent and Rosenbek, 1982; Ludlow and Bassich,

1984; Robin, Jordan, and Rodnitzky, 1986). These findings suggest difficulty with the rapid termination of voicing within utterances containing voiceless phonemes. Finally, McClean, Beukelman, and Yorkston's (1987) PD patients had difficulty varying vocal pitch to control a cursor in order to track a visually displayed sinusoidal target.

4. Laryngeal structure and movement. Hirose (1986) discussed electromyography (EMG) patterns in the thyroarytenoid muscle of a patient with PD with laryngoscopically confirmed limited vocal cord movement. Although neuromuscular discharges during phonation were not reduced and there were no pathologic discharge patterns, there was a loss of reciprocal suppression of the thyroarytenoid muscle during inspiration. This suggested that limited vocal cord motion may reflect a loss of appropriate reciprocal activity between agonist and antagonist muscles, rather than weakness. Relatedly, Gracco and others (1994) reported aerodynamic evidence of increased vocal tract resistance in a PD speaker, a finding suggestive of increased glottal or supraglottal muscle tension.

In a comprehensive telescopic cinelaryngoscopy study of 32 unselected patients with PD, Hanson, Gerratt, and Ward (1984) documented several laryngeal abnormalities. Among the most striking of the findings was that only two patients were free of "abnormal phonatory posturing," and those two had normal voices and no voice complaints. Vocal cord bowing during phonation, represented by a

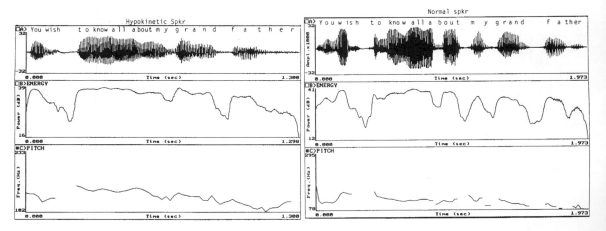

Figure 7–3 Raw waveform and energy and pitch (f_o) tracings for the sentence "You wish to know all about my grandfather" by a normal male speaker and a male with hypokinetic dysarthria. The normal speaker completes the sentence in ~ 2 secs, the hypokinetic speaker in 1.3 secs (66% of the normal speaker's rate, consistent with a perception of rapid rate). The energy tracing for the normal speaker has clearly defined syllables of varying duration; the hypokinetic speaker has few well-defined syllables, possibly reflecting the effects of rapid rate, continuous voicing, spirantization, and monoloudness. The speakers' pitch tracings are similar in contour, but the normal speaker has brief breaks in phonation during stop closure and voiceless consonants. The absence of breaks in phonation after the word "to" for the hypokinetic speaker probably reflect continuous voicing and spirantization.

significant glottic gap but with tightly approximated vocal processes, was observed in 30 patients; the increased glottal gap was correlated with perceived breathiness and reduced intensity. Tremulousness of the arytenoid cartilages was apparent during quiet breathing in some subjects, but the perception of voice tremor seemed more strongly related to the secondary effects of head tremor. Laryngeal structure asymmetries were apparent in many patients, with asymmetries occurring in vocal cord length, degree of bowing, and ventricular fold movements. Some patients exhibited approximation of the ventricular folds during phonation. In general, vocal cord closure was better in patients with hemiparkinsonism (that is, those with predominantly unilateral signs and symptoms). Voice was often better in patients with supraglottic contraction, which may have assisted adduction and reduced breathiness. The authors noted that the vocal cords appeared solid, in spite of bowing, in contrast to the hypotonicity that may be present with lower motor neuron (LMN) paralyses. The evidence of increased adductor contraction, asymmetric contraction, and vocal cord bowing inconsistent with LMN lesions, led to a conclusion that the abnormalities in phonatory postures were related to laryngeal muscle rigidity. These visual observations appear consistent with perceptual and acoustic features that imply abnormalities of laryngeal function in hypokinetic dysarthria.

In summary, acoustic and physiologic studies of phonatory attributes of hypokinetic dysarthria provide evidence of reduced laryngeal efficiency, flexibility, and control that are, for the most part, consistent with many perceived deviations in voice quality and prosody. Many of these abnormalities can be related to the underlying neuromuscular deficits of rigidity, reduced range of movement, and slowness of movement in the laryngeal muscles.

Resonance. Resonance abnormalities are not perceptually prominent, and this may explain why there have been few studies of velopharyngeal function in hypokinetic dysarthria. Mueller (1971) found no evidence of abnormal nasal airflow in his patients with hypokinetic dysarthria. In contrast, Hoodin and Gilbert (1989) did find increased nasal airflow in a study of parkinsonian patients. This finding did not correlate strongly with rated hypernasality and the authors speculated that resonance abnormalities may have been masked by phonatory abnormalities. They attributed increased nasal airflow rates to rigidity and reduced range of velopharyneal movements.

X-ray microbeam assessment of a small number of PD patients has demonstrated reduced degree

and velocity of velar movements during repetitive utterances (Hirose, Kiritani, and Sawashima, 1982b; Hirose and others, 1981). Hirose (1986) noted that velar displacement became limited and irregular at faster rates and that the velum tended to stay in an elevated posture. He suggested that this might be due to a loss of reciprocal suppression between functionally antagonistic muscle pairs (for example, velar-lowering resisted by action of velar-elevators). Finally, there is acoustic evidence that nasalization may spread across several consecutive syllables in some patients (Kent and Rosenbek, 1982; Robin, Jordan, and Rodnitzky, 1986).

To summarize, there is acoustic and physiologic evidence of velopharyngeal dysfunction, at least in some people with hypokinetic dysarthria. This seems to reflect the effects of slow movement, rigidity, or reduced range of movement. These can lead to the perception of hypernasality and weak intraoral pressure during pressure consonant productions.

Articulation—precision, rate, and range of movement. Acoustic and physiologic measures of articulatory dynamics provide considerable support for the perception of imprecise articulation in hypokinetic dysarthria. It appears that articulatory "undershoot," or failure to completely reach articulatory targets or sustain contacts for sufficient durations, play a significant role in imprecision.

A number of acoustic studies have detected evidence of *spirantization* during stop and affricate productions (Canter, 1965b; Kent and Rosenbek, 1982; Weismer, 1984; Ziegler and others, 1988). Spirantization, usually taken as evidence of articulatory undershooting, is characterized acoustically by the replacement of a stop gap with low intensity frication. It is attributed to a failure of complete articulatory closure for stop productions or the stop portion of affricates (Figure 7–3). Its effect is to reduce acoustic contrast and detail, a natural product of undershooting articulators and a reasonable explanation for some aspects of perceived imprecise articulation. Weismer (1984) considers spirantization of stops a unique characteristic of parkinsonian dysarthria.

Several physiologic studies provide evidence for reduced range and, sometimes, reduced speed of articulatory movements in hypokinetic speakers. Using a strain gauge transducer system, Hunker and Abbs (1984) and Hunker, Abbs, and Barlow (1982) have reported evidence of muscle stiffness or rigidity in the lips. Caliguiri (1989) found evidence of reduced amplitude and velocity of lip movements at conversational speech rates, and Gracco and others (1994) reported slowed lip movements during syllables with bilabial consonants. Netsell, Daniel, and Celesia (1975), in a study of upper lip movement (by EMG) and oral and nasal pressure during speech, found evidence of articulatory undershoot in the upper lip and, probably, velum. Lip muscle action potentials were decreased in duration and amplitude, suggesting a contribution of weakness (central, not peripheral) to inadequate lip movements. The overall pattern of results suggested that decreased range of movement in hypokinetic speech could be due to weakness of CNS control signals, rigidity, or acceleration of movements.

Studies of jaw movements yield similar results. Hirose (1986), examining activity of the anterior digastric (which lowers the jaw) and mentalis (which raises the jaw) muscles, noted that the temporal reciprocity between those muscle actions was not maintained on a speech repetition task. Similarly, Moore and Scudder (1989) found aberrant EMG patterns reflecting poorly defined reciprocal patterns of activity between jaw agonist and antagonistic muscles. That is, when jaw-elevating muscles were phasically active, the digastric was tonically active. Of interest, their most intelligible speaker had a severe breakdown of jaw muscle synergy. The authors interpreted this as evidence for differential impairment within the speech system, and the capacity of the system to compensate for deficits at some levels.

McClean, Beukelman, and Yorkston, (1987) found evidence of poor visuomotor tracking of a sinusoidal signal with both jaw and lip movements, although jaw control was better than lip control in their subjects. Zwirner and Barnes (1992) found acoustic evidence of decreased jaw stability (as reflected in first formant steadiness) during vowel prolongation in PD patients.

Hirose (1986) has stated that the physiologic mechanism of hypokinesia and rigidity may be based on persistent abnormal muscle contractions; that is, a problem with reciprocal adjustments of antagonistic muscles, or a loss of reciprocal suppression between functionally antagonist muscle pairs. Similar interpretations have been offered by Leanderson, Meyerson, and Persson (1972).

A number of physiologic studies have examined speech rate in hypokinetic dysarthria, a phenomenon of considerable interest because increased rate is often perceived. Results have been inconsistent, but illuminating, because they suggest that listener perceptions may not always reflect underlying movement dynamics.

Many studies demonstrate variability in rate across subjects, some being normal, some slow, and some fast. Several studies, however, have failed to find rate differences in speech AMRs or syllable repetition tasks, or during sentences (Connor, Ludlow, and Schulz, 1989; Ludlow, Connor, and Bassich, 1987; Canter, 1963, 1965b; Ewanowski, 1965; Tatsumi and others, 1979; Ziegler and others, 1988). Ludlow and Bassich (1984) found no group rate differences, but did note that their PD subjects had trouble increasing rate when requested. Although Canter (1963, 1965b) found no group differences in reading rate, he did note that some patients were very slow and some were very fast. Some had AMRs that could not be analyzed because they were too indistinct; others demonstrated "freezing."

Some studies have found evidence of reduced rate. Dworkin and Aronson (1986) and Ludlow, Connor, and Bassich (1987) found slow AMRs or slow syllable repetition rates in some subjects. Kruel (1972) documented slow reading rate, and Ludlow, Connor, and Bassich (1987) found reduced first and second formant transition rates, suggestive of decreased articulatory speed.

As might be expected from perceptual studies, some studies yield acoustic and physiologic evidence for increased speech rate. Hammen, Yorkston, and Beukelman (1989) reported faster overall speaking rate in four parkinsonian subjects; rate remained more rapid than normal when pauses were removed, suggesting that articulation rate was increased. Hirose and others (1981) and Hirose, Kiritani, and Sawashima (1982a,b) noted a tendency for increased rate and reduced range of lower-lip movement on syllable repetition tasks. Hirose (1986) likened abnormally fast speech rate to festinating gait, and speculated that this may reflect a disturbance of CNS inhibitory function, such as an abnormal release of an intrinsic oscillation mechanism. Similarly, Netsell, Daniel, and Celesia (1975) documented lip AMR rates of up to 13 per second (Figure 7–2), occurring in association with decreased range of movement. This extremely fast rate suggests a mode of speech over which there can be no voluntary control.

Weismer (1984) noted subtle decreases in segment durations and total utterance duration, but also noted that rates were comparable to those found in younger subjects. He suggested that the perception of fast rate could be partially due to age-related rate expectations of listeners (that is, expecting older speakers to be slower), as well as to articulatory imprecision and continuous voicing that reduce discrete acoustic contrasts; the resultant "blurring" of speech may also lead to a perception of increased rate. These are potentially valuable insights; clinicians may need to tune more finely their perceptual judgments when assessing speech rate in hypokinetic dysarthria.

Metter and Hanson (1986) found variable rates across subjects with PD, with both slow and fast rates represented. The tendency for rate to be abnormally fast or slow seemed to increase with increasing dysarthria severity.

Caliguiri (1989) reported decreased amplitude, movement time, and speed of labial movements at conversational speech rates, with a reduction of the abnormalities at slower rates. He noted that use of the term "hypokinetic" to describe speech deficits in PD has a physiologic basis, at least in the 5-syllable per second range. Finally, Ludlow, Connor, and Bassich's (1987) PD patients had trouble altering sentence and phrase durations when they were asked to speak at faster than conversational rates; that is, there was less of a difference between their conversational and fast rates in comparison to control speakers. The authors speculated that a major problem for these speakers is in controlling *alterations* in rate, even though the overall temporal organization of speech may be unaffected.

Stress, pause, and other durational characteristics. Findings of rate abnormalities and reduced frequency and intensity variability help explain some of the acoustic factors underlying the perception of prosodic insufficiency in hypokinetic dysarthria. Some additional factors, mostly related to stress, pause, and between-syllable durational differences, help to round out the disorder's prosodic features.

Although Canter (1963) found no differences between parkinsonian and control subjects in number of pauses or mean pause duration during reading, several studies have found such abnormalities. Parkinsonian subjects' pauses during speech have been shown to represent a higher percentage of the total time within speech samples (Hammen, Yorkston, and Beukelman, 1989; Metter and Hanson, 1986). Pauses may also occur slightly more frequently (Hammen, Yorkston, and Beukelman, 1989).

Illes and others (1988) found an increased frequency and duration of pauses that exceeded 200 milliseconds. These hesitations or pauses tended to be longer and occur more frequently at the beginning of sentences. There was also an increase in number of words between silent intervals, a finding that may be related to the perception of short rushes of speech. Finally, Ludlow and Bassich (1984) found reduced differences in word boundary durations between separate nouns and compound nouns (for example, the boundary between the syllables "sail" and "boats" in the sentences "They were sailboats" versus "They will sail boats") in parkinsonian speakers. This was correlated with perceptions of reduced stress.

Murry (1983) examined the ability to vary stress in the word initial and final position when answering questions with a standard sentence that established the point of emphasis (for example, responding "Bob bit Todd" in response to the question, "Who bit Todd?"). Normal subjects tend to increase frequency, intensity, and articulatory effort (for example, as measured by peak intraoral pressure) to signal stress in the word initial or final position. Murry's hypokinetic speaker demonstrated only minimal increases in frequency and intensity to signal stress, and this occurred at the expense of articulatory effort. Illes and others' (1988) hypokinetic speakers exhibited fewer interjections and "modalizations" (comments that bear on verbal behavior, such as "You know") during narrative speech. Combined with other findings, this suggests that hypokinetic speakers display silent pauses instead of fillers, and that this loss of verbal "asides" may be analogous to a reduction of the automatic movements that accompany purposeful movements in PD (that is, masked facial expression, reduced arm swing during walking, etc.).

Kent and Rosenbek (1982) have provided a useful summary of the acoustic "signature" of hypokinetic dysarthria. They label the pattern as *"fused,"* in which the contour across syllables within utterances is flattened or indistinct. This fused or flattened profile is characterized by: small and gradual fundamental frequency and intensity variations within and between syllables; continuous voicing; reduced variations in syllable durations; syllable reduction; indistinct boundaries between syllables because of faulty consonant articulation; and a spread of nasalization across consecutive syllables. In general, these features represent a reduced ability to use the full range of pitch, intensity, articulatory, and durational options that are available to the normal speaker (Figure 7–3).

Tremor. Voice tremor is not a prominent perceptual feature of hypokinetic dysarthria, and the tremor that can be detected seems not to differ substantially from the tremor in normal individuals (Phillipbar, Robin, and Luschei, 1989). However, underlying tremor within the speech system may nonetheless be important in hypokinetic dysarthria.

Hunker and Abbs (1984) found evidence of pathologic tremor in the jaw and lip at rest, during sustained postures, and during active and passive movement. They speculated that prolonged reaction times (that is, delayed initiation of movement) in PD may be due to an inability to initiate muscle contraction until it coincides with the involuntary burst of a tremor oscillation and that tremor rate may set limits on maximum rates of syllable production that can be attained without acceleration. Abbs, Hunker, and Barlow (1983) also observed lip and jaw tremor during nonspeech tasks involving muscle force. The lips and jaw were otherwise adequate in producing stable forces, although patients had difficulty producing stable tongue elevation forces. Putnam (1988), summarizing the relevant literature, noted that tremor may be involved in acceleration phenomena in hypokinetic dysarthria, and that patients may have to contend with the effect of tremor on phasic movements during speech.

The general observations derived from the acoustic and physiologic studies reviewed in this section are summarized in Table 7–6.

CASES

Case 7.1

A 69-year-old man presented with a five-year history of difficulty getting in and out of chairs, stiffness during walking, and difficulty turning in bed. He also had voice and handwriting difficulty. There was no history of encephalitis, toxic exposure, or drug use that might be related to his symptoms nor was there any family history of neurodegenerative disorder.

On neurologic exam, the armswing was diminished and the neck and extremities were rigid. He had a mild static tremor of the left hand and upper limb movements were bradykinetic. Facial expression was masked and postural reflexes were mildly impaired. An MRI scan was normal. He was referred for a speech assessment "to see if there are any clues in his voice as to the type of problem that he has."

Table 7–6 Summary of acoustic and physiologic findings in studies of hypokinetic dysarthria.*

Speech component	Acoustic or physiologic observation

Respiratory (or respiratory/ laryngeal)	Reduced:
	    Vital capacity
	    Amplitude of chest wall movements
	    Airflow volume during vowel prolongation
	    Intraoral pressure during AMRs
	    Syllables per breath group
	    Maximum vowel duration
	Increased:
	    Respiratory rate
	    Latency to begin exhalation
	    Latency to initiate phonation after exhalation initiated
	Irregular breathing patterns
	Paradoxic rib cage & abdominal movements
	Difficulty altering automatic breathing patterns for speech

Laryngeal	Bowed vocal cords in spite of solid, nonflaccid appearance
	Tremulousness of arytenoid cartilages
	Asymmetry of laryngeal structures & movements during phonation, especially in hemiparkinsonism
	Ventricular fold movement during phonation
	Decreased:
	    Intensity
	    Pitch & loudness variability
	    Speed to initiate phonation
	    Intensity peaks across syllables
	Increased f_o
	Increased glottal resistance
	Laryngealization
	Increased shimmer
	Continuous voicing in segments with voiceless consonants
	Voiceless transitions from vowels to following consonants
	Poor pitch control for visuomotor tracking

Velopharyngeal	Increased nasal airflow during nonnasal target productions Reduced velocity & degree of velar movement during speech Abnormal spread of nasalization across syllables

During speech examination, the patient described a one-year history of uncertainty if "words would come out." He believed his speech had become quieter and perhaps slower and that this was more obvious in the evening or after extended speaking. He reported occasional difficulty "getting going" with his speech even though he knew what he wished to say.

The jaw, lips, and tongue were mildly tremulous during sustained postures. Speech was characterized by breathy-hoarse voice quality (2), reduced loudness (1), and a tendency toward accelerated rate (0,1). Very infrequently, there were rapid repetitions or prolongations of initial phonemes. There was some nasal emission during production of pressure sound-filled sentences but he was not obviously hypernasal. Speech AMRs were normal. Prolonged "ah" was breathy-hoarse (1,2). Speech did not deteriorate during stress testing.

The speech clinician concluded "hypokinetic dysarthria, mild."

The neurologist concluded that the patient had parkinsonism. However, his symptoms were unresponsive to Sinemet. Because of this, the neurologist felt he might have striatonigral degeneration "which can appear much like Parkinson's disease at onset but is not Sinemet responsive."

Commentary. (1) Speech change is often associated with parkinsonism and may be among the signs encountered during initial neurologic evaluation. (2) Changes in voice quality and loudness are often among the initial complaints of patients with hypokinetic dysarthria. (3) Identification of hypokinetic dysarthria can provide confirmatory evidence for a diagnosis of parkinsonism.

Case 7.2

A 69-year-old man presented to neurology with a four-year history of progressive difficulty getting in and out of chairs and a two- to three-year history of speech difficulty. These had progressed to include slowness in walking and poor handwriting.

Neurologic examination disclosed generalized bradykinesia, some rigidity of the trunk and limbs, and abnormal pursuit and saccadic eye movements. "Severe

Table 7–6 Summary of acoustic and physiologic findings in studies of hypokinetic dysarthria.*—cont'd

Speech component	Acoustic or physiologic observation
Articulatory/ rate/prosody	Reduced: Amplitude & velocity of lip movement Amplitude & duration of lip muscle action potentials Jaw stability during vowel prolongation Tongue endurance & strength Spectrographic acoustic contrast & detail Speech rate Ability to increase rate on request First & second format transition rates (= slowness of movement) Syllable boundary durational differences between separate & compound nouns f_o, intensity, & articulatory effort increases to signal stress Variation in syllable duration Increased or accelerated: Connected speech & AMR rates Rate variability Frequency & duration of pauses during connected speech Articulatory undershoot of lip & velum Lip rigidity/stiffness Poor maintenance of temporal reciprocity between jaw depressors and elevators Poor visuomotor tracking with jaw and lip movements Abnormal jaw & lip tremor at rest, during sustained postures, & active & passive movement Spirantization of stops & affricates Continuous voicing Indistinct boundaries between syllables Spread of nasalization across syllables Small & gradual f_o & intensity variations within & between syllables

*Note that many of these observations are based on studies of only one or a few speakers, and that not all speakers with hypokinetic dysarthria will exhibit these features. Note also that these characteristics may not be unique to hypokinetic dysarthria; some may also be found in other motor speech disorders or non-neurologic conditions.

f_o, fundamental frequency.

speech hesitancy/stutters" was also apparent. He could barely walk and did so in slow shuffling steps.

During speech examination, the patient described himself as "stuttering" as a child, beginning at three years of age and resolving by his ninth year. This problem was mild and he had never had treatment for it. However, he noted that throughout his life he would "stutter" when excited, although his family had never noticed this. The patient had a brother who also reportedly stuttered as a child, with occasional dysfluencies in adulthood.

The tongue was tremulous on protrusion and during lateral movements. No other abnormalities were noted. Conversational speech, reading, and repetition were characterized by a remarkable degree of dysfluency, characterized by rapid repetition of initial sounds, syllables, and occasionally words and phrases. Sound and syllable repetitions occurred up to 30 to 40 repetitions per dysfluent moment. There was no evidence of associated struggle behavior during dysfluencies, although he did express frustration over them. In addition to the dysfluencies, articulation was moderately imprecise, pitch and loudness variability were reduced, and overall loudness was mildly reduced. Speech AMRs were rapid/accelerated. Prolonged "ah" was hoarse (2).

The clinician concluded, "Hypokinetic dysarthria. Marked-severe stuttering-like behavior associated with CNS disease, including some dysfluencies suggestive of palilalia. I strongly suspect the dysfluencies reflect a component of his hypokinetic dysarthria. In my opinion, this is a variant of hypokinetic dysarthria with associated dysfluencies and does not reflect the reemergence of his reported childhood stuttering."

During the patient's few days at the clinic, speech therapy was undertaken, primarily to modify his dysfluencies. Hand-tapping and use of pacing board were unsuccessful, because his limb movements were as accelerated/rapid as his speech. He did, however, respond very positively to delayed auditory feedback, with a significant reduction in speech rate and marked reduction of dysfluency. This greatly enhanced efficiency and intelligibility during conversation. The patient left the clinic with a recommendation to pursue therapy, with consideration given to acquiring a delayed auditory feedback device for use in conversation.

The neurologist concluded that the patient had idiopathic Parkinson's disease. Unfortunately, the patient did not respond to Sinemet.

Commentary. (1) Hypokinetic dysarthria may be among the prominent presenting signs of parkinsonism. (2) Dysfluencies occur commonly in hypokinetic dysarthria and palilalia may also occur. For some patients, dysfluencies may be the most debilitating component of their hypokinetic dysarthria. (3) The history of early childhood stuttering was of unknown significance in this case. However, recognizing that the patient had a hypokinetic dysarthria with associated dysfluencies helped establish that his speech deficit could probably not be attributed to a reemergence or persistence of childhood stuttering. Rather, it was related to the patient's neurologic disease. (4) Marked dysfluencies associated with hypokinetic dysarthria can be responsive to

speech therapy. These approaches will be discussed in Chapter 17.

Case 7.3

A 74-year-old woman presented to neurology with a four-year history of progressive "wobbling" when walking and a tendency to fall backwards. Neurologic examination initially suggested prominent proximal muscle weakness. Polymyositis, myasthenia gravis, and myopathy were suspected. Because she complained of "slurred" speech and "hesitation" when speaking, she was referred for speech assessment.

During speech examination, she stated, "When I speak, I don't know how it will come out. Sometimes words do not come out at all." Conversational speech was characterized by prolonged silent intervals, occasional whole word repetitions, and repeated syllables (for example, "I took dic-ta-ta-ta-ta-tion from him"). Rate was mildly accelerated and articulation was often mildly imprecise, with slighting of consonants when she spoke rapidly. Resonance was normal but voice quality was harsh. There was no evidence of speech deterioration during four minutes of continuous talking.

The clinician concluded, "Speech features are most suggestive of hypokinetic dysarthria. At times, the pattern is almost that of palilalia, also seen in parkinsonian patients. This is not a speech pattern of flaccid dysarthria; no suggestion of myasthenia gravis."

The speech diagnosis prompted additional neurologic investigation. Computed tomography scan was normal with the exception of mild generalized cerebral atrophy. Consultation with other neurologists ruled out peripheral nervous system disease and myopathy, and detected postural instability, slight rigidity, and brisk reflexes. Neurologic diagnosis was uncertain, but it was concluded that the patient had several parkinsonian symptoms, but without classic idiopathic PD. A diagnosis of PSP was entertained, but evidence for its diagnosis was considered equivocal.

Commentary. (1) Hypokinetic dysarthria is common in parkinsonism. (2) Diagnosis of hypokinetic dysarthria can be very helpful to neurologic diagnosis. In this case, it raised suspicions about CNS degenerative disease, and, specifically, parkinsonism. It helped focus attention on the central, as opposed to peripheral nervous system. (3) Dysfluencies and palilalia can be associated with hypokinetic dysarthria.

Case 7.4

A 29-year-old woman presented to the Rehabilitation Unit 14 months after cerebral anoxia that developed secondary to cardiac arrest during a tubal ligation. Neurologic examination revealed neck and left upper extremity rigidity, upper extremity dystonia, diffuse hyperactive reflexes, and weakness in all extremities. Gait was slow with short steps. She had difficulty with chewing and swallowing and frequently choked on solid foods.

Speech examination revealed: reduced loudness (3); imprecise articulation (3); accelerated speech rate (3); little variation in pitch, loudness, and syllable duration; reduced range of articulatory movement (3,4). Speech AMRs were "super fast and blurred."

The clinician concluded "hypokinetic dysarthria, severe." There was no evidence of aphasia but neuropsychologic assessment revealed deficits in attention, concentration, new learning, and short-term recall. She received speech therapy while on the Rehabilitation Unit, with subsequent improved speech intelligibility as long as she was cued to increase loudness and slow rate.

Commentary. (1) Hypokinetic dysarthria can occur in conditions other than parkinsonism and can be encountered in anoxic encephalopathy. In such cases, the dysarthria may not be distinguishable from hypokinetic dysarthria associated with idiopathic PD. (2) Cognitive deficits can be present in individuals with hypokinetic dysarthria.

Case 7.5

A 75-year-old man presented to neurology with a three- to four-year history of shuffling gait, stooped posture, loss of facial expression, tremor, and voice change. Neurologic examination confirmed the presence of these symptoms. The patient also admitted to occasional confusion and reduced memory. Neuropsychologic assessment revealed mild-to-moderate generalized organic cognitive decline consistent with mild dementia.

During speech examination, the patient complained of "hoarseness" and noted that his voice occasionally "gets to a whisper." Voice quality was characterized by: reduced loudness (1,2); continuous breathiness (1,2); monopitch and monoloudness (1,2). Articulation was equivocally fast during conversation. Speech AMRs were normal.

The clinician concluded, "Mild hypokinetic dysarthria, primarily characterized by reduced pitch and loudness variability, reduced volume, and breathiness." Because the patient cleared his throat frequently and had prominent dysphonia, he was referred for laryngeal examination; bowing of the vocal cords was observed.

The neurologist concluded that the patient had a degenerative CNS disease that did not fit well with classic idiopathic parkinsonism. Sinemet was prescribed. Two years later, although improved on Sinemet, the neurologic examination was unchanged and there was no other evidence of deterioration. Speech was also unchanged, with the exception that tongue tremulousness was apparent on protrusion.

Commentary. (1) Hypokinetic dysarthria frequently manifests itself as dysphonia and prosodic insufficiency. Such difficulties can remain the only speech symptoms for extended periods of time. (2) The dysphonia of hypokinetic dysarthria is frequently associated with bowing of the vocal cords. (3) Hypokinetic dysarthria is frequently associated with general cognitive impairments.

Case 7.6

A 51-year-old man presented to neurology for another opinion about his neurologic deficit. His difficulties began three years previously, over about a 10-day period, when he had several suspected myocardial infarctions. His symptoms at that time included speech difficulty and problems with gait.

Neurologic exam showed a loss of facial expression, generalized loss of associated movements, generalized bradykinesia, and generalized rigidity, greater on the left than right side.

During speech examination, the patient stated, "I can't talk in long sentences; I repeat myself; bad volume; out of breath fast." He had had three periods of speech therapy, benefiting from each, but only temporarily.

Examination revealed facial masking, reduced range of movement of the jaw, lips, and tongue, and, perhaps, mild left tongue weakness. Connected speech was characterized by: imprecise articulation (3); accelerated rate within utterances (2,3); monopitch and monoloudness (3,4); breathy-harsh-strained voice quality (2,3). In addition, during conversation he exhibited numerous phoneme and syllable repetitions and fairly frequent word and phrase repetitions, usually with associated accelerated rate, consistent with the characteristics of palilalia. At times, however, these repetitions appeared voluntary, based on his perception that he had not been understood, whereas at other times, they appeared involuntary. Speech AMRs were markedly imprecise and blurred. Intelligibility was significantly reduced, but improved with slowing of rate, which was facilitated by hand-tapping.

The clinician concluded, "Marked hypokinetic dysarthria and palilalia."

A recommendation was made that he resume speech therapy. It was felt that he might benefit from efforts to more consistently slow his rate and prepare himself respiratorily for each utterance. Development of a backup augmentative system was also recommended. The patient had been under the impression that speech therapy was intended to completely remediate his speech difficulty. During a lengthy discussion, the fact that speech therapy could not completely remediate his speech difficulty, but could focus on maximizing intelligibility, was stressed. The patient accepted this explanation, with disappointment, and did pursue additional speech therapy at a facility near his home.

Additional neurologic workup included an MRI scan that identified small lacunar infarcts in the right putamen and external capsule. The neurologist concluded that the patient had extrapyramidal disease as a result of a previous cerebrovascular event and, perhaps, diffuse cerebral ischemia that were secondary to an episode of hypotension of undetermined etiology. Although clinical findings were somewhat asymmetric and only a unilateral lesion was present on neuroimaging, the clinical picture appeared to reflect bilateral involvement of the basal ganglia.

Commentary. (1) Hypokinetic dysarthria and palilalia can result from cerebral ischemia and infarction. (2) Hypokinetic dysarthria can be among the most debilitating deficits stemming from basal ganglia disease. (3) Although neuroimaging evidence suggested only a unilateral lesion, the dysarthria and associated neurologic findings were strongly suggestive of bilateral involvement. (4) Dysarthric patients sometimes have unrealistic expectations about speech therapy. It is crucial that patients understand the goals of therapy when therapy is recommended. Counseling in this re-

gard is helpful to managing the patient's acceptance and understanding of their deficits and to developing an understanding of what may and may not be achieved with treatment.

SUMMARY

1. Hypokinetic dysarthria results from damage to the basal ganglia control circuit. It probably occurs at a rate comparable to that of other single dysarthria types. Its characteristics are most evident in voice, articulation, and prosody. The effects of rigidity, reduced force and range of movement, and slow individual and sometimes fast repetitive movements seem to account for many of its deviant speech characteristics.

2. Parkinsonism, the prototypic condition associated with hypokinetic dysarthria, is most often due to Parkinson's disease, a degenerative condition associated with a depletion of dopamine in the striatum of the basal ganglia. Several symptoms of the disease are often managed by medications that restore the balance between dopamine and acetylcholine within the basal ganglia. Several other neurodegenerative diseases may also cause parkinsonian symptoms and hypokinetic dysarthria.

3. Hypokinetic dysarthria may also result from nondegenerative conditions, most often including vascular disease, neuroleptic and illicit drugs, certain metabolic diseases, chronic exposure to heavy metals, trauma, and infection.

4. Patients frequently complain that their voice is weak or quiet, and sometimes that their rate is too rapid. They may also note dysfluencies and difficulty initiating speech. They often are aware of deterioration with fatigue or toward the end of an antiparkinsonian medication cycle. Drooling and swallowing complaints are common. Facial masking and a general reduction in the visible range of articulator movement during speech are common.

5. Several deviant speech characteristics combine to give many patients a distinctive flat, attenuated and sometimes accelerated speech pattern. This has been called prosodic insufficiency, and is characterized by monopitch, monoloudness, reduced stress, short phrases, variable rate, short rushes of speech, and imprecise articulation. Additional distinctive characteristics that may be present include inappropriate silences, breathy dysphonia, reduced loudness, and increased speech rate. Dysfluencies and palilalia may also be present.

6. In general, acoustic and physiologic studies have provided support for the auditory-perceptual characteristics of the disorder, have specified more precisely the disorder's acoustic and physiologic characteristics, and have documented the role of rigidity, reduced range of movement, slowness of movement, and acceleration phenomena during speech. Some data suggest that the perception of accelerated rate sometimes may be an artifact of listener expectations and reduced acoustic contrast.

7. Hypokinetic dysarthria can be the only, the first, or among the first and most prominent manifestations of neurologic disease. Its recognition can aid neurologic localization and diagnosis, and may contribute to the medical and behavioral management of the individual's disease and speech disorder.

REFERENCES

Abbs JH, Hunker CJ, and Barlow SM: Differential speech motor subsystem impairments with suprabulbar lesions: neurophysiologic framework and supporting data. In Berry WR, editor: Clinical dysarthria, San Diego, 1984, College-Hill.

Adams RD and Victor H: Principles of neurology, New York, 1991, McGraw-Hill.

Andrianopoulos MV, Duffy JR, and Kelly PJ: The effects on speech of ventral lateral thalamotomy for treatment of movement disorders (unpublished manuscript).

Arana GW and Hyman SE: Handbook of psychiatric drug therapy, ed 2, Boston, 1991, Little, Brown.

Aronson AE: Clinical voice disorders, ed 3, New York, 1991, Thieme.

Beal MF, Richardson EP, and Martin JB: Degenerative disease of the nervous system. In Wilson JD and others, editors: Harrison's principles of internal medicine, ed 12, New York, 1991, McGraw-Hill.

Berry WR: Clinical dysarthria, San Diego, 1983, College-Hill.

Boshes B: Voice changes in parkinsonism, J Neurosurg 24:286, 1966.

Brown DR: Neurosciences for allied health therapies, St Louis, 1980, Mosby–Year Book.

Brown JW: Aphasia, apraxia, and agnosia, Springfield, IL, 1972, Charles C. Thomas.

Caekebeke JFV and others: The interpretation of dysprosody in patients with Parkinson's disease, J Neurol Neurosurg Psychiatr 54:145, 1991.

Caligiuri MP: The influence of speaking rate on articulatory hypokinesia in parkinsonian dysarthria, Brain Lang 36:493, 1989.

Canter GJ: Speech characteristics of patients with Parkinson's disease: I. Intensity, pitch, and duration, J Speech Hearing Disord 28:221, 1963.

Canter GJ: Speech characteristics of patients with Parkinson's disease: II. Physiological support for speech, J Speech Hear Disord 30:44, 1965a.

Canter GJ: Speech characteristics of patients with Parkinson's disease: III. Articulation, diadochokinesis, and overall speech adequacy, J Speech Hear Disord 30:217, 1965b.

Connor NP, Ludlow CL, and Schulz GM: Stop consonant production in isolated and repeated syllables in Parkinson's disease, Neuropsychologia 27:829, 1989.

Critchley M: Arteriosclerotic parkinsonism, Brain 52:23, 1929.

Darkins AW, Fromkin VA, and Benson DF: A characterization of the prosodic loss in Parkinson's disease, Brain Lang 34:315, 1988.

Darley FL, Aronson, AE, and Brown JR: Clusters of deviant speech dimensions in the dysarthrias, J Speech Hear Res 12:462, 1969b.

Darley FL, Aronson AE, and Brown JR: Differential diagnostic patterns of dysarthria, J Speech Hear Res 12:246, 1969a.

Darley FL, Aronson AE, and Brown JR: Motor speech disorders, Philadelphia, 1975, WB Saunders.

Dworkin JP and Aronson AE: Tongue strength and alternate motion rates in normal and dysarthric subjects, J Commun Disord 19:115, 1986.

Ewanowski SJ: Selected motor-speech behavior of patients with parkinsonism, Ph.D. dissertation, University of Wisconsin , 1964.

Gracco LC and others: Aerodynamic evaluation of parkinsonian dysarthria: laryngeal and supralaryngeal manifestations. In Till JA, Yorkston KM, and Beukelman DR, editors: Motor speech disorders: advances in assessment and treatment, Baltimore, 1994, Paul H. Brookes.

Hammen VL, Yorkson KM, and Beukelman DR: Pausal and speech duration characteristics as a function of speaking rate in normal and dysarthric individuals. In Yorkston KM and Beukelman DR, editors: Recent advances in clinical dysarthria, Austin, TX, 1989, Pro-Ed.

Hanson DG, Gerratt BR, and Ward PH: Cinegraphic observations of laryngeal function in Parkinson's disease, Laryngoscope 94:348, 1984.

Hirose H: Pathophysiology of motor speech disorders (dysarthria), Folia Phoniatr Logop 38:61, 1986.

Hirose H and others: Patterns of dysarthric movement in patients with parkinsonism, Folia Phoniatr Logop 33:204, 1981.

Hirose H, Kiritani S, and Sawashima M: Patterns of dysarthric movement in patients with amyotrophic lateral sclerosis and pseudobulbar palsy, Folia Phoniatr Logop 34:106, 1982a.

Hirose H, Kiritani S, and Sawashima M: Velocity of articulatory movements in normal and dysarthric subjects, Folia Phoniatr Logop 34:210, 1982b.

Hoodin RB and Gilbert HR: Parkinsonian dysarthria: an aerodynamic and perceptual description of velopharyngeal closure for speech, Folia Phoniatr Logop 41:249, 1989.

Hunker CJ and Abbs JH: Physiological analyses of parkinsonian tremors in the orofacial system. In McNeil MR, Rosenbek JC, and Aronson AE, editors: The dysarthrias, Austin, TX, 1984, Pro-Ed.

Hunker C, Abbs J, and Barlow S: The relationship between parkinsonian rigidity and hypokinesia in the orofacial system: a quantitative analysis, Neurology 32:749, 1982.

Illes J and others: Language production in Parkinons's disease: acoustic and linguistic considerations, Brain Lang 33:146, 1988.

Jankovic J: Pathophysiology and clinical assessment of motor symptoms in Parkinson's disease. In Koller WC, editor: Handbook of Parkinson's disease, New York, 1992, Marcel Decker.

Judd LL: The therapeutic use of psychotropic medications. In Wilson JD and others, editors: Harrison's principles of internal medicine, ed 12, New York, 1991, McGraw-Hill.

Kammermeier MA: A comparision of phonatory phenomena among groups of neurologically impaired speakers, Ph.D. dissertation, University of Minnesota, 1969.

Kent RD and Rosenbek JC: Prosodic disturbance and neurologic lesion, Brain and Lang 15:259, 1982.

Kim R: The chronic residual respiratory disorder in post-encephalitic parkinsonism, J Neurol Neurosurg Psychiatry 31:393, 1968.

Koller WC: Diagnosis and treatment of tremors, Neurol Clin 2:449, 1984.

Kreul EJ: Neuromuscular control examination (NMC) for parkinsonism: vowel prolongations and diadochokinetic and reading rates, J Speech Hear Res 15:72, 1972.

LaPointe LL and Horner: Palilalia: a descriptive study of pathological reiterative utterances, J Speech Hear Res 46:34, 1981.

Laszewski A: Role of the department of rehabilitation in preoperative evaluation of parkinsonian patients, J Am Geriatr Soc 4:1280, 1956.

Leanderson R, Meyerson BA, and Persson A: Lip muscle function in parkinsonian dysarthria, Acta Otolaryngol 74:271, 1972.

Lehiste I: Some acoustic characteristics of dysarthric speech, Bibl Phonetica, Fasc. 2, Basel, Switzerland, 1965, S. Karger.

Leverenz J and Sumi SM: Prevalence of Parkinson's disease in patients with Alzheimer's disease, Neurology 34(suppl. 1):101, 1984.

Logemann JA and Fisher HB: Vocal tract control in Parkinson's disease: phonetic feature analysis of misarticulations, J Speech Hear Disord 46:348, 1981.

Logemann JA and others: Frequency and occurrence of vocal tract dysfunctions in the speech of a large sample of Parkinson patients, J Speech Hear Disord 43:47, 1978.

Ludlow CL and Bassich CJ: The results of acoustic and perceptual assessment of two types of dysarthria. In Berry W, editor: Clinical dysarthria, Boston, 1983, College-Hill.

Ludlow C and Bassich C: Relationship betweeen perceptual ratings and acoustic measures of hypokinetic speech. In McNeil J and Aronson A, editors: The dysarthrias: physiologic, acoustics, perception, management, Austin, TX, 1984, Pro-Ed.

Ludlow CL, Connor NP, and Bassich CJ: Speech timing in Parkinson's and Huntington's disease, Brain Lang 32:195, 1987.

Mayeux R, Stern Y, and Stanton S: Heterogeneity in dementia of the Alzheimer type: evidence of subgroups, Neurology 35:453, 1985.

McClean MD, Beukelman DR, and Yorkston KM: Speech-muscle visuomotor tracking in dysarthric and nonimpaired speakers, J Speech Hear Res 30:276, 1987.

Metter EJ and Hanson WF: Clinical and acoustical variability in hypokinetic dysarthria, J Commun Disord 19:347, 1986.

Mlcoch AG: Diagnosis and treatment of parkinsonian dysarthria. In Koller WC, editor: Handbook of Parkinson's disease, New York, 1992, Marcel Decker.

Moore CA and Scudder RR: Coordination of jaw muscle activity in parkinsonian movement: description and response to traditional treatment. In Yorkston KM and Beukelman DR, editors: Recent advances in clinical dysarthria, Austin, TX, 1989, Pro-Ed.

Mueller PB: Parkinson's disease: motor-speech behavior in a selected group of patients, Folia Phoniatr Logop 23:333, 1971.

Murdoch BE: Acquired speech and language disorders, New York, 1990, Chapman and Hall.

Murdoch BE and others: Respiratory function in Parkinson's subjects exhibiting a perceptible speech deficit: a kinematic and spirometric analysis, J Speech Hear Disord 54:610, 1989.

Murry T: The production of stress in three types of dysarthric speech. In Berry W, editor: Clinical dysarthria, Boston, 1983, College-Hill.

Netsell R, Daniel B, and Celesia GG: Acceleration and weakness in parkinsonian dysarthria, J Speech Hear Disord 40:170, 1975.

Olson WH and others, editors: Handbook of symptom-oriented neurology, Chicago, 1989, Mosby–Year Book.

Phillipbar SA, Robin DA, and Luschei ES: Limb, jaw, and vocal tremor in Parkinson's patients. In Yorkston KM and Beukelman DR, editors: Recent advances in clinical dysarthria, Boston, 1989, College-Hill.

Putnam AHB: Review of research in dysarthria. In Winitz H, editor: Human communication and its disorders, a review 1988, Norwood, NJ, 1988, Ablex Publishing.

Robin DA, Jordan LS, and Rodnitzky RL: Prosodic impairment in Parkinson's disease. Paper presented at the Clinical Dysarthria Conference, Tucson, AZ, 1986.

Smith E and Faber R: Effects of psychotropic medications on speech and language. Special Interest Division, ASHA, Neurophysiology and neurogenic speech and language disorders 2(2):4, 1992.

Solomon NP and Hixon TJ: Speech breathing in Parkinson's disease, J Speech Hear Res, 36:294, 1993.

Tatsumi IF and others: Acoustic properties of ataxic and parkinsonian speech, in syllable repetition tasks. Annual bulletin, Research Institute of Logopedics and Phoniatrics 13:99, 1979.

Tolosa ES and Santamaria J: Parkinsonism and basal ganglia infarcts, Neurology, 34:1516, 1984.

Weismer G: Articulatory characteristics of parkinsonian dysarthria: segmental and phrase-level timing, spirantization, and glottal-supraglottal coordination. In McNeil MR, Rosenbek JC, and Aronson AE, editors: The dysarthrias, Austin, TX, 1984, Pro-Ed.

Ziegler W and others: Accelerated speech in dysarthria after acquired brain injury: acoustic correlates, Br J Disord Commun 23:215, 1988.

Zwirner P and Barnes GJ: Vocal tract steadiness: a measure of phonatory and upper airway motor control during phonation in dysarthria, J Speech Hear Res 35:4, 1992.

8 Hyperkinetic Dysarthria

Hyperkinetic dysarthria is a perceptually distinguishable motor speech disorder that is most often
associated with diseases of the basal ganglia control circuit. It may be manifest in any or all of the
respiratory, phonatory, resonatory, and articulatory
levels of speech, and it often has prominent effects
on prosody. Unlike most central nervous system
(CNS)-based dysarthrias, it can result from abnormalities of movement at only one level of speech
production, sometimes only a few muscles at that
level. Its deviant speech characteristics are the
product of abnormal, rhythmic or irregular and
unpredictable, rapid or slow *involuntary* movements.

Involuntary movements are the theme that ties
together the manifestations of the disorder, but
there is considerable variability in their form and
locus. This heterogeneity could justify a formal
division of the disorder into subtypes under the
broad heading of hyperkinetic dysarthrias. Although the singular designation is used here, this
chapter's organization will reflect the necessity for
subdividing in order to capture some of the remarkable variability that may be encountered in
this type of dysarthria.

Hyperkinetic dysarthria is encountered as the
primary speech pathology in a large medical prac-

tice at a rate that is somewhat less than for other
major dysarthria types. From 1987 to 1990 at the
Mayo Clinic, hyperkinetic dysarthria accounted
for 6.0% of all dysarthrias and 5.5% of all motor
speech disorders seen in the Section of Speech
Pathology (Figure 1–3). However, these figures
do not reflect the occurrence of several disorders
that legitimately could be categorized as hyperkinetic dysarthrias but that, by convention, often
have not been. These disorders include spasmodic
dysphonias of neurogenic origin (for example,
those secondary to tremor or dystonia) and organic
voice tremor. If these disorders had been included
in the distribution estimates, hyperkinetic dysarthria would have accounted for approximately
26% of all dysarthrias and 24% of all motor
speech disorders!

Hyperkinetic dysarthria is perceptually distinguishable from other isolated dysarthria types, and
its diagnosis is often facilitated by observing the
visible abnormal orofacial, head, and respiratory
movements that underlie many of the speech abnormalities. The bizarreness of these involuntary
movements and resultant speech abnormalities frequently raise suspicions about psychogenic etiology, and proper recognition of the dysarthria can
be essential for accurate medical diagnosis. A

diagnosis of hyperkinetic dysarthria implies pathology in the basal ganglia, related portions of the extrapyramidal system, or sometimes the cerebellar control circuit. The diversity of lesion loci associated with hyperkinetic dysarthria (and movement disorders in general) reflects the diversity of abnormal movements that may occur in CNS disease and our limited understanding of their anatomy and pathophysiology.

The clinical features of hyperkinetic dysarthria illustrate the devastating effects on voluntary movement of involuntary movements and variations in muscle tone. Hyperkinetic speech often gives the impression that normal speech is being executed but then is interfered with by regular or unpredictable involuntary movements that distort, slow, or interrupt it.

ANATOMY AND BASIC FUNCTIONS OF THE BASAL GANGLIA CONTROL CIRCUIT

The anatomy and functions of the basal ganglia control circuit and other portions of the CNS that may be implicated in hyperkinetic dysarthria were discussed in Chapter 2 and reviewed in Chapter 7. The anatomy and functions of the circuit are the same as those discussed for hypokinetic dysarthria. They are briefly reviewed here with specific focus on the possible anatomic and pathophysiologic bases of hyperkinetic dysarthria.

The *ventrolateral nucleus* of the *thalamus* has a primarily excitatory effect on the cortex. The nuclei of the *basal ganglia* have complex interconnections that channel output to the cortex through the ventrolateral nucleus. The aggregate impulses from the basal ganglia have an inhibitory effect on the thalamus. As a result, they tend to inhibit cortical neuronal firing as well. Many hyperkinesias seem to result from a failure of these pathways to properly inhibit cortical motor discharges. This may happen in a number of ways. For example, the *subthalamic nucleus* normally exerts an inhibitory effect on the thalamus via its regulation of the *globus pallidus*. Destruction of the *subthalamic nucleus* causes reduced inhibitory output from the basal ganglia, with resultant increased thalamic and cortical firing. Consequently, uninhibited abnormal movement commands are "released" through the motor cortex to the corticospinal or corticobulbar pathways.

Other movement disorders may have similar explanations. For example, a loss of neurons in the *striatum*, which normally modulates the globus pallidus, can result in abnormal involuntary movements. Hyperkinesias can also result from a disruption of the normal equilibrium between *excitatory cholinergic (ACh)* and *inhibitory dopaminergic (dopamine)* neurotransmitters. That is, a rela-

tive increase in dopaminergic activity or a relative decrease in cholinergic activity within the circuit may result in hyperkinesia. Other neurotransmitters are also involved in functions of the basal ganglia control circuit and may be implicated in certain movement disorders, but their roles are not well understood (Adams and Victor, 1991). Finally, the basal ganglia control circuit's role in movement disorders is demonstrated by the outcome of neurosurgical lesions placed in the globus pallidus or ventrolateral nucleus of the thalamus. Such lesions abolish tremor, rigidity, and involuntary limb movements by interrupting the loop through which the abnormal movements are generated (Kelly and others, 1987).

Portions of the cerebellar control circuit can be similarly implicated in movement disorders and hyperkinetic dysarthria. For example, lesions in cerebellar structures such as the *dentate nucleus,* or in brainstem structures such as the *inferior olive* or *red nucleus,* can alter the circuit's discharge patterns to thalamocortical pathways. The resultant input to the cortex can ultimately lead to abnormal motor cortex discharges through the corticospinal and corticobulbar pathways, with subsequent abnormal, involuntary patterns of movement.

CLINICAL CHARACTERISTICS OF BASAL GANGLIA CONTROL CIRCUIT DISORDERS ASSOCIATED WITH HYPERKINETIC DYSARTHRIA

Some involuntary movements are normal. Startle reactions to loud noises, fear-induced tremor of the hands, shivering in response to cold, and jerking of body parts when falling asleep are all normal involuntary responses to certain intrinsic conditions or external stimuli. *Abnormal involuntary movements* are those that occur in conditions where motor steadiness is expected. They can occur at rest, during static postures, or during voluntary movement. They are usually abolished by sleep and exacerbated by anxiety and heightened emotions. In some cases they are triggered only by specific movements, such as speech, and they sometimes can be inhibited by adopting specific postures. The term *hyperkinesia* or *movement disorder* refers to these abnormal or excessive involuntary movements. The prefix "hyper" does not reflect excessive speed of voluntary movement; it indicates the presence of "extra" or involuntary movements that may range in rate from slow to fast. In fact, it is generally the case that *voluntary movements are slow* in those body parts that are affected by hyperkinesias.

The precise location and underlying pathophysiology of many movement disorders are poorly understood. As a result, classifications of them are descriptive, often based on the speed of the involuntary movements (that is, quick and slow hyperkinesias). Such divisions are often inadequate because quick and slow involuntary movements occur on a continuum and often reflect a mixture of slow and quick components. The trend to avoid these divisions is more evident today than in the past, but some descriptive terms can be useful because they convey something about the predominant character of the abnormal movement. In general, it is important to recognize that some hyperkinesias are rapid, unsustained, and unpatterned, whereas others are slower to develop, may be sustained for seconds (or longer), or may be prolonged to a degree that distorts posture in a constant or waxing and waning manner. Some individuals have combinations of these characteristics.

The varieties of movement disorders that are most relevant to understanding hyperkinetic dysarthrias are discussed in the following sections. Their basic characteristics are summarized in Table 8–1. Additional concepts that describe some

of the nonspeech motor behaviors in individuals with hyperkinetic dysarthria are also addressed.

Dyskinesia

Dyskinesia is a general term used to refer to abnormal, hyperkinetic, involuntary movements, regardless of etiology (Miller and Jankovic, 1990). It sometimes refers to abnormal movements that may be restricted to certain body parts (Adams and Victor, 1991; Jankovic, 1986).

Orofacial dyskinesias are involuntary movements of the mouth, face, tongue, and jaw that can occur without hyperkinesias elsewhere in the body. They are a common side effect of prolonged use of antipsychotic drugs, a condition known as *tardive dyskinesia.* Most hereditary and acquired diseases that cause orofacial dyskinesias are associated with basal ganglia pathology (Altrocchi and Forno, 1983).

Akathisia is a condition characterized by a subjective sense of motor restlessness and is

Table 8–1 Categories of abnormal movement and their predominant rate and rhythm characteristics and presumed anatomic substrate. All but the movements under "Other" may be associated with hyperkinetic dysarthria.

Designation	Speed	Rhythmicity	Anatomic substrate
Dyskinesia	Fast or slow	Irregular or rhythmic	Basal ganglia control circuit
Myoclonus	Fast or Slow	Irregular or rhythmic	Cortex to spinal cord
Palatopharyngolaryngeal	Slow	Regular	Brain stem (Guillain-Mollaret triangle)
Action	Fast	Irregular	Basal ganglia or cerebellar control circuit
Tics	Fast	Irregular but patterned	Basal ganglia control circuit
Chorea	Fast	Irregular	Basal ganglia control circuit
Ballism	Fast	Irregular	Area of subthalamic nucleus
Athetosis	Slow	Irregular	Basal ganglia control circuit
Dystonia	Slow	Irregular/sustained	Basal ganglia control circuit
Spasmodic dysphonia	Slow	Irregular/sustained	?
Spasmodic torticollis	Slow	Irregular/sustained	? Basal ganglia control circuit
Blepharospasm	Slow	Irregular	? Midbrain, cerebellum, facial nucleus
Spasm	Slow or fast	Irregular	? Basal ganglia control circuit
Hemifacial spasm	Fast	Irregular	Facial nucleus cerebellopontine angle, facial canal
Essential tremor	Slow or fast	Rhythmic	? Striatum
Organic voice	Slow	Rhythmic	Cerebellar control circuit
Spasmodic dysphonia	Slow	Rhythmic	?
Other*			
Fasiculations	Fast	Irregular	LMN
Synkinesis	Fast or Slow	Irregular	LMN
Facial myokymia	Intermediate	Rhythmic	LMN

*These abnormal movements may be visibly apparent in the speech muscles. However, they are not considered hyperkinesias because they do not, by themselves, interfere with voluntary movement. Fasiculations, synkinesis, and facial myokymia may be associated with flaccid, not hyperkinetic dysarthria, and are signs of LMN, not CNS pathology.
LMN, lower motor neuron.

often confused with psychotic agitation. It may be characterized by overt motor restlessness such as shifting position, pacing, and rubbing the scalp or limbs. It can occur in parkinsonism but is most often seen acutely in some patients taking neuroleptic drugs and some antihistamines. It occurs in about 25% of patients with tardive dyskinesia (Burke, 1984; Marsden and Fahn, 1987).

Myoclonus

Myoclonus is characterized by involuntary single or repetitive brief jerks of a body part; if repetitive, jerks can be rhythmic or nonrhythmic. They cannot be inhibited willfully. Myoclonic movements can be isolated to one group of muscles or they can be multifocal. They may occur spontaneously or they may be induced by visual, tactile, or auditory stimuli, or, sometimes, by voluntary movements. When brought on by movement, the condition is known as *action myoclonus* (*Clinical Examinations in Neurology,* 1991).

Myoclonus can be associated with lesions from the cortex to the spinal cord. It can occur in epilepsy, where it is considered a component of a seizure. Some forms are associated with cerebellar signs or dementia. A common form of acquired myoclonus is seen in the aftermath of cardiorespiratory arrest (*post anoxic myoclonus*).

Palatal myoclonus is a unique complex form of myoclonus associated with lesions in the area of the brain stem known as the *Guillain-Molaret triangle.* It can be associated with unique speech characteristics and will be discussed further in the section under Speech Pathology.

Hiccups (singultus) are a form of complex myoclonus produced by a brief spasm of the diaphragm with subsequent adduction of the vocal cords. They commonly result from irritation of the peripheral sensory nerves in the stomach, esophagus, diaphragm, or mediastinum, and may be associated with some toxic-metabolic conditions, such as uremia (*Clinical Examinations in Neurology,* 1991). Hiccupping may be a sign of medullary involvement in the region of the tractus solitarius, which has important respiratory control functions (Howard and others, 1992).

Tics

Tics are rapid, stereotyped coordinated or patterned movements that are under partial voluntary control. They tend to be associated with an irresistible urge to perform them and often can be voluntarily suppressed temporarily. Simple tics are difficult to distinguish from dystonia or myoclonus. Complex tics, however, are coordinated, and sometimes include jumping, noises, coprolalia, lip smacking, and touching. The prototypical tic condition is *Gilles de la Tourette's syndrome.* This syndrome will be discussed in more detail under the heading of Speech Pathology.

Chorea

Chorea is characterized by rapid, involuntary, random, purposeless movements of a body part. It may be present at rest and during sustained postures and voluntary movement. Choreiform movements may be subtle or they may grossly displace body parts. They are sometimes volitionally modified by the patient to make them appear intentional in order to cover them up and avoid embarrassment. Chorea can be inflammatory or infectious in origin (for example, Sydenham's chorea, encephalitis), or degenerative (for example, Huntington's chorea). It can result from metabolic and toxic conditions (for example, hepatic encephalopathy, phenothiazine and dopaminergic medications, Wilson's disease) and occasionally from vascular lesions of the lenticular nucleus or thalamus (Adams and Victor, 1991). It can also occur during pregnancy or as an idiopathic condition at any age (Darley, Aronson, and Brown, 1975).

Ballism

Ballism involves gross, abrupt contractions of axial and proximal muscles of the extremities that can produce flailing; when unilateral, the condition is called *hemiballismus.* Ballismus generally has the appearance of a very severe form of proximal chorea. Lesions causing ballism have been located within or near the subthalamic nucleus (*Clinical Examinations in Neurology,* 1991).

Athetosis

Athetosis is a relatively slow hyperkinesia that is characterized by an inability to maintain a body part in a single position because of superimposed slow, writhing, purposeless movements that tend to flow into one another. Athetosis is considered a major category of cerebral palsy. In adults, it may be caused by a variety of conditions. Athetotic and choreiform movements sometimes seem to combine with one another, hence the term *choreoathetosis.* The term "athetosis," especially when referring to an acquired condition, is often considered synonymous with dystonia (*Clinical Examinations in Neurology,* 1991).

Dystonia

Dystonia is a relatively slow hyperkinesia characterized by involuntary abnormal postures resulting from excessive co-contraction of antagonistic muscles. The primary abnormal movement tends to be slow and sustained, but there may be superimposed quick, even myocloniclike movements.

The abnormal posture may involve torsion of a body part. Dystonias probably reflect a combination of dopaminergic and cholinergic overactivity in the basal ganglia (Rosenfield, 1991).

Dystonia may involve only one segment of the body or contiguous regions (segmental). When only orofacial muscles are affected, the condition is often called *focal mouth dystonia* or *orofacial dyskinesia.* Many occupational cramp syndromes, such as writers cramp, are probably forms of dystonia. Dystonia may also be generalized, as in *dystonia musculorum deformans.*

Blepharospasm is characterized by a forceful, spasmodic, relatively sustained closure of the eyes. It can occur alone or with other dystonic disorders, particularly those involving orofacial muscles. Its biochemical and neuroanatomic mechanisms are poorly understood, but bilateral lid closure and blinking can be caused by stimulation of the midbrain and cerebellum. It may be related to denervation hypersensitivity of the facial nuclear complex or to disinhibition of the facial nucleus and brainstem reflexes (Jankovic and Patel, 1983).

Spasmodic torticollis is a segmental dystonia characterized by tonic or clonic spasms of the neck muscles, especially the sternocleidomastoid and trapezius. This causes deviation of the head to the right or left or, less frequently, backward (*retrocollis*) or forward (*antecollis*) (Brazis, Masdeu, and Biller, 1985). Torsion dystonias such as spasmodic torticollis are generally considered basal ganglia diseases. Although evidence is limited, focal lesions in the putamen, caudate, thalamus, and globus pallidus, or their connecting pathways, have been associated with the condition (Rothwell and Obeso, 1987).

Spasm

Spasm is a general descriptive term that designates a variety of muscular contractions. *Tonic spasms* are prolonged or continuous. *Clonic spasms* are repetitive, rapid in onset, and brief in duration.

Spasms are usually involuntary, even when they result from fear, anxiety, and conversion disorders. They often result in movement, but sometimes they limit motion (for example, when attempting to avoid back pain that may arise from movement). The term spasm is sometimes used to describe the abnormal postures seen in dystonia.

Hemifacial spasm is characterized by paroxysms of rapid, irregular clonic twitching of half of the face. The causative lesion affects the facial nerve in the cerebellopontine angle or facial canal, and is thought to result from a pulsating blood vessel (see Chapter 4). This interesting phenomenon illustrates that not all movement disorders result from primary lesions of the CNS control circuits or extrapyramidal system.

Tremor

Tremor is the most common involuntary movement. It involves the rhythmic (periodic) movement of a body part. It may be characterized as resting, postural, action, and terminal. *Resting tremor* occurs when the body part is in repose, *postural tremor* when the body part is maintained against gravity, *action tremor* during movement, and *terminal tremor* as the body part nears a target. Some clinically observable tremors are *physiologic,* meaning that they are exaggerations of the normal tremor that exists in muscle, becoming of sufficient amplitude to be visible under conditions of extreme fatigue or emotion. Physiologic tremor is in the 10 to 12 Hz range until the fifth decade, after which it progressively decreases with age (Koller, 1984).

Toxic tremors can be induced by endogenous toxic states, such as thyrotoxicosis and uremia, or by medications, toxins, or during withdrawal states from drugs or alcohol.

Essential (familial) tremor occurs with sustained posture and action and commonly affects the upper limbs, head, and voice. It tends to be reduced by alcohol.

Cerebellar tremor was discussed in Chapter 6; it occurs during postures and action, and terminally, and is primarily due to involvement of the dentatorubrothalamic pathway. *Wing-beating tremor* (occurring in Wilson's disease or hepatolenticular degeneration and not infrequently in multiple sclerosis) is a severe proximal postural tremor, and is considered a special type of cerebellar tremor. It has a wing-beating appearance when the arms are held in an outstretched or abducted position. It may be seen in any condition involving the dentatorubrothalamic pathways (*Clinical Examinations in Neurology,* 1991).

ETIOLOGIES

Hyperkinetic dysarthria can be caused by any process that can damage the basal ganglia control circuit or portions of the cerebellar control circuit or indirect activation pathways that can lead to hyperkinesias. These include degenerative, vascular, traumatic, inflammatory, toxic, and metabolic diseases. These broad etiologic categories are associated with hyperkinetic dysarthria with varying frequency, but the exact distribution of etiologies is unknown. Toxic-metabolic and idiopathic causes are probably the most frequent etiologies of isolated hyperkinetic dysarthria, however.

Some of the common neurologic conditions associated with hyperkinetic dysarthria with noticeably greater frequency than other dysarthria types are discussed below. Diseases that can be associated with the disorder but are more frequently associated with other dysarthria types (for example, Parkinson's disease) are discussed in chapters dealing with those dysarthrias.

Degenerative diseases

Huntington's disease, or *Huntington's chorea,* is an inherited autosomal dominant degenerative CNS disorder. Because it has complete penetrance, half of the offspring of individuals with the gene are affected. It usually begins insidiously by the fourth or fifth decade, with progression to death within about 15 years. Cellularly, there is severe loss of neurons in the caudate nucleus and putamen and diffuse neuronal loss in the cortex. Positron emission tomography (PET) may demonstrate decreased basal ganglia metabolism before structural changes are apparent on other neuroimaging studies (Breakfield and Bressman, 1987). Its most characteristic clinical feature is chorea, which can be generalized, but it is sometimes initially manifest in the cranial muscles. Dementia and personality changes are characteristic, and dysarthria and dysphagia are common.

Dystonia musculorum deformans usually results from autosomal dominant inheritance, with marked variation in clinical expression (Rosenberg and Pettegrew, 1991). It often is associated with postural deformities in the neck, trunk, and extremities. It usually begins in childhood as a focal dystonia and eventually spreads to affect other body parts. Neuronal loss has been reported in the dentate nucleus of the cerebellum and in the striatum and globus pallidus of the basal ganglia.

Movement disorders may also occur in degenerative diseases that primarily affect cognitive abilities. For example, the presence of orofacial dyskinesia in the elderly tends to be associated with dementia (D'Alessandro and others, 1986). Dyskinesia, especially orofacial dyskinesia, has been reported in 17% of individuals with a diagnosis of Alzheimer's disease (Mölsä, Marttila, and Rinne, 1984).

Toxic-metabolic conditions

Drugs are a very common cause of acute and delayed-onset dyskinesia and dystonia. *Neuroleptic* (meaning that which takes on the neuron) or *antipsychotic drugs* that block (antagonize) dopamine receptors are the most common cause of dyskinesia and dystonia (Miller and Jankovic, 1990). All antipsychotic drugs can cause movement disorders, but high potency neuroleptics such as fluphenazine (Prolixin) and haloperidol (Hal-

dol) are more likely to be associated with them than frequently used but lower potency agents such as chlorpromazine (Thorazine) and thioridazine (Mellaril) (Arana and Hyman, 1991). Other medications that affect the balance of neurotransmitters in the basal ganglia can also lead to movement disorders. These include dopaminergic drugs used in the treatment of Parkinson's disease and sometimes anticonvulsants used in the treatment of epilepsy (Fahn, Marsden, and Calne, 1987). Choreiform facial movements have also been associated with alcohol withdrawal and oral contraceptives, and in certain metabolic conditions, including anoxic or hepatic encephalopathy, hyperthyroidism, hypernatremia, hypoglycemia, choreocanthocytosis, and hypoparathyroidism (Adams and Victor, 1991; Jankovic, 1986). Postural tremor may be caused by alcoholism, thyrotoxicosis, and other toxic conditions (Darley, Aronson, and Brown, 1975). Dystonias have been associated with heavy metal intoxication (manganese) and hexosaminidase deficiency (Rosenfield, 1991).

Tardive dyskinesia (TD) is a condition that may develop after prolonged use of neuroleptic drugs, and is seen most commonly in patients with schizophrenia (Marsden, 1985); it develops in 20% of patients on long-term neuroleptics. It may also develop in response to drugs that can block dopamine, even if they are not used as antipsychotics. For example, TD has been reported in people taking metoclopramide for gastrointestinal disorders, phenothiazines for vertigo, certain antihistamines that are structurally related to phenothiazines, and tricyclic antidepressants that have anticholinergic properties (Marsden and Fahn, 1987). Although the first step in treating TD is drug withdrawal, the dyskinesia often worsens in the first weeks after withdrawal and sometimes does not emerge until drug use is stopped. Drug withdrawal may be associated with remission of the dyskinesias, perhaps in 60% of patients, but it may take three to five years (Marsden, 1985).

The most common manifestation of TD is a stereotyped *orobuccolingual dyskinesia* that can be characterized by stereotyped, repetitive, and involuntary lip smacking, pursing, puffing and retraction, tongue protrusion, and opening, closing, and lateral jaw movements.

TD may also affect respiratory function, with subsequent effects on speech (Casey and Robins, 1978; Faheem and others, 1982; Weiner and others, 1978). Portnoy (1979) has pointed out that changes in speech consistent with hyperkinetic dysarthria may be indicative of TD and that its early recognition may help prevent a permanent

TD if drug withdrawal or dosage modifications are possible.

Vascular disorders

Vascular lesions are not a common cause of hyperkinesias. However, infarcts in the basal ganglia control circuit, and sometimes the cerebellar control circuit, have been associated with movement disorders and hyperkinetic dysarthria, and stroke is the usual cause of hemichorea and hemiballism. Dystonia has been reported in cases with putaminal stroke and arteriovenous malformation (AVM) (Fross and others, 1987; Rosenfield, 1991). Chorea may result from vascular lesions of the lenticular nucleus or thalamus (Adams and Victor, 1991) and can occur in systemic lupus erythematosis (Rosenfield, 1991). Meige's syndrome (see "other") and palatal myoclonus have been reported in brainstem stroke (Day, Lefroy, and Mastaglia, 1986; Jankovic and Patel, 1983).

Infectious processes

Sydenham's chorea is a self-limiting condition that is usually associated with inflammation or infection such as streptococcal throat infections, scarlatina, or rheumatic fever. It occurs mostly in the young and usually resolves in a relatively short time (Warfel and Schlagenhauff, 1980). Chorea has also been associated with diphtheria and rubella (Rosenfield, 1991).

Neoplasm

Tumors of the basal ganglia and thalamus have been associated with chorea and dystonia (Rosenfield, 1991; Rothwell and Obeso, 1987).

Other

Meige's syndrome is a focal dystonia characterized by a combination of blepharospasm and oromandibular dystonia. It usually develops after age fifty. Etiology is often unknown, but it presumably involves the basal ganglia (Golper and others, 1983). Multiple sclerosis and hypoxic encephalopathy leading to rostral brainstem or diencephalic lesions have been reported as causing blepharospasm (Day, Lefroy, and Mastaglia, 1986; Jankovic and Patel, 1983).

Gilles de la Tourette's syndrome is a disorder the primary characteristics of which are motor and vocal tics. Its symptoms are always apparent before adulthood and most cases are probably hereditary. Its pathophysiology is not understood but it may be related to striatal dopamine receptor abnormalities (Kurlan, 1989). Its vocal and speech characteristics will be discussed in the section on Speech Pathology.

Abnormalities of the dental arch in edentulous elderly people has been associated with involuntary chewing movements (D'Alessandro and others, 1986). Disruption of dental proprioception has been suggested as a general explanatory mechanism (Jankovic, 1986).

Facial dyskinesias may be observed in schizophrenic individuals, and they can occur prior to the introduction of antipsychotic drugs (Jankovic, 1986).

Chorea gravidarum is a benign choreiform disorder that occurs during pregnancy and usually disappears after pregnancy (Warfel and Schlagenhauff, 1980).

SPEECH PATHOLOGY
Distribution of etiologies, lesions, and severity in clinical practice

The box on page 196 summarizes the etiologies for 86 quasirandomly selected cases seen at the Mayo Clinic with a primary speech pathology diagnosis of hyperkinetic dysarthria. Cases with organic voice tremor and neurogenic spasmodic dysphonia were not included in the review because their etiology is nearly always unknown. The cautions expressed in Chapter 4 about generalizing these data to the general population of patients with hyperkinetic dysarthria or to all speech pathology practices also apply here.

The data establish that hyperkinetic dysarthria can result from several medical conditions. The distribution of the etiologies is quite different from that associated with most other dysarthria types. Fifty-nine percent of the cases were of undetermined etiology, with toxic or metabolic causes accounting for an additional 17% of the cases. These percentages illustrate the elusive nature of the neuroanatomic bases of movement disorders, and they suggest that their causes may often lie in neurochemical abnormalities rather than structural lesions.

The nature and muscular locus of involuntary movements of unknown etiology illustrate the heterogeneity that exists in this group of speech disorders. The abnormal movements were given numerous descriptive labels, including dyskinesia, dystonia, torticollis, retrocollis, antecollis, chorea, tremor, myoclonus, action myoclonus, and action dystonia. In some cases the neurologic diagnosis was limited to general labels such as "movement disorder," "extrapyramidal syndrome," and "acquired basal ganglia disorder."

The largest single diagnosis for the 86 cases was orofacial dyskinesia of unknown etiology (21%). This means that the patients' movement disorders were confined to the face, jaw, tongue, pharynx, or

ETIOLOGIES OF DYSARTHRIA FOR 86 QUASIRANDOMLY SELECTED CASES WITH A PRIMARY SPEECH PATHOLOGY DIAGNOSIS OF HYPERKINETIC DYSARTHRIA AT THE MAYO CLINIC FROM 1969–1990. PERCENTAGE OF CASES UNDER EACH BROAD ETIOLOGIC HEADING IS GIVEN IN PARENTHESES. CASES WITH ORGANIC VOICE TREMOR AND NEUROGENIC SPASMODIC DYSPHONIA WERE NOT INCLUDED IN THE SAMPLE BECAUSE ETIOLOGY IS NEARLY ALWAYS IDIOPATHIC IN THOSE DISORDERS.

Unknown (59%)
　Orofacial dyskinesia (21%)
　　(described as: oral dyskinesia, oromandibular dystonia, lingualmandibular dystonia, buccolingual dyskinesia, extrapyramidal facial movement disorder, focal dystonia)
　Spasmodic torticollis/retrocollis/antecollis (9%)
　Face/neck/axial dyskinesia (7%)
　Chorea (3%)
　Meige's syndrome (2%)
　Torticollis and facial dystonia (2%)
　Segmental dystonia and tremor (1%)
　Thoracolaryngeal dystonia (1%)
　Abdominal myoclonus (1%)
　Action dystonia (1%)
　Focal seizure disorder (1%)
　Other (8%)
　　Movement disorder, dyskinesia, extrapyramidal syndrome, acquired basal ganglia disorder, myoclonus, indeterminate brainstem lesion

Toxic/Metabolic (17%)
　Tardive dyskinesia (9%)
　Drug-induced dyskinesia (3%)
　Dialysis encephalopathy (2%)
　Hepatic encephalopathy (1%)
　Hypoparathyroidism (1%)

Degenerative (9%)
　Huntington's chorea (5%)
　Unspecified degenerative CNS disease (2%)
　Dystonia musculorum deformans (1%)

Multiple (5%)
　Multiple sclerosis + drug-induced parkinsonism (1%)
　Familial ataxia + alcoholism (1%)
　Senile chorea + stroke (1%)
　Tardive dyskinesia + stroke + anxiety (1%)

Other (3%)
　Tourette's syndrome (1%)
　Myoclonic epilepsy (1%)
　No neurologic diagnosis (1%)

Infectious (2%)
　Sydenham's chorea

Trauma (1%)
　Post cerebellar tumor removal (ataxia and palatal myoclonus)

Vascular (1%)
　Brainstem stroke

CNS, central nervous system.

larynx. This highlights the predilection of many movement disorders for the orofacial muscles, the likelihood that many generalized movement disorders may be manifest first in the orofacial area, and the importance of recognizing the meaning of abnormal orofacial movements and hyperkinetic dysarthria as signs of neurologic disease. The prevalence of movement disorders that are limited to the head and neck muscles in people with hyperkinetic dysarthria is further illustrated by the relatively high frequency of cases with face/neck/axial dyskinesia (7%), spasmodic torticollis, retrocollis, or antecollis (9%), and tardive dyskinesia (9%). Therefore, about 85% of the 86 cases had a hyperkinetic dysarthria in which the underlying movement disorder was not evident in the limbs (this percentage would be even higher if organic voice tremor and neurogenic spasmodic dysphonias were included in the sample).

Most cases with toxic/metabolic etiology were drug-related, most often involving neuroleptic or anticonvulsive medications. Although most were delayed in onset (tardive), some occurred soon after medication was started. In contrast to the distribution of etiologies for other dysarthria types, drugs were the most frequent *known* cause of hyperkinetic dysarthria in this sample.

Huntington's chorea was the most frequent degenerative disease (5% of the entire sample). The remaining etiologic categories (infectious, trauma, vascular) were not frequently represented, but did contain conditions with established and prominent associations with hyperkinesias (that is, Tourette's syndrome, myoclonic epilepsy, Sydenham's chorea, palatal myclonus).

To what extent was dysarthria the only manifestation of an involuntary movement disorder? Forty-one percent of the sample had involuntary movements that were confined to the orofacial muscles but that were present at rest or during nonspeech movements. Five cases (6%) had a hyperkinetic dysarthria in which the hyperkinesia was action-induced, and was not present during orofacial movements other than speech (this percentage would be considerably higher if cases with organic voice tremor and neurogenic spasmodic dysphonia were included). Therefore, speech sometimes can be the only manifestation of a movement disorder. Such cases are often diagnosed as psychologic in origin, and they may have a painfully long history of repeated psychiatric assessments and treatment, without any connection emerging between psychopathology and the speech disorder, and without benefit from psychotherapy, behavioral interventions, or psychotropic medications. Such cases illustrate a lack of understanding about the possible connection between speech disorders and neurologic disease, especially when speech is the presenting and only obvious physical problem.

What speech structures were involved in these cases, and how often was only a single structure involved? Table 8–2 summarizes the percentage of cases in which a clear indication was given about involvement of the jaw, face, tongue, palate, larynx, and respiratory muscles and the percentage of cases in which only one of those structures was affected. It is clear that more than one speech structure is involved in most cases, and that face, tongue, and jaw involvement are most frequently recognized (note again that organic voice tremor and spasmodic dysphonia were not included in the sample, so laryngeal involvement is underrepresented). Combined jaw, face, and tongue hyperkinesia was the most frequently recognized combination of involved structures. It is also apparent that only a single speech structure may be involved in hyperkinetic dysarthria. Nine cases (10%) had only one structure affected; the palate was the only structure not affected in isolation. In a few cases, involuntary movement in the singly involved structure was induced only by speech; for example, two patients with jaw dystonia had abnormal jaw movements only during speech. Therefore, these data suggest that involuntary movements underlying hyperkinetic dysarthria usually involve more than a single speech structure, but they sometimes affect only a single speech structure, and sometimes occur only during speech.

Precise anatomic localization of lesions for the patients in this sample, as predicted by the high frequency of undetermined etiologies, was sparse. Only about 65% of the sample had computed tomography (CT) scans or magnetic resonance imaging (MRI). For those who did, 65% had no identifiable pathology. Detected abnormalities were often nonfocal or not necessarily related to the movement disorder. For example, several cases

Table 8–2 Percentage of patients with involvement of the jaw, face, tongue, palate, larynx, and respiratory muscles—singly and in combination—for 86 cases with hyperkinetic dysarthria (excluding organic voice tremor and spasmodic dysphonia).

Structure involved	% in combination with other structures	% isolated
Jaw	52	3
Face	67	1
Tongue	56	3
Palate	13	0
Larynx	44	1
Respiratory	7	1

had evidence of general cerebral or cerebellar atrophy, bilateral white matter changes, or ventricular dilatation. A few had evidence of cortical lesions, but there was no common site among them. Five patients (9% of those with neuroimaging studies) had evidence of basal ganglia pathology, two patients had evidence of cerebellar pathology, and one had evidence of a thalamic lesion. Even in cases with identifiable lesions in the basal ganglia, cerebellum, and thalamus, it was sometimes concluded that they were not directly responsible for the movement disorder (for example, one patient's movement disorder was most likely due to tardive dyskinesia). Therefore, although neuroimaging studies (at least CT and MRI) sometimes yield evidence of pathology, the connection between the identifiable lesion and the movement disorder is not always clear.

This retrospective review did not permit a clear delineation of dysarthria severity. However, in those patients for whom a judgment of intelligibility was explicitly stated (51% of the sample), *30% had reduced intelligibility.* The degree to which this figure accurately estimates the frequency of intelligibility impairments in the population with hyperkinetic dysarthria is unclear. It is likely that many patients for whom an observation of intelligibility was not made had normal intelligibility, but the sample probably contains a larger number of mildly impaired patients than is encountered in the typical rehabilitation setting. In addition, reduced intelligibility is only one measure of deficit and may not accurately represent degree of handicap or disability. For example, many hyperkinetic dysarthrias significantly reduce efficiency (speed) of communication without affecting intelligibility, and the visible involuntary and bizarre movements that are responsible for many aspects of the dysarthria can have devastating social and emotional consequences. The relatively low frequency of intelligibility impairments in this dysarthria is fortunate, but to conclude that it usually does not have a significant impact on verbal and nonverbal communication (and emotional and social consequences) probably grossly underestimates its impact on affected individuals.

Finally, movement disorders and hyperkinetic dysarthria can occur in conditions that also affect cognitive functions (for example, Huntington's chorea). Of the patients in the sample whose cognitive abilities were explicitly commented on or formally assessed (67% of the sample), *36% had some impairment of cognitive ability.*

Patient perceptions and complaints

Patient complaints are often dependent on the type of movement disorder and the level of the speech system it affects. Those with nonrhythmic hyperkinesias (for example, chorea, dystonia) affecting the jaw, face, tongue, and larynx tend to describe their speech as slurred, slow, halting, or "hard to get out." Somewhat surprisingly, those with hyperkinesia at several levels of the speech system may not be aware of the abnormal movements (Burke, 1984), even when they are visibly apparent to the examiner. They may, however, recognize their inability to maintain a steady jaw, face, or tongue posture when asked to by the examiner. Failure to spontaneously complain about orofacial hyperkinesias is more frequent in patients whose hyperkinesia is apparent only during speech, chewing, or swallowing (that is, they complain of difficulty with speech but not the underlying abnormal movement). Chewing and swallowing complaints are common in chorea and dystonia.

Patients whose hyperkinesia is limited to a single or a few structures may complain of abnormal movements, both at rest and during speech. Complaints about abnormal movements at rest may predominate in patients whose hyperkinesias are mild or can be suppressed temporarily during speech. These complaints include feelings of tightness in affected structures, an inability to move a structure, an inability to control or inhibit abnormal movements, or a sense that the structure simply "doesn't work right." Some patients report being able to suppress the abnormal movements for a time but find that they return with a vengeance when their efforts cease.

Patients with prominent laryngeal hyperkinesias (usually associated with tremor or dystonia) often complain that their voices are shaky, tight, close off, or don't want to come out. Because of increased resistance to air flow with laryngeal spasm during speech, patients may complain of shortness of breath or physical exhaustion during speech and associate it with respiratory difficulty. When the problem is isolated to the larynx, however, the patient usually does not note similar fatigue during strenuous nonspeech physical activities. Patients with respiratory hyperkinesias that are triggered only by speaking may be unaware of the locus of the problem, even when they are acutely aware of their abnormal speech.

Some patients learn that the severity of orofacial dystonic posturing or movements can be reduced or eliminated by certain tactile or proprioceptive *sensory tricks.* For example, patients with torticollis may learn that bringing the hand to the chin or the back of the head will allow them to posture the head more normally; patients with involuntary jaw opening may learn that lightly touching the hand to the jaw may prevent the movement. With increasing severity or duration of the disorder,

however, the facilitory effect of these tricks dimin-
ishes. It should be noted that the term "sensory
tricks" is descriptive, and the real mechanism for
their effect is unknown (Fahn, Marsden, and
Calne, 1987). Nonetheless, patient reports of previously successful sensory tricks, or observation of
them during examination, are very useful diagnostically because they are rarely developed in other
dysarthria types or in psychogenic speech disorders characterized by abnormal movements.

Chorea

Nonspeech oral mechanism. The jaw, face,
tongue, and palate are usually normal in size,
strength, and symmetry. The gag reflex is often
normal. Pathologic oral reflexes may not be
present. Drooling is occasionally observed, and
chewing and swallowing difficulties are not uncommon.

The most striking abnormality is motor unsteadiness and, often, easily observed choreiform
movements. At rest or during attempts to maintain
lip retraction and rounding, mouth opening, or
tongue protrusion, quick, unpredictable, involuntary movements may occur. They can range from
subtle exaggerations of facial expression to movements that are so pervasive and prominent that
affected structures seem never to be at rest (Figure
8–1 A, B). Difficulty recognizing these movements as hyperkinesias occurs when movements

are subtle and infrequent because they may be
difficult to distinguish from normal unsteadiness;
and when patients display motor impersistence or
cognitive impairments that raise doubts about their
ability to sustain adequate effort on the task.

Speech. Conversation, reading, and speech alternating motion rates (AMRs) are very useful for
eliciting the unpredictable breakdowns of articulation and the abnormalities of rate and prosody that
may predominate. Vowel prolongation is indispensable because it provides an opportunity to observe
fluctuations in the steady state of the vowel induced
by choreiform movements. The open vowel "ah" is
particularly useful because adventitious movements of the jaw, face, tongue, and palate can be
easily observed and heard during it.

Careful visual observation of the patient during
speech is important. It provides confirmatory evidence of abnormal movements as the source of the
speech deficit, and permits the identification of at
least some of the structures involved in the movement disorder.

Table 8–3 summarizes the neuromuscular deficits presumed by Darley, Aronson, and Brown
(1969a & b, 1975) to underlie the hyperkinetic
dysarthria of chorea. Nearly all aspects of movement may be disturbed. The direction and rhythm
of movement may be altered by involuntary movements, and rate is generally slowed by them. Force
and range of individual and repetitive movements

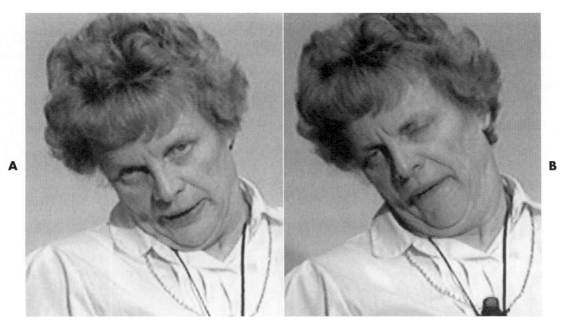

A   **B**

Figure 8–1 Quick, involuntary head, jaw, face, lip, and eye movements in a woman with
generalized chorea. The depicted movements in panels **A** and **B** were very brief and separated from
each other by < 1 second.

Table 8–3 Neuromuscular deficits associated with hyperkinetic dysarthria associated with dystonia and chorea.

Disorder	Direction	Rhythm	Rate		Range		Force	Tone
	Individual movements	Repetitive movements	Individual movements	Repetitive movements	Individual movements	Repetitive movements	Individual movements	Muscle tone
Dystonia	Inaccurate due to slow involuntary movements	Irregular	Slow	Slow	Reduced to normal	Reduced to normal	Normal	Excessive (biased)
Chorea	Inaccurate due to quick > slow involuntary movements	Irregular	Slow	Slow	Reduced to excessive	Reduced to excessive	Reduced to excessive	Often excessive (biased)

Adapted from Darley FL, Aronson AE, and Brown JR: Clusters of deviant speech dimensions in the dysarthrias, J Speech Hear Res 12:462, 1969b.

may vary from reduced to normal to excessive depending on the presence or absence of choreic movements at the moment and the relationship of their direction to that of the intended voluntary speech gesture. Muscle tone may be excessive and, when it is, it tends to be biased. The relationship of these characteristics to specific deviant speech characteristics are discussed below, as are findings from relevant acoustic and physiologic studies.

Clusters of deviant dimensions and prominent deviant speech characteristics. Darley, Aronson, and Brown (1969b) identified several clusters of deviant speech dimensions in their 30 patients with chorea, but a complete review of each of them is unnecessary to appreciate the major features of the disorder. Only those clusters that are most prominent and distinctive of the hyperkinetic dysarthria of chorea will be addressed. Here we will focus primarily on the most deviant or unique speech characteristics and their relationship to movement abnormalities at each level of the speech system. These characteristics are useful to understanding the disorder's underlying neuromuscular deficits, the components of the speech system that tend to be most prominently involved, and the features that help to distinguish this presentation of hyperkinetic dysarthria from other dysarthria types. The most deviant speech characteristics encountered in the hyperkinetic dysarthria of chorea are summarized in Table 8–4.

Respiration. Choreiform movements affecting respiration during speech can be reflected in sudden *forced involuntary inspiration or expiration.* Although not pervasive, and not necessarily severe, this feature was not encountered by Darley, Aronson, and Brown (1975) in any other dysarthria type.

Phonation. Patients may exhibit *harsh voice quality, excess loudness variations,* and a *strained-strangled voice quality.* These features correlated with one another in Darley, Aronson, and Brown's subjects to form the cluster of *phonatory stenosis,* presumably resulting from relatively brief, random hyperadductions of the vocal cords (excess loudness variations could also result from choreic respiratory movements). Phonatory stenosis may be sufficient to cause *voice stoppages* in some patients. Acoustic analysis of patients with Huntington's disease has documented the presence of increased fundamental frequency variability, reflecting instability of laryngeal movements during speech (Zwirner and Barnes, 1992).

Although infrequent, some patients may exhibit *transient breathiness.* This may occur as a result of brief, involuntary vocal cord abduction, poor timing between expiration and phonation, or possibly

in response to, or in compensation for, the physically exhausting effects of phonatory stenosis.

Resonance. Chorea may lead to *hypernasality* in some patients, although it is rarely constant or severe. Hypernasality was correlated with *imprecise consonants* and *short phrases* in Darley, Aronson, and Brown's subjects, forming the cluster of *resonatory incompetence.* This suggests that air wastage through the velopharyngeal port may at least partially explain the occurrence of imprecise consonants and short phrases in some speakers.

Articulation. Imprecise articulation is the most prominent, but not the most distinguishing feature of the hyperkinetic dysarthria of chorea. It tends to

Table 8–4 The most deviant speech dimensions encountered in the hyperkinetic dysarthria of *chorea* by Darley, Aronson, and Brown (1969a) listed in order from most to least severe. Also listed is the component of the speech system associated with each characteristic. The component "prosodic" is listed when several components of the speech system may contribute to the dimension. Characteristics listed under "Other" include speech features not among the most deviant but which may occur and are not typical of most other dysarthria types.

Dimension	Speech component
Imprecise consonants	Articulatory
Prolonged intervals*	Prosodic
Variable rate*	Prosodic
Monopitch	Phonatory-prosodic
Harsh voice quality	Phonatory
Inappropriate silences*	Prosodic
Distorted vowels	Articulatory-prosodic
Excess loudness variations*	Respiratory-phonatory-prosodic
Prolonged phonemes*	Prosodic
Monoloudness	Phonatory-prosodic
Short phrases	Prosodic
Irregular articulatory breakdowns	Articulatory
Excess and equal stress	Prosodic
Hypernasality	Resonatory
Reduced stress	Prosodic
Strained-strangled quality	Phonatory
Other	
Sudden forced inspiration or expiration*	Respiratory-prosodic
Voice stoppages*	Phonatory-prosodic
Transient breathiness*	Phonatory

*Tend to be distinctive or more severely impaired than in any other single dysarthria type.

co-occur with *distorted vowels* and hypernasality, and in Darley, Aronson, and Brown's patients these features formed the cluster of *articulatory-resonatory incompetence. Irregular articulatory breakdowns* also occur frequently. All of these features are presumably the result of various combinations of choreiform movements of the jaw, face, tongue, and palate. Acoustic analysis has provided support for this conclusion. Zwirner and Barnes (1992), examining the stability of steady state vowels, found abnormal variability in the first formant (suggestive of abnormal jaw movements) and second formant (suggestive of abnormal tongue position and shape) in speakers with Huntington's disease.

Prosody. Prosodic disturbances are prominent. They may reflect the primary effects of chorea on speech as well as the individual's response to the unpredictable movements. As Darley, Aronson, and Brown stated, "The flow of speech is often jerky, generated in fits and starts. As they proceed, patients are seemingly on guard against anticipated speech breakdowns, making compensation from time to time as they feel the imminence of glottic closure, respiratory arrest, or articulatory hindrance" (1975, p. 207).

The most prominent cluster of speech characteristics in Darley, Aronson's, and Brown's study was *prosodic excess,* comprised of *prolonged intervals, inappropriate silences, prolonged phonemes,* and *excess and equal stress.* Patients also exhibited *prosodic insufficiency,* characterized by *monopitch, monoloudness, reduced stress,* and *short phrases.* Many patients also had *variable rate,* possibly reflecting their efforts to complete phrases quickly before the next involuntary movement. The co-occurrence of the seemingly mutually exclusive clusters of prosodic excess and prosodic insufficiency attests to the moment-to-moment variability that occurs in this form of dysarthria, and the unpredictability of the effects of relatively quick and variable involuntary movements on speech. They probably also reflect the combined effects of the primary motor disturbance and the individual's compensatory or cautious response to it.

What features of the hyperkinetic dysarthria of chorea help identify and distinguish it from other motor speech disorders? Most apparent is the transient and unpredictable nature of the deviant speech characteristics, the most obvious of which are *hypernasality, strained-harshness, transient breathiness, articulatory distortions and irregular articulatory breakdowns, loudness variations,* and *sudden forced inspiration or expiration.* These features, often in combination with the speaker's attempt to avoid or compensate for them, lead to *prolonged intervals and phonemes, variable rate,*

inappropriate silences, voice stoppages, and *excessive or insufficient stress patterns.* The primary and distinguishing speech and speech-related findings in this form of hyperkinetic dysarthria are summarized in Table 8–5.

Dystonia

Nonspeech oral mechanism. As in chorea, the oral mechanism is often normal in size, strength, and symmetry, and reflexes may be normal. Drooling may occur, and chewing and swallowing complaints are common. Patients frequently complain that food gets stuck in the throat or that chewing is difficult because of jaw or tongue movements (Golper and others, 1983). The striking features of the nonspeech oral mechanism exam are most evident at rest or during attempts to maintain steady facial postures. Dystonic movements are slower than those of chorea, and have a waxing and waning character. Blepharospasm and facial grimacing may be present, as may intermittent, relatively sustained spasms that lead to mouth opening and closing, lip pursing or retraction, and

Table 8–5 Primary distinguishing speech and speech-related findings in the hyperkinetic dysarthria of *chorea.*

Perceptual	
Phonation-respiration	Sudden forced inspiration-expiration, voice stoppages, transient breathiness, strained-harsh voice quality, excess loudness variations
Resonance	Hypernasality (intermittent)
Articulation	Distortions and irregular breakdowns, slow and irregular AMRs
Prosody	Prolonged intervals and phonemes, variable rate, inappropriate silences, excessive-inefficient-variable patterns of stress
Physical	Quick, unpatterned involuntary head/neck, jaw, face, tongue, palate, pharyngeal, laryngeal, thoracic-abdominal movements at rest, during sustained postures and movement Dysphagia
Patient complaints	Effortful speech, inability to "get speech out," involuntary orofacial movements Chewing and swallowing problems

AMR, alternating motion rate.

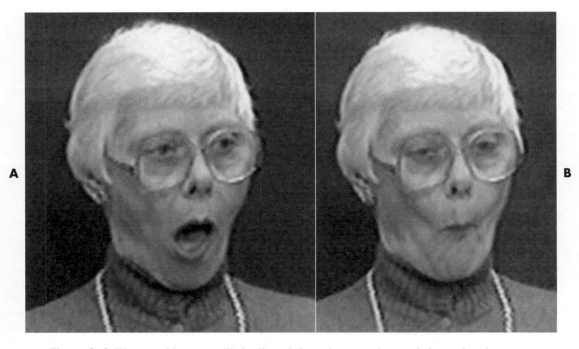

Figure 8-2 Woman with oromandibular-lingual dystonia attempting to sit in a relaxed posture, with **A** relatively slow involuntary jaw opening and tongue lateralization and protrusion and **B** involuntary lip pursing.

protrusion or rotary movements of the tongue (Figure 8-2, A, B). Affected neck muscles may cause elevation of the larynx; torsion of the neck may be marked in patients with torticollis. As in chorea, recognition of dystonia is most difficult when movements are subtle or when cognitive or other motor deficits make valid observations difficult.

Patients may use sensory tricks to inhibit dystonic movements, and it is important to ask if they are aware of such tricks when they do not use them spontaneously. These often involve pressure or light touch to the jaw, cheek, or back of the neck; some patients will hold a pipe in the mouth because it inhibits jaw, lip, or tongue dystonias.

In some cases, the nonspeech oral mechanism examination may be entirely normal, dystonic movements being triggered only by speech. There is a tendency for such patients to have very focal dystonic movements that may involve only the jaw, tongue, pharynx, larynx, or respiratory muscles.

Speech. Conversational speech or reading, speech AMRs, and vowel prolongation are useful when assessing the hyperkinetic dysarthria of dystonia. Careful visual observation of the patient during speaking is similarly important.

Table 8-3 summarizes the neuromuscular deficits presumed by Darley, Aronson, and Brown (1969a & b, 1975) to underlie the dysarthria of dystonia. Nearly all aspects of movement may be disturbed. Direction and rhythm of movement may

be altered by dystonic movements, and rate is generally slow. Range of individual and repetitive movements may be normal but can be reduced by excessive and biased muscle tone. The relationship of these characteristics to specific deviant speech characteristics is discussed in the next section, as are findings from relevant acoustic and physiologic studies.

Clusters of deviant dimensions and prominent deviant speech characteristics. Darley, Aronson, and Brown (1969b) found several clusters of deviant speech dimensions in their 30 patients with dystonia. Only those that are most prominent and distinctive will be addressed here; the focus will be on the most deviant or distinctive speech characteristics and their relationship to movement abnormalities at each level of the speech system.* The most deviant speech characteristics encountered in the hyperkinetic dysarthria of dystonia are summarized in Table 8-6.

Respiration. The dystonic speakers in Darley, Aronson, and Brown's study did not exhibit speech characteristics that clearly reflected respiratory dystonia. However, some did demonstrate *excess loudness variations,* and a small number had mild *alternating loudness.* These features

---

*Golper and others (1983) found a pattern of speech deficits very similar to Darley, Aronson, and Brown's dystonic patients in a group of 10 patients with focal cranial dystonia (Meige's syndrome).

Table 8–6 The most deviant speech dimensions in the hyperkinetic dysarthria of *dystonia* encountered by Darley, Aronson, and Brown (1969a), listed in order from most to least severe. Also listed is the component of the speech system associated with each characteristic. The component "prosodic" is listed when several components of the speech system may contribute to the dimension. Characteristics listed under "Other" include speech features not among the most deviant but which may occur and are not typical of most other dysarthria types.

Dimension	Speech component
Imprecise consonants	Articulatory
Distorted vowels*	Articulatory-prosodic
Harsh voice quality*	Phonatory
Irregular articulatory breakdowns*	Articulatory
Strained-strangled quality*	Phonatory
Monopitch	Phonatory-prosodic
Monoloudness	Phonatory-prosodic
Inappropriate silences*	Prosodic
Short phrases	Prosodic
Prolonged intervals	Prosodic
Prolonged phonemes	Prosodic
Excess loudness variations*	Respiratory-phonatory-prosodic
Reduced stress	Prosodic
Voice stoppages*	Phonatory-prosodic
Slow rate	Articulatory-prosodic
Other	
Audible inspiration*	Phonatory-respiratory
Voice tremor*	Phonatory
Alternating loudness*	Respiratory-phonatory-prosodic

*Tend to be distinctive or more severely impaired than in any other single dysarthria type.

could reflect abnormal respiratory movements or respiratory movements made in an effort to overcome phonatory stenosis. Golper and others (1983) found similar characteristics and noted respiratory dyskinesia in two of their patients.

Phonation. Several phonatory deviations may be present, including *harshness, strained-strangled voice quality, excess loudness variations,* and *voice stoppages.* Combined with *short phrases,* these characteristics combined in Darley, Aronson, and Brown's dystonic speakers to form the cluster of *phonatory stenosis,* a cluster also found in speakers with chorea. All of these characteristics can be related to dystonic or spasmodic hyperadduction of the vocal cords during phonation.

Some patients exhibit *audible inspiration,* probably secondary to involuntary vocal cord adduc-

tion during inhalation. With the exception of patients with flaccid dysarthria and vocal cord abductor weakness, this feature is rarely encountered in other dysarthria types.

Although not prominent in frequency of occurrence or severity, *voice tremor* may be present. In fact, voice tremor was more evident in speakers with dystonic speech than in any other dysarthric group studied by Darley, Aronson, and Brown.

Resonance. Although dystonic movements can affect velopharyngeal function during speech, hypernasality is not a pervasive characteristic and is usually rated as mild when present (Darley, Aronson, and Brown, 1969a).

Articulation. Imprecise consonants, distorted vowels, and irregular articulatory breakdowns may be prominent when dystonia affects articulators. These features formed the cluster *articulatory inaccuracy* in Darley, Aronson, and Brown's dystonic speakers. They logically reflect the effects on articulation of adventitious involuntary jaw, face, lip, or tongue movements (Figures 8–3 and 8–4). This conclusion receives support from acoustic analyses that have identified excessive second formant fluctuations during steady state vowels in patients with tardive dyskinesia (Gerratt, 1983). This acoustic variability reflects reduced vocal tract stability induced by orofacial dyskinesia (Figure 8–5).

Prosody. Prosodic disturbances are prominent and are similar to those encountered in chorea. *Monopitch, monoloudness, short phrases,* and *reduced stress* may be present, and in Darley, Aronson, and Brown's speakers they combined to form the cluster of *prosodic insufficiency.* Also commonly heard are *prolonged intervals, prolonged phonemes,* and *slow rate,* features that combined to form the cluster of *prosodic excess. Inappropriate silences* and *excess and equal stress* may also be detected and they contribute to the general perception of exaggerated stress patterns. All of these deviant speech features may reflect the effect of slowness of movement or interruptions in the flow of normal movements during speech.

Similar to chorea, the co-occurrence of clusters of prosodic excess and prosodic insufficiency may reflect the variable nature of dystonia with its underlying co-occurring slowness and its reduced range of movement, and the speaker's compensatory or cautious response to the primary disorder.

What features of the hyperkinetic dysarthria of dystonia help identify and distinguish it from other motor speech disorders? Most apparent is the variable nature of the deviant speech characteristics, the most prevalent of which are *imprecision and irregular breakdowns of articulation, inappropriate variability of loudness and rate, strained*

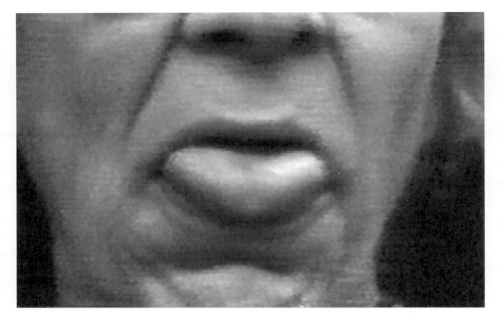

Figure 8–3 Woman with predominantly lingual dyskinesia during normally rapid production of alternating motion rates for /pʌ/; involuntary tongue protrusion prevents bilabial closure.

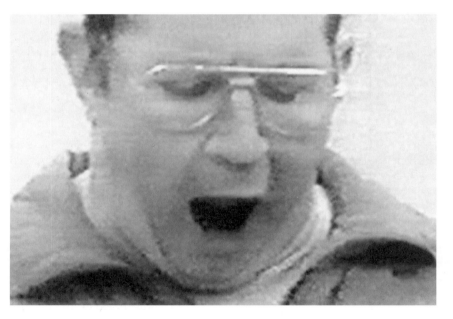

Figure 8–4 Man with jaw opening dystonia during production of the /æ/ in "grand." Excessive jaw opening and lingual retraction occurred only during speech and were associated almost exclusively with production of open vowels or velar consonants (see *Case 8.2* for complete description).

harshness, transient breathiness, and *audible inspiration.* These features, often in combination with the speaker's attempt to avoid or compensate for dystonic movements, may lead to *slow rate, prolonged intervals and phonemes, inappropriate silences,* and prosodic features that lead to both *excessive and insufficient stress patterns.* The primary and distinguishing speech and speech-related

findings in this form of hyperkinetic dysarthria are summarized in Table 8–7.

Athetosis

Although athetosis is a major subcategory of cerebral palsy, the term "athetosis" is rarely used to describe movement disorders acquired in adulthood (possibly because many neurologists consider

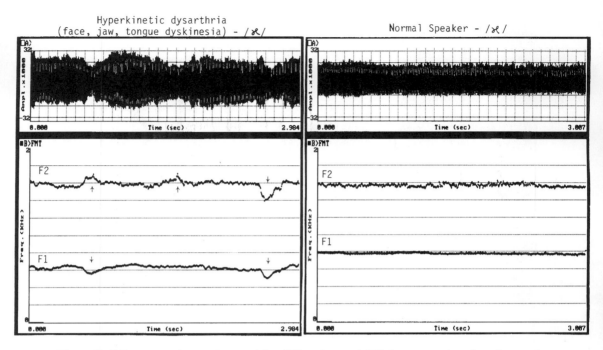

Figure 8–5 Raw acoustic waveform and first (*F1*) and second (*F2*) formant tracings for a 3-second prolongation of the vowel /æ/ by a man with face, jaw, and tongue dyskinesia (*left side*) and a normal male speaker (*right side*). Maintenance of steady vocal tract posture is reflected in all tracings for the normal speaker. In contrast, the hyperkinetic speaker's abnormal movements are reflected in the raw waveform and in the relatively sustained (∼ 230 to 280 ms) fluctuations in F1 and F2 (*see arrows*). The fluctutations are sometimes apparent in F1 and F2 simultaneously, but not always, and there is variability in their amplitude and direction. The fluctuations reflect auditorily perceptible abnormal movements of the tongue, lips, or jaw.

athetosis to be synonymous with dystonia). As a result, the literature on the dysarthria of athetosis is based exclusively on studies of children or adults with cerebral palsy. The results of such studies suggest that the speech characteristics of athetosis are probably captured within the descriptions of dysarthria associated with dystonia, and perhaps chorea, that have already been addressed. Because of this apparent overlap, and because the focus of this book is on acquired motor speech disorders, the literature on the speech of individuals with athetotic cerebral palsy will not be discussed here.*

Spasmodic torticollis (cervical dystonia)

Spasmodic torticollis (ST) affects the cervical neck muscles and not the cranial nerve innervated speech muscles (but facial spasms are not infrequent in patients with ST [Couch, 1976]).

---

*The interested reader is referred to reviews or comprehensive descriptive studies by Darley, Aronson, and Brown (1975); Hardy (1983); Kent and Netsell (1978); Nielson and O'Dwyer (1984); Platt and others (1980); Platt, Andrews, and Howie (1980); and Putnam (1988).

Unless accompanied by dystonia that directly affects the speech muscles, any ST-related speech abnormalities are presumably secondary to the effects of neck postural deviations on primary speech muscle activity, or to alterations in the shape of the subglottic, glottic, or supraglottic vocal tract induced by abnormal neck postures (Figure 8–6 *A, B*). Given the severe distortions of neck posture that may occur in ST, it is surprising that speech is not affected more frequently and dramatically.

The most detailed study of speech in patients with ST was reported by LaPointe, Case, and Duane (1994). They analyzed the speech of 70 individuals with ST and compared them to 20 age-matched controls. A number of group differences emerged from their acoustic analyses, with the ST group demonstrating: reduced reading rate (STs' 165 wpm versus controls' 195 wpm); reduced speech AMRs and sequential motion rates (SMRs) (STs' 4 to 5/sec versus controls' 5 to 7/sec); reduced maximum duration of /s/, /z/, and vowel prolongation (STs' 15 to 19 secs versus controls' 20+ secs); reduced habitual pitch, highest pitch, and pitch range in females; and reduced

Table 8–7 Primary distinguishing speech and speech-related findings in the hyperkinetic dysarthria of *dystonia.*

Perceptual	
Phonation-Respiration	Strained-harsh voice quality, voice stoppages, audible inspiration, excess loudness variations, alternating loudness, voice tremor
Resonance	Hypernasality
Articulation	Distorted vowels, irregular articulatory breakdowns, slow irregular AMRS
Prosody	Inappropriate silences, excess loudness variations, excessive-inefficient-variable patterns of stress
Physical	Relatively slow, waxing and waning head-neck, jaw, face, tongue, palate, pharyngeal, laryngeal, thoracic-abdominal movements Present at rest, during sustained postures and movement, but sometimes only during speech Improvement with "sensory tricks" Dysphagia
Patient complaints	Effortful speech, inability to "get speech out," involuntary orofacial movements "Tricks" that improve speech temporarily Chewing and swallowing problems (food "sticks" in throat)

AMR, alternating motion rate.

phonation reaction time. Intelligibility ratings were also reduced for the ST group, although the authors stated the overall impression "was that it was functional and intelligible, even if subtly different along some parameters" (p. 62). Focusing specifically on indices of vocal steadiness, Zraik and others (1993) found evidence of increased vocal jitter and shimmer and decreased harmonic-to-noise ratio during vowel prolongation in 24 speakers with ST who were compared to matched control speakers.

These effects seem predominantly laryngeal and articulatory in character, with possible secondary effects on prosody. In general, these acoustic findings suggest that the speech of some speakers with ST *may* be perceived as: *slowly initiated; reduced in maximum duration of utterances; re-*

duced in pitch and *pitch variability* (at least in females), *dysphonic,* and *reduced in rate.* These deficits, when present, are usually mild, and intelligibility is usually maintained. The exact manner in which ST affects speech movements or vocal tract configurations is unclear. The speech characteristics of the disorder deserve further study, however, as much to establish how speakers adapt so well to abnormal head/neck postures, as to understand the physiologic bases of the speech abnormalities that may occur. The primary speech and speech-related findings associated with ST are summarized in Table 8–8.

Palatopharyngolaryngeal myoclonus

Palatopharyngolaryngeal myoclonus (PM) is a rare disorder that is characterized by relatively abrupt rhythmic or semirhythmic unilateral or bilateral movements of the soft palate, pharyngeal walls, and laryngeal muscles. The lesion causing it has been localized to the area of the brain stem and cerebellum known as the Guillain-Mollaret triangle, encompassing the loop among the dentate nucleus, red nucleus, and inferior olive (the dentatorubroolivary tracts). Palatopharyngolaryngeal myoclonus is regarded by some as the prototypic hyperkinetic movement disorder that depends on a central pacemaker that generates myoclonic jerks that are time-locked in different muscles. The inferior olive is thought to be the pacemaker, and hypertrophic degeneration of it is a very common autopsy finding in people with the condition (Deuschl and others, 1990).

Palatopharyngolaryngeal myoclonus is usually caused by a brain stem or cerebellar vascular event, but tumor, encephalitis, multiple sclerosis, and other degenerative diseases affecting the same general areas have been reported as causes (Aronson, 1990; Deuschl and others, 1990). When caused by an acute lesion there may be a delay of several months-to-years before the PM emerges (Matsuo and Ajax, 1978).

Palatopharyngolaryngeal myoclonus can also be idiopathic. Deuschl and others (1990) found 27% of 287 cases with PM to have unknown etiologies. They referred to this condition as "essential rhythmic palatal myoclonus," similar to other benign extrapyramidal conditions of undetermined origin, such as essential tremor (which includes essential or organic voice tremor). Patients with this idiopathic condition had a much higher frequency of "earclicks" (see explanation below) and a slower rate of myoclonus (< 120 per minute) than patients with symptomatic PM (that is, PM with established etiology), were generally under 40 years of age at onset, and frequently also had myoclonus of the chin or perioral area.

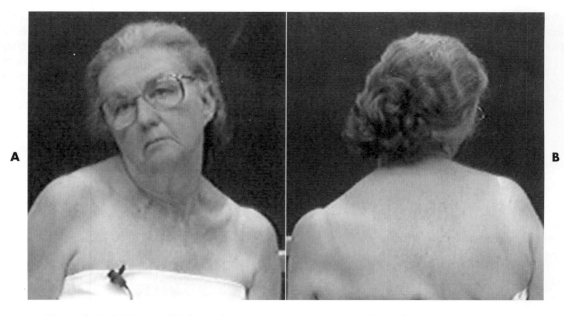

Figure 8–6 A, Front and **B,** back views of a woman with spasmodic torticollis attempting to sit in a normal resting posture. The neck rotation and head turning are sustained and involuntary.

Table 8–8 Primary distinguishing speech and speech-related findings in the hyperkinetic dysarthria of *spasmodic torticollis.*

Perceptual	
Phonation-respiration	Reduced pitch and pitch variability
	Dysphonia
Articulation-prosody	Reduced rate, delayed speech initiation, slow AMRs
Physical	Relatively sustained deviation of head to right or left, forward or back
	Sensory tricks reduce abnormal posturing
Patient complaints	Speech often reported as normal
	Complaints related to neck movement and pain
	Occasional dysphagia
	Aware of sensory tricks that reduce spasm temporarily

Nonspeech oral mechanism. Palatopharyngolaryngeal myoclonus is present at rest, during sustained postures and movement, and during sleep. In some cases, the eyeballs, diaphragm, tongue, lips, and jaw are also involved. The most common finding in PM is abrupt, rhythmic, beating-like elevation of the soft palate at a rate of 60 to 240 per minute. Pharyngeal contractions also may be apparent and, because of activity of the tensor veli palatini, may produce opening and closing of the eustachian tube with an associated clicking sound that sometimes can be heard by others (Aronson, 1990). Deuschl and others (1990) reported that these "earclicks" were a very frequent complaint in patients with idiopathic PM and were rare in symptomatic PM.

Myoclonic movements of the larynx can sometimes be seen on the external surface of the neck, and patients may complain of a clicking sensation in the larynx or a sensation of laryngeal spasm (Aronson, 1990). It is important to distinguish myoclonic movements in the external neck from carotid pulses, which are usually slower and do not visibly displace the laryngeal cartilages. Myoclonic movements of the lips and even the nares are sometimes present. Apparent lingual myoclonus may be seen, but lingual jerks may be secondary to laryngeal myoclonus.

Speech. The effects of PM on speech, even when it affects the jaw, lips, tongue, palate, pharynx, and larynx, are not very apparent under most circumstances and may not be detectable at all during conversational speech because they are so brief and relatively low in amplitude. If apparent during connected speech, it is perceived as a slow voice tremor and, less frequently, as *intermittent hypernasality* (Darley, Aronson, and Brown, 1975). However, the effects of PM can usually be heard during vowel prolongation as *momentary rhythmic arrests* or *tremorlike variations* at a rate that matches the rate of palatal myoclonus. Myoclonic variations can be distinguished from those of essential voice tremor by their slower frequency and the relatively abrupt character of each cycle (voice tremor has a slower, more sinusoidal, waxing and waning character). Rarely, a *clicking noise* is audible, reflecting eustachian tube opening. There may be occasional *prolonged silent intervals* or *inappropriate silences* if myoclonic vocal cord adduction occurs before inhalation at phrase boundaries is completed (Aronson, 1990). If the diaphragm is involved, there may be momentary interruptions in phonation due to interrupted air flow.

The hyperkinetic dysarthria of PM is probably rare as an isolated or "pure" speech disturbance. Except in cases of idiopathic PM, the disorder is usually accompanied by other signs of posterior fossa damage. As a result, PM probably most often occurs as one part of a speech disturbance that may include spastic, ataxic, flaccid, or unilateral upper motor neuron (UMN) dysarthria. Table 8–9 summarizes the primary speech and speech-related findings associated with PM.

Action myoclonus

The effect of action myoclonus on speech has received little attention, but it has been established that dysarthria can result from it (Aronson, O'Neill

Table 8–9 Primary distinguishing speech and speech-related findings in the hyperkinetic dysarthria of *palatopharyngolaryngeal myoclonus.*

Perceptual	
Phonation-respiration	Often no apparent abnormality. Momentary voice arrests during contextual speech when severe Voice arrests or myoclonic beats at 60 to 240 Hz during vowel prolongation
Resonance	Usually normal, but occasional intermittent hypernasality
Articulation-prosody	Usually normal, but brief silent intervals if myoclonus interrupts inhalation or initiation of exhalation, phonation, or articulation
Physical	Myoclonic movements of palate, pharynx, and larynx, and sometimes lips, nares, tongue, and respiratory muscles Laryngeal/pharyngeal myoclonus sometimes observable beneath neck surface
Patient complaints	Earclicks Patient often unaware of myoclonic movements and usually doesn't complain of speech difficulty

and Kelly, 1984). The character of action myoclonus is quite different from that of PM, and its effects can have a greater functional impact on speech than does PM.

Dysarthria is apparently common in patients with action myoclonus in nonspeech muscles. Fahn, Davis, and Rolland (1979), in a review of 59 cases, noted that at least 40% had dysarthria; it is unclear, however, whether the dysarthria was due to the action myoclonus or another co-occurring neuromuscular deficit.

Action myoclonus is distinguished from other myoclonic conditions because it is induced by muscle activity and is less generalized and rhythmic than other forms. In a classic description of four cases, Lance and Adams (1963) noted that "the essential clinical picture was that of an arhythmic fine or coarse jerking of a muscle or group of muscles in disorderly fashion, excited mainly by muscular activity when a conscious attempt at precision was required, worsened by emotional arousal, suppressed by barbiturates, and superimposed on a mild cerebellar ataxia" (p. 119). The jerks were typically < 200 msec in duration, and occurred singly or in series. Each patient had slow and "slightly slurred" speech.

Action myoclonus is often associated with cerebellar, basal ganglia, and pyramidal system involvement. Lance and Adams (1963) suggested that it may be a product of unrestrained synchronous or repetitive firing of thalamocortical neurons in the ventrolateral thalamus, the main relay nucleus from the cerebellum to the cortex. These abnormal discharges are then relayed in the cortex to the corticospinal and corticobulbar tracts where they result in action myoclonus. Abnormal thalamocortical activity may be explained by inadequate control from the pontine reticular formation, or by abnormally synchronous impulses through dentatothalamic pathways.

The most common etiology of action myoclonus is *anoxic encephalopathy* (in which the principle findings have been degeneration of cells and fibers in the globus pallidus, hippocampus, deep folia in the cerebellum, and the deep layers of the cerebral cortex, especially the parietal and occipital lobes (Lance and Adams, 1963). Multiple other causes also have been documented, including idiopathic and progressive myoclonic epilepsy, toxic-metabolic disturbances, infectious processes (for example, encephalitis), paraneoplastic cerebellar degeneration, stroke, and multiple sclerosis (Lance, 1986).

By definition, action myoclonus is not present at rest, and nonspeech oral mechanism examination may be entirely normal unless deficits in addition to the action myoclonus are present. Aronson, O'Neill, and Kelly (1984) have presented the only specific description of the dysarthria of action myoclonus. The disorder appears to have its primary perceptual effects on articulation (labial) and phonation. Their four cases were described as having stable orofacial muscles at rest, but quick, gross or fine jerky movements during attempts to speak. *"Repetitive fluctuation of phonation"* and *adductor voice arrests* that were synchronous with *myoclonic spasms of the lips* were characteristic. *Slow speech rate* was apparent in each case and the myoclonic movements *worsened with increased speech rate.* Slow rate could be compensatory, although the authors noted that, consistent with the general physiology of myoclonus, it could also reflect brief periods of inability to contract muscles following myoclonic jerks. These observations suggest that patients suspected of having the disorder should be asked to speak at slow, average, and rapid rates. Noticeable deterioration of voice quality or articulatory adequacy with increased rate, or the emergence of myoclonic facial movements with increased rate, would help confirm the diagnosis because other dysarthrias are generally not triggered by increases in rate (intelligibility may improve at slowed rates, but the underlying disordered movements are generally not altered). Speech AMRs may be particularly useful for making such observations. Table 8–10 summarizes the primary speech and speech-related findings associated with the hyperkinetic dysarthria of action myoclonus.

Table 8–10 Primary distinguishing speech and speech-related findings in the hyperkinetic dysarthria of *action myoclonus.*

Perceptual	
Phonation-respiration	Occasional adductor voice arrests
Articulation-prosody	Slow rate, decreased precision with increased rate Marked deterioration of AMR regularity with increased rate
Physical	Normal at rest unless other neuromuscular deficits present Quick, gross, or fine jerky movements of orofacial muscles during speech—especially lips—worsening with increased rate
Patient complaints	Awareness of imprecise speech and inability or reluctance to speak at normal or rapid rates

AMR, alternating motion rate.

Tics—Gilles de la Tourette's syndrome

Tics may occur as an isolated, nonspecific disorder, but Gilles de la *Tourette's syndrome* (TS) is the prototypic tic disorder. It is defined operationally in the *Diagnostic and Statistical Manual of Mental Disorders* (DSM-IIIR, 1987) as including: multiple motor tics; one or more vocal tics; onset before 21 years of age; and duration of more than one year. Although traditionally viewed as a severe and disabling condition, TS is now recognized as a clinically heterogeneous disorder with motor and behavioral features that vary along a severity continuum (Kurlan, 1989).

Tourette's syndrome, which affects mostly males (4:1 ratio) (Breakfield and Bressman, 1987), may be accompanied by a number of behavioral disorders. About 50% have obsessive-compulsive disorders or attention deficit hyperactivity disorder. Stuttering, dyslexia, conduct disorder, panic attacks, multiple phobias, depression, and mania are reportedly much more common in TS than in control subjects (Comings, 1987), although an etiologic association between TS and those problems has not been established (Kurlan, 1989).

It is now generally accepted that most cases of TS are genetically determined. Kurlan (1989), in his summary of current concepts of the disorder, indicates that TS occasionally has been linked to chronic neuroleptic exposure, carbon monoxide poisoning, head trauma, and viral encephalitis.

Tics are brief involuntary movements or sounds that occur over a background of normal motor activity (Kurlan, 1989). When simple, they are brief and isolated (for example, eyeblink, head twitch, facial grimace). When complex, they may consist of coordinated movements that seem purposeful (for example, touching, jumping, or obscene gestures). Some patients experience "sensory tics" that are somatic sensations, such as pressure, tickling, and temperature changes, that may lead to movements intended to relieve the sensation, such as tightening or stretching of muscles (Kurlan, 1989). Tics are often bizarre-appearing and are frequently misinterpreted as signs of psychiatric disease.

In addition to motor tics and behavioral disorders, TS is characterized by *vocal tics* that may be isolated or embedded within voluntary verbal utterances. Vocal tics are unique because they represent the only dysarthria in which *specific* sounds or spoken words represent the disorder.

Simple vocal tics include noises and sounds that are made repetitively, and sometimes can be suppressed temporarily. The most common of these are *throat clearing* and *grunting,* followed in nonexhaustive descending order by *yelling-screaming, sniffing, barking, snorting, coughing, spitting, squeaking,* and *humming* (Comings,

1990). These sounds are usually executed rapidly, and some of them may reflect a response to a sensation in the larynx or throat (Kurlan, 1989). More complex vocal tics may include *echolalia* (repetition of other's utterances), *palilalia* (discussed in Chapter 7), and *coprolalia.*

Coprolalia (copro = feces; lalia = lips), or involuntary, compulsive, repetitive, almost ritualistic swearing is one of the most dramatic, although not universally present, features of TS (the words "fuck," "shit," and "piss" are the most common scatalogical utterances, according to Comings, 1990). The words are often said softly or incompletely and are sometimes accompanied by throat clearing or other noises, possibly reflecting a partially successful attempt to suppress or mask them. They may emerge independent of any volitional verbal expression, or at the start of or within volitional utterances. They sometimes may appear socially acceptable or even humorous, but the social and psychological consequences for the patient are often tragic. Why coprolalia occurs is not entirely clear, but the reason may lie in explanations of TS as a disorder of disinhibition (Comings, 1990), possibly secondary to striatal dopamine receptor supersensitivity, which is the current prevailing neurobiologic explanation

Table 8–11 Primary distinguishing speech and speech-related findings in the hyperkinetic dysarthria of *Gilles de la Tourette syndrome.*

Perceptual	
Phonation-respiration	Coughing, grunting, throat clearing, screaming, moaning, etc.
Resonance	Sniffing
Articulation-prosody	Humming, whistling, lip smacking, echolalia, palilalia, coprolalia
Physical	Multiple motor tics (for example, eyeblinks, head twitch, facial grimacing, jumping, touching, obscene gestures)
Patient complaints	Awareness of vocal and motor tics, compulsion to perform them, and inability to inhibit them for sustained periods Behavioral and psychiatric disorders may be present (for example, obsessive-compulsive, phobias, hyperactivity and attention deficit disorder, learning disability)

for tics (Kurlan, 1989).

The primary speech and speech-related characteristics of TS are summarized in Table 8–11.

Organic voice tremor

Organic or essential voice tremor is often viewed as a disorder separate from other motor speech disorders. However, it occurs in about 20% of patients with essential tremor (Jankovic, 1990) and can be classified as a hyperkinetic dysarthria of tremor.*

Essential tremor is the most common of the movement disorders and is considered a benign, autosomal dominant condition with variable penetrance (Findley and Koller, 1987; Jankovic, 1986). About 50% of cases are familial, and most of the remaining cases are idiopathic (essential). It can begin at any age, but average age of onset is in the fifth decade. Although generally benign, a focal presentation of the disorder (such as voice tremor) sometimes spreads to include other body parts (Koller, 1984). It is sometimes a precursor to, or associated with, other movement disorders such as focal dystonias, dystonia musculorum deformans, and spasmodic torticollis (Findley and Koller, 1987).

The localization of essential voice tremor (and essential tremor in general) is unknown, but it is probably related to a CNS oscillatory abnormality. Rhythmic neuronal firing has been recorded in the ventrolateral thalamus in patients with essential tremor, and essential tremor in the limbs (but generally not the voice) can be abolished by ventrolateral thalamotomy. Abnormalities have been reported in the caudate nucleus and putamen, brain stem, and cerebellum (Aronson, 1990). These observations suggest that the oscillation may be generated by activity in the cerebellorubrothalamocortical circuit (Findley and Koller, 1987).[†]

The onset of organic voice tremor can be gradual or sudden, but is acute in a minority of cases (Brown and Simonson, 1963). When mild, patients may not be aware of its presence. Those

---

*Essential tremor can affect the tongue, sometimes in isolation, but essential lingual tremor is probably rare in comparison to essential voice tremor. Patients with lingual tremor are usually unaware of it. It occurs at a rate of 4 to 8 Hz, is generally apparent on protrusion but not at rest, and is often alcohol-responsive (Biary and Koller, 1987). Its effects on speech are unclear.

[†]Patients with cerebellar disease sometimes have voice tremor. The tremor frequency is in the range of 3 Hz, similar in frequency to other forms of cerebellar postural tremor (Ackerman and Ziegler, 1991). This is lower than that of essential voice tremor and usually occurs with an ataxic dysarthria. Although its frequency is in the general range of palatolaryngeal myoclonus, it can occur without evidence of myoclonic movements.

who are aware often note that it worsens with fatigue and psychologic stress and that it often improves with alcohol intake; although not all patients with essential tremor respond positively to alcohol, other forms of tremor usually do not, so the presence of an alcohol effect is helpful to differential diagnosis. Organic voice tremor can occur as an isolated problem, but is often accompanied by head or extremity tremor (Aronson and Hartman, 1981; Brown and Simonson, 1963). When monosymptomatic, it is frequently misdiagnosed as a psychogenic disorder (Aronson, 1990).

Oral mechanism. Lingual tremor may be apparent at rest or on protrusion in patients with organic voice tremor. When present during phonation, it may represent genuine lingual tremor or be secondary to vertical oscillations of the larynx. Tremorous movements of the jaw and lips are often apparent at rest, during sustained postures, and during vowel prolongation. Palatal and pharyngeal tremor are often obvious during sustained "ah," synchronous with the perceived voice tremor. Fiberscopic observation of the larynx may reveal rhythmic vertical laryngeal movements, and adductor and abductor oscillation of the vocal folds, synchronous with the perceived voice tremor (Aronson, 1990; Tomoda and others, 1987). Vertical oscillations of the larynx also can often be seen on the external neck during vowel prolongation. Tomoda and others (1987) recorded EMG evidence of tremor in the cricothyroid muscle and expiratory muscles (rectus abdominus) in three patients with organic voice tremor, synchronous with voice tremor. They suggested that voice tremor may be an action tremor of voluntary expiratory muscles that affect phonatory function. Although respiratory tremor should be considered a possible source of voice tremor, it is probably not a primary factor in most cases of organic voice tremor.

Speech. Aronson (1990) describes three effects of essential tremor on voice: (1) a "typical" organic voice tremor when the adductor and abductor vocal cord tremor components are relatively equal, (2) an adductor spastic dysphonia when the adductor component is predominant, and (3) an abductor spastic dysphonia when the abductor component is predominant. Only the typical voice tremor will be addressed here (spasmodic dysphonias will be discussed in the following section).

Voice tremor may not be apparent during contextual speech, especially when mild, which may be why some patients are unaware of it. It is *most easily perceived during vowel prolongation.* To rule out a respiratory contribution to the voice tremor, it is often useful to have the patient prolong /s/ and /z/. If a respiratory tremor is present, rhythmic fluctuations in the quality of both sounds should be apparent; if the /s/ is steady, and the /z/ or vowel contains tremor, a prominent respiratory contribution to the voice tremor is probably not present.

Organic voice tremor most often occurs at a *frequency of 4 to 7 Hz,* most often in the 5 to 6 Hz range with a tendency for tremor frequency to be slower with increasing age (Aronson and Hartman, 1981; Brown and Simonson, 1963). The tremor has a *sinusoidal, quavering,* or *rhythmic waxing and waning character* during vowel prolongation, presumably due to rhythmic alterations in pitch or loudness (Figure 8–7). When severe, there may be *abrupt, staccato voice arrests* that, in most cases, are rhythmic (Aronson, Brown, Litin, and Pearson, 1968). The tremor may, however, lose its rhythmic character when voice arrests are present, possibly because of the person's efforts to avoid or otherwise compensate for them; in such cases, having them prolong a vowel at a higher pitch may abort the arrests and allow the tremor to be heard more easily. Patients with marked-to-severe organic voice tremor may have a *reduced speech rate* secondary to phonatory interruptions; speech rate may also be reduced secondary to jaw, lip, and tongue tremor. The primary speech and speech-related characteristics associated with organic voice tremor are summarized in Table 8–12.

Spasmodic dysphonia (spastic dysphonia)

Spasmodic dysphonia (SD), or spastic dysphonia, designates a group of isolated or relatively isolated voice disorders that are characterized by strained or breathy voice qualities resulting from adductor or abductor laryngospasm. They can have several causes.

Concepts of the disorder have an interesting history. For a number of years SD was thought to be a manifestation of psychopathology, usually stemming from psychologic trauma, stress, or anxiety. Neurologic etiologies were rarely considered. Today, the etiologic pendulum has swung to a point where many investigators and clinicians assume that the disorder is always neurogenic, with only lesion loci and the specific neurophysiologic nature of the disorder in question. Along with this trend has come a shift from use of the term "spastic" to the term "spasmodic" to characterize the dysphonia. This latter trend is probably useful. Although the term "spastic" describes the strained character of the adductor form of the disorder, it does not appear that spasticity (in the physiologic sense) is responsible for most cases of SD. The term "spasmodic" retains some descriptive power and at the same time suggests that spasm (or dystonia) is the basis for at least some

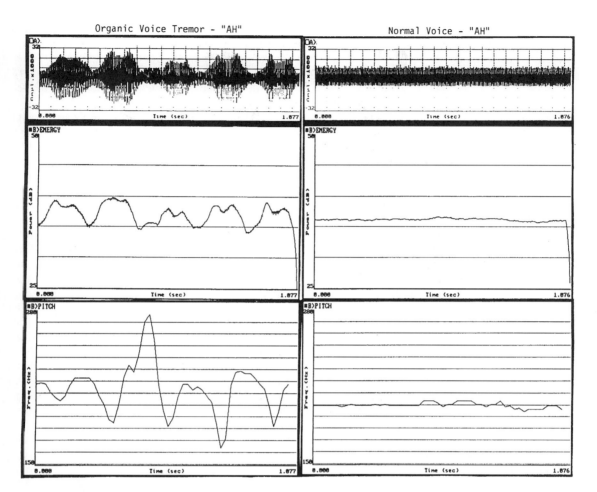

Figure 8–7 Raw acoustic waveform, energy, and pitch contours for a ~1 second prolongation of /a/ by a female speaker (see *Case 8.5* for full clinical description) with a ~5 Hz organic voice tremor (*left side*) and a normal female speaker (*right side*). The fairly regular tremor is apparent in all tracings and stands in marked contrast to the steady maintenance of the same parameters by the normal speaker.

forms of the disorder. From the practical standpoint, however, the labels spastic dysphonia and spasmodic dysphonia can be considered synonymous.

Aronson (1990) has argued that a diagnosis of SD should be modified to specify likely etiology. There are three broad etiologic possibilities: *neurogenic, psychogenic,* and *idiopathic.* This recognizes that SD can have at least two etiologies—neurogenic and psychogenic—and that etiology sometimes cannot be specified with any degree of confidence (hence, is idiopathic). It is important to recognize that psychogenic and neurogenic SD often cannot be distinguished on the basis of auditory perceptual characteristics; the distinction is often made on the basis of history and other examination findings. Evidence that SD can have a psychogenic etiology will be discussed in Chapter 14. Here we will address only neurogenic varieties of SD, which justifiably can be included among the hyperkinetic dysarthrias.

It is also important to establish if SD is *adductor, abductor,* or *mixed* in form. *Ad*ductor SD, the much more common variety, is characterized by adductor laryngospasms that give the voice a strained, tight character. *Ab*ductor SD is characterized by abductor laryngospasms that give it an intermittent breathy or aphonic character. And, some patients have a combination of the two, with both intermittent strained and breathy qualities. There is no evidence that these symptomatic types vary in distribution as a function of neurogenic versus psychogenic etiology. Cannito and Johnson (1981) have suggested that adductor and abductor SD occur on a continuum and are not really separate disorders (they may, however, be managed differently).

Ignoring possible etiologic differences, SD has an average age of onset of about 45 to 50 years, but it can develop anywhere from the third to

Table 8–12 Primary distinguishing speech and speech-related findings in the hyperkinetic dysarthria of *organic voice tremor.*

Perceptual	
Phonation-respiration	Quavering, rhythmic, waxing and waning tremor, most evident on vowel prolongation, at a rate of approx. 4 to 7 Hz. Voice arrests may occur in severe forms but may disappear if pitch is raised.
Articulation	Usually normal, but rate may be slowed
Prosody	Normal pitch and loudness variability may be restricted or altered by the voice tremor
Physical	Rhythmic, vertical laryngeal movements and adductor and abductor oscillations of the vocal cords synchronous with voice tremor. Tremor of jaw, lips, tongue, and palate/pharynx may be present, especially during phonation. Lingual and jaw tremor may be secondary to laryngeal tremor
Patient complaints	Shaky or jerky voice Worse with fatigue or anxiety Improves with alcohol Frequent family history of tremor

eighth decades. Male:female ratio ranges from 1:1 to 1:4. It may develop suddenly, but usually begins insidiously, taking about a year to develop into its full-blown state. Remissions are rare when the cause is neurologic (Aronson, 1990; Izdebski, Dedo, and Boles 1984). It is not unusual for the disorder to begin during a flulike illness, or during a period of acute or chronic psychologic stress (Aronson, 1990); this may be the case even when SD is clearly neurogenic in origin.

A number of factors influence SD, and wide intraindividual fluctuations are often noted. Emotional stress, anxiety, depression, and sometimes physical exertion can make symptoms worse; voice may also worsen when the person concentrates on speech. These effects are superficially suggestive of psychogenic etiology, but it should be noted that many of them are active in people with unambiguous neurogenic movement disorders and are common complaints in many patients with dysarthrias. In contrast to most other dysar-

thria types, however, voice in SD may be normal during singing or laughter and under conditions of surprise or quickly emitted "automatic" utterances. In general, the movement disorder underlying neurogenic SD is *action-induced,* the triggering action being volitional speech.

Tremor and dystonia have a strong association with SD. This suggests that SD is related to extrapyramidal system dysfunction in the broad sense, more specifically to dysfunction in the basal ganglia or cerebellar control circuits. Spastic dysphonia may be an isolated, focal manifestation of tremor or dystonia, or may coexist with more full-blown manifestations of them.

The theory that tremor or dystonia can be focal to the larynx receives support from other focal manifestations of tremor and dystonia, and the fact that the basal ganglia seem to have a somatotopic organization. Jankovic (1990) notes that the somatotopic organization of the basal ganglia plays an important role in the muscular distribution of hyperkinesias and the preferential involvement of head and orofacial structures in them.

In an extensive review of evidence for the neurologic underpinnings of SD, Cannito (1991) concluded that SD probably results from an impairment of the volitional motor system, rather than the limbic or lower brainstem centers for vocal control. He based this conclusion on evidence from several studies of: a relatively high incidence of extrapyramidal and pyramidal motor signs in patients with SD; neuroimaging evidence for such lesions (Finitzo and Freeman, 1989)*; the tendency for the disorder's manifestations to be greater for complex than simple verbal activities; and a strong association between SD voice and speech characteristics and those found in spastic dysarthria and the hyperkinetic dysarthrias of dystonia and chorea. He tied these data to models of hyperkinesias that implicate cortical premotor-striatal-pallidal-thalamic control circuits that are normally involved in the control of complex, voluntary sequential movements.

Spastic dysphonia of essential voice tremor presumably occurs when: the adductor component of the tremor predominates and causes adductor laryngospasms and squeezing of the glottis (adductor SD of essential voice tremor); when the abductor component of the tremor predominates and causes abductor laryngospasm and widening of the glottis (abductor SD of essential voice

---

*The interested reader is referred to the work of Finitzo and Freeman (1989) and an exchange of letters between Aronson and Lagerlund (1991) and Finitzo and others (1991) for a comprehensive and critical overview of approaches to establishing the neurologic locus of SD, and the methodologic and interpretive challenges and controversies faced by such efforts.

tremor); or when the tremor amplitude is relatively balanced in adductor and abductor muscles but sufficient to cause both abductor and adductor laryngospasm (mixed adductor and abductor SD of essential voice tremor). Therefore, there appears to be a continuum within which a diagnosis of essential voice tremor can "spill over" into a diagnosis of SD. The continuum seems to include severity as well as the balance of muscle forces involved in adductor and abductor laryngeal activity. In addition to perceptual evidence, a link between SD and essential tremor comes from evidence of nonlaryngeal tremor in patients with SD. For example, about one-third of patients with SD have evidence of essential tremor elsewhere (Jankovic, 1990). Aronson and Hartman (1981) found a similar tremor frequency between patients with essential voice tremor and patients with SD and voice tremor, and their SD patients had a high incidence of tremor elsewhere in the body.

Spastic dysphonia can also be a manifestation of a focal laryngeal dystonia, a logical possibility given the well-established fact that dystonias can be focal to other muscle groups (for example, blepharospasm, oromandibular, torticollis). The association of SD with dystonia is also established by its co-occurrence with Meige's syndrome (Marsden and Sheehy, 1982) and the occurrence of laryngospasm in patients with focal cranial dystonia (Golper and others, 1983) and spasmodic torticollis (Aronson, 1990).

Nonspeech oral mechanism. Spastic dysphonia patients may have normal oral mechanism examinations. If associated with generalized or other orofacial tremor or dystonia, Meige's syndrome, or spasmodic torticollis, manifestations of those problems will be apparent. Sometimes, soft neurologic signs such as facial or palatal asymmetry, mild weakness, and pathologic oral reflexes are present. None of these findings seem directly relevant to the SD, however, and it should be kept in mind that because SD is an *action-induced* disorder, the only evidence for it may be found during voluntary speech.

Speech (adductor SD). The primary perceptual feature of adductor SD is a *strained, jerky, grunting, squeezed, groaning,* and *effortful* voice quality. When mild, there may be no more than a mild *strained quality.* These qualities can be *intermittent or relatively continuous.* Silent articulatory *movements* or *sound repetitions,* presumably as a result of unanticipated laryngospasms, may be present. When tremor underlies adductor SD, there may be a *staccato quality* or an obvious *tremor or rhythmic character* to the laryngospasms. This is heard most easily during vowel prolongation; when voice arrests are prominent, having the patient phonate at a higher pitch may attenuate the

arrests and permit perception of the tremor. There may be associated head, jaw, lip, tongue, palatal, pharynx, and thoracic tremor during vowel prolongation. When dystonia underlies the laryngospasm, the spasmodic voice may be continuous or arrests may be unpredictable. Speech *rate may be slow* (Merson and Ginsberg, 1979). Although slowed rate may be secondary to laryngospasm, Cannito, Kondraske, and Johns (1991) found evidence of slowed SMRs, even when they were whispered, suggesting possible involvement of supralaryngeal muscles. The possibility of supralaryngeal involvement is also raised by Cannito's (1989) finding of reduced second formant steadiness during vowel prolongation when laryngeal activity was presumably eliminated by the use of an electrolarynx to produce voice.

Videofluoroscopy and videofiberoptic laryngoscopy of the larynx during speech may reveal rhythmic, arrhythmic, or relatively sustained adductor spasms of the true vocal folds and arytenoids, but as severity increases spasm of the false cords and even the inferior pharyngeal constrictor muscles may be observed (Finitzo and Freeman, 1989; McCall, Skolnick, and Brewer, 1971; Parnes, Lavarato, and Myers, 1979). In some cases, the entire larynx may move upward, implicating spasmodic activity in the extrinsic laryngeal muscles as well. High amplitude muscle burst activity in the 6 to 7 Hz range, synchronous with fluctuations in the speech waveforem, have been observed in the thyroarytenoid and levator palatini muscles (Finitzo and Freeman, 1989; Watson and others, 1991). Jerky and dysrhythmic movements of the thorax and abdomen may be apparent during speech, synchronous with strained voice and voice arrests; these are probably a secondary effect of uncontrolled glottic closure. When severe, there may be facial grimacing, associated neck contractions, and movements of the shoulder girdle and upper arms. The overall picture may be one of extreme physical effort during speech; this may be one of the primary complaints of patients with the disorder, sometimes exceeding their dissatisfaction with the voice itself.

Spectrographic analyses have also documented a breakdown in formant structure, abnormal intensity fluctuations, and widely spaced vertical striations at irregular intervals (reflecting reduced fundamental frequency and aperiodicity of phonation), interruptions in articulation, separation of sounds in syllables, and delayed onset of phonation in vowels (Wolfe and Bacon, 1976; Ludlow and Connor, 1987). A tendency toward reduced fundamental frequency and loudness has also been documented (Ludlow and Connor, 1987). These acoustic attributes are generally consistent with and further refine perceptual descriptions of the disorder.

Speech (abductor SD). In abductor SD, voice is interrupted by brief inappropriate *breathy or aphonic segments* that are most easily triggered by unvoiced consonants in the beginning of an utterance or syllable. During these segments *air flow increases.* There is evidence that *speech rate may be slowed* (Merson and Ginsberg, 1979). Spectrographic analysis has revealed increased aspiration time for initial stops, a loss of energy in the higher formants, and intensity fluctuations (Wolfe and Bacon, 1976). Direct observation of the larynx may show abduction of the vocal folds during phonation, resulting in a wide glottal chink; these coincide with breathy releases. If tremor is present, abductor movements may be rhythmic. Electromyography has identified increased activity in the thyroarytenoid and posterior cricoarytenoid muscles in speakers with this form of SD (Watson and others, 1991). There is a breakdown of formant structure or superimposed noise on vertical striations in spectrograms of speakers with abductor SD (Wolfe and Bacon, 1976). The primary speech and speech-related findings associated with SD are summarized in Table 8–13.

CASES

Case 8.1

A 73-year-old man presented with a five-month history of "hesitation" in speech, which had initially worsened for a few months and then plateaued. There was no dysphagia and no changes in mental status. He had never taken phenothiazines. Neurologic examination was normal with the exception of abnormal orofacial movements. Computed tomography scan and electroencephalogram (EEG) were normal. Routine laboratory studies and screening for heavy metal poisoning were within normal limits.

During speech examination, the patient complained of halting and slurred speech as well as involuntary mouth movements. Examination revealed tremor of the lips at rest and on lip rounding, and semirhythmic movement of the tongue at rest. A regular voice tremor was present during vowel prolongation. Contextual speech was interrupted by relatively rapid chewing and smacking and rounding movements of the lips. They were noticeably reduced if the patient spoke while biting on a tongue depressor or with some pressure at the angle of the mouth.

The clinician concluded that the patient had a "hyperkinetic dysarthria associated with orofacial dyskinesia with an accompanying tremor component."

The patient was advised to speak while holding a pipestem in his mouth and biting down, and he was given some practice at doing it. The neurologist recommended a trial of Inderal for the movement disorder. Several weeks later, the patient wrote to indicate that the Inderal had significantly reduced, but not eliminated, his facial grimacing. He also noted that "a pipe held between my teeth is definitely effective, and socially acceptable."

Table 8–13 Primary distinguishing speech and speech-related findings in the hyperkinetic dysarthria of *spasmodic dysphonia.*

Perceptual *Phonation-respiration*	*Adductor:* Continuous or intermittent strained, jerky, squeezed, effortful quality, with voice arrests when severe. If tremor-based, voice tremor may be apparent, especially during vowel prolongation at higher pitches
	Abductor: Brief, breathy, or aphonic segments, most obvious at beginning of utterances or in voiceless consonant environments
Resonance	*Adductor:* Usually normal
	Abductor: Usually normal, but occasional intermittent hypernasality and nasal emission
Articulation-prosody	*Adductor:* Inappropriate silences, silent articulatory movements, and sound repetitions, especially when voice, are prominent. Contextual speech and AMRs may be slowed secondary to laryngospasms
	Abductor: Phrases may be short due to air wastage through glottis during abductor spasms.
Physical	Nonlaryngeal muscles are usually normal, unless tremor or dystonia is present elsewhere (for example, head/limb tremor, orofacial dyskinesia, torticollis)
	Rhythmic or arrhythmic spasms of true cords and arytenoids, and sometimes false cords and pharyngeal constrictors, usually only during speech
	Jerky and arrhythmic thoracic/abdominal movements, usually secondary to adductor laryngospasm
	Facial grimacing and neck/shoulder movements secondary to severe adductor laryngospasms
Patient complaints	*Adductor:* Tight, strained voice
	Abductor: Intermittent, weak, breathy, aphonic voice
	Adductor and abductor: Increased physical effort and fatigue associated with speaking. Occupational, social, and emotional impact may be significant. Voice may improve with alcohol when tremor-based.

Commentary. (1) Orofacial dyskinesias/focal mouth dystonias often develop without a clear etiologic explanation. They can be present in the absence of any other neurologic symptoms and in the absence of abnormalities on neuroimaging studies. (2) Orofacial dyskinesias can affect speech. (3) Sensory tricks, such as biting down or exerting some pressure on the cheek, are often effective (temporarily) in relieving abnormal movements and improving speech.

Case 8.2

A 53-year-old man presented to neurology with an 18-month history of speech difficulty and a right upper and lower limb movement disorder. The course was one of gradual onset and progression. A question had been raised about manganese intoxication, possibly secondary to exposure when welding, or from materials used in refinishing a boat.

Neurologic evaluation revealed the presence of torsion dystonia of the right foot during walking and right upper extremity cogwheel rigidity. A jaw opening dystonia during speech was also apparent. He was referred for speech evaluation.

The patient was aware of abnormal jaw movements during speech but was unaware of difficulty at other times, including during chewing and swallowing. His speech tended to worsen when he was anxious or excited, and with alcohol consumption. Speech was better in the morning, following relaxation exercises, and when writing or drawing while speaking; he felt this latter activity distracted his attention from speech.

Oral mechanism examination at rest and during nonspeech sustained postures was normal. During speech he had intermittent marked jaw opening and tongue retraction. Superficially, these movements were random but careful analysis established that they were strongly associated with the occurrence of open vowels and velar consonants (that is, sounds requiring jaw opening or back of tongue elevation). Speech improved somewhat during whispering and noticeably when he clenched his jaw during speaking. It improved moderately when he wrote while talking. His jaw opening dystonia was often sufficient to arrest speech, with continuation possible only after the dystonic interval passed.

Magnetic resonance imaging (MRI) and single photon emission computed tomography (SPECT) scans were normal. Additional laboratory and radiologic studies were negative. An electromyogram revealed normal blink and facial nerve conduction and a normal masseter-inhibiting reflex. There was no evidence of abnormal activity in the lateral pterygoid muscles and digastric muscles at rest or during chewing and drinking, but tonic spasms of 500 to 3,000 milliseconds were seen in those muscles during speech.

It was concluded that the patient had a progressive extrapyramidal disorder of unclear etiology. It was recommended that he avoid welding, painting, and other heavy metal exposure. Sinemet was prescribed. There was some improvement in the patient's limb symptoms but no change in speech. Subsequent examination of the paint and several metals to which the patient had been exposed failed to provide convincing evidence that his disorder was due to heavy metal intoxication.

Commentary. (1) Dystonia affecting speech can be specific to small groups of muscles (jaw and tongue in this case) and, in fact, may be present only during speech. In some cases, focal, speech-induced dystonias can be relatively phoneme-specific; in this case they were triggered by open vowels and back of tongue elevation. (2) Focal speech-induced dystonias sometimes improve with altered postures and distraction and are generally better under conditions of relaxation. The worsening of dystonia or speech difficulty under conditions of anxiety do not establish anxiety as a cause of the dysarthria. (3) Perhaps more frequently than any other dysarthria type, the cause of hyperkinetic dysarthria may be indeterminate.

Case 8.3

A 49-year-old woman presented to neurology with a one-year history of ataxia and movement difficulties, including speech. Her problems had begun suddenly with a severe headache and "drunken" speech. Within days she noticed some twitching of the right facial muscles and shaking and twitching in her hands. Medical workup shortly after onset suggested a diagnosis of myoclonic epilepsy of cortical origin.

During speech examination she complained of slurred speech. She noted a feeling of "tightness" in her face and neck intermittently when speaking. Oral mechanism examination was normal at rest. Myoclonic or tremor-like movements of the tongue were obvious during protrusion and lateral movements. There was no obvious palatal or pharyngeal myoclonus. Jaw and perioral myoclonus were more apparent during sustained phonation than when her mouth was open without phonation. Traces of nasal emission were apparent during pressure sound production. Some dystonic-like perioral movements were also apparent during speech. Her speech was characterized by reduced rate (3), and imprecise articulation (3), with difficulty achieving bilabial closure during connected speech, apparently secondary to dystonic lip contractions. Voice quality was strained-hoarse (2,3) with monopitch and monoloudness (3). Prosody was characterized by excess and equal syllabic stress. Prolonged "ah" was unsteady (2). Speech AMRs were regular when produced at a rate of l per second but markedly irregular when she attempted to maximize rate. Intelligibility was reduced.

The clinician concluded that the patient had a "hyperkinetic dysarthria of action myoclonus. In addition, there appear to be some dystonic perioral movements during speech that make it difficult for her to achieve bilabial closure. Speech clearly worsens during attempts to increase speech rate and she has consciously reduced her rate because of this." Some suspicion was raised about accompanying ataxic and spastic components to her dysarthria, although it was felt that her scanning prosody and strained voice could well be secondary to efforts at compensation for her hyperkinetic dysarthria.

Neurologic evaluation indicated the presence of ataxia in the limbs, hyperreflexia, and action-induced myoclonus of the trunk, extremities, and face.

A complete work-up confirmed a diagnosis of myoclonic epilepsy of cortical origin. Etiology was unclear;

there was no evidence for a hereditary basis. An undiagnosed viral illness was felt to be the most likely cause.

Commentary. (1) Some movement disorders may be speech specific. (2) Action myoclonus can cause dysarthria, one whose manifestations are noticeably exacerbated by increased speaking rate. In some cases, the myoclonus is associated with dystoniclike movements.

Case 8.4

A 35-year-old woman presented to neurology with a two-year history of gradual mental deterioration, handwriting difficulty, reduced ability to concentrate, and reduced personal hygiene. She complained of speech difficulty, stating, "Nobody can understand me." There was a family history of Huntington's disease, most convincingly present in the patient's father, who died at age 45. Neurologic evaluation identified difficulty with balance and the presence of involuntary movements, generalized motor impersistence, mild cogwheel rigidity, and probable dementia. Neuropsychological assessment confirmed the presence of significant cognitive/memory limitations.

Magnetic resonance imaging showed an abnormality in the right putamen that could have represented iron deposition that is sometimes seen in Huntington's disease. Mild generalized atrophy was also present.

During speech examination, rapid, unsustained, choreiclike movements of the lower face, jaw, and tongue were present at rest. Involuntary tongue clicking was noted. She had difficulty maintaining a protruded tongue, open mouth, and lip retraction, as much because of motor impersistence as involuntary movements. Speech was characterized by: accelerated rate (1,2); imprecise articulation with irregular articulatory breakdowns (1,2); dysprosody (2); variable rate (1,2). Choreiform movements tended to delay the initiation of speech or delay continuation of speech at phrase boundaries. Vowel prolongation was characterized by a low amplitude tremor. Speech AMRs were irregular (1,2). Pitch and loudness variability were reduced, but they occasionally varied inappropriately.

The clinician concluded, "hyperkinetic dysarthria associated with dyskinetic/choreiform movements of the lower face, jaw, and tongue. Her tendency toward accelerated rate and monopitch and monoloudness raise the possibility of an accompanying hypokinetic component, although it is possible that those characteristics are secondary to efforts to 'race through' speech before the next occurrence of orofacial involuntary movements." The clinician also noted that, although there was no evidence of aphasia, the patient appeared to be impaired cognitively, and often responded impulsively. She was seen for one session of speech therapy during which she demonstrated an ability to slow her rate and improve articulatory precision. She was unable to do this without constant reminders, however.

The family was counseled about the best strategy to use when they were unable to understand the patient; this focused primarily on cueing her to reduce speech rate.

Commentary. (1) Hyperkinetic dysarthria and orofacial choreiform movements may be among the presenting signs of Huntington's chorea. (2) Cognitive deficits and personality changes often accompany the hyperkinetic dysarthria of Huntington's chorea. (3) People with chorea affecting speech will sometimes accelerate rate in order to complete a statement before the next involuntary movement. This may give the appearance of an accompanying hypokinetic component to their dysarthria; the distinction between hypokinetic dysarthria and such compensatory efforts can be difficult to make in such cases.

Case 8.5

A 70-year-old woman presented to Ear, Nose, and Throat with a one-year history of voice difficulty. She denied chewing or swallowing difficulty. She had never smoked and did not have a history of alcohol abuse. Ear, Nose, and Throat examination was normal. She was referred for speech evaluation.

During speech assessment, the patient reported a one-year history of gradually developing voice difficulty that she described as "a quiver." This worsened under conditions of stress and fatigue. She denied other speech difficulties and difficulties with chewing and swallowing. She felt self-conscious about her voice and it occasionally made her reluctant to speak. She reported that her father had "parkinsonism" and that her 71-year-old brother had some "shaking in his hands."

Oral mechanism exam was normal in size, strength, and symmetry. There was a subtle low amplitude tremor of her lips at rest, and tremor of her jaw, tongue, palate and pharynx were quite apparent during vowel prolongation. Articulation and resonance were normal. During conversation, a voice tremor with occasional voice interruptions was apparent. The tremor was particularly apparent during vowel prolongation. There was no evidence of respiratory tremor during prolonged voiceless fricatives or prolonged audible exhalations.

The clinician concluded, "Organic voice tremor with tremor frequency in the 5 to 8 Hz range. No other speech-language abnormalities detected. There are no other deviant speech characteristics to suggest the presence of hypokinetic dysarthria which might reflect early Parkinson's disease." This impression was discussed with the patient who was relieved to have a diagnosis. She expressed concern, however, that her voice difficulty might reflect Parkinson's disease. She was referred for neurologic assessment to rule out Parkinson's disease. Neurologic examination was normal, with the exception of her voice tremor. There was no evidence of parkinsonism. Propranolol was prescribed in an effort to reduce the voice tremor, but was ineffective.

Commentary. (1) Voice tremor can be an isolated manifestation of a hyperkinetic dysarthria. (2) Laryngeal tremor may not be apparent (or may be missed) during laryngeal examination, and correct diagnosis is often made solely on the basis of perception of voice tremor. (3) Organic voice tremor can occur in the absence of other neurologic signs. (4) In addition to voice tremor's effect on communication ability, it often raises concerns in the patient about more serious neurologic disease. In this case, the patient could be reassured that her condition was probably benign. The speech pathologist's impression was confirmed during neurologic evaluation. (5) In some cases, the most effective management of a speech problem is correct diagnosis. This patient expressed relief about her diagnosis and a relative lack of concern about the minor difficulties her voice problem was causing her in some social situations.

Case 8.6

A 73-year-old woman presented to neurology with a 10-year history of voice difficulty that was present upon awakening one day, without obvious explanation. The problem worsened, but had been stable for three to four years. She had had several periods of speech therapy, without benefit. Neurologic evaluation identified the presence of a head tremor, postural upper extremity tremor, and "spastic speech." A cause for these abnormal movements was not identified during a complete neurologic work-up.

During speech examination, the patient associated onset of her voice problem with a period of considerable psychological stress (her adopted son was having difficulty with drugs and was in the process of attempting to locate his biologic parents). She also noted that her voice worsened when she was anxious or spoke in group situations. She noted mild improvement in her voice when she had a glass of wine.

Her voice was characterized by a tremor that consistently interrupted her voice and mildly slowed speech rate. Prolonged "ah" contained consistent, somewhat irregular and strained voice interruptions. At higher pitches, voice interruptions disappeared and a tremor became apparent. Tremor was not apparent during prolongation of voiceless fricatives.

The clinician concluded, "Adductor spasmodic dysphonia of essential voice tremor, moderate-marked in severity."

Botox injection (discussed in Chapter 17) was recommended. Her voice improved significantly after several weeks of a weak-breathy dysphonia and very mild swallowing difficulty. She noted a marked reduction in physical effort to speak and was very pleased with her voice quality. Voice quality was indeed markedly improved, although evidence of mild voice tremor persisted, but without voice interruptions.

Commentary. (1) Adductor spasmodic dysphonia can develop in association with organic voice tremor. Voice tremor may be accompanied by tremor elsewhere in the body, particularly in the jaw, face, tongue, palate, and pharynx. (2) The onset of spasmodic dysphonia is often associated with psychological stress, even when examination reveals an organic basis for the problem. The relationship between psychological stress and neurogenic spasmodic dysphonia is unclear, but the presence of psychological stress at the time of onset does not rule out the possibility of neurogenic etiology for persisting voice difficulty. (3) Proper diagnosis of adductor spasmodic dysphonia can lead to fairly effective treatment of the disorder.

SUMMARY

1. Hyperkinetic dysarthria is usually associated with dysfunction of the basal ganglia control circuit, but may also be related to involvement of the cerebellar control circuit or other portions of the extrapyramidal system. It probably occurs somewhat less frequently in speech pathology practices than other dysarthria types, but if organic voice tremor and neurogenic spasmodic dysphonias are included in such comparisons, the disorder may be more prevalent than all other single dysarthria types. Its characteristics can be manifest in the respiratory, phonatory, resonatory, and articulatory levels of speech, and prosody is often prominently affected. The deviant speech characteristics of hyperkinetic dysarthria reflect the effects on speech of abnormal rhythmic or irregular and unpredictable, rapid or slow involuntary movements.

2. Hyperkinetic dysarthria is a heterogenous disorder, both in terms of the variety of abnormal movements that can lead to it, and the particular speech muscles affected by the involuntary movements. The movement disorders underlying it are often categorized by the degree to which they vary in speed and rhythmicity. The most common abnormal movements associated with hyperkinetic dysarthria include myoclonus, tics, chorea, athetosis, dyskinesia, dystonia, spasm, and tremor.

3. The cause of hyperkinetic dysarthria is very often unknown, and this appears particularly true when the movement disorder is limited to the speech and cervical muscles. Toxic and metabolic conditions are frequent causes of the disorder, antipsychotic or neuroleptic medications representing the most frequent toxic cause. Orofacial dyskinesias and hyperkinetic dysarthria are often the first or only manifestation of drug toxicity and tardive dyskinesia. Hyperkinetic dysarthria is not uncommonly associated with degenerative neurologic conditions. Infection, neoplasm, trauma, and stroke are possible but infrequent causes.

4. The jaw, face, and tongue are frequently affected by hyperkinesias, usually in combination. Occasionally, hyperkinetic dysarthria is associated with involuntary movement in only a single speech structure, such as the jaw. Organic voice tremor and spasmodic dysphonias very frequently have speech abnormalities that are perceptually limited to phonatory functions. Sometimes the involuntary movements are action-induced and occur only during speech. In such cases, the dysarthria is frequently misdiagnosed as psychogenic in origin.

5. Patient complaints and specific deviant speech characteristics associated with hyperkinetic dysarthria are quite variable, and are dependent on the type of involuntary movement and the

specific levels of the speech system affected. Distinctions can generally be made among hyperkinetic dysarthrias that are due to chorea, dystonia, spasmodic torticollis, palatopharyngolaryngeal myoclonus, action myoclonus, tics, organic voice tremor, and spasmodic dysphonias. These distinctions justify consideration of hyperkinetic dysarthria as a plural disorder, with subtypes based on the nature of the underlying involuntary movement.

6. In general, acoustic and physiologic studies have provided support for the auditory-perceptual characteristics of hyperkinetic dysarthria, have specified more precisely the disorder's acoustic and physiologic characteristics, and have established approaches to documenting and quantifying relevant parameters of the disorder.

7. Hyperkinetic dysarthria can be the only, the first, or among the first and most prominent manifestations of neurologic disease. Its recognition can aid neurologic localization and diagnosis and may contribute to the medical and behavioral management of the individual's disease and speech disorder.

REFERENCES

Ackerman H and Ziegler W: Cerebellar voice tremor: an acoustic analysis, J Neurol Neurosurg Psychiatry 54:74, 1991.

Adams RD and Victor M: Principles of neurology, New York, 1991, McGraw-Hill.

Altrocchi PH and Forno LS: Spontaneous oral-facial dyskinesia: neuropathology of a case, Neurology 33:802, 1983.

Arana GW and Hyman SE: Handbook of psychiatric drug therapy, ed 2, Boston, 1991, Little Brown.

Aronson AE: Clinical voice disorders, New York, 1990, Thieme.

Aronson AE, O'Neill BP, and Kelly JJ: The dysarthria of action myoclonus: a new clinical entity. Paper presented at the Clinical Dysarthria Conference, February, 1984.

Aronson AE and Hartman DE: Adductor spastic dysphonia as a sign of essential (voice) tremor, J Speech Hear Disord 46:52, 1981.

Aronson AE, Brown JR, Litin EM, and Pearson JS: Spastic dysphonia. II. Comparison of essential (voice) tremor and other neurologic and psychogenic dysphonias, J Speech Hear Disord 33:219, 1968.

Aronson AE and Lagerlund TC: Neuroimaging studies do not prove the existence of brain abnormalities in spastic (spasmodic) dysphonia, J Speech Hear Res 34:801, 1991.

Biary N and Koller WC: Essential tongue tremor, Mov Disord 2:25, 1987.

Brazis P, Masdeu JC, and Biller J: Localization in clinical neurology, Boston, 1985, Little-Brown.

Breakfield XO and Bressman S: Molecular genetics of movement disorders. In Fahn S and Marsden ED, editors: Movement disorders two, London, 1987, Butterworths.

Brown JR and Simonson J: Organic voice tremor: a tremor of phonation, Neurology 13:520, 1963.

Burke RE: Tardive dyskinesia: current clinical issues, Neurology 34:1348, 1984.

Cannito MP: Neurobiological interpretations of spasmodic dysphonia. In Vogel D and Cannito MP, editors: Treating disordered speech motor control, Austin, Texas, 1991, Pro-Ed.

Cannito MP: Vocal tract steadiness in spasmodic dysphonia. In Yorkston KM and Beukelman DR, editors: Recent advances in clinical dysarthria, Boston, MA, 1989, College-Hill.

Cannito M and Johnson J: Spastic dysphonia: a continuum disorder, J Commun Disord 14:215, 1981.

Cannito MP, Kondraske GV, and Johns DF: Oral-facial sensorimotor function in spasmodic dysphonia. In Moore CA, Yorkston KM, and Beukelman DR, editors: Dysarthria and apraxia of speech: perspective on management, Baltimore, MD, 1991, Brooks Publishing.

Casey DE and Robins P: Tardive dyskinesia as a life-threatening illness, Am J Psychiatry 135:486, 1978.

Clinical examinations in neurology, ed 3, Philadelphia, 1991, WB Saunders.

Comings DE: A controlled study of Tourette syndrome. VII. Summary: a common genetic disorder causing disinhibition of the limbic system, Am J Hum Genet 41:839, 1987.

Comings DE: Tourette syndrome and human behavior, Durate, CA, 1990, Hope Press.

Couch JR: Dystonia and tremor in spasmodic torticollis. In Eldridge R and Fahn S, editors: Advances in neurology, vol 14, New York, 1976, Raven Press.

D'Alessandro R and others: The prevalence of lingual-facial-buccal dyskinesias in the elderly, Neurology 36:1350, 1986.

Darley FL, Aronson AE, and Brown JR: Motor speech disorders, Philadelphia, PA, 1975, WB Saunders.

Darley FL, Aronson AE, and Brown JR: Differential diagnostic patterns of dysarthria, J Speech Hear Res 12:246, 1969a.

Darley FL, Aronson AE, and Brown JR: Clusters of deviant speech dimensions in the dysarthrias, J Speech Hear Res 12:462, 1969b.

Day TJ, Lefroy RB, and Mastaglia FL: Meige's syndrome and palatal myoclonus associated with brain stem stroke: a common mechanism? J Neurol Neurosurg Psychiatry, 49:1324, 1986.

Deuschl G, Mischke G, Schenk E, et al: Symptomatic and essential rhythmic palatal mycoclonus, Brain, 113:1645, 1990.

Diagnostic and statistical manual of mental disorders, ed 3, (revised), Washington, DC, 1987, American Psychiatric Association.

Faheem DA and others: Respirator dyskinesia and dysarthria from prolonged neuroleptic use: tardive dyskinesia? Am J Psychiatry, 139:517, 1982.

Fahn S, Davis JM, and Rolland LP: Cerebral hypoxia and its consequences. In Fahn S, David JM, and Rolland, editors: Advances in neurology, New York, 1979, Raven Press.

Fahn S, Marsden C, and Calne DB: Classification and investigation of dystonia. In Marsden CD and Fahn S, editors: Movement disorders 2, London, 1987, Butterworths.

Findley LJ and Koller WC: Essential tremor: a review, Neurology 37:1194, 1987.

Finitzo T and Freeman F: Spasmodic dysphonia, whether and where: results of seven years of research, J Speech Hear Res 32:541, 1989.

Finitzo T and others: Whether and wherefore: a response to Aronson and Lagerlund, J Speech Hear Res 34:806, 1991.

Fross RD and others: Lesions of the putamen: their relevance to dystonia, Neurology 37:1125, 1987.

Gerratt BR: Formant frequency fluctuation as an index of motor steadiness in the vocal tract, J Speech Hear Res 26:297, 1983.

Golper LA and others: Focal cranial dystonia, J Speech Hear Disord 48:128, 1983.

Hardy JC: Cerebral palsy, Englewood Cliffs, NJ, 1983, Prentice-Hall.

Howard RS and others: Respiratory involvement in multiple sclerosis, Brain 115:479, 1992.

Izdebski K, Dedo HH, and Boles L: Spastic dysphonia: a patient profile of 200 cases, Am J Otolaryngol 5:7, 1984.

Jankovic J: Cranial-cervical dyskinesias. In Appel SH, editor: Current neurology, vol 6, Chicago, 1986, Mosby–Year Book Publishers.

Jankovic J and Patel SC: Blepharospasm associated with brainstem lesions, Neurology 33:1237, 1983.

Kelly PJ and others: Computer-assisted stereotactic ventralis lateralis thalamotomy with microelectrode recording control in patients with Parkinson's disease, Mayo Clinic Proceedings 62:655, 1987.

Kent R and Netsell R: Articulatory abnormalities in athetoid cerebral palsy, J Speech Hear Disord 43:353, 1978.

Koller WC: Diagnosis and treatment of tremors, Neurol Clin 2:499, 1984.

Kurlan R: Tourette's syndrome: current concepts, Neurology 39:1625, 1989.

Lance JW: Action myoclonus, Ramsay Hunt syndrome, and other cerebellar myoclonic syndromes. In Fahn S, editor: Advances in neurology, vol 43, myoclonus, New York, 1986, Raven Press.

Lance JW and Adams RD: The syndrome of intention or action myoclonus as a sequel to anoxic encephalopathy, Brain 87:111, 1963.

LaPointe LL, Case JL, and Duane DD: Perceptual-acoustic speech and voice characteristics of subjects with spasmodic torticollis. In Till JA, Yorkston KM, and Beukelman DR, editors: Motor speech disorders: advances in assessment and treatment, Baltimore, 1994, Paul H. Brookes.

Ludlow CL and Connor NP: Dynamic aspects of phonatory control in spasmodic dysphonia, J Speech Hear Res 30:197, 1987.

Marsden CD: Is tardive dyskinesia a unique disorder? In Casey DE, Chase TN, Christensen AV, and Gerlach J, editors: Dyskinesias: research and treatment, New York, NY, 1985, Springer-Verlag.

Marsden CD and Fahn S, editors: Problems in the dykinesias, Movement disorders 2, London, England, 1987, Butterworths.

Marsden CD and Sheehy MP: Spastic dysphonia, Meige disease, and torsion dystonia, Neurology 32:1202, 1982.

Matsuo F and Ajax ET: Palatal myoclonus and denervation supersensitivity in the central nervous system, Ann Neuro 5:72, 1978.

McCall GN, Skolnick ML, and Brewer DW: A preliminary report of some atypical movement patterns in the tongue, palate, hypopharynx, and larynx of patients with spasmodic dysphonia, J Speech Hear Disord 37:466, 1971.

Merson RM and Ginsberg AP: Spasmodic dysphonia: abductor type; a clinical report of acoustic, aerodynamic and perceptual characteristics, Laryngoscope 89:129, 1979.

Miller LG and Jankovic J: Drug-induced dyskinesias. In Appel SH, editor: Current neurology volume 10, Chicago, IL, 1990, Mosby–Year Book.

Mölsä PR, Marttila RJ, and Rinne UK: Extrapyramidal signs in Alzheimer's disease, Neurology 34:1114, 1984.

Nielson P and O'Dwyer N: Reproducibility and variability of speech muscle activity in athetoid dysarthria of cerebral palsy, J Speech Hear Res 27:502, 1984.

Parnes SM, Lavarato AB, and Myers EN: Study of spastic dysphonia using videofiberoptic laryngoscopy, Ann Otol Rhinol Laryngol 87:322, 1979.

Platt LJ and others: Dysarthria of adult cerebral palsy: I. Intelligibility and articulatory impairment, J Speech Hear Res 23:28, 1980.

Platt LJ, Andrews G, and Howie P: Dysarthria of adult cerebral palsy: II. Analysis of articulation errors, J Speech Hear Res 23:41, 1980.

Portnoy RA: Hyperkinetic dysarthria as an early indicator of impending tardive dyskinesia, J Speech Hear Disord 44:214, 1979.

Putnam AHB: Review of research in dysarthria. In Winitz H, editor: Human communication and its disorders, a review 1988, Norwood, NJ, 1988, Ablex Publishing.

Rosenberg RN and Pettegrew JW: Genetic neurologic disease. In Rosenberg RN, editor: Comprehensive neurology, New York, NY, 1991, Raven Press.

Rosenfield DB: Pharmacologic approaches to speech motor disorders. In Vogel D and Cannito MP, editors: Treating disordered speech motor control, Austin, TX, 1991, Pro-Ed.

Rothwell JC and Obeso JA: The anatomical and physiological basis of torsion dystonia. In Marsden CF and Fahn S, editors: Movement disorders 2, London, England, 1987, Butterworths.

Tomoda H and others: Voice tremor: dysregulation of voluntary expiratory muscles, Neurology 37:117, 1987.

Warfel JH and Schlagenhauff RE: Understanding neurologic disease: a textbook for therapists, Baltimore, MD, 1980, Urban and Schwarzenberg.

Watson BC and others: Laryngeal electromyographic activity in adductor and abductor spasmodic dysphonia, J Speech Hear Res 34:473, 1991.

Weiner WJ and others: Respiratory dyskinesias: extrapyramidal dysfunction and dyspnea, Ann Int Med 88:327, 1978.

Wolfe VI and Bacon M: Spectrographic comparison of two types of spastic dysphonia, J Speech Hear Disord, 41:325, 1976.

Zraik RI and others: Acoustic correlates of voice quality in individuals with spasmodic torticollis, J Med Speech Lang Pathol 1(4):261, 1993.

Zwirner P and Barnes GJ: Vocal tract steadiness: a measure of phonatory and upper airway motor control during phonation in dysarthria, J Speech Hear Res 35(4):761, 1992.

9 Unilateral Upper Motor Neuron Dysarthria

Chapter Outline

Unilateral upper motor neuron (UUMN) dysarthria is a distinguishable motor speech disorder that is associated with damage to the upper motor neurons (UMNs) that carry impulses to the cranial and spinal nerves that supply the speech muscles. It is primarily a disorder of articulation. Its deviant characteristics most likely reflect the effects of weakness, and perhaps incoordination, on speech.

In contrast to other dysarthria types, the label for this dysarthria is anatomic rather than pathophysiologic. This is because its pathophysiology and perceptual characteristics have received little systematic investigation, thereby limiting the degree to which clinical manifestations can be related to pathophysiology. It is well-documented, however, that dysarthria can result from UUMN lesions. Although there is some intuitive support for calling this dysarthria a "flaccid dysarthria" of UUMN origin, it seems best to withhold such a designation until its clinical characteristics and physiologic underpinnings are better defined, and to restrict its label to what is most certain about it; hence, its designation as UUMN dysarthria.

Why has UUMN dysarthria received so little attention? One reason is that it usually has been considered a mild and temporary problem (Darley, Aronson, and Brown, 1975; Metter, 1985). Disorders that are subtle in their clinical manifestations and short-lived are naturally difficult to study. In addition, UUMN dysarthria often co-occurs with aphasia or apraxia of speech when the lesion is in the left hemisphere, and with other cognitive and, perhaps, nondysarthric speech deficits when the lesion is in the right hemisphere. Such disorders can be devastating in their effects on communication; as a result, a dysarthria may be masked by them or made more difficult to study because of their presence. In general, therefore, UUMN dysarthria has probably received little attention because of its presumed mildness, short duration, and frequent co-occurrence with deficits that may mask or overwhelm its manifestations, thereby minimizing its functional importance and making it difficult to isolate and study.

It should be recognized, however, that UUMN dysarthria is sometimes the patient's most obvious communication disorder and sometimes the only manifestation of neurologic disease. Its recognition is especially important when it is a relatively isolated symptom; when the case, the lesion tends to be small and may escape detection by sophisticated neuroimaging techniques, especially early postonset. An understanding of its characteristics is also important because it may co-occur and be difficult to distinguish from other speech disorders that are associated with unilateral cerebral disease, such as apraxia of speech (left hemisphere lesions) and "aprosodia" (right hemisphere lesions).

Unilateral upper motor neuron dysarthria is encountered as the primary speech pathology in a large medical practice at a rate comparable to that for the other major single dysarthria types. From 1987 to 1990 at the Mayo Clinic, it accounted for 9.9% of all dysarthrias and 9% of all motor speech disorders seen in the section of Speech Pathology. This is almost certainly an underestimate of its true frequency in clinical practice, however, because it occurs frequently as a secondary diagnosis in patients with aphasia and apraxia of speech.

The clinical features of UUMN dysarthria probably primarily reflect the effects of weakness and maybe incoordination on the side of the face and tongue opposite the UMN lesion. The pattern of speech gives the impression that weakness limits the precision with which speech can be produced and sometimes that articulation is not well coordinated.

ANATOMY AND BASIC FUNCTIONS OF THE UPPER MOTOR NEURON SYSTEM

The UMN system includes the *direct and indirect activation pathways.* It was described in detail in Chapter 2 and was reviewed again in Chapter 5 when the effects on speech of bilateral UMN lesions (spastic dysarthria) were discussed. It is reviewed here only with reference to its implications for the deficits encountered in UUMN dysarthria and the neurologic deficits that frequently accompany it. Its relevant anatomy and functions can be summarized as follows:

1. The UMN system is bilateral, half of it originating in the right hemisphere, the other half in the left hemisphere.
2. The *direct activation pathway* passes rather directly as *corticobulbar* and *corticospinal tracts* to the cranial and spinal nerves, respectively, mostly to the side opposite their origin. It emerges from the *cerebral cortex* and begins its descent in the *corona radiata.* The corona radiata converges into the *internal capsule* in the vicinity of the basal ganglia and thalamus (corticobulbar fibers are grouped primarily in the *genu,* or midportion, of the internal capsule). From there it descends to the brain stem where corticobulbar fibers cross to the opposite side just before reaching the cranial nerve nuclei they are to innervate; corticospinal fibers cross in the pyramids of the medulla. The impulses traveling in the direct pathway appear *crucial for finely coordinated, skilled movements.*
3. The *indirect activation pathway* of the UMN system has the same contralateral destinations and it crosses in the brain stem in the same general areas as the direct activation pathway. However, along its route it has synaptic connections in the *basal ganglia, cerebellum, reticular formation,* and other *brainstem nuclei.* This pathway appears *crucial for regulating reflexes and controlling posture and tone* upon which skilled movements may be superimposed.
4. In the bulbar speech muscles of most people, the general *principle of contralateral innervation holds true only for the lower face and, to a lesser extent, the tongue.* The trigeminal nerve, the fibers of the facial nerve going to the upper face, and the glossopharyngeal, vagus, and accessory nerves receive both contralateral and ipsilateral UMN innervation. This bilateral input to most of the speech cranial nerves, and the fact that the tongue—as a midline structure—receives bilateral UMN input, provides a degree of redundancy that helps to preserve breathing, feeding, and motor speech

---

PRIMARY CLINICAL FEATURES OF UUMN LESIONS. ALL FEATURES ARE PRESENT ON THE SIDE OF THE BODY CONTRALATERAL TO THE SIDE OF THE LESION.

Direct activation pathway (pyramidal tract)
Hemiplegia or hemiparesis
Loss/impairment of fine, skilled movements
Absent abdominal reflex
Babinski sign
Hyporeflexia
Central facial weakness at rest and during voluntary movement
Lingual weakness

Indirect activation pathway (extrapyramidal tract)
Increased muscle tone
Spasticity
Clonus
Hyperactive stretch reflexes
Decerebrate or decorticate posturing
Central facial weakness apparent during emotional expression

UUMN, unilateral upper motor neuron.

functions when UMN lesions are confined to one side of the brain.

CLINICAL CHARACTERISTICS PRODUCED BY UNILATERAL UPPER MOTOR NEURON LESIONS

The distinctive effects of UUMN lesions affecting the direct and indirect activation pathways are summarized in the box above.* Briefly, such lesions are often associated with contralateral hemiplegia or hemiparesis. A combination of weakness and spasticity is usually present in the affected limbs; *weakness, hyporeflexia, and hypotonia tend to predominate shortly after the onset of acute lesions,* with *spasticity, hyperactive stretch reflexes, and increased muscle tone emerging over time.* A *Babinski reflex* is usually present on the affected side. Corticobulbar involvement is often manifest by a *contralateral lower facial weakness* (often called a "central" facial weakness to distinguish it from peripheral VIIth nerve lesions, which usually affect the upper and lower face).

A combination of direct and indirect pathway lesion effects are usually present, at least in the limbs. Depending on the specific site of lesion, however, the upper or lower limb or bulbar

---

*These features were discussed in more detail in Chapter 5.

muscles may be relatively spared. For example, some lesions affect only the bulbar muscles and hand.

ETIOLOGIES

Unilateral upper notor neuron dysarthria can be caused by any process that can damage UMNs unilaterally. Because degenerative, inflammatory, and toxic-metabolic diseases usually produce diffuse effects, they are rarely associated with focal unilateral signs. Trauma can produce focal deficits, including UUMN dysarthria, although its typical multifocal, bilateral, or diffuse effects usually are associated with other dysarthria types. Tumors confined to one side of the central nervous system (CNS) can cause UUMN dysarthria when they invade or produce mass effects on UMN structures and pathways unilaterally.

Stroke is by far the most common cause of UUMN damage. It is, therefore, appropriate to review a few of the vascular conditions that can produce relatively isolated UMN deficits.

Left carotid or middle cerebral artery occlusions are the most common causes of infarcts that lead to UMN deficits that are also accompanied by aphasia or apraxia of speech. Right carotid or middle cerebral artery occlusions are the most common cause of infarcts that lead to UMN deficits that are also accompanied by neglect and cognitive disturbances characteristic of right hemisphere pathology. Unilateral infarcts in the distribution of the posterior cerebral, basilar, and, less frequently, anterior cerebral arteries can also cause UUMN deficits.

Sometimes small infarcts occur in cortical or subcortical areas of the cerebral hemispheres or in the brain stem as the result of occlusion of the small penetrating branches of the large cerebral arteries. These small infarcts are often called *lacunes* or *lacunar infarcts* because, in healing, they leave behind a small cavity (lacune).* They most often involve the lenticulostriate branches of the anterior and middle cerebral arteries, the thalamoperforant branches of the posterior cerebral arteries, and the paramedian branches of the basilar artery.

The most common sites of lacunar infarcts are the putamen, caudate nucleus, thalamus, pons, internal capsule, and white matter below the cerebral cortex (Fisher, 1982). These locations estab-

lish the importance of lacunes as a mechanism for producing UUMN dysarthria (and spastic dysarthria, when lesions are bilateral); that is, most of them are part of the UMN pathways.*

Because of their location, lacunes often are not associated with aphasia, neglect, visual field deficits, severe memory impairment, or alterations in consciousness. Their signs are primarily motor or sensorimotor in most cases.

Fisher (1982) has outlined a number of "lacunar syndromes." Several of them have dysarthria resulting from a unilateral lesion among their defining characteristics. The most relevant of these are:

1. *Pure motor hemiparesis*—a pure motor stroke involving the face, arm, and leg on one side in the absence of sensory deficit, homonymous hemianopia, aphasia, agnosia, or apraxia. The lesion may be in the corona radiata, internal capsule, cerebral peduncle, or pons. The vascular origin, therefore, is usually a branch of the middle cerebral artery or vertebrobasilar system.

2. *Ataxic hemiparesis*—this involves signs of pure motor hemiparesis plus cerebellar dysmetria in the affected limbs. The lesion is often in the pons (at the junction of the upper one-third and inferior two-thirds of the basis pontis) or the internal capsule or corona radiata (Fisher, 1978; Huang and Lui, 1984). It has also been reported in patients with thalamic hemorrhage (Verma and Maheshwari, 1986).

3. *Dysarthria clumsy hand syndrome*—facial weakness, dysarthria, and dysphagia are prominent, but there is also slight weakness and clumsiness of the hand. The lesion is usually in the genu or posterior limb of the internal capsule or the adjacent corona radiata, and sometimes in the pons (Koppel and Weinberger, 1987). This syndrome may account for 6% of lacunar infarcts (Chamorro and others, 1991).

4. *Pure dysarthria*—the sudden onset of dysarthria without other signs (except for face and tongue weakness). This syndrome was found in about 1% of 670 consecutive cases of stroke (Arboix and others, 1991). The genu of the internal capsule or the adjacent corona radiata are probably the most frequent lesion sites in cases of pure dysarthria resulting from a unilateral stroke (Bogousslavsky and Regli, 1990; Ichikawa and Kageyama, 1991; Ozaki and others, 1986, 1991).

---

*Lacunes account for about 25% of all strokes in some clinical practices (Chamorro and others, 1991). They range in size from 0.2 to 15 cu mm; the smallest of them may escape detection by computed tomography scan (Mohr, 1982). Approximately 90% of patients with lacunes have a history of systemic arterial hypertension (Fisher, 1982).

---

*Dysarthria has been found in 25% of patients with lacunar infarcts (Arboix, Marti-Vilalta, and Garcia, 1991). Fries and others (1993) noted dysarthria in 7 out of 23 (30%) patients with capsular stroke.

SPEECH PATHOLOGY

Unfortunately, the neurology literature's description of the dysarthria in patients with UUMN lesions rarely extends beyond applying the label of dysarthria. Description is usually limited to vague terms such as "slow dysarthria," "slurred," "unintelligible," "defective articulation," or "thick."

There has been no systematic large group prospective study of UUMN dysarthria. However, a few studies do permit a rough picture of it to be pieced together, one that must be considered tentative until more systematic studies are undertaken. Here, the results of a relatively large retrospective study of 56 patients with a speech pathology diagnosis of UUMN dysarthria (Duffy and Folger, 1986)* will serve as a vehicle for describing the disorder. Findings from other studies will be used to supplement and modify the observations of that study as appropriate.

Distribution of etiologies, lesions, and severity in clinical practice

Etiology. The etiology of the dysarthria in Duffy and Folger's patients was stroke in 91% of the cases. Seven percent had tumors. The remaining one patient had cerebritis.

The predominance of stroke as an etiology is consistent with most studies that have attempted to describe the dysarthria. For example, in the only published study specifically designed to examine the dysarthria associated with UUMN lesions, Hartman and Abbs' (1992) group of six patients all had had strokes.[†]

Lesion loci. The lesion sites for the sample are summarized in the box on page 226. The distribution is consistent with that predicted from the anatomy of the UMN system, its vascular supply, and the literature on the locus of lacunar infarcts that may produce dysarthria.

Lesions were supratentorial in about 95% of the cases. The internal capsule and pericapsular region were the most common lesion sites. Larger lesions of the cerebral hemispheres usually were limited to or included the frontal lobes. A few patients had lesions in the thalamus, midbrain, or pons.

Regarding side of lesion, 61% had lesions in the left hemisphere and 34% had lesions in the right hemisphere. The difference in the distribution between right and left hemisphere lesions probably does not represent dominance of the left hemisphere for functions that go awry in UUMN dysarthria.* The distribution does indicate that UUMN dysarthria can result from lesions on either side of the brain.

Severity. The severity of dysarthria in Duffy and Folger's patients could not always be ascertained from their records. However, it was probably mild in many cases. For example, speech therapy was judged unnecessary for 21% of the patients. An additional 29% were not treated for unstated reasons; it is likely that therapy also was considered unnecessary for many of them. Half of the patients did receive therapy and 92% improved during treatment. These observations are in general agreement with those of Hartman and Abbs (1992) who found mild reductions in intelligibility based on perceptual judgments and an intelligibility test (single word intelligibility ranged from 81 to 93% in their six patients). However, marked-to-severe dysarthria has been reported in some cases, including patients with right hemisphere lesions in whom the deficit could not be attributed to accompanying aphasia or apraxia of speech (Ropper, 1987; Spertell and Ransom, 1979).

Twenty-three percent of Duffy and Folger's patients were more than one month postonset when evaluated, and 9% were more than one year postonset. Therefore, UUMN dysarthria can persist beyond the immediate postonset period, contrary to suggestions that it is a transient problem[†] (Benke and Kertesz, 1989; Darley, Aronson and

---

*Duffy and Folger's patients were selected on the basis of their speech diagnosis and clinical or neuroimaging evidence of only a single lesion confined to one side of the brain. Patients with parkinsonism and cerebellar lesions were excluded, as were all patients with apraxia of speech. Patients with aphasia that was severe enough to preclude obtaining a sufficient speech sample also were not included (18% of the sample were aphasic, but usually only mildly so).

[†]The exclusive stroke etiology may reflect the authors' desire to study patients with small, focal lesions rather than the natural distribution of etiologies of the disorder. Small strokes are ideal for investigating unilateral upper motor neuron dysarthria because their anatomic boundaries are easier to define than those of diseases with more difficult to localize effects, such as traumatic brain injuries, tumor, or infection.

---

*There is no reason to expect a lateralization effect to exist. The greater percentage of cases with left hemisphere lesions could simply reflect referral bias (for example, many patients may have been referred primarily because of their aphasia) or differences in the distribution of left- and right-sided strokes that come to medical attention. Relatedly, some studies of the consequences of subcortical stroke report that dysarthria occurs more frequently or is more pronounced when the lesion is in the right than in the left hemisphere (Fromm and others, 1985).

[†]Recovery of limb motor function following unilateral capsular stroke is generally very good. Limb motor recovery from unilateral stroke is less adequate when multiple motor areas or their descending pathways are affected (Fries and others, 1993).

PRIMARY ORAL MECHANISM, CLINICAL NEUROLOGIC FINDINGS, AND CONFIRMED OR PRESUMED LESION LOCUS FOR 56 CASES WITH A PRIMARY SPEECH DIAGNOSIS OF UUMN DYSARTHRIA (DUFFY AND FOLGER, 1986). PERCENTAGE OF CASES IS GIVEN IN PARENTHESES.

Oral mechanism findings

Unilateral lower facial weakness (82%)
Unilateral lingual weakness (52%)
Unilateral palatal weakness (5%)

Clinical neurologic findings

Hemiplegia/hemiparesis (79%)
Sensory deficits (20%)
Dysarthria and clumsy hand only (13%)
Dysarthria and bulbar weakness only (lower face or tongue) (5%)

Lesion locus*

Internal capsule (34%)
Lobar (cortical and subcortical, usually frontal) (29%)
Pericapsular (11%)
Lobar, cortical (usually frontal) (7%)
Lobar, subcortical (usually frontal) (7%)
Pericapsular, subcortical, lobar (5%)
Internal capsule or pons (4%)
Brain stem (2%)
Thalamus and midbrain (2%)

---

*Lobar—region affecting all or portions of a lobe in a cerebral hemisphere, divisible into cortical and subcortical subcategories when possible; *pericapsular*—region of the internal capsule plus adjacent structures projecting to or from the cerebral cortex, including the corona radiata.

Brown, 1975; De Jong, 1986; Yorkston, Beukelman, and Bell, 1988).

These observations suggest that UUMN dysarthria is usually mild and that significant recovery takes place in many cases. However, it sometimes requires speech therapy, it may reduce speech intelligibility, and it may persist beyond the period of spontaneous recovery following stroke.

Patient perceptions and complaints

Patients with UUMN dysarthria are usually aware of their speech difficulty. They may minimize its effects, however, especially when intelligibility is preserved. When the etiology is stroke, by the time they are seen for formal speech assessment patients are often more impressed with the improvement they have made than the degree of deficit that remains. When the dysarthria is more severe, patients may express distress over its effect on their intelligibility or efficiency of communication. They often describe their speech as *slurred, thick,* or *slow,* or they may complain that words "just don't come out right."

Patients frequently complain of *drooling* or a *heavy feeling* on the affected side of the face or corner of the mouth and sometimes of heaviness or thickness in the tongue, especially when speaking.

Chewing and swallowing difficulty are not unusual (Horner and Massey, 1988), especially early post-onset. Many complain of drooling from the affected side of the mouth.

Patients with clinically apparent aphasia or apraxia of speech often will not complain of their dysarthria because its functional effects are overwhelmed by the language and motor programming deficits. As with most other dysarthria types, patients tend to complain that their speech deteriorates under conditions of physical fatigue or psychological stress.*

Clinical findings

The lesions leading to UUMN dysarthria usually produce a constellation of physical signs and symptoms on the side of the body contralateral to the lesion (see the box on page 223). For example,

---

*Brodal (1973), an anatomist, made observations following his own right capsular stroke that provide sophisticated testimonial support for many common patient complaints. He spoke of feelings of decreased force of innervation and problems with skilled movements, as if they were no longer automatic, requiring increased volitional energy to generate movement. Even six months after his stroke, he felt his speech deteriorated under conditions of fatigue.

79% of Duffy and Folger's patients had hemiplegia or hemiparesis and 20% had sensory deficits (see the box on page 226). Language and other cognitive disturbances may be present and often have a greater impact on spoken communication than the dysarthria. When aphasia results from left subcortical lesions, an accompanying dysarthria is very frequently reported (Damasio and others, 1982; Metter and others, 1983; Naeser and others, 1982).

Thirteen percent of Duffy and Folger's patients had dysarthria and a clumsy hand, and 5% had dysarthria and face and tongue weakness as their only neurologic abnormality. Dysarthria, frequently with accompanying facial weakness, has been reported as the only sign of unilateral lesion in the internal capsule or corona radiata (Huang and Broe, 1984; Ichikawa and Kageyama, 1991; Ozaki and others, 1991).

Nonspeech oral mechanism. The box on page 226 summarizes the primary oral mechanism findings in Duffy and Folger's patients. Unilateral lower "central" facial weakness was present in a large percentage of cases. This weakness is often apparent at rest and during movement. If components of both the direct and indirect activation pathways are involved, weakness will be apparent during voluntary and emotional facial movements. If the indirect pathway is relatively spared, however, emotional facial expression, such as smiling, may be relatively symmetric, reflecting the ability of the indirect pathways to drive emotional expression even when voluntary control is impaired. This mismatch between voluntary and emotional facial expression is not unusual in UUMN dysarthria.

Unilateral tongue weakness was apparent in about half of Duffy and Folger's patients. It is usually reflected in deviation of the tongue to the weak side on protrusion. It can also be detected on attempts to lateralize the tongue, or on lateral strength testing. Difficulty turning or pushing the tongue to one side is sometimes detectable when tongue deviation on protrusion is not apparent.

The jaw is usually normal or weakness goes unnoticed on clinical examination, but contralateral weakness is occasionally apparent clinically (Bogousslavsky and Regli, 1990) and has been demonstrated electrophysiologically (Cruccu, Fornarelli, and Manfredi, 1988; Hartman and Abbs, 1992). Palatal asymmetry is unusual but is evident in some cases. Vocal cord weakness is presumably rare or nonexistent, but the vocal cords have not been systematically examined in patients with UUMN lesions.*

In a comprehensive study of 100 patients with unilateral stroke, all of whom had unilateral limb weakness, Willoughby and Anderson (1984) made the following observations of the oral mechanism: the jaw opened normally in 98% of patients (jaw clenching was weak on the affected side in 15%); unilateral lower face weakness was present in 75%, with voluntary weakness greater than weakness on emotional expression in 21%; unilateral palatal asymmetry or weakness was present in only 2%; the tongue protruded in the midline in 88%. Sixty percent of the sample had a dysarthria that was usually mild or moderate. Dysarthria occurred in both right and left hemisphere lesions. Melo and others (1992), in a study of 225 consecutively admitted cases with stroke and hemiparesis, found lower facial weakness in 79% and dysarthria in 29%. Forty-seven percent had deep hemispheric lesions, 25% had cortical lesions (usually in the anterior distribution of the middle cerebral artery), and 4% had lesions in the brain stem. Ninety-three percent of the dysarthric patients had facial weakness. The results of both of these studies are in general agreement with those of Duffy and Folger, in spite of the fact that in neither of them were patients selected for the presence of dysarthria. They establish that dysarthria occurs frequently in unilateral lesions of the cerebral hemispheres. Willoughby and Anderson point out that the high incidence of dysarthria with such lesions is often ignored in neurology texts.

It has been well-documented that dysphagia, as well as audible or silent aspiration, can occur with UUMN lesions (for example, Bogousslavsky and Regli, 1990: Horner and others, 1988; Horner and Massey, 1988; Meadows, 1973). Similar to the dysarthria, these problems are often mild, and recovery is good.

Speech. The speech characteristics of UUMN dysarthria, as identified by Duffy and Folger, are summarized in the box on page 228. Studies by Hartman and Abbs (1992), Benke and Kertesz (1989), and Ropper (1987) also provide some data about the disorder's features.*

The most pervasive deficit, present in 95% of patients, was *imprecise consonants.* A smaller percentage of patients had *irregular articulatory breakdowns* in contextual speech, and about one-third

---

*Bogousslavsky and Regli (1990) reported hypotonia and decreased movement of the vocal cord contralateral to an internal capsule lesion in one patient.

---

*Hartman and Abbs studied six patients with unilateral upper motor neuron lesions and dysarthria. Benke and Kertesz studied 35 patients with left hemisphere lesions and 35 patients with right hemisphere lesions and speech deficits (for our purposes, the Benke and Kertesz findings are confounded by the presence of apraxia of speech and aphasia, and perhaps "aprosodia," in their patients). Ropper described 10 patients with severe dysarthria resulting from right hemisphere lesions.

DEVIANT SPEECH CHARACTERISTICS IN 56 CASES WITH A PRIMARY SPEECH DIAGNOSIS OF UUMN DYSARTHRIA (DUFFY AND FOLGER, 1986). ONLY THOSE CHARACTERISTICS NOTED IN TWO OR MORE CASES ARE SHOWN. PERCENTAGE OF CASES EXHIBITING EACH CHARACTERISTIC IS GIVEN IN PARENTHESES.

Articulation (98%)*[†][‡]
Imprecise consonants (95%)*[†][‡]
Irregular articulatory breakdowns (14%)

Abnormal speech AMRs (91%)*
Slow (72%)*
Imprecise (33%)
Irregular (33%)*

Phonation (57%)*[†]
Harshness (39%)*[‡]
Reduced loudness (9%)[†][‡]
Strained-harshness (5%)

Rate and prosody (23%)*[†]
Slow rate (18%)*[†][‡]
Increased rate in segments (4%)
Excess and equal stress (4%)

Resonance (14%)[†]
Hypernasality (11%)[†]

* Also noted by Hartman and Abbs (1992).
[†] Also noted by Benke and Kertesz (1989).
[‡] Also noted by Ropper (1987).
AMRs, alternating motion rates.
UUMN, unilateral upper motor neuron.

had *irregular alternating motion rates (AMRs).* Imprecision was also apparent in AMRs of a number of patients. When severity of these characteristics was noted, it was usually rated as mild, although some patients had moderate-marked imprecision. Imprecise articulation is often attributed to the unilateral lower facial and tongue weakness that are apparent in so many patients with the disorder (Aronson, 1990).

Irregular articulatory breakdowns and irregular AMRs are usually associated with ataxic dysarthria.* The reasons for their presence in UUMN dysarthria are unclear. They could reflect clumsiness that occurs as a normal by-product of weakness (Landau, 1988) or an imbalance of muscle forces in midline structures (jaw, tongue) or structures that move synchronously (right and left face) when unilateral weakness is present. They could also reflect ataxic-like incoordination resulting from damage to cerebellocortical fibers that intermingle with UMN fibers in white matter pathways.*

The second most prominent deviant feature was *slow AMRs,* which were usually mildly slowed. Such slowness was not as striking in contextual speech, where it was noted in only 18% of patients. The reasons for slowness are not entirely clear, but weakness or compensatory efforts to maintain precision and regularity are possible explanations.

Surprisingly, 39% of patients had a mild-moderate dysphonia, which was described as

---

*It is interesting in this regard that Ropper's (1987) description of dysarthria in patients with right hemisphere lesions noted that "the overall pattern had some resemblance to the speech of an intoxicated individual" (p. 1061).

*The internal capsule and white matter pathways between the thalamus and cortex, for example, contain cerebellocortical and proprioceptive pathways that might, when damaged, contribute to ataxic-like movements. Attig (1994) and Mori and others (1984) have suggested that limb ataxia induced by capsular or corona radiata lesions may reflect disruption of cerebellocortical or thalamocortical projections. Brodal (1973) stated that "it is extremely likely that the interruption of pathways other than the direct corticobulbar pathways is of importance ... the cerebrocerebellar pathways are presumably important and involved in achieving smooth movements" (p. 685).

harsh or, infrequently, *strained-harshness.* Nine percent of the patients had *reduced loudness,* possibly also reflecting phonatory or respiratory-phonatory dysfunction. These findings are surprising in light of the common assumption that the vocal cords are spared from deficits because the Xth nerve receives bilateral UMN input.* The dysphonia could reflect: the effect of subtle vocal cord weakness, mild spasticity from the UUMN lesion† or, possibly, spasticity from an undetected lesion on the other side; an artifact of the increased frequency of dysphonia in the elderly, the most frequent victims of stroke; other factors unrelated to the specific effects of UUMN lesions on speech (for example, the general effects of illness or inactivity). Relative to the first two possibilities, it might be the case that the UMN supply to the Xth nerve is not always completely bilateral in some individuals, making their laryngeal (and velopharyngeal) muscles more susceptible to the effects of unilateral lesions. At this point, it is important to recognize the somewhat perplexing occurrence of dysphonia in some people with UUMN dysarthria. However, because we do not understand its neurologic basis, it is probably premature to consider dysphonia a necessary or salient or distinguishing feature of this type of dysarthria.

Mild *hypernasality* was present in 11% of patients, again somewhat surprising in light of the presumed bilateral UMN supply to the Xth nerve. The reasons for its occurrence may be similar to those offered in the previous paragraph for the occurrence of dysphonia.

Prosodic abnormalities were infrequent, and most often reflected in mildly *slowed rate.* A few patients had increased rate in segments or excess

Table 9–1 Primary clinical speech and speech-related findings in UUMN dysarthria.

Perceptual	
Articulation and prosody	Imprecise articulation
	Irregular articulatory breakdowns
	Slow rate
	Slow AMRs
	Imprecise AMRs
	Irregular AMRs
*Phonation**	Harshness
	Decreased loudness (infrequent)
*Resonance**	Hypernasality (infrequent)
Physical	Unilateral lower facial weakness
	Unilateral lingual weakness
Patient complaints	Slurred speech/difficulty with pronunciation
	Drooping lower face/"heavy" lower face
	"Thick" or heavy tongue
	Drooling
	Mild swallowing difficulty
	May not complain of dysarthria if aphasia is present and more predominant

*The neurologic bases of these features, if any, are unclear.
AMRs, alternating motion rates.
UUMN, unilateral upper motor neuron.

and equal stress. The presence of irregular articulatory breakdowns may also have altered prosody in some cases.

Finally, in addition to the features noted in the box on page 228, Hartman and Abbs (1992) also found monopitch, monoloudness, low pitch, and short phrases to be among their patients' most deviant speech characteristics; breathiness was present in a few subjects. In contrast to Duffy and Folger's observations, they noted that harshness and irregular articulatory breakdowns were not prominent features in their subjects (although harshness was present to a mild degree in some of their subjects, and irregular AMRs were identified during acoustic analysis).

The primary clinical speech and speech-related characteristics associated with UUMN dysarthria are summarized in Table 9–1. The prominent deviant speech characteristic is *imprecise articulation,* but *slowed rate* and *irregular articulatory breakdowns* may also be apparent. *Harshness, reduced loudness,* and *hypernasality* may be present in some cases. In general, these characteristics are mild-moderate in severity, although they may be worse in some patients.

---

*Metter's (1985) clinical description of unilateral upper motor neuron dysarthria included breathiness and hypophonia, and sometimes reduced loudness. Reduced loudness, breathiness, and hoarseness have also been noted in studies of aphasia resulting from unilateral subcortical lesions (for example, Alexander and LoVerme, 1980; Damasio and others, 1982, 1984; Metter and others, 1986). The lesions in these studies usually include the basal ganglia, thalamus, internal capsule, or corona radiata.

Dysphonia may be an important marker of dysphagia in patients with UUMN lesions. For example, Horner and Massey (1988) found dysphonia in 91% of their aspirating patients with UUMN lesions. Dysphonia was less frequently present in nonaspirating patients.

†It has been shown that cerebral blood flow can be diminished in the hemisphere contralateral to a unilateral stroke (Dobkin and others, 1989). This evidence of "transhemispheric diaschisis" might explain the presence of a strained-harsh voice quality in some people with UUMN lesions, especially early postonset.

Hartman and Abbs (1992) noted that a number of the deviant features present in their subjects are found in spastic dysarthria, but they felt that the pattern of deficits in their patients was unlike that encountered in spastic, flaccid, or ataxic dysarthria. This also seems to be the case in Duffy and Folger's patients and other reports in the literature. That some speech characteristics that are often associated with weakness, spasticity, and incoordination are present in this dysarthria makes sense on the basis of damaged structures and their presumed functions. Because its anatomic substrate is confined to one side of the brain, however, it also makes sense that UUMN dysarthria is not identical to other dysarthria types that have already been discussed.

Acoustic and physiologic findings

As might be expected, acoustic and physiologic studies of patients with UUMN dysarthria are limited. In fact, the work of Hartman and Abbs (1992) is the only such published study. A few papers have examined some physiologic parameters of components of the speech system during nonspeech tasks, but without regard to the presence of dysarthria.

Hartman and Abbs (1992) obtained electromyographic (EMG) and strength and nasal pressure measures from the jaw, lip, tongue, and nares of six patients with UUMN lesions and dysarthria. Tongue force and nasal pressure data did not clearly distinguish the dysarthric from control subjects. EMG measures were reduced in magnitude on the side of the jaw contralateral to the lesion and reduced force of jaw movement was present in most of the patients.* Most also had reduced activity and/or strength in the lower lip contralateral to their lesion. These findings are in agreement with clinical observations of lower facial weakness in many patients with UUMN lesions and dysarthria, and the presence of unilateral jaw weakness in some.

Acoustic measures of speech AMRs demonstrated slowed and abnormally irregular AMRs.

---

*Crucci, Fornarelli, and Manfredi (1988) found evidence of reduced electromyographic activity of the masseter at maximum strength on the side of the jaw contralateral to the lesion in 15 hemiplegic patients. They concluded that even though the masticatory nucleus of the Vth nerve receives bilateral upper motor neuron input, the contralateral hemisphere exerts predominant control of voluntary activity.

Przedborski and others (1988) have presented data that document presence of abnormalities of parasternal intercostal muscle activity during voluntary respiratory activities shortly after the onset of middle cerebral artery strokes. They suggest that voluntary respiratory activities of intercostal muscles and the diaphragm are predominantly controlled by contralateral corticospinal pathways.

The slow AMRs were matched by perceptual ratings of AMRs, but irregular AMRs were not perceived in their patients (irregular AMRs were noted in some of Duffy and Folger's patients).

CASES

Case 9.1

A 55-year-old right-handed man was admitted to the hospital with a four-day history of progressive right hemiparesis and dysarthria. Neurologic evaluation revealed dysarthria and a dense right hemiparesis and mild sensory loss in the right face and upper limb. Computed tomography (CT) scan showed evidence of an infarct in the posterior limb of the left internal capsule.

Speech evaluation two and a half weeks after onset revealed a right central facial weakness. Speech was characterized by: imprecise articulation (2,3); harsh voice quality (0,1); slow speech AMRs (−1,2). Intelligibility was moderately reduced. There was no evidence of aphasia or any other cognitive disturbance.

The clinician concluded, "Flaccid dysarthria, UUMN type." The patient was seen for only one session of speech therapy before his discharge from the hospital. He did not return for follow-up.

Commentary. (1) UUMN dysarthria commonly affects articulation and sometimes voice quality. (2) It can be associated with moderate reductions of speech intelligibility. (3) The internal capsule is a common site for lesions that cause UUMN dysarthria. Isolated internal capsule lesions in the dominant hemisphere are rarely, if ever, associated with aphasic language impairment or other cognitive disturbances.

Case 9.2

A 70-year-old right-handed man was admitted to the hospital with the sudden onset of inability to express himself, a right facial droop, and weakness in his right upper extremity. History and clinical evaluation were consistent with a middle cerebral artery stroke. Computed tomography scan identified an area of decreased attenuation in the left frontal lobe consistent with recent infarction.

Speech and language evaluation three days postonset revealed a mild-moderate aphasia with deficits apparent in verbal formulation and comprehension, as well as reading and writing. Verbal communication, however, was functional. Right facial and tongue weakness were apparent. There was no evidence of apraxia of speech. The patient's speech was characterized by: imprecise articulation (1); reduced loudness (0,1); hoarseness (1,2). Speech intelligibility was normal. The patient began speech-language therapy. Within one week his dysarthria had resolved and the only evidence of aphasia was infrequent word-finding difficulties.

Commentary. (1) UUMN dysarthria associated with dominant hemisphere lesions is frequently associated with aphasia. In this case, the dysarthria and aphasia were about equal in severity at onset. (2) UUMN dysarthria frequently resolves rapidly and completely (in this case, within one week postonset). (3) The frontal lobe is most often implicated when UUMN dysarthria is the result of a cortical lesion.

Case 9.3

A 73-year-old right-handed man was admitted to the hospital with a one-day history of slurred speech and difficulty using his right hand. Neurologic examination demonstrated only dysarthria and mild right upper extremity weakness and clumsiness. The neurologist felt the patient's presentation was consistent with a "dysarthria-clumsy hand syndrome." Subsequent CT scan demonstrated a lacunar infarct in the area of the left lateral basal ganglia and centrum semiovale.

Speech examination the following day identified very mild right lower central facial weakness and mild deviation of the tongue to the right on protrusion. Speech was characterized by: breathy-hoarse voice quality (0,1); reduced loudness (−1,2); irregular articulatory breakdowns (2); monopitch and loudness (1,2); and equivocal acceleration of speech rate. Speech AMRs were normal in rate but imprecise (1,2) and irregular (2). Speech intelligibility was moderately reduced. There was no evidence of aphasia or apraxia of speech.

The clinician concluded that the patient had "a moderately severe UUMN dysarthria." Speech therapy was recommended and improvement in speech was noted prior to discharge several days later. There was no evidence of aphasia or apraxia of speech.

Commentary. (1) UUMN dysarthria can be the only or among only a few symptoms of unilateral neurologic disease. (2) UUMN dysarthria is often associated with subcortical lesions.

Case 9.4

A 57-year-old man was seen in the clinic for evaluation of residual symptoms stemming from a "stroke" about three years earlier. Neurologic examination revealed dysarthria and left hemiparesis. The neurologist concluded that the patient had a "pure motor hemiparesis, almost like a capsular infarct."

Speech evaluation revealed mild left lower face and tongue weakness. Speech was characterized by: imprecise articulation and imprecise AMRs (1). Articulatory precision improved noticeably with a moderate slowing of speech rate. Phonation and resonance were normal.

The clinician concluded that the patient demonstrated a "mild UUMN dysarthria." Some time was spent demonstrating to the patient the advantages of slowing his speech rate. He appreciated the benefits of this speaking strategy but did not believe speech therapy was necessary. The clinician agreed.

Commentary. (1) UUMN dysarthria can result from lesions on the right or the left side of the brain. (2) It can persist long after the spontaneous recovery period. (3) Persisting UUMN dysarthria is often mild and usually does not require speech therapy.

Case 9.5

An 81-year-old right-handed man was admitted to the hospital with a two-day history of "garbled speech" and left facial weakness. Neurologic examination revealed left facial weakness and mild left upper extremity

weakness. Computed tomography scan one week after onset revealed a lesion in the right posterior frontal lobe that was consistent with an area of recent infarct. A complete neurologic work-up led to a right carotid endarterectomy two weeks later, without any deterioration in neurologic status.

Speech evaluation 12 days after surgery demonstrated a left central facial weakness (2,3) and deviation of the tongue to the left on protrusion. The patient wore loose-fitting dentures. Speech was characterized by: hoarse-rough voice quality (2); imprecise articulation (1); occasional acceleration of speech rate (1,2); slowed and imprecise AMRs (0,1). Speech intelligibility was, at worst, mildly reduced. The patient believed his speech was quite adequate and did not wish speech therapy. His wife and daughter felt that his speech was almost back to his pre-stroke level and they had only occasional mild difficulty understanding him. Although the clinician felt that he might benefit from speech therapy, the patient was not pushed to pursue it.

Commentary. (1) UUMN dysarthria can affect voice quality as well as articulation in some cases. (2) The effects of dysarthria on intelligibility can be exacerbated by nonneurologic factors, such as loose-fitting dentures. Problems with dentures frequently become more pronounced after a stroke that affects oromotor function and can present additional barriers to adequate articulation. (3) Recommendations for speech therapy must consider both the patient's needs and wishes, as well as the clinician's judgment about the need for therapy.

Case 9.6

A 66-year-old right-handed man with a 20-year history of hypertension was admitted to the hospital after the sudden onset of right hemiplegia, right facial weakness, and inability to speak. A CT scan three weeks postonset showed an area of low attenuation in the left centrum semiovale that extended down into the adjacent lentiform nucleus, consistent with an infarct.

Language examination three weeks postonset was normal. The patient had a right lower facial weakness. The tongue was normal on protrusion but lateral movements were mildly slowed. Voice quality was harsh-breathy (1). Articulation was imprecise (1). In addition, the patient occasionally repeated the first phoneme of a word and was mildly hesitant, but there were no obvious trial-and-error misarticulations or clear-cut substitutions of sounds. The clinician concluded that the patient had a "flaccid, UUMN dysarthria." The possible presence of an accompanying apraxia of speech was mentioned but evidence for it was considered equivocal. The patient received four sessions of speech therapy that focused on improving articulation through increased self-monitoring and slowing of rate. He improved and asked that therapy be terminated so that he could devote more time to physical therapy.

Commentary. (1) UUMN dysarthria is often associated with subcortical lesions. (2) When the lesion is in the presumed dominant hemisphere, questions about the presence of aphasia and apraxia of speech often arise. There was no evidence of aphasia in this patient, but he did exhibit a few speech characteristics that were *suggestive of apraxia of speech. Although it was concluded that apraxia of speech was not present, this case illustrates the difficulty that may be encountered in distinguishing between dysarthria and apraxia of speech. Both disorders can co-occur in patients with unilateral left hemisphere lesions. (3) Improvement in speech is usually noted in patients with UUMN dysarthria. It is not unusual for patients to terminate therapy on their own once speech becomes intelligible and sufficiently efficient. Evidence of dysarthria may persist, however.*

SUMMARY

1. UUMN dysarthria results from unilateral damage to the UMN pathway. Its diagnosis as a primary communication disorder occurs at a frequency comparable to that of other major single dysarthria types. It is primarily manifest in articulation, but phonation and prosody may also be affected.
2. The anatomic designation of this dysarthria type is based on the locus of lesions associated with it. The fact that its clinical characteristics and pathophysiologic underpinnings are not well described or understood prevents a pathophysiologic designation for the disorder at this time. It is possible, however, that its deviant characteristics reflect the effects of weakness and perhaps incoordination of tongue and lower face movements during speech.
3. Stroke is the most common cause of UUMN dysarthria. Lesions on either side of the brain anywhere along the UMN pathway from the cortex to the brain stem can cause it, but the majority of lesions are in the cerebral hemispheres, most often in the posterior frontal lobe or the internal capsule or related white matter pathways.
4. Lower facial weakness and hemiparesis very often accompany UUMN dysarthria. Contralateral lingual weakness is not uncommon, and drooling and dysphagia may occur.
5. UUMN dysarthria is usually only mild to moderate in severity and recovery from it is often quite good. However, it sometimes is marked in severity and can persist as a significant deficit beyond the period of spontaneous recovery.
6. The most common deviant speech characteristics are imprecise articulation and irregular articulatory breakdowns, both of which may be apparent during contextual speech and AMRs. Speech rate may be slow. Dysphonia may be present in the form of harshness and reduced loudness, and mild hypernasality is present in some cases.
7. Physiologic studies have documented unilaterally reduced strength and force of jaw and lip movements, and acoustic analyses have confirmed reduced rate and irregular AMRs.
8. UUMN dysarthria can be the only or among the first and most prominent signs of neurologic disease. Its recognition and correlation with UUMN dysfunction can aid the localization and diagnosis of neurologic disease. Improved understanding of this dysarthria may assist efforts to study other speech and communication deficits that may be associated with unilateral neurologic disease, disorders whose manifestations may be masked, compounded, or comfounded by UUMN dysarthria.

REFERENCES

Alexander M and LoVerme S: Aphasia after left intracerebral hemorrhage, Neurology 30:1193, 1980.

Arboix A and Martí-Vilalta JL: Lacunar infarctions and dysarthria, Arch Neurol 47:127, 1990.

Arboix A, Martí-Vilalta JL, and Garcia JH: Clinical study of 227 patients with lacunar infarcts, Stroke 21:842, 1990.

Arboix A, Massons J, Oliveres M, and Titus F: Isolated dysarthria, Stroke 22(6):531, 1991.

Aronson AE: Clinical voice disorders, New York, 1990, Thieme.

Attig E: Parieto-cerebellar loop impairment in ataxic hemiparesis: proposed pathophysiology based on an analysis of cerebral blood flow, Can J Neurol Sci 21:15, 1994.

Benke T and Kertesz A: Hemispheric mechanisms of motor speech, Aphasiology 3:627, 1989.

Bogousslavsky J and Regli F: Capsular genu syndrome, Neurology 40:1499, 1990.

Brodal A: Self-observations and neuro-anatomical considerations after a stroke, Brain 96:675, 1973.

Chamorro A and others: Clinical-computed tomographic correlations of lacunar infarction in the Stroke Data Bank, Stroke 22:175, 1991.

Cruccu G, Fornarelli M, and Manfredi M: Impairment of masticatory function in hemiplegia, Neurology 38:301, 1988.

Damasio AR and others: Aphasia with nonhemorrhagic lesions in the basal ganglia and internal capsule, Arch Neurol 39:15, 1982.

Damasio H, Eslinger P, and Adams HP: Aphasia following basal ganglia lesions: new evidence, Semin Neurol 4:151, 1984.

Darley FL, Aronson AE, and Brown JR: Motor speech disorders, Philadelphia, 1975, WB Saunders.

DeJong RN: Case taking and the neurologic examination. In Baker AB and Joynt RJ, editors: Clinical neurology, vol 1, Philadelphia, 1986, Harper and Row.

Dobkin JA and others: Evidence for transhemispheric diaschisis in unilateral stroke, Arch Neurol 46:1333, 1989.

Duffy JR and Folger WN: Dysarthria in unilateral central nervous system lesions. Paper presented at the annual convention of the American Speech-Language-Hearing Association, Detroit, November 1986.

Fisher CM: Ataxic hemiparesis, Arch Neurol 35:126, 1978.

Fisher CM: Lacunar strokes and infarcts: a review, Neurology 32:871, 1982.

Fries W and others: Motor recovery following capsular stroke, Brain 116:369, 1993.

Fromm D and others: Various consequences of subcortical stroke: prospective study of 16 consecutive cases, Arch Neurol 42:943, 1985.

Hartman DE and Abbs JH: Dysarthria associated with focal unilateral upper motor neuron lesion, Eur J Disord Commun 27:187, 1992.

Horner J and Massey W: Silent aspiration following stroke, Neurology 38:317, 1988.

Horner J and others: Aspiration following stroke: clinical correlates and outcome, Neurology 38:1359, 1988.

Huang C and Broe G: Isolated facial palsy: a new lacunar syndrome, J Neurol Neurosurg Psychiatry 47:84, 1984.

Huang CY and Lui FS: Ataxic-hemiparesis, localization and clinical features, Stroke 15:363, 1984.

Ichikawa K and Kageyama Y: Clinical anatomic study of pure dysarthria, Stroke 22:809, 1991.

Koppel BS and Weinberger G: Pontine infarction producing dysarthria-clumsy hand syndrome and ataxic hemiparesis, Eur Neurol 26:211, 1987.

Landau WM: Ataxic hemiparesis: special deluxe stroke or standard brand? Neurology 38:1799, 1988.

Meadows JC: Dysphagia in unilateral cerebral lesions, J Neurol Neurosurg Psychiatry 36:853, 1973.

Melo TP and others: Pure motor stroke: a reappraisal, Neurology 42:789, 1992.

Metter EJ: Speech disorders: clinical evaluation and diagnosis, Jamaica, NY, 1985, Spectrum Publications.

Metter EJ and others: Comparison of metabolic rates, language, and memory in subcortical aphasias, Brain Lang 19:33, 1983.

Metter EJ and others: Left hemisphere intracerebral hemorrhages studied by (F-18)-fluorodeoxyglucose PET, Neurology 36:1155, 1986.

Mohr JP: Lacunes, Stroke 13:3, 1982.

Mori E and others: Ataxic hemiparesis from small capsular hemorrhage: computed tomography and somatosensory evoked potentials, Arch Neurol 41:1050, 1984.

Naeser MA and others: Aphasia with predominantly subcortical lesion sites: description of three capsular/putaminal aphasia syndromes, Arch Neurol 39:2, 1982.

Ozaki I and others: Capsular genu syndrome, Neurology 41:1853, 1991.

Ozaki I and others: Pure dysarthria due to anterior internal capsule and/or corona radiata infarction: a report of five cases, J Neurol Neurosurg Psychiatry 49:1435, 1986.

Przedborski S and others: The effect of acute hemiplegia on intercostal muscle activity, Neurology 38:1882, 1988.

Ropper AH: Severe dysarthria with right hemisphere stroke, Neurology 37:1061, 1987.

Spertell RB and Ransom BR: Dysarthria-clumsy hand syndrome produced by capsular infarct, Ann Neurol 6:263, 1979.

Verma AK and Maheshwari MC: Hypesthetic-ataxic-hemiparesis in thalamic hemorrhage, Stroke 17:49, 1986.

Willoughby EW and Anderson NE: Lower cranial nerve motor function in unilateral vascular lesions of the cerebral hemisphere, Brit Med J 289:791, 1984.

Yorkston KM, Beukelman D, Bell K: Clinical management of dysarthric speakers, San Diego, 1988, College-Hill.

10 Mixed Dysarthrias

Imposing functional and anatomic divisions on the nervous system helps our attempts to understand the brain's operations. It also establishes a framework for localizing and categorizing nervous system diseases. Unfortunately, no rule of nature obligates neurologic disease to restrict itself to the divisions we impose upon it. As a result, the effects of neurologic disease can be "mixed" and spread across two or more divisions of the nervous system.

The frequent refusal of neurologic disease to be focal and compartmentalized applies to its effects on speech. Chapters 4 through 9 focused on "pure" dysarthrias that reflect damage to only one of the divisions of the motor speech system. For practical clinical purposes at least, many people do have only a single type of dysarthria. However, dysarthria often is not pure because the damage that has caused it is not limited to a single motor system disturbance. Therefore, many people with dysarthria have a *mixed dysarthria,* that is, a combination of two or more of the pure types that have already been discussed.

Mixed dysarthrias are common. They are encountered as the primary speech pathology in a large medical practice at a rate considerably higher than that for any of the single dysarthria types. From 1987 to 1990 at the Mayo Clinic, mixed dysarthrias accounted for 34.7% of all dysarthrias and 31.6% of all motor speech disorders seen in the section of speech pathology (Figure 1–3).

Does the fact that many dysarthrias are mixed minimize the value of categorizing them into types? No. In fact, because dysarthrias reflect underlying neuropathology, recognition of the mixed forms is also valuable to neurologic localization and diagnosis. For example, a patient with a diagnosis of Parkinson's disease (PD) who has a mixed hypokinetic-ataxic dysarthria may not have PD, or may have more than PD, because PD should not be associated with ataxic dysarthria. Therefore, the recognition of each component of a mixed dysarthria may help to rule out certain neurologic diagnoses or make other diagnoses more likely.

Mixed dysarthrias represent a heterogeneous group of speech disorders and neurologic diseases. Virtually any combination of two or more of the pure dysarthria types is possible, and in any particular mix any one of the components may predominate. In spite of its heterogeneity, and the fact that sorting out the various components of mixed dysarthrias can be quite difficult, many mixed dysarthrias are perceptually distinguishable. And, like pure forms, they may be the first or among the first signs of neurologic disease.

In this chapter, common etiologies of mixed dysarthrias will be reviewed, with an emphasis on diseases that are frequently encountered in neurology and medical speech pathology practices. The most common types of mixed dysarthrias and their relation to specific neurologic diseases also will be addressed. Finally, the mixed dysarthrias that are encountered in several specific neurologic diseases will be discussed because they have been studied sufficiently to permit clinical descriptions of their most salient characteristics. Their descriptions will help document that they are lawfully derived from diseases that affect more than one component of the nervous system.

ETIOLOGIES

Mixed dysarthrias can be caused by many conditions within each of the broad categories of neurologic disease. More than any other dysarthria type, mixed dysarthrias can result from the occurrence of more than one neurologic event (for example, multiple strokes) or the co-occurrence of two or more neurologic diseases (for example, stroke plus Parkinson's disease). Moreover, they occur commonly in a number of degenerative diseases that affect more than one portion of the nervous system.

In this section, attention will be given to conditions that may cause mixed dysarthrias more frequently than any single dysarthria type. The definitions and descriptions of conditions whose speech manifestations have been studied in some detail will be emphasized. The specific speech characteristics associated with several of these disorders will be addressed in the section covering speech pathology.

Degenerative diseases

A number of degenerative diseases are commonly associated with mixed dysarthrias because they tend to affect more than one portion of the motor system. Some of these diseases primarily affect motor functions; others are more diffuse in their effects, producing sensory, autonomic, and cognitive deficits as well.

Motor neuron disease: amyotrophic lateral sclerosis. Motor neuron diseases (MNDs) are a group of disorders that primarily affect motor neurons or anterior horn cells. They include spinal muscle atrophy, progressive bulbar palsy, and amyotrophic lateral sclerosis (ALS), all of which appear to be variations of the same disorder (Rowland, 1991; Williams and Windebank, 1991).*

Spinal muscle atrophy is a syndrome of limb wasting and weakness, with or without cranial nerve weakness and without evidence of upper motor neuron (UMN) involvement. Because it does not usually affect speech, and is associated with flaccid and not mixed dysarthria when it does, it will not be discussed further.

Progressive bulbar palsy (PBP) is a syndrome dominated by LMN weakness of cranial nerve muscles. Dysarthria and dysphagia are its predominant signs. The UMN signs in the bulbar muscles may or may not be present (Rowland,

1991). When PBP is confined to the LMNs, it is associated with flaccid, not mixed dysarthria. In this chapter, the term *amyotrophic lateral sclerosis* is preferred to PBP (in a sense, PBP can be thought of as ALS without limb involvement).

Amyotrophic lateral sclerosis is characterized by UMN and LMN signs that may affect the limbs and the bulbar muscles (Rowland, 1980). The terms ALS and MND are often used interchangeably, but ALS is preferred here. Because ALS represents a mixed UMN and LMN disease that often affects the bulbar muscles, it has a natural and common association with mixed *spastic-flaccid* dysarthria.

The incidence of ALS is about 1.3 per 100,000 (Kurtzke, 1991). Males are affected more than females (2:1). It is usually difficult to establish time of onset of ALS because more than half of anterior horn cells must be lost before weakness is apparent and because patients may adapt well to weakness (Mulder, 1982). About 80% of affected individuals develop symptoms between 40 and 70 years of age. Median age of onset is about 55 years, and peak rate of occurrence is between 60 and 70 years (Kurtzke, 1991; Mulder, 1982; Rowland, 1980). The course of the disease is usually 1 to 5 years, with median survival of about 3 years, although some patients survive for 10 to 20 years (Mulder, 1982). It usually occurs sporadically, so most cases probably have one or more exogenous, environmental causes. Viral and immunologic theories are numerous. About 5% of cases are familial, with a pattern suggestive of autosomal dominance (Rowland, 1991).

The diagnosis of ALS is made on the basis of its clinical profile and electrophysiologic confirmation. Clinical features include fatigue, cramping, fasciculations, weakness, and muscle atrophy, as well as hyperactive deep tendon reflexes with spasticity (weakness is often focal initially). Eye movements, bowel and bladder control, and autonomic and cognitive functions are usually spared, although some patients have an accompanying dementia (Caselli and others, 1993; Mulder, 1982). Electromyographic (EMG) findings of denervation (fibrillations) and reinervation (large polyphasic motor unit action potentials) from two or more extremities (with the bulbar muscles counted as an extremity) are considered diagnostic of the disease (Rowland, 1991).

Although its first signs and symptoms are usually in the limbs, about *30% of patients have their initial problems in the bulbar muscles* (Rose, 1977), *most often represented by dysarthria and dysphagia*. Patients with bulbar deficits as the first symptoms tend to have a more rapid course because dysphagia and airway obstruction represent

---

Primary lateral sclerosis (PLS) is sometimes grouped with motor neuron diseases, and it may be difficult to distinguish from ALS. It is characterized by corticospinal and corticobulbar tract signs but has no lower motor neuron involvement. It may be associated with spastic dysarthria and was discussed in Chapter 5.

major threats to life. If respiratory muscles are prominently involved, decreased ventilation is also life-threatening. Death from ALS usually is related to respiratory failure or infection (Mulder, 1982).

Neuropathologically, ALS is associated with selective loss of motor neurons. This is evident in the large pyramidal cells in the precentral and postcentral cortex, the corticospinal tracts, motor nuclei of cranial nerves, and anterior horns of the spinal cord. Atrophic large myelinated and unmyelinated peripheral nervous system (PNS) fibers and evidence of denervation are also present (Hughes, 1982; Williams and Windebank, 1991).

Multiple sclerosis. Multiple sclerosis (MS) is the most common of acquired demyelinating central nervous system (CNS) diseases. Its cause is unknown, but evidence suggests that an exogenous agent (a virus) may be important in triggering demyelination (Rodriguez, 1989).

The reported incidence of MS is 58 per 100,000. It affects women more frequently than men. It usually begins between 20 and 40 years of age, with onset unusual before age 20 and after age 60 (Smith and Scheinberg, 1985).

Multiple sclerosis can produce a great variety of signs and symptoms because the lesions associated with it are often multiple and disseminated. Problems with gait and sphincter control are common, as are visual and other sensory difficulties. Cerebellar dysfunction is often, although not invariably, associated with MS; dysarthria, nystagmus, and intention tremor are some of its major manifestations. Cranial nerve abnormalities may occur and can include trigeminal neuralgia, Bell's palsy, and facial myokymia.

Cognitive deficits, previously thought to be uncommon, may occur in as many as 25% of patients with progressive MS (Smith and Scheinberg, 1985). Memory and conceptual abilities may be preferentially impaired. Psychiatric problems are not unusual. They most often involve affective disorders, which may be a direct consequence of the demyelinating process or a reaction to the disability caused by the disease (Petersen and Kokmen, 1989). Aphasia and apraxia of speech are rare but have been reported (Henderscheê, Stam, and Derix, 1987; Olmos-Lau, Ginsberg, and Geller, 1977; Poser, 1978), as have difficulties with higher-level language functions that are not specifically aphasic in character (Lethlean and Murdoch, 1993).

Diagnosis can be quite difficult, and approximately 10% of MS patients are misdiagnosed (Herndon, 1990). Its distinction from brain tumors and psychiatric disturbances can be particularly difficult; for example, MS is sometimes misdiag-

nosed as hysteria (Herndon and Brooks, 1985; Schiffer and Slater, 1985).

Diagnostic criteria generally include evidence of lesions in two or more CNS locations, primarily affecting white matter, and evidence of two or more episodes that are a month or more apart, or a 6-month history of progressive signs and symptoms (Smith and Scheinberg, 1985). Magnetic resonance imaging (MRI) may provide the best evidence of MS because of its sensitivity to white matter lesions, but cerebrospinal fluid examination, visual and auditory evoked potentials, and computed tomography (CT) scanning are also helpful in diagnosis (Sibley, 1985).

The course of MS is unpredictable. Some patients have a benign course, experiencing a single episode or only a few attacks, with complete or nearly complete remission. Others have an exacerbating-remitting course, with episodes of deterioration followed by near-complete recovery, a pattern that may persist for years. Still others have a remitting-progressive course with a slow accumulation of deficits. Finally, some have a progressing course, with the insidious onset and slow progression of disease without remission (Smith and Scheinberg, 1985).

Multiple sclerosis affects scattered areas of the nervous system, with a predilection for white matter and periventricular areas, the brainstem, spinal cord, and optic nerves. Myelinated fibers in gray matter may also be affected (Herndon, 1985). Multiple sclerosis plaques are characterized by primary demyelination (destruction of myelin sheaths with preservation of axons) and death of oligodendrocytes (the cells that produce myelin) in the center of the lesion (Rodriguez, 1989). Some lesions may be acute, with active myelin breakdown, whereas others reflect chronic, inactive demyelinated glial scars. In acute plaques, edema occurs in the area of affected nerve fibers. Resolution of edema may explain some of the recovery from deficits after an exacerbation.

Dysphagia is relatively uncommon in patients who are ambulatory but does occur in others (Matthews and others, 1985). Dysarthria tends to be uncommon at the onset of the disease but sometimes is the presenting symptom (see Chapter 6 for a discussion of paroxysmal ataxic dysarthria). When present, dysarthria may reflect nearly any *single type or combination of single types.* A *spastic-ataxic* dysarthria may be the most common mixed dysarthria associated with MS, but it should not be considered *the* dysarthria of MS.

Friedreich's ataxia. Friedreich's ataxia is an inherited degenerative disease that is predominantly spinocerebellar, but it may also be associated with spasticity, lower motor neuron (LMN) weakness, and extrapyramidal movement disorders. It was discussed in Chapter 6 (Ataxic Dysarthria), but it clearly can be associated with mixed dysarthria, most often *ataxic* and *spastic* dysarthria.

Progressive supranuclear palsy. Also known as Steele-Richardson-Olszewski syndrome, progressive supranuclear palsy (PSP) is a nonfamilial, degenerative neurologic disease. It is often mistaken for PD or, less frequently, Alzheimer's disease or a multiinfarct state. It typically develops in the sixth decade, with death usually occurring within 10 years (Jankovic, 1984).

Supranuclear ophthalmoparesis (paralysis of vertical gaze, especially downgaze) is the distinguishing feature of PSP, but the gaze palsy is not always the first symptom (Kleinschmidt-DeMasters, 1989). Initial complaints often include gait difficulty and postural instability and falling. The constellation of vertical gaze palsy, parkinsonian symptoms (bradykinesia and rigidity), postural instability, and pseudobulbar palsy usually suggest the diagnosis (Jankovic, 1984; Lees, 1987). Unlike PD, tremor is usually absent in PSP.

Most patients with PSP develop dysarthria, dysphagia, drooling, and pseudobulbar affect. Behavioral changes, including irritability and depression, as well as cognitive changes, are not uncommon. Cognitive changes tend to be related to prefrontal lobe impairments (Grafman and others, 1990; Maher, Smith, and Lees, 1985).

Pathologically, PSP is associated with neuronal atrophy, especially in the brain stem and cerebellum. Ventricular dilatation and neurofibrillary tangles are typically present. The most severely affected areas include the subthalamic nucleus, red nucleus, substantia nigra, globus pallidus, superior colliculi, and, often, a number of brainstem nuclei. The cranial nerves and the cerebral cortex, with the exception of the frontal lobes, are usually spared (Lees, 1987).

The clinical signs and pathology of PSP are indicative of multisystem degeneration. Several dysarthria types are possible, and mixed dysarthria frequently occurs, most often in the form of various combinations of *hypokinetic, spastic,* and *ataxic* types.

*Shy-Drager syndrome.** Shy-Drager syndrome (SDS) is a progressive neurologic disease of un-

known etiology that affects the motor components of the autonomic and somatic divisions of the CNS. Its earliest signs are usually orthostatic hypotension (a decrease in blood pressure upon standing), incontinence, decreased respiration, and impotence, all which reflect autonomic nervous system involvement. Additional signs may include gait disturbance, generalized weakness, limb tremor, dysarthria and dysphagia, and laryngeal stridor. The various motor manifestations of the disease can occur singly or in combination. If the autonomic manifestations go undetected, the disease may be misdiagnosed as cerebellar degeneration or PD.

The most common types of dysarthria associated with SDS are *hypokinetic, ataxic, spastic,* and *flaccid.*

Olivopontocerebellar atrophy. Olivopontocerebellar atrophy (OPCA) is a degenerative neurologic disease that usually begins in the fifth decade. Its essential features are cerebellar dysfunction and extrapyramidal, parkinsonian features. Corticospinal tract signs and peripheral neuropathy, including the bulbar cranial nerve nuclei, can be present (Konigsmark and Weiner, 1970; Landis and others, 1974). Some of the more variably present deficits include dementia and palatal myoclonus (Duvoisin, 1987).

Degeneration in the middle cerebellar peduncles, cerebellar white matter and Purkinje cells, and pontine, olivary, and arcuate nuclei is usually extensive (Adams and Victor, 1991; Duvoisin, 1987). The disease appears closely related to a condition known as *spinocerebellar degeneration,* in which corticospinal features also occur (Adams and Victor, 1991). Olivopontocerebellar atrophy may be difficult to distinguish from PD (see Chapter 7) and striatonigral degeneration (discussed in the next section).

Dysarthria has received little attention although it occurs commonly in OPCA (Landis and others, 1974). Considering the areas of the motor system that may be affected, however, various combinations of *ataxic, spastic, hypokinetic,* and *flaccid* dysarthria seem possible.

Striatonigral degeneration. Striatonigral degeneration is closely related to PD, but it has a different pathologic basis and can have different clinical manifestations. It is usually initially associated with unilateral rigidity, stiffness, and akinesia, which then spread to the other side and progress. A flexed posture, slowness of movement, poor balance, a tendency to faint, and dysarthria are often noted. There are usually no cerebellar signs and no tremor or involuntary movements. Postmortem examination reveals degenerative

---

*Patients with a combination of symptoms of Shy-Drager syndrome, olivopontocerebellar atrophy, and striatonigral degeneration are not uncommon. Because of this overlap, it has been argued that these disorders should be grouped under the single heading of *multiple systems atrophy* (Quinn, 1989).

changes and neuronal loss in the putamen and caudate nucleus, and also in the substantia nigra (Adams and Victor, 1991).

The dysarthrias of striatonigral degeneration have not been investigated. At the least, *hypokinetic* dysarthria would be anticipated, but the co-occurrence of *hyperkinetic* and perhaps *spastic* dysarthria might be possible.

Corticobasal degeneration. Corticobasal degeneration is a progressive disease of unknown etiology that is characterized by variable combinations of rigidity, tremor, spasticity, mild cerebellar signs, and significant difficulty with the voluntary control of movement (apraxia). Cognitive changes may occur in later stages of the disease. Postmortem examination reveals cortical atrophy (usually frontal motor, premotor, and parietal) and nerve cell loss in the substantia nigra, thalamus, lentiform, subthalamic, and red nuclei, midbrain tegmentum, and locus ceruleus (Gibb, Luthert, and Marsden, 1989). The disorder is sometimes asymmetric in its presentation and course (Adams and Victor, 1991).

The motor speech disorders associated with corticobasal degeneration have not been studied, but dysarthria may be fairly common. For example, Riley and others (1990) reported its presence in 7 of their 15 patients, and Gibb, Luthert, and Marsden (1989) reported its presence in two of their three patients. Clinical observations suggest that *hypokinetic, spastic, ataxic,* and, perhaps, *hyperkinetic* dysarthria, singly or in combination, may occur. *Apraxia of speech* may also be present, either as the sole motor speech disorder or in combination with dysarthria.

Toxic-metabolic conditions

When toxic and metabolic diseases alter neurologic functions, their effects tend to be diffuse. When they affect the motor system, they commonly affect more than one of its components. When motor speech is affected, the result is often a mixed dysarthria. Some toxic-metabolic conditions that may be associated with mixed dysarthrias are described in this section.

Wilson's disease. Wilson's disease (WD) is a rare autosomal recessive genetic metabolic disorder associated with inadequate processing of dietary copper. It is also known as *hepatolenticular degeneration* or *progressive lenticular degeneration* to indicate liver involvement and the consistent postmortem findings of degeneration in the lenticular nuclei of the basal ganglia. The metabolic inadequacy in WD leads to a build-up of copper in the liver, brain, and cornea of the eye, with the appearance of neuromotor signs by late adolescence or early adulthood. Patients who go

untreated may become anarthric. It can be fatal if it goes undiagnosed (Adams and Victor, 1991).

Wilson's disease may present with a hepatic (liver) or neurologic disturbance or less frequently as a psychiatric illness (Topaloglu and others, 1990). The one pathognomonic sign of WD is a golden brown ring (Kayser-Fleischer rings) around the cornea of the eyes, reflecting copper deposits. Its classic neurologic manifestations are confined to motor systems and include a bizarre, wing-beating tremor when the arms are outstretched, trunkal rigidity and slowness of movement, drooling, dysphagia, dysarthria, ataxia, and facial masking or a grinning, vacuous smile (Adams and Victor, 1991). Basal ganglia symptoms usually predominate, but cerebellar deficits are sometimes most obvious (Menkes, 1989). A CT scan may show enlarged lateral ventricles, widening of cerebellar sulci, a shrunken-appearing brain stem, and hypodensity in the area of the basal ganglia and thalamus (Adams and Victor, 1991; Menkes, 1989). The basal ganglia are usually the most severely affected structures. If diagnosed before permanent damage occurs, a low copper diet, potassium sulfide (to minimize copper absorption), and a chelating agent called D-penicillamine (to promote urinary excretion of copper) can restore a proper copper balance and reverse many of the neurologic manifestations (Menkes, 1989).

Abnormalities of the bulbar muscles are very common (Sternlieb, Giblin, and Scheinberg, 1987). *Dysarthria is considered a cardinal feature of WD,* and it may be its initial sign (Oder and others, 1991; Topaloglu and others, 1990). The most common types of dysarthria associated with WD are *hypokinetic, spastic,* and *ataxic.*

Hepatocerebral degeneration. Hepatocerebral degeneration can occur in people who have survived several episodes of hepatic coma or in patients with chronic liver disease. Common clinical manifestations include limb tremor, chorea or choreoathetosis in the face and limbs, unsteady gait, ataxia, and dysarthria. Corticospinal signs and mental deterioration may also be present. Pathologically, abnormalities are noted in the cerebral cortex, the lenticular nuclei, thalamus, and a number of brainstem nuclei. The lesions are similar to those encountered in Wilson's disease (Adams and Victor, 1991).

The dysarthrias associated with this condition have not been studied. The presence of *hyperkinetic, ataxic, spastic,* or *hypokinetic* forms seems possible.

Hypoxic encephalopathy. Hypoxic encephalopathy is a diffuse neurologic condition resulting from a lack of oxygen to the brain because of failure of the heart and circulation or failure of the lungs and respiration. There are many possible causes for these failures, but they most often involve suffocation (as from drowning or strangulation), carbon monoxide poisoning, diseases that paralyze respiratory muscles (such as Guillain-Barré), or damage the CNS diffusely (as in traumatic brain injury), myocardial infarction, or cardiac arrest.

In general, when consciousness is lost and oxygen deprivation exceeds 5 minutes, permanent neurologic damage occurs. If consciousness and responsiveness are regained, several posthypoxic syndromes may emerge, including dementia with or without signs of extrapyramidal involvement, visual agnosia, a parkinsonian syndrome with dementia, choreoathetosis, cerebellar ataxia, and action myoclonus (Adams and Victor, 1991).

The dysarthrias associated with hypoxic encephalopathy have not been investigated. The involvement of cortical, extrapyramidal, and cerebellar structures predicts the possible emergence of a number of dysarthria types that could include, at the least, *hypokinetic, hyperkinetic,* and *ataxic* forms, either singly or in combination.

Central pontine myelinolysis. Central pontine myelinolysis (CPM) is a serious metabolic condition characterized by destruction of myelin in the base of the pons. It also can affect the thalamus, subthalamus, amygdala, striatum, internal capsule, lateral geniculate bodies, white matter of the cerebellum, and deep layers of the cerebral cortex and adjacent white matter.

It is often associated with alcoholism and other conditions related to malnutrition, and it may occur in people with chronic liver or kidney disease. It is believed that the basis pontis and other affected structures may be especially susceptible to some acute metabolic fault, such as rapid correction or overcorrection of a profound electrolytic disturbance like hyponatremia (Adams and Victor, 1991; Mancall, 1989).

A variety of neurologic signs are possible in CPM, but quadriplegia, spasticity, dysarthria or anarthria, and pseudobulbar palsy are not uncommon.

The dysarthrias of CPM have not been studied. Clinical experience suggests that *spastic, ataxic,* and *hyperkinetic* forms, at the least, can occur.

Vascular disorders

Multiple cerebral infarcts that affect various components of the motor system have a natural association with mixed dysarthrias. They can literally produce any combination of mixed dysarthrias. Single brainstem strokes can also result in mixed dysarthrias because of the close proximity of pyramidal and extrapyramidal fibers, the cerebellar control circuit, and cranial nerve nuclei in that area of the brain. As a result, various combinations of *spastic, ataxic,* and *flaccid* dysarthria are not uncommon in brainstem infarcts. *Hyperkinetic* dysarthria (for example, secondary to palatal myoclonus) can also occur.

Trauma

The diffuse or multifocal lesions associated with closed head injuries (CHI) can produce virtually any combination of mixed dysarthrias. Trauma from neurosurgery, especially if it involves posterior fossa structures, can also result in a variety of mixed dysarthrias.

Tumor

Tumors, especially in the brain stem, can cause mixed dysarthrias because they can invade or produce mass effects on multiple components of the nervous system. Brainstem tumors can be associated with various combinations of *spastic, ataxic,* and *flaccid* dysarthria.

Infectious diseases

The diffuse or multifocal effects of infectious diseases such as meningitis, encephalitis, and AIDS can be associated with a wide variety of mixed dysarthrias. A specific example of one such infectious disease is *progressive multifocal leukoencephalopathy (PML).**

Progressive multifocal leukoencephalopathy is a rare, usually viral, demyelinating CNS disease that tends to occur in people with autoimmune disorders (for example, in AIDS and malignancies such as lymphoma and chronic lymphocytic leukemia) and in people who are immunocompromised by immunosuppressive therapy. The predominantly white matter lesions in PML are most prominent in cerebral subcortical areas and the corticomedullary junction. The cerebellum, optic nerves, and spinal cord can also be affected. Clinical features include hemiparesis, ataxia, visual and other sensory deficits, and speech, language, and cognitive problems (Krupp and others, 1985; Lethlean and Murdoch, 1993).

The dysarthrias of PML have not been studied in any detail. Lethlean and Murdoch (1993) described the language deficits of one woman with PML and noted the presence of severe dysarthria; its type was not identified, but its clinical features suggest it was mixed, possibly with spastic and ataxic components.

Kimmel and Schutt (1993) and Hook and others (1992) have described four cases with multifocal leukoencephalopathy in response to chemotherapy

---

*Leukoencephalopathy is also discussed briefly in Chapter 5.

(5-fluorouracil and levamisole) for colon cancer. Lesions were multiple and scattered throughout the cerebral cortex and brain stem. Of interest, the dysarthria (not described further) was among the initial manifestations of the condition, along with ataxia, diplopia, and confusion. The multiple lesion sites make it quite possible that the dysarthrias were mixed. The pathogenesis of the PML was unclear, but because patients improved when chemotherapy was discontinued, the investigators believed the syndrome reflected a toxic effect of chemotherapy. The course and outcome for the patients suggest that recognition of a developing dysarthria may be an early indication of neurotoxicity in this type of chemotherapy.

SPEECH PATHOLOGY

Sorting out the individual components of a mixed dysarthria can be difficult. Clinical uncertainty about all or some of the components of a mixed dysarthria probably occurs much more frequently than for the diagnosis of any single dysarthria type. It is not unusual, for example, to identify with confidence one of the components of a mixed dysarthria but to be uncertain if a second or third or fourth component is also present. Diagnostic impressions such as "the patient has an unambiguous mixed spastic-ataxic dysarthria, possibly with an accompanying flaccid component" or "ataxic dysarthria versus mixed spastic-ataxic dysarthria" are not unusual in clinical practice. This uncertainty probably reflects combinations of the shortcomings of perceptual (and acoustic and physiologic) methods, the natural overlap among manifestations of disease in different portions of the motor system, and the "true" equivocal presence of certain neurologic signs in some cases. The need to draw equivocal or qualified conclusions can be unsettling to the clinician's desire for certainty and precision, but there is little choice when uncertainty reflects clinical reality. It may be reassuring (or equally as unsettling) to know that clinical neurologic examinations frequently reach similar tenuous interpretations of signs and symptoms.

Table 10–1 summarizes the types of dysarthria that may be encountered in a number of neurologic diseases that can produce mixed dysarthrias. It may be useful for setting a range of expectations for types of dysarthria that may be present when a neurologic diagnosis is relatively unambiguous and for identifying mixed dysarthrias that may be incompatible with particular neurologic diagnoses. Chapter 15, which addresses differential diagnosis, will summarize distinctive features of each of the single dysarthria types in a manner that helps identify each of the components that make up a mixed dysarthria (in particular, see Tables 15–3 and 15–4).

In the remainder of this section, common etiologies of mixed dysarthrias and the most common mixed dysarthrias encountered in clinical practice will be discussed. The dysarthrias encountered in specific neurologic diseases, the speech characteristics of which have been studied in some detail will also be summarized.

Distribution of etiology, types, and severity in clinical practice

Etiologies. The box on p. 242 summarizes the etiologies for 300 quasirandomly selected cases seen at the Mayo Clinic with a primary speech pathology diagnosis of mixed dysarthria. The cautions expressed in Chapter 4 about generalizing these data to the general population or all speech pathology practices apply here as well.

The data establish that mixed dysarthrias can be caused by a wide variety of neurologic conditions. More than 60% of the cases were accounted for by degenerative diseases, and more than 80% were accounted for by degenerative, demyelinating, and vascular diseases.

By far, ALS was the most frequent degenerative neurologic disease associated with mixed dysarthria (41% of all cases).* Nine percent of cases clearly had degenerative CNS disease, but the diagnosis was otherwise nonspecific. The remaining degenerative cases were spread across nearly all of the neurologic degenerative diseases that were discussed earlier in this chapter.

Demyelinating diseases accounted for 6% of the cases. The majority of them had MS.

Multiple strokes accounted for about half of the vascular cases (12% of all cases). The sites of the strokes were widely distributed within the CNS and included both hemispheres, the brain stem, and cerebellum. The location of single strokes causing mixed dysarthria was nearly always in the brain stem.

Closed head injuries accounted for most of the traumatic etiologies. Lesions, when identifiable, were widely distributed in the brain, most often in subcortical areas, brain stem, or cerebellum. Tumors accounted for 4% of the cases; a majority of the tumors were located in the posterior fossa.

A combination of diseases accounted for about 4% of the cases. These included various combinations of vascular, inflammatory, degenerative, trau-

---

*Although this figure may approximate that encountered in large tertiary medical care centers, it is almost certainly an overestimate of the percentage of cases seen in speech pathology practices in rehabilitation or primary care settings.

Table 10–1 Types of dysarthria that may be present in neurologic diseases that can produce mixed dysarthrias.

	Dysarthria					
Disease	Flaccid	Spastic	Ataxic	Hypokinetic	Hyperkinetic	UUMN
Degenerative						
ALS	++	++	?	–	–	–
MS	+	+/++	+/++	+	+	+
Friedreich's ataxia	?	+	++	–	–	–
PSP	–	++	+	++	–	–
Shy-Drager syndrome	+	+/++	++	++	–	–
OPCA*	+	++	++	+/?	–	–
Striatonigral degeneration*	–	+/?	–	++	+/?	–
Corticobasal degeneration*†	–	+/++	+	+/++	?	?
Toxic-metabolic						
Wilson's disease	–	+/++	+/++	++	–	–
Hepatocerebral degeneration*	–	+/++	+/++	+/++	+/++	–
Hypoxic encephalopathy*	–	?	+/++	+/++	+/++	–
CPM*	–	++	+/++	–	+/++	–
Vascular†	+	+/++	+/++	+	+	+/++
Tumor*†	+	+	+	+/?	+/?	+
Infectious*†	+	+	+	+	+	+
Traumatic*†	+	+/++	+/++	+/++	+	+

Dysarthria is not inevitably present in all patients with these diseases; the list of diseases is not exhaustive.

ALS, amyotrophic lateral sclerosis; *CPM,* central pontine myelinolysis; *MS,* multiple sclerosis; *OPCA,* olivopontocerebellar atrophy; *PSP,* progressive supranuclear palsy.

++. Very often present when dysarthria is present and may be quite typical for a particular disease; +, sometimes present, but not necessarily "typical" for a particular disease; ?, very uncommon *or* of uncertain presence; –, not present.

* The dysarthria has not been explicitly studied in the particular disorder.

† Apraxia of speech may also be present.

matic and toxic-metabolic conditions. Toxic-metabolic and inflammatory etiologies, by themselves, were responsible for mixed dysarthrias in a small percentage of cases. Finally, about 4% of cases had undetermined neurologic diagnoses. The indeterminate nature of these disorders ranged from unexplained signs and symptoms (for example, dysarthria, dystonia, blepharospasm) to identifiable lesions of undetermined etiology (for example, undetermined posterior fossa lesion).

Types of mixed dysarthrias. A great variety of combinations of single types of dysarthria were encountered in the sample. A combination of two dysarthrias represented 84% of all cases of mixed dysarthria, 14% contained three dysarthria types, and 2% contained a combination of four types. The dominance of two dysarthria types in mixed dysarthria reflects either the "reality" of localization of neurologic disease in the sample or the limitations on auditory perceptual abilities to detect more than two dysarthria types in any one

person; a combination of these explanations is most likely.*

Table 10–2 summarizes the frequency of occurrence of each single dysarthria type within the sample. Because ALS was so prominent in the sample, the distributions for the entire sample and that portion of the sample exclusive of ALS cases are given.

For the entire sample, spastic dysarthria was the most common single type encountered; it was present in 91% of the cases. Flaccid and ataxic dysarthria were present in 54% and 43% of the cases, respectively. Hypokinetic and hyperkinetic dysarthria were encountered less frequently, in 21% and 13% of the cases, respectively.

*The difficulty that can be encountered in sorting out types in mixed dysarthrias is highlighted by the fact that one component of the mixed dysarthria was considered questionably or equivocally present in about 6% of the 300 cases. This uncertainty was associated with flaccid, spastic, ataxic, and hypokinetic types.

ETIOLOGIES FOR 300 QUASIRANDOMLY SELECTED CASES WITH A PRIMARY SPEECH PATHOLOGY DIAGNOSIS OF MIXED DYSARTHRIA AT THE MAYO CLINIC, 1969 TO 1990. PERCENTAGE OF CASES UNDER EACH BROAD ETIOLOGIC HEADING IS GIVEN IN PARENTHESES.

Degenerative (63%)
ALS (including diagnoses of ALS, MND, and progressive bulbar palsy) (41%)
Nonspecific CNS degenerative disease (9%)
PSP (2%)
OPCA (2%)
Cerebellar degeneration (2%)
Spinocerebellar degeneration (2%)
Parkinsonism (2%)
Shy-Drager syndrome (1%)
Multiple systems atrophy (1%)
Other (Wilson's disease, hepatocerebral degeneration, Creutzfeldt-Jakob disease, PD versus
    Shy-Drager disease, PD versus PSP) (2%)

Vascular (12%)
Multiple strokes (6%)
Single stroke (5%)

Demyelinating (6%)
Multiple sclerosis (4%)
Other (2%)

Traumatic (5%)
CHI (4%)
Surgical (<1%)

Tumor (4%)
Mass (mostly posterior fossa) (3%)
Paraneoplastic (<1%)

Undetermined (4%)

Multiple causes (4%)
Various combinations of stroke, encephalopathy, cerebellar degeneration, Shy-Drager syndrome, postthalamotomy or other neurosurgery, PD, drug toxicity, CHI, primary lateral sclerosis

Toxic/metabolic (1%)
Hypothyroidism, central pontine myelinolysis, neuroleptic toxicity, hypoxic encephalopathy, hepatic encephalopathy, undetermined metabolic disease

Inflammatory (1%)
Postviral encephalopathy, progressive encephalopathy, spongioform encephalopathy

ALS, amyotrophic lateral sclerosis; *CHI,* closed head injury; *CNS,* central nervous system; *MND,* motor neuron disease; *OPCA,* olivopontocerebellar atrophy; *PD,* Parkinson's disease; *PSP,* progressive supranuclear palsy.

When cases of ALS were excluded, spastic dysarthria remained the most frequently encountered type (85% of cases). Ataxic dysarthria was present in nearly two thirds of the cases. Flaccid, hypokinetic, and hyperkinetic dysarthrias were each encountered in approximately 20% to 35% of cases. In general, therefore, spastic dysarthria was the most frequent single type of dysarthria encountered in patients with mixed dysarthrias, even when diagnoses of ALS were excluded. Ataxic

dysarthria was present quite frequently in mixed dysarthrias that did not include a diagnosis of ALS. Flaccid dysarthria was encountered in more than half of cases, if diagnoses of ALS were included, but in only about one quarter of cases if ALS diagnoses were excluded. Hypokinetic and hyperkinetic dysarthrias were found within mixed dysarthrias, but less frequently than other types.

Table 10–3 summarizes the most common types of mixed dysarthria for the sample of 300 patients. The most common neurologic diagnosis for each mixed type is also given. Mixed flaccid-spastic dysarthria was the most frequent mixed dysarthria, accounting for 42% of the entire sample. The vast majority (88%) of these cases

had ALS. This suggests that gradual onset and progression of a mixed flaccid-spastic dysarthria should generate a high index of suspicion about ALS. The association of ALS with mixed flaccid-spastic dysarthria represents the strongest association of any mixed dysarthria with a specific neurologic disease in the sample.

Mixed ataxic-spastic dysarthria accounted for 23% of the mixed dysarthrias. Neurologic diagnoses were quite variable, with a majority of cases associated with vascular, demyelinating (usually MS), degenerative, and inflammatory etiologies.

Hypokinetic-spastic dysarthria accounted for 7% of the mixed dysarthrias. Again, neurologic diagnoses were quite variable, although about 50% were associated with PSP or undefined degenerative CNS diseases.

Mixed ataxic-flaccid-spastic dysarthria accounted for 6% of the mixed dysarthrias. Of interest, 59% of these cases had a neurologic diagnosis of ALS, which supports the clinical

Table 10–2 Distribution of individual dysarthria types encountered in a sample of 300 patients with a primary speech pathology diagnosis of mixed dysarthria. Percentages are given for the entire sample and the portion of the sample without a diagnosis of ALS.

Type	Entire sample	Sample without ALS
Flaccid	54%	25%
Spastic	91%	85%
Ataxic	43%	66%
Hypokinetic	21%	35%
Hyperkinetic	13%	21%

ALS, amyotrophic lateral sclerosis.

Table 10–3 The most common types of mixed dysarthria and the most frequent neurologic diagnoses in a sample of 300 patients with a primary speech pathology diagnosis of mixed dysarthria.

Type (% of entire sample)	Neurologic diagnosis (% of category)
Flaccid-spastic (42%)	ALS (88%) Vascular (5%) Tumor (2%) Other (5%)
Ataxic-spastic (23%)	Vascular (17%) Demyelinating disease (13%) CNS degenerative disease (12%) Inflammation (9%) Tumor (6%) Trauma (6%) Cerebellar degeneration (7%) Spinocerebellar degeneration (6%) Other (24%)
Hypokinetic-spastic (7%)	Degenerative CNS disease (30%) PSP (20%) Vascular (20%) Other (15%) Multiple (15%)
Ataxic-flaccid-spastic (6%)	ALS (59%)* Vascular (18%) Other (23%)
Hyperkinetic-hypokinetic (3%)	Parkinson's disease (67%)† Other (33%)
Other types (19%)	—

* The ataxic component was equivocal in about half of these cases.
† Often associated with on-off medication effects.
ALS, amyotrophic lateral sclerosis; CNS, central nervous system; PSP, progressive supranuclear palsy.

impression that ataxic or ataxic-like dysarthria may be perceived in individuals with ALS, particularly when their dysarthria is mild. This will be discussed further when the specific speech characteristics of ALS are addressed.

Mixed hyperkinetic-hypokinetic dysarthria accounted for 3% of the mixed dysarthrias. About two thirds of these cases had a diagnosis of PD. It appears that the mixed dysarthria for many of these patients was associated with on-off medication effects.

Many other mixed dysarthrias were encountered. In fact, in this sample of 300 patients, a total of 29 different combinations of single dysarthria types were documented. Other than the mixed types just discussed, however, none of the other mixed types occurred very frequently.

Severity and other characteristics. This retrospective review did not permit a precise delineation of dysarthria severity. However, in the sample of 300 patients, intelligibility was specifically commented on in 68%; in those cases, *76% had reduced intelligibility.* The degree to which this figure accurately estimates intelligibility impairments in mixed dysarthrias is unclear. It is likely that many patients for whom an observation of intelligibility was not made had normal intelligibility. However, the sample probably contains a larger number of mildly impaired patients than is encountered in a typical rehabilitation setting.

Because of its association with damage to more than one portion of the nervous system, it is reasonable to expect that some patients with mixed dysarthrias have cognitive disturbances. For the patients in this sample whose cognitive abilities were explicitly judged or formally assessed (77% of the sample), *28% exhibited some impairment of cognitive ability. Excluding patients with ALS from the sample, a much higher percentage of patients were cognitively impaired (68% of the sample).*

Finally, in spite of the fact that mixed dysarthria reflects involvement of more than one portion of the motor system, dysarthria was nonetheless the initial symptom in 20% of the sample and among the initial symptoms in 25% of the sample. Perhaps more important, for 12% of the sample, dysarthria (sometimes with accompanying dysphagia) was the only complaint and neurologic finding at the time the patient presented for neurology and speech pathology diagnosis.

Motor neuron disease: amyotrophic lateral sclerosis

Dysarthria may be the first manifestation of ALS, and it usually develops at some point during the disease's course (Gubbay and others, 1985). When dysarthria and dysphagia are the initial symptoms of ALS, they tend to remain the most functionally limiting symptoms as the disease progresses (Yorkston and others, 1993). Saunders, Walsh, and Smith (1981) reported that 47% of those with ALS who were receiving hospice care had reduced speech intelligibility, and that 25% became anarthric. Only 25% were intelligible just prior to death. Sitver and Kratt (1982) found that those who required augmentative communicative devices needed them an average of three years following diagnosis, and that such devices were used for an average of two years.

It is important to recognize that dysarthria in ALS may not be perceived as mixed at all points during the disease. It may present as either flaccid or spastic dysarthria; when mixed, one type may predominate.

Nonspeech oral mechanism. Oral mechanism findings are generally consistent with those encountered in patients with flaccid or spastic dysarthria of any etiology. Therefore, if spasticity is present, jaw jerk and sucking reflexes, a hyperactive gag reflex, slow orofacial movements, and pseudobulbar affect may predominate. If LMNs are affected, the gag reflex may be reduced, the cough weak, and the face lacking in tone. Lingual fasciculations may present early, and atrophy may be prominent. Fasciculations may also be apparent in the chin and corners of the lips. Dysphagia may be present on upper or lower motor neuron bases. It is not unusual for ALS patients with flaccid-spastic dysarthria to have an audible reflexive dry swallow.

Carrow and others (1974) found that tongue atrophy and dysphagia were the two most common signs in ALS patients with reduced intelligibility; 83% of their patients with reduced intelligibility had tongue atrophy. This is probably more than coincidental, for atrophy means that fewer muscle fibers are available for contraction, and force of movement is reduced in all directions.

Speech. Darley, Aronson, and Brown (1969a & b) studied 30 patients with ALS and found a combination of the deficits that were present in their groups with flaccid dysarthria alone and spastic dysarthria alone. The primary speech dimensions and clusters of deviant speech dimensions for these ALS patients are summarized in Table 10–4. It is apparent in the table that some features are clearly associated with spastic or flaccid dysarthria and that others can be attributed to either type. In addition, three features were present that were not found in flaccid or spastic dysarthria alone: *prolonged intervals, prolonged phonemes,* and *inappropriate silences.* These mainly prosodic features may reflect a summation of flaccid and spastic influences on speech. The

Table 10–4 The clusters and most deviant speech dimensions, ranked from most to least severe, associated with the mixed flaccid-spastic dysarthria of ALS, as well as the degree to which the flaccid versus spastic component probably contributes to each feature.

Dimension/cluster	Component
Dimensions	
Imprecise consonants	Either or both
Hypernasality	Flaccid > spastic
Harshness	Spastic > flaccid
Slow rate	Spastic
Monopitch	Either or both
Short phrases	Either or both
Distorted vowels	Spastic
Low pitch	Spastic
Monoloudness	Spastic > flaccid
Excess and equal stress	Spastic
Prolonged intervals*	Combined
Reduced stress	Spastic
Prolonged phonemes*	Combined
Strained-strangled quality	Spastic
Breathiness	Flaccid > spastic
Audible inspiration	Flaccid
Inappropriate silences*	Combined
Nasal emission	Flaccid
Clusters	
Prosodic excess	Spastic
Prosodic insufficiency	Spastic
Articulatory-resonatory incompetence	Spastic
Phonatory stenosis	Spastic
Phonatory incompetence	Flaccid
Resonatory incompetence	Flaccid

*Not a prominent dimension in either flaccid or spastic dysarthria. May represent the combined effects of both dysarthria types.
Data from Darley FL, Aronson AE, and Brown JR: Clusters of deviant speech dimensions in the dysarthrias, J Speech Hear Res 12:462, 1969a; and Darley FL, Aronson AE, and Brown JR: Differential diagnostic patterns of dysarthria, J Speech Hear Res 12:246, 1969b.

combined effects of UMN and LMN deficits on speech are also reflected in the finding that distorted vowels, slow rate, short phrases, and imprecise consonants were rated as more severe in the ALS group than in any other group studied by Darley, Aronson, and Brown. The six clusters of deviant dimensions that were identified match with clusters found in spastic and flaccid dysarthria and provide further support to the types of dysarthria that are prominent in the disorder.

The prominence of phonatory features in speakers with ALS is supported by Carrow and others (1974). Of their patients 80% had harsh voices,

65% were breathy, 63% had tremor, 60% had strained-strangled quality, 41% had audible inhalation, and 46% had abnormally high or low pitch (75% were hypernasal).

The finding of tremor in Carrow and others' patients is curious because tremor is not a finding in flaccid or spastic dysarthria. However, Aronson (1990) has discussed the presence of a rhythmic, 9 to 12 Hz rapid tremor or "*flutter*" in some patients with ALS. It is detectable during vowel prolongation but usually not during connected speech. The presence of vocal flutter is generally interpreted as an LMN characteristic rather than as a "central" tremor.

The vocal harshness in patients with ALS and mixed flaccid-spastic dysarthria often has a "*wet*" or "*gurgly*" character. It is presumably due to turbulence during speech from saliva that has accumulated in the pyriform sinuses and on the vocal cords because of reduced frequency of swallowing.

Occasionally, when the dysarthria is mild, a patient with ALS exhibits irregular articulatory breakdowns during contextual speech leading to a perception of *ataxic or ataxic-like dysarthria*. The reasons for this are unclear, but they may be similar to those offered in Chapter 9 for the ataxic-like characteristics that may be perceived in unilateral upper motor neuron dysarthria.

The work of the Kents and their colleagues has shed some light on the articulatory abnormalities that contribute most to reduced intelligibility in ALS. Using their word intelligibility test (see Chapter 3), several studies of men and women with ALS and varying degrees of intelligibility impairment (Kent and others, 1990, 1992) have found that the most disturbed phonetic features tend to be related to velopharyngeal function (nasal-oral distinctions); lingual functions for articulatory manner contrasts (stop versus affricate); syllable shape; voicing contrasts; regulation of tongue height for vowels; and production of syllable final consonants. In general, these results refine less precise perceptual analyses showing that hypernasality, imprecise consonants, and harshness are frequent characteristics in ALS. They also demonstrate that all speech functions are not affected uniformly and that some lingual functions are affected less than others; for example, front versus back vowel, long versus short vowel, and general place of articulation distinctions were particularly resistant to intelligibility problems.

To summarize, the dysarthria of ALS may be *flaccid, spastic,* or, most often, *mixed flaccid-spastic.* The overall pattern of the mixed form, beyond mild degrees of impairment, is one of *labored, slowly produced speech with short phrases and intervals between words and phrases, grossly defective articulation, hypernasality, strained-strangled and groaning voice quality, and monopitch and monoloudness.*

Physiologic and acoustic findings. The physiologic and acoustic characteristics of speech in ALS have received some attention. Findings have confirmed or modified perceptual hypotheses and extended our understanding of the disorder. The primary findings of these studies are summarized in Table 10–5.

Hirose, Kiritani, and Sawashima (1982), using x-ray microbeam technology, studied articulatory patterns in two ALS patients and confirmed the presence of very slow single and repetitive articulatory movements, limited range of movement, and difficulty maintaining velar elevation for sequences requiring velopharyngeal closure. Maximum velocity of articulator movement was reduced, but regularity of repetitive movements was preserved. Of interest, lip and tongue movements were often accompanied by excessive jaw displacement. They called this apparent compensatory jaw movement "jaw dependency" and related it to the relative preservation of the Vth nerve and jaw function in ALS. In general, the overall movement characteristics seemed consistent with the resultant imprecise articulation, vowel distortions, hypernasality, and nasal emission commonly perceived in speakers with ALS.

Studies examining maximum strength of voluntary jaw, lip, and tongue contraction in ALS speakers have documented weakness in all muscles, and the tongue is usually the most affected structure (DePaul and Brooks, 1993; DePaul and others, 1988; Dworkin, Aronson, and Mulder, 1980; Langmore and Lehman, 1994). Some of these studies have found a significant relationship between the measured weakness and the perceived severity of the dysarthria, but some have not. It seems that the relationship between weakness and speech disability in ALS is neither simple nor direct. This may be partially attributable to the ability of some muscle groups to compensate for weakness in others. For example, DePaul and others (1988) noted that speech problems in their patients were exacerbated when the jaw was fixed during speech, suggesting that the jaw may have been compensating for weakness in other articulators during unrestricted speaking conditions. The complex relationship may also be related to the fact that only about 10% of the maximum contraction force in muscles studied are

Table 10–5 Summary of acoustic and physiologic findings in studies of ALS.

Speech component	Acoustic or physiologic observation
Respiratory	Reduced vital capacity Chest wall muscle weakness
Laryngeal	Abnormal f_o (too high or low) Abnormal jitter, shimmer, harmonic-noise ratio Decreased maximum vowel duration
Velopharyngeal	Difficulty maintaining velar elevation
Articulation, rate, prosody	Slow single and repetitive articulatory movements Reduced range of articulatory movements Reduced maximum velocity of articulation Reduced maximum force of tongue, lip, and jaw movements Excessive jaw movement (probably compensatory) Increased stop-gap duration Blurring of voiced-voiceless VOT distinctions (articulatory-laryngeal) Increased vowel duration within syllables Reduced/shallow/flattened F2 slope within words Exaggerated formant trajectories at vowel onset within syllables Frequency and/or amplitude fluctuations during vowel prolongation related to perceived vocal flutter

*Note that some of these findings are based on only a few speakers and that not all speakers with ALS (or mixed spastic-flaccid dysarthria) exhibit these features. Note also that these characteristics may not be unique to ALS or mixed spastic-flaccid dysarthria; some may be found in other motor speech disorders or other neurologic or nonneurologic conditions.
ALS, amyotrophic lateral sclerosis; f_o, fundamental frequency; *F2,* second formant; *VOT,* voice onset time.

generated during speech, thus permitting significant decrements in maximum force without decrements in speech (Kent and others, 1989).

Putnam and Hixon (1984) studied chest wall kinematics in 10 ALS patients who complained of shortness of breath when supine. Vital capacity was reduced in the upright position in several subjects. Overall findings were generally indicative of chest wall muscle weakness, particularly in inspiratory muscles. Patients tended to generate higher lung volumes for loud reading only when compelled, suggesting that such activity was effortful and difficult to perform repetitively. Putnam and Hixon pointed out that low lung volumes can be a liability to utterance length and loudness and might explain reduced loudness and stress contrasts, short phrases, and reduced power for coughing in patients with respiratory weakness.

Several investigations have examined the acoustic attributes of ALS speakers. Among the common findings are abnormal fundamental frequency (too high or low); abnormal jitter, shimmer, and harmonic-noise ratio; longer stop-gap durations (time from cessation of acoustic energy in a preceding vowel to the onset of acoustic energy from the articulatory burst for a subsequent initial stop-plosive); longer vowel duration in syllables; decreased maximum vowel duration; short phrase duration (Caruso and Burton, 1987; Kent and others, 1991, 1992; Ramig and others, 1990; Turner and Weismer, 1993). Some investigators have documented a blurring of the voice onset time (VOT) distinctions between initial voiced and voiceless stops (Seikel, Wilcox, and Davis, 1991), but others have not (Caruso and Burton, 1987), and not all studies have found abnormalities in jitter, shimmer, and harmonic-noise ratio (Kent and others, 1991). In general, these findings are indicative of slow lingual or laryngeal movements, aperiodicity or instability of movements, and weakness of movements during speech.

Perhaps the most reliable and potentially useful acoustic findings are those to emerge from studies of the slope of the second formant (F2) in intelligibility test words. The F2 slope seems to be a sensitive index of lingual function—and perhaps speech proficiency in general—for people with ALS. The F2 slope may reflect the rate at which lingual movements occur and, by inference, the rate at which motor units can be recruited. The slope of F2 has been found by the Kents and others (1989, 1991, 1992) to decline along with reductions in intelligibility in single subjects followed longitudinally and in groups of men and women with a range of intelligibility impairments (Figure 10–1). Kent and others (1989) noted that

the F2-intelligibility relationship may not be linearly correlated across the range of possible intelligibility scores (the relationship may be curvilinear). Measures other than F2 may be required to predict the full range of intelligibility scores in patients with ALS.*

Weismer and others (1992) found shallower slopes of formant transitions, exaggerations of formant trajectories at the onset of vocalic nuclei, and greater interspeaker variability in ALS speakers than in control subjects. Patients who were less than 70% intelligible had more aberrant trajectory characteristics than those with better intelligibility. Poorly intelligible speakers tended to have flat trajectories or very shallow slopes. It appears that measures of formant transitions, particularly F2, may be a useful index for monitoring the course of ALS and for making predictions about intelligibility impairments.

Finally, Aronson and others (1992) examined the acoustic characteristics of the vocal "flutter" that is present in some people with ALS. Vowel prolongations with perceptible flutter[†] were analyzed by fast fourier transformation (FFT) after the signal was demodulated into frequency and amplitude components. Multiple frequency and amplitude modulations were present, and the modulations were more prominent in ALS than in control subjects. The prominent frequencies spanned the range from 0 to 25 Hz but most had peaks in the 6 to 12 Hz range. These findings provide some acoustic support for the perception of a rapid tremor or flutter in some ALS patients, but they do not clarify the basis for the phenomenon. The authors speculated that the flutter is probably not central because tremor is not typically heard in spastic dysarthria alone, the only obvious CNS dysarthria present in ALS. They noted that patients with peripheral neuropathy can have tremor in the 8 to 12 Hz range. In addition, the tremor could be a sign of loss of motor units, resulting in an intermittent absence of motor unit firing that, when it affects intrinsic laryngeal muscles, might be perceived as a tremor or flutter.

Multiple sclerosis

Dysarthria is the most common communication disorder associated with multiple sclerosis (MS) (Beukelman, Kraft, and Freal, 1985). The type and

---

*Yorkston and others (1993) present data that suggest that reductions in speaking and alternating motion rates in people with ALS may be precursors of reduced intelligibility.
[†]They also noted tremorous movements of the true cords and supraglottic muscles on fiberscopic examination of ALS patients with vocal flutter.

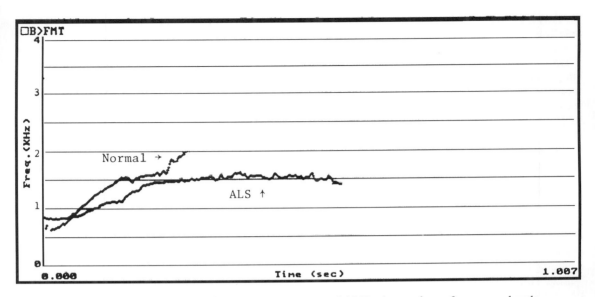

Figure 10–1 Second formant (F2) tracings for the vowel /ӕ/ in the word *wax* for a normal male speaker and a man with mixed spastic-flaccid dysarthria associated with ALS (analysis based on method described by Kent and others, 1989). Relative to the normal speaker, the F2 slope for the dysarthric speaker is only about half as steep, covers a smaller frequency range, and takes about twice the time to complete. This long and flattened F2 trajectory is an acoustic correlate of slow speaking rate and slowed and restricted range of articulatory movements that can underly mixed spastic-flaccid dysarthria.

severity of the dysarthria is variable, an observation compatible with the variable presentations of the disease in general.

Darley, Aronson, and Goldstein (1972) studied 168 patients with a diagnosis of MS. The group had a variable distribution of spinal, cerebellar, brainstem, and cerebral involvement. Fifty-nine percent of the patients had essentially normal speech, and an additional 28% were only "minimally" impaired. Severity of dysarthria was related to overall severity of neurologic deficit and to the number of neurologic systems involved (for example, cerebellar, brainstem, cerebral). These results are roughly compatible with Beukelman, Kraft, and Freal's (1985) survey of 656 patients with MS. Only 23% reported having communication disorders, and only 3% of those with such disorders reported that it interfered with their employment. The frequency of communication disorders increased with increased restrictions in mobility imposed by the disease. Ninety-six percent had no difficulty communicating with strangers, but 28% with such difficulty used augmentative communication devices. Therefore, dysarthria may or may not be present in MS. When present, it is often mild, but severity tends to be related to overall severity of the disease, and it can be severe enough to require augmentation of verbal communication.

Nonspeech findings in MS that have implications for speech production include the occasional presence of reduced vital capacity and inadequate ventilation (Darley, Aronson, and Goldstein, 1972; Howard and others, 1992). Respiratory complications are frequent in the terminal stages of MS and may also occur during disease relapses. Such impairments can include generalized or diaphragmatic respiratory muscle weakness, disordered regulation of automatic and voluntary breathing, and bulbar weakness leading to aspiration and infection. Some patients have obstructive sleep apnea, and some require mechanical respiratory support (Howard and others, 1992). Facial paralysis similar to Bell's palsy occurs in about 10% of patients with MS, and facial myokymia and trigeminal neuralgia may also be present (Smith and Scheinberg, 1985).

Table 10–6 summarizes the deviant speech characteristics and some of the related dysfunctions found in Darley, Aronson, and Goldstein's (1972) study of patients with MS. The presence of impaired loudness and pitch control and sudden articulatory breakdowns are suggestive of ataxic dysarthria, but the dysarthria was spastic in some patients. The presence of spastic dysarthria in MS is also suggested by the findings of Farmakides and Boone (1960) who reported hypernasality, reduced pitch variability, and slow rate in some of their 82 patients with MS.

Darley, Aronson, and Goldstein pointed out that "scanning speech" is not characteristic of MS. For

Table 10-6 Speech deviations and related functions in a sample of 168 patients with MS.

Deviation	% of sample
Speech	
Impaired loudness control	77
Harshness	72
Defective articulation	46
Impaired emphasis	39
Impaired pitch control	37
Hypernasality	24
Inappropriate pitch level	24
Breathiness	22
Sudden articulatory breakdowns	9
Related functions	
Decreased vital capacity	35
Nasal escape (on oral manometer)	2
Inadequate ventilation	2

Based on Darley FL, Aronson AE, and Goldstein NP: Dysarthria in multiple sclerosis, J Speech Hear Res 15:229-245, 1972.
MS, multiple sclerosis.

example, only a small percentage of patients had increased stress on unstressed syllables, the rated feature that is most relevant to a perception of scanning speech (most who did have this feature had cerebellar involvement). This finding should temper previous tendencies to describe scanning speech as *the* speech of MS.

It seems reasonable to conclude that *ataxic* and *spastic dysarthria* and *mixed ataxic-spastic dysarthria* are among the most frequent dysarthria types encountered in MS. Perhaps more than in any other of the degenerative diseases discussed here, however, the dysarthrias of MS are unpredictable. It is prudent to consider virtually any dysarthria type or combination of types as possible in patients with the disease.

Friedreich's ataxia

The few studies of speech in Friedreich's ataxia (FA) establish that, despite the disease's label, its associated dysarthria is not always ataxic and that the dysarthria can be mixed. This is a logical consequence of the disease's capacity to affect more than cerebellar structures.

Joanette and Dudley (1980) studied the contextual speech of 22 patients with FA and rated speech on 16 of the dimensions used in the Darley, Aronson, and Brown (1969a & b) studies. The most deviant dimensions included monopitch, hypernasality, imprecise consonants, monoloudness, harshness, inappropriate pitch level, excess loudness variation, distorted vowels, excess and equal stress, prolonged phonemes, abnormal rate, irregu-

lar articulatory breakdowns, inappropriate silences, prolonged intervals, and pitch breaks. These characteristics suggest more than a single dysarthria type, and the study's additional analyses support such a conclusion. Factor analysis and a Q-factoring procedure revealed two primary factors and separated subjects into three groups according to various combinations of the two factors. The factors that emerged were called a "general dysarthria factor" and a "phonatory stenosis" factor. The general factor appeared to reflect ataxia with predominant effects on articulation, and the phonatory stenosis factor seemed to have predominant effects on phonatory function (it is likely that the phonatory factor reflected a spastic dysarthria, although the authors did not label it as such).

Gilman and Kluin (1984) studied the connected speech, alternating motion rates (AMRs), and vowel prolongations of three individuals with FA and cerebellar findings, explicitly noting that no subject had corticobulbar or LMN involvement on nonspeech examination. The primary deviant speech features included audible inspiration, abnormal respiratory synchrony, fluctuating pitch, transient explosiveness, harshness, breathiness, alternating loudness, mild hypernasality, occasional imprecise consonants, irregular articulatory breakdowns, slow rate, excess and equal stress, and prolonged phonemes and intervals. Voice quality was strained-strangled, and speech AMRs were slow. Although the authors concluded that ataxic dysarthria is *the* dysarthria of FA, this requires some qualification. First, the patients reportedly did not have corticobulbar involvement, which can occur in FA; in fact, the presence of strained-strangled voice quality, and perhaps hypernasality and slow AMRs, suggests a spastic component may have been present. Second, the patients had mild deficits, so the results should not be generalized to more severe levels of impairment or advanced stages of the disease. Therefore, although these patients seem to have had an ataxic dysarthria, it is not clear that they did not have another dysarthria type as well (perhaps spastic) or that it can be concluded that FA is associated only with ataxic dysarthria.

Gentil (1990) acoustically analyzed the speech of 14 individuals with FA. The AMRs and vowel prolongations were more variable, word durations were longer, and speech AMRs were slower than normal. The overall acoustic pattern was described as slow, irregular, variable in fundamental frequency and intensity, and abnormal in prosody. Unfortunately, the perceptual characteristics of speech were not well described, and clinical judgments about type of dysarthria were not made. The acoustic findings are suggestive of ataxic dysarthria but are ambiguous relative to other types that might have been present.

To summarize, perceptual and acoustic studies of FA, as well as the known sites of nervous system degeneration in people with the disease, suggest that *ataxic dysarthria* may be the most frequently encountered dysarthria in FA but that other types may also be present, particularly *spastic dysarthria*. Thus, it can be concluded that mixed dysarthria can be present in FA and inferred that the most common mix is an *ataxic-spastic dysarthria*.

Progressive supranuclear palsy

Dysarthria is probably the least well-described clinical sign of progressive supranuclear palsy (PSP), in spite of its being a frequent early and prominent manifestation of the disease (Lees, 1987; Lu, Duffy, and Maraganore, 1992; Metter and Hanson, 1991; Podoll, Schwarz, and Noth, 1991). Given the predilection of the disease to produce parkinsonian, pseudobulbar, and sometimes ataxic features, it is reasonable to predict the possible presence of several types of dysarthria in PSP.

Oral mechanism examination can also reveal various confirmatory signs encountered in patients with hypokinetic, spastic, and ataxic dysarthria. Although orofacial manifestations of parkinsonism (for example, facial masking) are most frequent, evidence of pseudobulbar palsy (for example, pseudobulbar affect, hyperactive jaw jerk) are common. In addition, in contrast to the flexed neck posture often seen in PD, patients with PSP may exhibit neck extension, with the head pointed upward (Lees, 1987). Dysphagia is not unusual (Lees, 1987; Podoll, Schwarz, and Noth, 1991; Pillon and others, 1986). Kluin and others (1993) found dysphagia in 73% of their 44 patients with PSP; they noted, however, that dysphagia occurred less frequently than dysarthria.

The dysarthrias of PSP have received some delineation in a few studies. Metter and Hanson (1991) studied 15 consecutive patients with PSP whose most prominent neurologic findings were rigidity and bradykinesia; spasticity and ataxia were also present in some patients. As often occurs, many of their patients had a diagnosis of PD, and a few had a diagnosis of cerebellar degeneration before a diagnosis of PSP was made. Four patients had spastic dysarthria, 10 had hypokinetic dysarthria, and one had a mixed spastic-ataxic dysarthria. In addition, "ataxic speech features were reported occasionally among patients in both the hypokinetic and spastic dysarthria groups" (p. 131), implying that mixed hypokinetic-ataxic dysarthria was present in some pa-

tients. The authors also noted that dysarthria was frequently an early sign or symptom of PSP and that palilalia was a prevalent symptom.

In a study of 44 patients with PSP who were unselected for type of speech disorder, Kluin and others (1993) reported that all had a mixed dysarthria that was judged as moderate in 68% and severe in 23% of patients. Dysarthria types included hypokinetic, spastic, and ataxic; 68% of patients had all three types. For the group as a whole, spastic dysarthria was judged the most severe component, followed by hypokinetic and then ataxic. The ataxic component was present least frequently but nonetheless present in 68% of patients. Of interest, palilalia was present in 11% of patients, "acquired stuttering" in 20%, and echolalia in 7%. Metter and Hanson (1991) also observed palilalia as a prevalent symptom in their patients, and its presence in PSP has also been commented on by others (Lebrun, Devreux, and Rousseau, 1986; Lees, 1987).

Lu, Duffy, and Maraganore (1992) retrospectively reviewed the records of 40 randomly selected patients with complete speech pathology evaluations and a neurologic diagnosis of PSP. They compared the speech findings with those for a similarly selected group of patients with PD. The results provided a description of the dysarthrias of PSP and some interesting contrasts with the dysarthria encountered in PD. Dysarthria was among the earliest symptoms and signs of disease in 35% of the patients with PSP, more frequently than in patients with PD (14%). Virtually all of the PSP patients exhibited dysarthria at the time of diagnosis of PSP, compared to 91% of patients with PD. Various types of dysarthria were present in the group with PSP, including hypokinetic (20%), spastic (20%), mixed hypokinetic-spastic (50%), mixed hypokinetic-spastic-ataxic (7%), and anarthria (3%). All of the patients with PD who were dysarthric had an isolated hypokinetic dysarthria.

Several speech findings seemed to distinguish the PSP group from those with PD. Characteristics found more frequently in those with PSP than PD included monopitch, hoarseness, nasal emission, excess and equal stress, hypernasality, imprecise articulation, and slow rate. Characteristics found more frequently in PD than PSP included vocal flutter, reduced loudness, reduced stress, tremor, breathiness, and rapid rate. These differences are logically related to the exclusivity of features of hypokinetic dysarthria in the PD group and the frequent added presence of features of other dysarthria types in PSP, particularly spastic dysarthria. The investigators concluded that the presence of a dysarthria type other than hypokinetic in patients with a neurologic diagnosis of PD should raise questions about the accuracy of the PD diagnosis and suggest the possibility that PSP is present instead. This distinction may be particularly important for a disease like PSP, which is often misdiagnosed as PD (Jankovic, 1984).

To summarize, observations establish that (1) mixed dysarthria is common and tends to appear early in PSP; (2) *hypokinetic* and *spastic* dysarthria—or a mix of the two—are most commonly present, but *ataxic* dysarthria, usually in combination with hypokinetic or spastic dysarthria, can also occur; and (3) recognition of mixed dysarthria in patients with suspected PSP or PD may be particularly helpful to differential diagnosis. Information to date suggests that the presence of hypokinetic dysarthria or a mixed dysarthria with a hypokinetic component (perhaps with associated palilalia) early in the course of disease might be more strongly associated with PSP than other degenerative neurologic diseases, such as PD.

Shy-Drager syndrome

There has been little systematic investigation of the dysarthrias associated with Shy-Drager syndrome (SDS), although Linebaugh (1979) has established at least some of the types that may be encountered. He reviewed 80 patients with a diagnosis of SDS who were seen at the Mayo Clinic over a 14-year period. Thirty-five (44%) had dysarthria. Of those with dysarthria, 43% had ataxic dysarthria, 31% had hypokinetic dysarthria, and 26% had various combinations of mixed dysarthrias. Thus, dysarthria occurs frequently in SDS, and single or mixed types may be present.

Three forms of mixed dysarthria were present: *hypokinetic-ataxic, ataxic-spastic,* and *spastic-ataxic-hypokinetic.* The isolated dysarthrias and each of the mixed forms are consistent with the involvement of direct and indirect motor systems and the basal ganglia and cerebellar control circuits that occurs in the disease. Because SDS can masquerade as conditions that are associated with more limited involvement of the nervous system (such as PD or cerebellar degeneration), the recognition of a mixed versus single dysarthria can contribute to differential diagnosis. Consultation requests such as "Is this SDS or PD? Do speech characteristics fit better with one or the other diagnosis?" reflect an awareness that the presence of a mixed dysarthria would be inconsistent with a diagnosis of PD and, depending on the mix, would not be inconsistent with a diagnosis of SDS.

Some SDS patients develop *laryngeal stridor,* which presents as excessive snoring and stridor, and sometimes sleep apnea. Bannister and others (1981) reported autopsy findings for three patients that documented the presence of posterior cri-

coarytenoid weakness, without obvious pathology in other laryngeal muscles. They concluded that the nucleus ambiguus (at least that portion supplying the posterior cricoarytenoid) is at risk in multiple-systems atrophy (SDS), along with the pyramidal, extrapyramidal, and cerebellar systems.

If inhalatory stridor is perceptible on inhalation prior to speaking or at phrase boundaries during speech, it technically represents evidence of a *flaccid dysarthria.* Although Linebaugh did not note the presence of inhalatory stridor in his patients, it is encountered clinically. In fact, the presence of inhalatory stridor without significant adductor vocal cord weakness in patients with various combinations of spastic, ataxic, and hypokinetic dysarthria is probably rare in degenerative diseases other than SDS. In other words, the presence of a mixed hypokinetic-ataxic-spastic dysarthria plus a flaccid dysarthria represented by inhalatory stridor should raise suspicions about the presence of SDS.

Olivopontocerebellar atrophy

The dysarthria that may occur in olivopontocerebellar atrophy (OPCA) has received little attention. Gilman and Kluin (1984) examined the reading, vowel prolongations, and speech AMRs of three patients with OPCA. Each had neuroimaging and clinical neurologic evidence of cerebellar involvement plus corticobulbar findings suggestive of UMN spasticity (for example, pseudobulbar affect, active gag reflex, slow facial movements). The primary speech findings included occasional audible inspiration, occasional abnormal respiratory synchrony, low pitch, monopitch, strained-strangled harshness, alternating loudness, low volume, hypernasality, imprecise articulation, irregular articulatory breakdowns, distorted vowels, slow rate, equalized and occasional excessive stress, and prolonged phonemes and intervals. Overall severity was mild in one patient and moderate in two. The authors concluded that the overall speech patterns were consistent with a mixed ataxic-spastic dysarthria. With the exception of audible inspiration (which raises the possibility of a flaccid component associated with LMN posterior cricoarytenoid weakness), the perceptual results appear compatible with such a conclusion.

Hartman and O'Neill (1989) discussed a man with a clinical diagnosis of OPCA whose predominant deviant speech characteristics included articulatory distortions, slow speaking rate, slow and irregular AMRs, strained-strangled hoarseness, vocal flutter, decreased loudness, hypernasality, and nasal emission. (He also had stuttering-like dysfluencies that may or may not have reflected a reemergence of developmental stuttering.) The speech diagnosis was mixed flaccid-spastic dysarthria.

To summarize, the presence of *ataxic* or *spastic* or *flaccid dysarthria,* or various combinations of the three, is consistent with the sites of degeneration in OPCA, the few clinical reports in the literature, and anecdotal clinical experience. Because OPCA also may be associated with parkinsonian features, it can be presumed that a *hypokinetic dysarthria* is also possible. Additional study is required to delineate more completely the nature of the dysarthrias that may be encountered in OPCA.

Wilson's disease

Wilson's disease (WD) often affects the bulbar muscles. Dysarthria is one of the most frequent and sometimes the only manifestation of the disorder (Sternlieb, Giblin, and Scheinberg, 1987; Topaloglu and others, 1990). Oral mechanism findings in patients with WD can be similar to those encountered in patients with hypokinetic, ataxic, or spastic dysarthria. Dystonia also may be present and is considered responsible for the inappropriate and fixed "pseudo smile" exhibited by some patients (Sternlieb, Giblin, and Scheinberg, 1987). Dysphagia and drooling are not unusual.

Berry and others (1974a) have conducted the only systematic investigation of the speech characteristics associated with WD. They examined 20 patients with various combinations of ataxia, rigidity, and spasticity. Patients' speech was perceptually analyzed using the methods of Darley, Aronson, and Brown (1969a & b). The most prominent deviant speech characteristics and clusters of speech characteristics (based on factor analysis) derived from the study are summarized in Table 10–7.

Within the group, speech characteristics and clusters of deviant characteristics suggestive of hypokinetic, ataxic, and spastic dysarthria were found. Many of the perceived deviant characteristics occur in more than one of the dysarthria types. However, inappropriate silences, found in hypokinetic dysarthria, were present and are not shared with any other dysarthria type. Features of ataxic dysarthria that are not shared with hypokinetic or spastic dysarthria included irregular articulatory breakdowns, prolonged phonemes, and prolonged intervals. Features of spastic dysarthria that are not shared with hypokinetic or ataxic dysarthria included hypernasality, strained voice quality, and short phrases. Berry and his colleagues concluded that the dysarthria of WD can be mixed, containing various combinations of *hypokinetic, ataxic,* and *spastic,* but they noted that pure forms of each of those dysarthrias can be present in some patients.

Berry and others (1974b) monitored patients undergoing penicillamine and low copper diet management of their WD and found a correlation

Table 10–7 Prominent deviant characteristics and clusters of speech characteristics associated with Wilson's disease.

Features	Hypokinetic	Ataxic	Spastic
Characteristics			
Reduced stress	x		x
Slow rate		x	x
Excess and equal stress		x	x
Low pitch	x		x
Irregular articulatory breakdowns		x	
Hypernasality			x
Inappropriate silences	x		
Prolonged phonemes		x	
Prolonged intervals		x	
Strained voice			x
Short phrases			x
Clusters (based on factor analysis)			
Prosodic insufficiency	x		x
Phonatory stenosis			x
Prosodic excess		x	
Articulatory-resonatory incompetence	x		x

Based on Berry WR and others: Dysarthria in Wilson's disease, J Speech Hear Res 17:169, 1974a.
Only those characteristics that are *not* common to all three dysarthria types are listed; see the original study for a listing of all deviant characteristics.

between improvement in deviant speech characteristics and general neurologic improvement during treatment. This establishes that careful monitoring of speech during medical treatment of WD can serve as an index of the effectiveness of treatment for the disease.

CASES

Case 10.1

A 68-year-old man presented to neurology, stating "I don't know what's the matter with me. If you have a cure, I'd be delighted." During the previous 4 years, he developed the insidious onset of impotence, occasional stumbling and falling, dysphagia with aspiration of liquids, and occasional laryngeal stridor. He had recently developed urinary urgency and clumsiness in his hand.

On neurologic exam, he exhibited axial rigidity, poor station, orthostatic hypotension, reduced upward gaze, and dysarthria. An EMG revealed evidence of a mild, predominantly motor peripheral neuropathy. Autonomic reflex testing demonstrated a generalized autonomic neuropathy. Laryngeal examination revealed left vocal cord paresis.

During speech examination, he noted a one-year history of a "higher and weaker" voice and a sense that his speech was "clumsy." He reported choking on liquids and occasional "laryngospasms" during sleep. He was no longer able to play the trumpet or flute because of respiratory fatigue and stated, "I get out of breath for no good reason." Finally, he complained that his lips were "tight and being stretched across my mouth."

Oral mechanism examination revealed a slight left lower facial droop, equivocal bilateral reduction in tongue strength, a weak cough and glottal coup, and inhalatory laryngeal stridor at phrase boundaries during speech and when inhaling rapidly. His speech was characterized by accelerated rate (1); monopitch and monoloudness (3); imprecise articulation (1); reduced loudness (1). Pitch was mildly elevated. Vowel prolongation was strained-harsh (1) and unsteady (1,2). A vocal "flutter" was sometimes detected. Speech AMRs were irregular (1,2) and occasionally accelerated or "blurred."

The clinician concluded the patient had, "mixed dysarthria in which a hypokinetic component is most prominent. His mildly irregular AMRs and vocal unsteadiness suggest an ataxic component. The subtle strained component to his voice could represent a mild spastic component, although there are no other features of spasticity. His laryngeal stridor suggests posterior cricoarytenoid weakness and his vocal flutter may reflect weakness of laryngeal adductors as well."

Pulmonary function tests were abnormal but nonspecific. An MRI of the head showed moderate cerebellar atrophy, predominantly vermian, and periventricular atrophy.

The neurologist concluded that the patient had multiple-systems atrophy that most closely corresponded to Shy-Drager syndrome. Several drugs whose action would stimulate dopamine receptors were recommended. The patient was counseled about the likely course of his disease. He declined a need for speech therapy at the time but was told that therapy might be effective in maintaining intelligibility or helping to develop augmentative means of communication if that became necessary.

Commentary. (1) Mixed dysarthria occurs commonly in degenerative neurologic disease. (2) A number of dysarthria types may be perceptually evident in mixed dysarthria. This patient had unequivocal hypokinetic and flaccid dysarthria, probable ataxic dysarthria, and possible spastic dysarthria. All of these types were compatible with the diagnosis of multiple-systems atrophy, especially Shy-Drager syndrome. (3) Many patients with obvious dysarthria decline speech therapy when intelligibility and speech efficiency are relatively well maintained.

Case 10.2

A 35-year-old woman with a 10-year history of chronic progressive MS presented for consideration of thalamotomy to control a severe bilateral upper limb tremor. Clinical neurologic examination revealed hyperreflexia; pathologic reflexes; bilateral weakness, spasticity, and impaired coordination; severe resting, postural, and movement tremor of upper and lower extremities; nystagmus; and optic neuritis. Neuropsychologic assessment demonstrated severe impairment of new learning and memory and a generalized loss of intellectual abilities.

During speech evaluation, the patient noted a one-year history of progressive speech difficulty. Oral mechanism examination demonstrated reduced face and lingual strength and a sucking reflex. Speech was characterized by slow rate (3); irregular articulatory breakdowns (2); breathy-hoarse voice quality (2); hypernasality with nasal emission (2). Speech intelligibility was significantly reduced.

The clinician concluded that the patient had a "mixed spastic-ataxic dysarthria of moderate severity."

Unfortunately, the presence of abnormal somatosensory evoked potentials precluded adequate localization within the thalamus for lesion placement to abolish her tremor. Surgery was not recommended. The patient was not motivated to pursue speech therapy.

Commentary. (1) Mixed dysarthria is not uncommon in patients with MS who are dysarthric. Mixed spastic-ataxic dysarthria may be the most common mixed dysarthria encountered in MS. (2) Cognitive deficits may be present in MS, and they can compound difficulties with communication. (3) In spite of reduced intelligibility, not all patients are motivated or interested in speech therapy.

Case 10.3

A 49-year-old woman was referred by her internist for evaluation of a speech problem of 2 months' duration that her family interpreted as a response to psychological stress. During speech evaluation, the patient admitted to considerable family stress but felt she was handling it well. Her voice difficulty began with a cold, and she described its initial character as "nasal." She had also developed swallowing difficulty, characterized by food sticking in her throat after a swallow had been initiated and the necessity to swallow several more times to get it down. She had recently begun to choke on liquids. She admitted that food occasionally squirreled in her cheeks and that she sometimes needed to use her fingers to remove it. She had begun to gag when brushing her teeth and swallowing saliva and reported "crying a lot," even when she did not wish to do so. She admitted to some "twitching" around her eyes and left upper lip.

Oral mechanism examination revealed bilateral lower face and tongue weakness and reduced lateral tongue AMRs. Nasal emission occurred on pressure consonants. Her gag reflex was hyperactive, but her cough and glottal coup were weak. A sucking reflex was present.

Contextual speech was characterized by groaning and strained voice quality (1); reduced loudness (−2); hypernasality (2); imprecise and weak pressure consonants (2,3); reduced rate (2); short phrases and monopitch and monoloudness (2,3). Speech AMRs were slow but regular (2,3). Vowel prolongation was mildly strained and breathy.

The clinician concluded that the patient had a "mixed flaccid-spastic dysarthria of moderate severity." The patient declined a recommendation for speech therapy because her primary concern was diagnosis. She was referred for neurologic evaluation.

Neurologic examination showed evidence of hyperreflexia and pathologic reflexes in all limbs and weakness in her face. An EMG examination failed to provide evidence for LMN disease in the limbs; CT scan of the head was normal.

Her speech continued to worsen. Two months later she was writing to communicate much of the time. She had moderate bilateral lower facial weakness, equivocal jaw weakness, markedly reduced tongue strength, and possible lingual atrophy. Gag reflex was hyperactive, and cough and glottal coup were markedly weak. A sucking reflex was present. She had an audible reflexive swallow and inhalatory stridor. Connected speech was characterized by strained-hoarseness (2), reduced loudness (2), hypernasality (2), and imprecise articulation (3). Rate was slow (2,3) and phrases short, with monopitch and monoloudness (3). Inhalatory stridor was present at phrase boundaries. Vowel prolongation was strained-harsh-wet. Speech AMRs were slow (3). She displayed pseudobulbar crying.

Speech therapy was recommended. Speech intelligibility improved for about 1 month, but then deteriorated. An EMG 1 month later demonstrated abnormalities in all limbs consistent with motor neuron disease. The patient communicated fairly efficiently with writing until her death from respiratory and cardiac arrest about 6 months later.

Commentary. (1) Dysarthria can be the initial manifestation of neurologic disease and fairly frequently is the presenting sign of ALS. It may be present and progress for some time before diagnosis is confirmed.

(2) Initial signs of neurologic disease are sometimes misinterpreted as responses to psychological stress. When the symptom is speech difficulty, careful examination can help distinguish a motor speech disorder from a psychogenic speech disturbance. (3) Mixed spastic-flaccid dysarthria is the "prototypic" mixed dysarthria of ALS. Its effects on intelligibility can be dramatic and often lead to a need for augmentative or alternative forms of communication.

Case 10.4

A 77-year-old woman was hospitalized for an apparent exacerbation of myasthenia gravis. The disease had been present for 46 years, but she had recently developed difficulty with speech, swallowing, and right leg and left arm weakness. Her prior symptoms of myasthenia gravis had been predominantly ophthalmic and the disease had been well controlled with pyridostigmine (Mestinon). An increase in pyridostigmine dose as well as a course of steroids had done nothing to improve her dysarthria and dysphagia. Her lack of response to these drugs raised the possibility that myasthenia gravis might not be the only cause of her dysarthria.

During speech evaluation, the patient reported a three-month history of speech and swallowing problems. She was frequently choking, with occasional nasal regurgitation. She also complained of increased ease of crying, even when she did not feel sad. She did not complain of progressive worsening of her speech during the day or with extended talking.

Oral mechanism examination revealed mild jaw and lower facial weakness. The tongue was weak bilaterally, but neither fasciculations nor atrophy was present. Palatal movement during vowel prolongation was minimal. A gag reflex could not be elicited. A sucking reflex was present. She had a prominent audible reflexive swallow. Her speech was characterized by slow rate (3); reduced phrase length, never exceeding two syllables; strained-harsh voice quality (3); hypernasality (3), with audible nasal emission on pressure sounds; monopitch and monoloudness (3). Speech AMRs were slow (3), slower than expected for her degree of weakness. Vowel prolongation was strained-hoarse and occasionally characterized by flutter.

The clinician concluded that the patient had, "Mixed spastic-flaccid dysarthria. I believe the spastic component predominates and that respiratory weakness generates the most significant flaccid component. The spastic component, and her pseudobulbar affect, are suggestive of UMN involvement and cannot be explained on the basis of weakness secondary to myasthenia gravis. On the basis of this examination, it is not possible to determine if the LMN component of her dysarthria is secondary to neuromuscular junction disease or some other disturbance in LMN function. However, there is no significant deterioration of her speech with stress testing."

Based on the speech evaluation, EMG studies were conducted. They failed to show evidence of ALS. A CT scan of the head showed moderate diffuse cerebral and cerebellar atrophy and a small lacunar infarct in the left basal ganglia. The neurologist concluded that the patient's difficulties were probably due to a combination of myasthenia gravis and pseudobulbar palsy of undetermined origin. However, multiple small infarctions were suspected as the cause of her pseudobulbar palsy.

Commentary. (1) By definition, mixed spastic-flaccid dysarthria identifies the presence of upper and lower motor neuron dysfunction. In this case, the speech diagnosis helped establish that myasthenia gravis could not be the sole explanation for the patient's difficulties. (2) Mixed dysarthrias can result from the co-occurrence of two or more diseases. In this case, the patient had a confirmed diagnosis of myasthenia gravis and, possibly, vascular disease leading to multiple CNS infarcts.

Case 10.5

A 55-year-old woman presented to Ear, Nose, and Throat with a nine-month history of cervical pain and hoarseness following a motor vehicle accident. Her ENT examination was normal. She was referred to speech pathology for evaluation of her hoarseness.

During speech evaluation, the patient noted that her dysphonia developed immediately after her motor vehicle accident and that vocal cord polyps were identified and removed by laser four months later. Her voice gradually returned to normal over the next few months, but hoarseness then returned, with an occasional "slurry" quality to her speech. She denied swallowing difficulty or problems with emotional expressiveness.

Oral mechanism examination revealed equivocal lingual weakness but bilateral lingual fasciculations. There was significant nasal emission during production of pressure-filled sentences, although the palate was symmetric and mobile. Speech was characterized by hypernasality (1); imprecise articulation (0,1); hoarse-rough voice quality (1,2) with occasional diplophonia. Vowel prolongation was breathy-hoarse-rough-strained (1). Speech AMRs were normal, except for equivocal slowing on "tuh." There was a very subtle vocal "flutter" during vowel prolongation.

The clinician concluded, "I believe the patient has a flaccid dysarthria that includes the Xth nerve, above the pharyngeal branch, and the XIIth nerve. A component of her dysphonia may indeed be due to excessive musculoskeletal tension in the laryngeal area, perhaps due to efforts to compensate for laryngeal trauma or weakness. However, findings are very suspicious for Xth and XIIth nerve weakness. Neurologic examination is strongly recommended."

On neurologic examination, in addition to her speech and cranial nerve findings, phrenic nerve weakness was suspected because she complained of shortness of breath when lying supine. On EMG, the phrenic nerve was normal; there were mild neurogenic changes in the tongue bilaterally, of indeterminate duration and origin.

Eight months later the patient returned for follow-up assessment. She had had increased episodes of choking, and it had become "more difficult to form words and letters" when speaking. She complained that her swallow was often audible and that she swallowed more slowly. She also noted, "When I cry, my mouth wants to start laughing." Oral mechanism exam revealed bilateral chin fasciculations, lower face weakness, lingual

weakness, fasciculations and atrophy, nasal escape during pressure sound production, and a weak cough and glottal coup. A sucking reflex and subtle "on the verge of crying" facial expression were present. Speech was characterized by slow rate (1,2); excess and equal stress (1,2); hypernasality with nasal emission (1); vocal "flutter;" strained-harsh voice quality (1); reduced pitch (2). Vowel prolongation was characterized by flutter and a rough-strained voice quality. Speech AMRs were slow (1). Speech intelligibility was normal.

The clinician concluded, "Mixed flaccid-spastic dysarthria, with clear worsening of speech difficulty and the emergence of a spastic component since she was last seen. Strongly suspect mixed bilateral upper and lower motor neuron dysfunction." The patient denied a need for speech therapy, and the clinician concurred. She was advised to seek reevaluation if her speech problems worsened.

Subsequent neurologic evaluation identified the presence of diffuse hyperreflexia and pathologic reflexes and weakness in her upper and lower extremities. An EMG showed widespread denervation in three extremities, as well as the tongue, consistent with ALS.

Commentary. (1) Dysphonia may be the first sign of neurologic disease. It can co-occur or be mistaken for vocal abuse or musculoskeletal tension-related dysphonias. (2) Dysarthria associated with ALS does not always present as a mixed dysarthria. (3) When dysarthria is present in ALS, it usually is eventually mixed flaccid-spastic in character.

Case 10.6

A 51-year-old woman presented with a 13-year history of PD with marked fluctuations in her neurologic signs and symptoms during her parkinsonian medication cycle. Neurologic examination revealed dysarthria, right arm dystonia and rigidity, bradykinesia, and left arm and leg tremor.

The patient was seen for speech evaluation 1.5 hours after her last carbidopa-levodopa (Sinemet) dose. Severe limb, torso, and head dyskinesias were present. The oral mechanism was normal in size, strength, and symmetry. Dyskinetic movements of her jaw, face, and tongue were apparent but not prominent during speech. Her speech was characterized by accelerated rate (2,3); reduced loudness (1,2); imprecise articulation (1,2); monopitch and monoloudness (1,2); variable rate (1,2); occasional inappropriate silences (1). Vowel prolongation was unsteady and intermittently mildly strained. Speech AMRs were irregular (1). Speech intelligibility was judged as very mildly reduced.

The clinician concluded that the patient had a "moderately severe mixed hypokinetic-hyperkinetic dysarthria, with the hypokinetic component predominating." It was recognized that her speech probably fluctuated with carbidopa-levodopa effects, and the patient was quite certain that it was more difficult to talk when her medication wore off. Speech therapy was undertaken, and the patient was quite successful in slowing her speech rate, with subsequent improvement in intelligibility and quality. With some adjustments in medication dosage and timing, there were fewer fluctuations in her speech and other neurologic signs.

Commentary. *(1) A mixed hypokinetic-hyperkinetic dysarthria can occur in PD, reflecting the direct effects of the disease on speech and its interaction with medication effects. (2) Fluctuations in the severity and nature of dysarthria in patients with PD can occur, sometimes dramatically, as a result of "on and off" effects associated with fluctuating medication effects. (3) Careful monitoring of speech can be a useful way to monitor medication effects in certain neurologic diseases.*

Case 10.7

A 61-year-old woman presented to neurology with a 6-year history of progressive coordination difficulty and an 18-month history of dysarthria. Clinical neurologic examination confirmed the presence of gait ataxia, upper limb incoordination, slowed and ataxic eye movements, and dysarthria.

During speech evaluation, the patient described speaking as a "real effort." She stated that she had to speak more slowly to be understood but admitted that she was unable to talk more rapidly. She had no chewing or swallowing complaints and denied drooling or difficulty with emotional control. Oral mechanism examination was essentially normal, with the exception that her cough and glottal coup were poorly coordinated. Speech was characterized by slow rate (2); irregular articulatory breakdowns (2); excess and equal stress (2); abnormal alterations in pitch, loudness, and duration of words and syllables (3); strained voice quality (1). Vowel prolongation was hoarse and unsteady. Speech AMRs were slow and irregular (2).

The clinician concluded that the patient had a "mixed dysarthria, predominantly ataxic, but with a mild spastic component." Intelligibility was minimally compromised, and the patient denied a need or desire for speech therapy. She was advised to pursue reassessment if her speech difficulty worsened.

Head CT scan demonstrated cerebellar and pontine atrophy. The neurologist concluded that the patient had OPCA (the patient's mother probably had a similar disease).

Commentary. *(1) Often OPCA is associated with a mixed dysarthria, in this case a mixed ataxic-spastic dysarthria with the ataxic component predominating. This mix logically reflects the sites of neurologic degeneration in the disease, and the dysarthria was a confirmatory sign for the neurologic diagnosis. (2) Mixed ataxic-spastic dysarthria is not diagnostic of any particular neurologic disease. As in most cases, the speech diagnosis is contributory to localization, rather than establishing underlying pathology.*

SUMMARY

1. Mixed dysarthrias reflect various combinations of flaccid, spastic, ataxic, hypokinetic, hyperkinetic, and unilateral UMN dysarthria. They occur more frequently than any of the single dysarthria types, highlighting the fact that dysarthria often reflects damage to more than one component of the speech motor system.

2. Mixed dysarthrias can be caused by many conditions that can damage more than one portion of the nervous system, but degenerative diseases are probably their most frequent cause. Single vascular events and single neoplasms leading to mixed dysarthrias tend to occur in the posterior fossa. Mixed dysarthrias resulting from toxic-metabolic conditions, infection, multiple vascular events, and trauma may be the product of diffuse or multifocal damage in many portions of the nervous system.

3. Because a number of diseases are associated with damage to specific parts of the nervous system, the types of mixed dysarthrias encountered in them are somewhat predictable. This is best exemplified by the mixed spastic-flaccid dysarthria that is classically associated with ALS. Overall, most mixed dysarthrias help identify the locus of their causative underlying lesions and sometimes whether they are consistent with specific neurologic diagnoses; they do not, by themselves, usually indicate their specific etiology.

4. Spastic dysarthria is probably the most frequently occurring type of dysarthria encountered within mixed dysarthrias. Flaccid and ataxic dysarthrias also occur fairly frequently. Hypokinetic, hyperkinetic, and unilateral UMN dysarthria are also encountered in mixed dysarthrias, but less frequently than the other dysarthria types.

5. Intelligibility is often affected in mixed dysarthrias. Patients with mixed dysarthrias, excluding those with ALS, frequently also have associated cognitive deficits.

6. In spite of the fact that mixed dysarthria reflects damage to more than one component of the motor system, it is fairly frequently the presenting complaint or among the earliest manifestations of neurologic disease. Thus, accurate recognition of the components of mixed dysarthrias can aid the localization and diagnosis of neurologic disease and may contribute to the medical and behavioral management of affected individuals.

REFERENCES

Adams RD and Victor M: Principles of neurology, New York, 1991, McGraw-Hill.

Aronson AE: Clinical voice disorders, New York, 1990, Thieme.

Aronson AE and others: Rapid voice tremor, or "flutter," in amyotrophic lateral sclerosis, Ann Otol Rhinol Laryngol 101:511, 1992.

Bannister R and others: Laryngeal abductor paralysis in multiple system atrophy: a report on three necropsied cases, with observations on the laryngeal muscles and the nuclei ambigui, Brain 104:351, 1981.

Berry WR and others: Dysarthria in Wilson's disease, J Speech Hear Res 17:169, 1974a.

Berry WR and others: Effects of penicillamine therapy and low-copper diet on dysarthria in Wilson's disease (hepatolenticular degeneration), Mayo Clin Proc 49:405, 1974b.

Beukelman DR, Kraft GH, and Freal J: Expressive communication disorders in persons with multiple sclerosis: a survey, Arch Phys Med Rehabil 66:675, 1985.

Carrow E and others: Deviant speech characteristics in motor neuron disease, Arch Otolaryngol 100:212, 1974.

Caruso AJ and Burton EK: Temporal acoustic measures of dysarthria associated with amyotrophic lateral sclerosis, J Speech Hear Res 30:80, 1987.

Caselli RJ and others: Rapidly progressive aphasic dementia and motor neuron disease, Ann Neurol 33:200, 1993.

Darley FL, Aronson AE, and Brown JR: Clusters of deviant speech dimensions in the dysarthrias, J Speech Hear Res 12:462, 1969a.

Darley FL, Aronson AE, and Brown JR: Differential diagnostic patterns of dysarthria, J Speech Hear Res 12:246, 1969b.

Darley FL, Aronson AE, and Brown JR: Motor speech disorders, Philadelphia, 1975, WB Saunders.

Darley FL, Aronson AE, and Goldstein NP: Dysarthria in multiple sclerosis, J Speech Hear Res 15:229-245, 1972.

DePaul R and Brooks R: Multiple orofacial indices in amyotrophic lateral sclerosis, J Speech Hear Res 36:1158, 1993.

DePaul R and others: Hypoglossal, trigeminal, and facial motoneuron involvement in amyotrophic lateral sclerosis, Neurology 38:281, 1988.

Duvoisin RC: The olivopontocerebellar atrophies. In Marsden CD and Fahn S, editors: Movement disorders 2, Boston, 1987, Butterworths.

Dworkin JP, Aronson AE, and Mulder DW: Tongue force in normals and dysarthric patients with amyotrophic lateral sclerosis, J Speech Hear Res 23:828, 1980.

Farmakides MN and Boone DR: Speech problems of patients with multiple sclerosis, J Speech Hear Disord 25:385, 1960.

Gentil M: Dysarthria in Friedreich disease, Brain Lang 38:438, 1990.

Gibb WRG, Luthert PJ, and Marsden CD: Corticobasal degeneration, Brain 112:1171, 1989.

Gilman S and Kluin D: Perceptual analysis of speech disorders in Friedreich disease and olivopontocerebellar atrophy. In Bloedel JR and others, editors: Cerebellar functions, New York, 1984, Springer-Verlag.

Grafman J and others: Frontal lobe function in progressive supranuclear palsy, Arch Neurol 47:553, 1990.

Gubbay SS and others: Amyotrophic lateral sclerosis: a study of its presentation and prognosis, J Neurol 232:295, 1985.

Hartman DE and O'Neill BP: Progressive dysfluency, dysphagia, dysarthria: a case of olivopontocerebellar atrophy. In Yorkston KM and Beukelman DR, editors: Recent advances in dysarthria, Boston, 1989, College-Hill.

Henderscheê D, Stam J, and Derix MMA: Aphemia as a first symptom of multiple sclerosis, J Neurol Neurosurg Psychiatry 50:499, 1987.

Herndon RM: Pathology and pathophysiology of multiple sclerosis, Semin Neurol 5:99, 1985.

Herndon RM: Multiple sclerosis. In Johnson RT, editor: Current therapy in neurologic disease, Philadelphia, 1990, BC Decker.

Herndon RM and Brooks B: Misdiagnosis of multiple sclerosis, Semin Neurol 5:94, 1985.

Hirose H, Kiritani S, and Sawashima M: Patterns of dysarthric movement in patients with amyotrophic lateral sclerosis and pseudobulbar palsy, Folia Phoniatr Logop 34:106, 1982.

Hook CC and others: Multifocal inflammatory leukoencephalopathy with 5-fluorouracil and levamisole, Ann Neurol 31:262, 1992.

Howard RS and others: Respiratory involvement in multiple sclerosis, Brain 115:479, 1992.

Hughes JT: Pathology of amyotrophic lateral sclerosis. In Rowland LP, editor: Advances in neurology, vol 36, human motor neuron diseases, New York, 1982, Raven Press.

Jankovic J: Progressive supranuclear palsy, clinical and pharmacological update, Neurol Clin 2:473, 1984.

Joanette J and Dudley JG: Dysarthric symptomatology of Friedreich's ataxia, Brain Lang 10:39, 1980.

Kent RD and others: Quantitative description of the dysarthria in women with amyotrophic lateral sclerosis, J Speech Hear Res 35:723, 1992.

Kent RD and others: Relationship between speech intelligibility and the slope of second-format transitions in dysarthric subjects, Clin Linguistics Phonetics 3:347, 1989.

Kent RD and others: Impairment of speech intelligibility in men with amyotrophic lateral sclerosis, J Speech Hear Disord 55:721, 1990.

Kent RD and others: Speech deterioration in amyotrophic lateral sclerosis: a case study, J Speech Hear Res 34:1269, 1991.

Kimmel DW and Schutt AJ: Multifocal leukoencephalopathy: occurrence during 5-fluorouracil and levamisol therapy and resolution after discontinuation of chemotherapy, Mayo Clin Proc 68:363-1993.

Kleinschmidt-DeMasters BK: Early progressive supranuclear palsy: pathology and clinical presentation, Clin Neuropathol 8:79, 1989.

Kluin KJ and others: Perceptual analysis of speech disorders in progressive supranuclear palsy, Neurology 43:563, 1993.

Konigsmark BW and Weiner LP: The olivopontocerebellar atrophias: a review, Medicine 49:227, 1970.

Krupp LB and others: Progressive multifocal leukoencephalopathy: clinical and radiographic features, Ann Neurol 17:344, 1985.

Kurtzke JF: Risk factors in amyotrophic lateral sclerosis. In Rowland LP, editor: Advances in neurology, vol 56, New York, 1991, Raven Press.

Landis DM and others: Olivopontocerebellar degeneration: clinical and ultra structural abnormalities, Arch Neurol 31:295, 1974.

Langmore SE and Lehman ME: Physiologic deficits in the orofacial system underlying dysarthria in amyotrophic lateral sclerosis, J Speech Hear Res 37:28, 1994.

Lebrun Y, Devreux F, and Rousseau J: Language and speech in a patient with a clinical diagnosis of progressive supranuclear palsy, Brain Lang 27:247, 1986.

Lees AJ: The Steele-Richardson-Olszewski syndrome (progressive supranuclear palsy). In Marsden CD and Fahn S, editors: Movement disorders 2, Boston, 1987, Butterworths.

Lethlean BJ and Murdoch BE: Language dysfunction in progressive multifocal leukoencephalopathy: A case study, J Med Speech-Lang Pathol 1:27, 1993.

Lethlean JB and Murdoch BE: Language problems in multiple sclerosis, J Med Speech-Lang Pathol 1:47, 1993.

Linebaugh C: The dysarthrias of Shy-Drager syndrome, J Speech Hear Disord, 44:55, 1979.

Lu FL, Duffy JR, and Maraganore D: Neuroclinical and speech characteristics in progressive supranuclear palsy and Parkinson's disease: a retrospective study. Paper presented at the Conference on Motor Speech, Boulder, CO, April 1992.

Ludlow CL and others: Site of penetrating brain lesions causing chronic acquired stuttering, Ann Neurol 22:60, 1987.

Maher ER, Smith EM, and Lees AJ: Cognitive deficits in the Steele-Richardson-Olszewski syndrome (progressive supranuclear palsy), J Neurol Neurosurg Psychiatry 48:1234, 1985.

Mancall EL: Central pontine myelinolysis. In Rowland LP, editor: Merritt's textbook of neurology, Philadelphia, 1989, Lea and Febiger.

Matthews WB and others: McAlpine's multiple sclerosis, New York, 1985, Churchill Livingstone.

Menkes JH: Disorders of metal metabolism. In Rowland LP, editor: Merritt's textbook of neurology, Philadelphia, 1989, Lea and Febiger.

Metter EJ and Hanson WR: Dysarthria in progressive supranuclear palsy. In Moore CA, Yorkson KM, and Beukelman DR, editors: Dysarthria and apraxia of speech: perspectives on management, Baltimore, 1991, Paul H Brookes.

Mulder DW: Clinical limits of amyotrophic lateral sclerosis. In Rowland LP, editor: Advances in neurology, vol 36, human motor neuron diseases, New York, 1982, Raven Press.

Oder W and others: Neurologic and neuropsychiatric spectrum of Wilson's disease: a prospective study of 45 cases, J Neurol 238:281, 1991.

Olmos-Lau N, Ginsberg MD, and Geller JB: Aphasia in multiple sclerosis, Neurology 27:623, 1977.

Petersen RC and Kokmen E: Cognitive and psychiatric abnormalities in multiple sclerosis, Mayo Clin Proc 64:657, 1989.

Pillon B and others: Heterogeneity of cognitive impairment in progressive supranuclear palsy, Parkinson's disease, and Alzheimer's disease, Neurology 36:1179, 1986.

Podoll K, Schwarz M, and Noth J: Language functions in progressive supranuclear palsy, Brain 114:1457, 1991.

Poser S: Multiple sclerosis, New York, 1978, Springer-Verlag.

Putnam AHB and Hixon TJ: Respiratory kinematics in speakers with motor neuron disease. In McNeil MR, Rosenbek JC, and Aronson AE, editors: The dysarthrias: physiology, acoustics, perception, management, San Diego, 1984, College-Hill.

Quinn N: Multiple system atrophy—the nature of the beast, J Neurol Neurosurg Psychiatry (special suppl):78, 1989.

Ramig LO and others: Acoustic analysis of voice in amyotrophic lateral sclerosis: a longitudinal case study, J Speech Hear Res 55:2, 1990.

Riley DE and others: Cortical-basal ganglionic degeneration, Neurology 40:1203, 1990.

Rodriguez M: Multiple sclerosis: basic concepts and hypothesis, Mayo Clin Proc 64:570, 1989.

Rose FC: Motor neuron disease, New York, 1977, Grune and Stratton.

Rowland LP: Motor neuron diseases: the clinical syndromes. In Mulder DW, editor: The diagnosis and treatment of amyotrophic lateral sclerosis, Boston, 1980, Houghton Mifflin.

Rowland LP: Ten central themes in a decade of ALS research. In Rowland LP, editor: Advances in neurology, vol 56, New York, 1991, Raven Press.

Saunders C, Walsh T, and Smith M: Hospice care in the motor neuron diseases. In Saunders C and Teller JC, editors: Hospice: the living idea, Dunton Green, UK, 1981, Edward Arnold Publishers.

Schiffer RB and Slater RJ: Neuropsychiatric features of multiple sclerosis, Semin Neurol 5:127, 1985.

Seikel JA, Wilcox KA, and Davis J: Dysarthria of motor neuron disease: longitudinal measures of segmental durations, J Commun Disord 24:393, 1991.

Sibley WA: Management of the patient with multiple sclerosis, Semin Neurol 5:134, 1985.

Sitver MS and Kratt A: Augmentative communication for the person with amyotrophic lateral sclerosis (ALS), ASHA 24:783, 1982.

Smith CR and Scheinberg LC: Clinical features of multiple sclerosis, Semin Neurol 5:85, 1985.

Sternlieb I, Giblin DR, and Scheinberg H: Wilson's disease. In Marsden CD and Fahn S, editors: Movement disorders 2, Boston, 1987, Butterworths.

Topaloglu H and others: Tremor of tongue and dysarthria as the sole manifestation of Wilson's disease, Clin Neurol Neurosurg 92:295, 1990.

Turner GS and Weismer G: Characteristics of speaking rate in the dysarthria associated with amyotrophic lateral sclerosis, J Speech Hearing Res 36:1158, 1993.

Weismer G and others: Formant trajectory characteristics of males with amyotrophic lateral sclerosis, J Acoust Soc Am 91:1085, 1992.

Williams DB and Windebank AJ: Motor neuron disease (amyotrophic lateral sclerosis), Mayo Clin Proc 66:54, 1991.

Yorkston KM and others: Speech deterioration in amyotrophic lateral sclerosis: implications for the timing of intervention, J Med Speech-Lang Pathol 1:35, 1993.

11 Apraxia of Speech

We now turn our attention to a category of motor speech disorders that is different from the dysarthrias. Its designation, *apraxia of speech (AOS),* distinguishes it from the neuromuscular problems represented by the dysarthrias, as well as from linguistically based speech errors associated with aphasia. The clinical manifestations of AOS are believed to reflect a disturbance in the *programming of movements* for speech. Unlike the dysarthrias,* AOS can exist without clinically apparent impairments in the speech muscles for nonspeech tasks. Unlike aphasia, in which there are nearly always multimodality impairments of language, AOS can exist independent of impairments in verbal comprehension, reading comprehension, and writing, as well as independent of verbal errors that are unrelated to articulation and prosody. Although AOS often coexists with dysarthria and aphasia, the distinctiveness of its clinical characteristics, its apparent nature as a motor programming disturbance, and its occasional emergence as the only disturbance of speech justify its identification as a unique type of speech disorder. Its distinction from other motor speech disorders is additionally warranted because it is nearly always the result of pathology in the left cerebral hemisphere.

Apraxia of speech is encountered as the primary speech pathology in a large medical practice at a rate comparable to that of several of the major single dysarthria types. From 1987 to 1990 at the Mayo Clinic, it accounted for 9% of the motor speech disorders seen in the Section of Speech Pathology (Figure 1–3). It also occurs very frequently as a secondary diagnosis in patients with left (dominant) hemisphere lesions whose primary communication difficulties are due to aphasia. It may also be a secondary diagnosis in patients whose primary diagnosis is dysarthria or some other neurogenic disturbance of communication ability. Therefore, AOS is present in far more than 9% of patients who have communication disorders associated with left hemisphere pathology.

The clinical features of AOS convey the impression that muscles are capable of normal function and that the appropriate message has been formulated, but that it is either difficult to enact the planned message or that the perceptual characteristics of the sounds that emerge are not what is intended. Careful study of AOS can illustrate the distinctions between motor speech programming and the neuromsucular execution of speech, and between motor speech programming and the formulation and organization of the linguistic units that are spoken. Such study also highlights the difficulty often encountered in attempts to make such distinctions.

In this chapter, the functions and location of motor speech programming mechanisms will be summarized. Some of the theoretical and clinical debate about the existence and nature of AOS will be reviewed but not dwelled upon. Emphasis will be placed on the clinical milieu in which AOS is encountered, its auditory and visible perceptual attributes, relevant acoustic and physiologic data, and some clinical case studies. The distinction between AOS and dysarthria and aphasia will be addressed in some detail in Chapter 15, which focuses on differential diagnosis.

---

*With the possible exception of speech-induced movement disorders, such as certain dystonia-based hyperkinetic dysarthrias.

ANATOMY AND BASIC FUNCTIONS OF THE MOTOR SPEECH PROGRAMMER

Motor speech control involves the interactive participation of all components of the motor speech system, as well as higher level activities related to conceptualization, language, and motor planning. The motor programming component of these activities is sometimes referred to as the *motor speech programmer (MSP)* (Darley, Aronson, and Brown, 1975). The MSP is influenced by sensory feedback, the basal ganglia and cerebellar control circuits, the reticular formation and thalamus, the limbic system, and the right hemisphere. From this perspective, motor speech programming involves widespread areas of the central nervous system (CNS). However, for the purpose of understanding the highest levels of speech programming—pathways and structures that specify the patterns and sequences of movements for speech—the *left cerebral hemisphere* can be thought of as the location of the MSP and the locus of lesions that lead to AOS.

The MSP has a primary role in establishing the motor program for achieving the cognitive and linguistic goals of spoken messages. It organizes the motor commands that ultimately result in the production of temporally sequenced sounds, syllables, words, and phrases at particular rates and patterns of stress and rhythm. The primary left hemisphere functions of the MSP seem to be more strongly tied to the linguistic aspects of speech (phonologic, semantic, syntactic, morphologic, and linguistic components of stress) than to its emotional or affective components, the latter components perhaps being more strongly influenced by contributions from the limbic system and right hemisphere. The linguistic input to the MSP comes largely from the left hemisphere's perisylvian area, which includes temporoparietal cortex and posterior portions of the frontal lobe, and, in a less definitive way, from the basal ganglia and thalamus. The anatomic proximity or overlap of these language areas with those of the MSP make it likely that damage to the perisylvian language zone often results in a co-occurrence of language-related deficits (aphasia) and AOS. In clinical reality this indeed is very often the case.

When a phonologic representation of a portion of a verbal message has been formulated (presumably most crucially in the temporoparietal cortex), the MSP must be activated to organize and activate a plan for its motor execution. This seems to involve the transformation of the abstract phonemes to a neural code that is compatible with the operations of the motor system. Execution of this motor program results in the activation of muscles in patterns that generate an acoustic signal compatible with the speaker's linguistic and communicative goals. Because speech is produced so quickly and without conscious effort by adults, it is reasonable to assume that the MSP selects, sequences, activates, and controls *preprogrammed movement sequences* (well-established subroutines, or "macros," to use computer terminology) that, through learning and practice, can be run off somewhat automatically. This permits rapid speech rates and greater allocation of resources to the more conscious formulation and monitoring of the cognitive and linguistic goals of communication.

The MSP relies heavily on *premotor areas,* of which *Broca's area* apparently has special importance. Broca's area seems to contribute to the specification of speech movements based on input from sensory modalities and areas involved in linguistic formulation. These premotor areas are linked to the basal ganglia and cerebellar control circuits and have reciprocal connections with the primary motor cortex that puts into effect the motor speech program.

The *supplementary motor area* is also involved in the activities of the MSP, although it may be further removed than Broca's area from the actual specification of specific speech movements. It has connections with the primary motor cortex and Broca's area, the basal ganglia by way of the thalamus, and the limbic system. It seems to be tied to cognitive and emotional processes that drive or motivate action and may play an important role in the initiation of propositional speech, as well as in its control. In general, however, it is not a common site of lesions associated with AOS.

The *parietal lobe somatosensory cortex* and the *supramarginal gyrus* are also implicated in the activities of the MSP and may be particularly important in integrating sensory information necessary for skilled motor activity. In addition, the *insula* appears to play a role in motor speech programming, at least from the standpoint that it is a frequent site of lesion in patients with AOS (Dronkers and others, 1993. Tognola and Vignolo, 1980). Finally, the basal ganglia, consistent with its known role in motor control, seems active in the activities of the MSP; lesions of the striatum have been associated with AOS (see, for example, Kertesz, 1984).

In general, conclusions about the presumed anatomy and functions of the MSP are supported by clinical findings. That is, lesions that produce AOS are usually located in the left posterior frontal or parietal lobe, in the insula, or in the basal ganglia. This reasoning is admittedly circular, however. On the one hand, much of the data upon which notions of motor speech programming for speech are derived are from the study of patients who presumably had AOS. On the other hand, the speech characteristics of people with lesions in the aforementioned areas are distinguishable from those associated with the dysarthrias. It is also clinically apparent that AOS can exist in people whose speech muscles perform normally for nonspeech activities and who are normally able to express language through nonspeech channels (for example, writing). Careful observation and analysis of their speech suggest that something is awry with the programming of speech movements. This disturbance has come to be called AOS by clinicians and investigators who recognize its distinctiveness, its value in contributing to our understanding of the neurology of speech and the localization of disease, and the unique demands it places on patients and clinicians who try to minimize its effects on communication.

NONSPEECH, NONOROMOTOR, AND NONLINGUISTIC CHARACTERISTICS OF PATIENTS WITH APRAXIA OF SPEECH

Apraxia of speech is frequently accompanied by physical speech mechanism findings, oromotor behaviors, and disorders of language that testify to the presence of dominant hemisphere pathology. These characteristics will be discussed in the speech pathology section later in this chapter.

Several additional clinical findings commonly accompany AOS. They usually reflect damage to the left frontal or parietal lobe or to left subcortical pathways and structures associated with the direct and indirect activation pathways. Many patients have varying degrees of right-sided weakness and spasticity, and some have associated sensory deficits. A Babinski sign and hyperactive stretch reflexes are also common. A hyperactive gag reflex and pathologic oral reflexes (suck, snout, jaw jerk) are not commonly present unless there are bilateral upper motor neuron (UMN) lesions, a condition not required for the presence of AOS.

Patients sometimes have *limb apraxia (LA),* a disorder also associated with left hemisphere pathology and characterized by deficits in the performance of purposive limb movements without impairment of strength, mobility, sensation, or coordination. It tends to affect movement control of both the right and left limbs, even though LA in the right extremity is often masked by right hemiplegia. It has been more widely accepted in neurology as a distinct clinical entity than has AOS, in spite of approaches to its clinical diagnosis that are highly variable and subjective. The psychological, physiologic, and anatomic bases of LA have been addressed extensively in the neurologic literature, even before the early part of this century when Liepman (1900) presented his historically dominant and widely accepted conceptualization of apraxia.

A comprehensive review of LA is beyond the scope of this chapter.* From the theoretical standpoint, it is important to recognize that there are important historical and conceptual similarities and differences between notions of apraxia as it affects the limbs versus speech. Anyone interested in in-depth study of AOS also should be familiar with theoretical and clinical issues associated with LA. From the clinical standpoint, it is important to recognize that patients with left hemisphere pathology may have difficulty organizing movements of both their right and left extremities, sometimes only on formal testing, but in some cases during activities of daily living. Of special relevance for issues related to communication, LA may interfere with writing as well as with propositional nonverbal communication (such as pantomime and sign language).[†] This is an important consideration for patients with severe AOS who may be in need of an augmentative or alternative form of communication.

ETIOLOGIES

Apraxia of speech can be caused by any process that damages dominant hemisphere structures involved in motor speech programming. Because inflammatory and toxic-metabolic diseases usually produce diffuse effects, only rarely are they associated with an isolated AOS. Tumors and trauma (especially surgical trauma) are more likely to cause focal unilateral signs. When they affect the left hemisphere, AOS may result.

Vascular lesions are the most common cause of AOS. There is nothing unique about the nature of the vascular disturbances (or inflammatory, toxic-metabolic, tumor, or traumatic etiologies, for that matter) that cause AOS, except that they are localized to dominant hemisphere speech programming structures and pathways.

Degenerative neurologic diseases are uncommonly associated with AOS, but sometimes they

---

*Overviews of theoretical and clinical assessment and diagnostic issues in limb apraxia can be found in a number of sources. For example, brief basic summaries can be found in Brookshire (1992); Wertz, LaPointe, and Rosenbek (1984); and Mesulam (1985). More detailed reviews and discussion can be found in DeRenzi (1985), Duffy and Duffy (1989, 1990a), Heilman (1979), Roy and Square-Storer (1990), and Square-Storer and Roy (1989).

[†]Aphasia also is related to difficulty in expressing propositional or symbolic meanings through pantomime and sign language (for example, see Duffy and Duffy, 1981, 1990b; and Duffy, Watt, and Duffy, 1981).

present as focal motor disturbances, one of which can be AOS. For example, although rare, AOS can occur in *multiple sclerosis (MS)*. Because *corticobasal degeneration* can be asymmetric in its presentation and often produces apraxia for many voluntary movements, AOS is sometimes the sole or primary motor speech disorder and can be among the presenting signs of the disease (Rosenfeld and others, 1991). Corticobasal degeneration and MS were discussed in Chapter 10.

A few additional degenerative conditions deserve mention because AOS can be among their prominent and presenting signs. *Primary progressive aphasia (PPA)* or *slowly progressive aphasia* is a disorder of insidious onset and slow, gradual progression that can exist in the absence or relative absence of generalized cognitive impairment. It reflects a degenerative condition that presumably predominantly affects the left perisylvian area of the brain (Duffy, 1987; Duffy and Petersen, 1992). It is not clear if PPA represents a distinct pathologic entity or a relatively longstanding focal manifestation of entities such as Alzheimer's disease, Pick's disease, focal spongiform degeneration, or nonspecific cellular degeneration, but Duffy and Petersen (1992) concluded that it has been described frequently enough to be considered a distinct clinical-behavioral entity. Their review of 54 cases reported in the literature from 1977 to 1990 also led them to conclude that PPA can be nonfluent or Broca-like in character, at least sometimes with an accompanying AOS. This author's clinical observations also suggest that AOS can be, for a considerable period of time, the only manifestation of degenerative neurologic disease, perhaps justifying its designation as "primary progressive AOS."

It may be that PPA (with AOS) is a variant of disorders that recently have been called *asymmetric cortical degenerative syndromes*. Three permutations of slowly progressive focal degenerative neurologic symptoms have been discussed by Caselli and others (1992) and Caselli and Jack (1992)—aphasia (PPA) associated with evidence of left hemisphere dysfunction, perceptuomotor dysfunction associated predominantly with bilateral (but often right greater than left hemisphere) parietal dysfunction, and neuropsychiatric dysfunction associated with frontal lobe dysfunction. These investigators presented illustrative cases demonstrating that the locus of cortical atrophy or hypoperfusion predicted by the behavioral deficits was confirmed by neuroimaging techniques. Therefore, it appears that degenerative disease—perhaps representing a variety of underlying pathologies—can present with focal manifesta-

tions and that AOS and aphasia can be among such manifestations.

Creutzfeldt-Jakob disease (CJD), also designated *subacute spongiform encephalopathy*, is a rapidly progressive (death usually occurring in 1 to 2 years), untreatable infectious degenerative disease with onset in early adulthood or midlife. It is characterized by dementia, cerebellar ataxia, fasciculations, pyramidal and extrapyramidal signs, myoclonic jerks, and a characteristic electronencephalogram (EEG) pattern (Adams and Victor, 1991; Mumenthaler, 1990). A variety of dysarthria types may be present, but dysarthrias in CJD have not been studied systematically. Signs and symptoms are rarely unilateral but three case reports (Mandell, Alexander, and Carpenter, 1989; Shuttleworth, Yates, and Paltan-Ortiz, 1985; Yamanouchi, Budka, and Vass, 1986) document that CJD can announce itself focally as aphasia. Review of these cases suggests that some of the patients probably also had AOS.

To summarize, AOS encountered in most clinical settings has usually been caused by stroke, and sometimes by tumor or trauma. Although uncommon, the insidious development of AOS in the absence of vascular disease, trauma, or evidence of tumor may be the presenting sign of a degenerative central nervous system (CNS) disease.

SPEECH PATHOLOGY
Terminology and theory

Someone once said, "When knowledge is lacking, a name comes to take its place." Different beliefs about the nature of AOS, efforts to achieve compatibility with embraced models of language, ego, nationalism, and the politics of academia and medicine have all probably contributed to the abundance of terms that have been applied to the disorder. Some of the terms summarized in the box on page 263 are rarely encountered in clinical practice today; they survive only as vehicles for tracing the history of study of AOS. A number of labels are still used in addition to AOS. The most common are *speech apraxia, oral verbal apraxia, Broca's aphasia, aphemia,* and *aphasic phonologic impairment*. Speech apraxia, oral verbal apraxia, and perhaps aphemia are synonymous with AOS. Broca's aphasia probably includes but encompasses more than AOS, and aphasic phonologic impairment may resemble but is different than AOS.

The debate about the nature of AOS has traditionally centered on whether it is distinguishable from aphasia. The frequent co-occurrence of aphasia with AOS and the overlap of anatomic regions that are crucial to language and motor speech

TERMS USED IN THE LITERATURE TO DESIGNATE SPEECH DISTURBANCES ASSOCIATED WITH APRAXIA OF SPEECH.

Afferent motor aphasia	Speech apraxia
Anarthria	Peripheral motor aphasia
Aphemia	Phonematic aphasia
Apraxic dysarthria	Phonetic disintegration
Articulatory dyspraxia	Primary verbal apraxia
Ataxic aphasia	Pure motor aphasia
Broca's aphasia	Secondary verbal apraxia
Little Broca's aphasia	Sensorimotor impairment
Cortical dysarthria	Speech sound muteness
Efferent motor aphasia	Subcortical motor aphasia
Expressive aphasia	Word muteness
Oral verbal apraxia	

Derived primarily from reviews by Darley FL, Aronson AE, and Brown JR (1975); Square-Storer PA and Roy EA (1989); and Wertz RT, LaPointe LL, and Rosenbek JC (1984).

programming naturally fuel such debate and predict that resolution will be difficult to achieve. Remarkably perhaps, there now seems to be general agreement that (1) at least some of the speech sound abnormalities of some aphasic patients are attributable to motor programming rather than linguistic deficits and that (2) a disorder of speech motor programming can result from left cerebral lesions that may or may not also cause difficulties with language. The support for these conclusions comes from studies of patients with AOS but normal language in nonspeech modalities, careful clinical perceptual descriptions, and acoustic and physiologic studies, sometimes with comparisons to aphasic and dysarthric speakers.*

It is beyond the scope of this chapter to review the details of the literature on the nature of AOS, particularly its distinction or lack thereof from aphasia. Some basic questions that frequently arise in clinical practice that reflect this debate should be addressed, however, because they bear on differential diagnosis and the use of terminology in clinical practice.

First, *is the term AOS synonymous with Broca's or nonfluent aphasia?* The answer is no, but requires explanation. Most definitions of Broca's and nonfluent aphasia do not give overt recogni-

tion to the existence of a motor speech programming deficit.* They do, however, describe patients' speech as slow, labored, or effortful, "dysarthric," reduced in phrase length, abnormal in prosody, and having poor "articulatory agility." These characteristics are consistent with those of speakers with AOS. If patients with Broca's aphasia truly are *also* aphasic, their speech usually is also characterized by grammatic and syntactic errors and problems with word retrieval, as well as problems with verbal comprehension, reading, and writing.

It is reasonable to conclude that people with Broca's and nonfluent aphasia usually have an accompanying AOS. In fact, McNeil and Kent (1990) argue that AOS may be an integral part of the syndrome of Broca's aphasia and that its presence may be required for its diagnosis. But, AOS is not synonymous with Broca's aphasia because the aphasic component of the syndrome includes deficits that are not explainable by AOS. They also are not synonymous because AOS can occur without any manifestations of aphasia.

Because of the strong association between AOS and Broca's aphasia, many studies of AOS have examined patients with Broca's aphasia. The review of acoustic and physiologic studies later in this chapter has included studies of people with Broca's aphasia under the assumption that many (perhaps most) of their speech deficits are reflections of AOS rather than aphasic phonologic deficits.

---

*Questions have recently arisen about the distinction between AOS and dysarthria. The distinction may be as difficult in some respects as those between motor programming deficits and aphasia (see, for example, the work of McNeil and others, 1990b; McNeil, Caliguiri, and Rosenbek, 1989; and Weismer and Liss, 1991). Perceptual, acoustic, and physiologic comparisons between AOS and the dysarthrias (particularly ataxic and unilateral UMN dysarthrias) will probably receive more attention in the near future.

---

*Representative procedures for identifying Broca's aphasia are included in frequently used tests of aphasia, such as the *Boston Diagnostic Aphasia Examination* (Goodglass and Kaplan, 1983) and the *Western Aphasia Battery* (Kertesz, 1982).

Are all sound level errors made by aphasic patients manifestations of AOS? Again, the answer is no, but with qualifications. This question is motivated by the presence of sound level errors in people with Wernicke's and conduction aphasia. Their speech, by definition, is usually perceived as fluent, easily produced, and prosodically normal. Many of their perceived sound substitutions, omissions, and additions probably reflect problems at the phonologic level of language; that is, their errors represent inadequate selection and sequencing of phonologic units but with subsequent adequate programming of them for execution by the MSP (as opposed to correctly selected phonemes being produced abnormally in those with AOS).

Ease of production and normal prosody appear to be major clues to distinguishing aphasic phonologic errors from those attributable to AOS. However, McNeil and Kent (1990) point out that some patients with Wernicke's and conduction aphasia make detectable phonetic-level errors. Differences, therefore, may be those of degree, with motor level deficits predominating in speakers with AOS (and Broca's or nonfluent aphasia) and phonologic deficits, when they are present, predominating in Wernicke's, conduction, and other fluent aphasias.

Are there subtypes of AOS? Many theories of apraxia suggest that breakdowns at different stages of motor programming may lead to different types of apraxia. For example, Rosenbek, Kent, and LaPointe (1984) state that "we might imagine errors in planning to be distinct from errors in serial ordering, which in turn could be distinct from errors in execution or implementation" (p. 22). Square-Storer and Roy (1989) state that "several subtypes of apraxia of speech may exist in that several cortical and subcortical sites appear responsible for the programming of spatial and temporal information requisite for normal motor speech production" (p. 25). Rosenbek, Kent, and LaPointe (1984) conclude, however, that whether the concept of different types of AOS is useful is a matter of disagreement.*

Notions about AOS subtypes center around divisions by lesion loci and variations in prosody and types of articulatory errors. In general, one type of AOS has been described as characterized by relatively well-formed articulatory errors (frank substitutions) with periods of normal prosody. It contrasts with another type of AOS characterized by distorted approximations of phonetic targets with relatively pervasive rate and prosodic abnormalities. The former type is associated with poste-

rior lesions (parietal-temporal), the latter with frontal or subcortical lesions.

There are some clinical data that suggest differences in AOS characteristics based on lesion site. Square, Darley, and Sommers (1982), for example, found that patients with parietal lesions had a predominance of frank substitution errors (and considerable dysfluency), while a patient with a basal ganglia lesion had a predominance of distortions. Deutsch (1984) found that apraxic speakers with parietal or temporal lesions made a greater number of sequencing errors (for example, transpositions of phonemes or syllables) than apraxic speakers with frontal lesions. Square-Storer and Apeldoorn (1991) reported that two AOS patients with subcortical lesions had increased word durations and excessive stress on unstressed syllables in contrast to an AOS patient with biparietal lesions who did not have increased durations. They argued that a criterion for AOS diagnosis of dysprosody unrelieved by periods of normal stress, rhythm, and intonation may not be valid because some speakers with AOS can have normal durations and prosody. They suggested that the presence or absence of unrelieved abnormal prosody might distinguish subcortical from cortical AOS or that the pervasive dysprosody might actually reflect the presence of AOS with an accompanying UMN dysarthria.

In general, therefore, *if* there are types of AOS, one type may be associated with a preponderance of articulatory substitutions and transposition errors with a prosodic pattern that is not pervasively abnormal. The other type may be predominated by articulatory distortions and unrelieved abnormal rate and prosody, a pattern more consistent with the characteristics of AOS to be described in this chapter.

Most clinicians would agree that these patterns of speech disturbance exist among people with left hemisphere lesions. What they represent, however, is not clear. They might reflect breakdowns at different levels of the motor programming process, warranting subdividing AOS into types. Alternatively, they could reflect the blurred boundaries between disorders of language and motor planning and programming, and between motor planning and programming and motor execution; that is, one "type" might actually reflect a linguistic phonologic disorder such as that encountered in Wernicke's or conduction aphasia (or an aphasic phonologic disorder plus AOS), and the other "type" a dysarthria (or an AOS plus dysarthria). If the latter explanation is true, then there may not be types of AOS, only AOS versus aphasia or dysarthria, or AOS plus aphasia or dysarthria. At this time, it seems inappropriate to subdivide AOS until the common features of the disorder are better delineated and understood.

*See Buckingham (1979), Luria (1980), Rosenbek, Kent, and LaPointe (1984), and Square-Storer and Roy (1989) for discussions of this issue.

ETIOLOGIES FOR 107 QUASIRANDOMLY SELECTED CASES WITH A PRIMARY SPEECH PATHOLOGY DIAGNOSIS OF AOS AT THE MAYO CLINIC FROM 1969 TO 1990. PERCENTAGE OF CASES UNDER EACH BROAD ETIOLOGIC HEADING IS GIVEN IN PARENTHESES.

Vascular (58%)
Single left hemisphere stroke (48%)
Multiple strokes, including left hemisphere (10%)

Degenerative (16%)
Unspecified degenerative CNS disease (9%)
Alzheimer's disease or dementia (4%)
Other: PPA; CJD; leukoencephalopathy (3%)

Traumatic (15%)
Neurosurgical (e.g., left hemisphere tumor resection, aneurysm or AVM repair, hemorrhage evacuation) (13%)
Closed head injury (2%)

Tumor, left hemisphere (6%)

Other (5%)
AOS or "expressive aphasia" of undetermined etiology (4%)
Seizure disorder (1%)

Multiple causes (1%)
Left hemisphere stroke + dementia

AOS, apraxia of speech; *AVM*, arteriovenous malformation; *CJD*, Creutzfeldt-Jakob disease; *CNS*, central nervous system; *PPA*, primary progressive aphasia.

The reader should note that the following descriptions of the clinical milieu, perceptual features, and acoustic and physiologic correlates of AOS are based largely on studies of patients with *pure* AOS; that is, they had no evidence of aphasia or dysarthria. This should contribute to understanding the attributes of AOS as it exists in "pure culture," but the clinical reality is that AOS errors often are intermixed with aphasic or dysarthric errors; the clinician may frequently struggle with the interpretation of errors as apraxic versus aphasic or dysarthric in nature. Differential diagnosis between AOS and aphasia and between AOS and dysarthria will be addressed in Chapter 15.

Distribution of etiologies, lesions, and associated deficits in clinical practice

The box above summarizes the etiologies for 107 quasirandomly selected cases seen at the Mayo Clinic with a primary speech pathology diagnosis of AOS.* The cautions expressed in Chapter 4 about generalizing these findings to the general population or to all speech pathology practices apply here as well.

The data establish that AOS can result from a number of medical conditions, the distribution of which is quite different from several dysarthria types but somewhat similar to those for spastic and unilateral UMN dysarthrias. Nearly 90% of the cases were accounted for by vascular, degenerative, or traumatic etiologies. Nearly 60% were accounted for by vascular etiologies alone.

Single strokes in the left hemisphere middle cerebral artery distribution accounted for most of the vascular causes. This is consistent with the prominence of stroke as an etiology of focal neurologic signs and the localization of crucial speech programming functions in the left hemisphere. The remainder of the vascular cases had multiple strokes in which at least one of the lesions was in the left hemisphere.

The localization of left hemisphere strokes for patients who had computed tonography (CT) or magnetic resonance imaging (MRI) scans that identified a lesion was generally consistent with notions about lesion localization in AOS. The frontal lobe was most frequently included in the lesion distribution but not much more often than the parietal lobe. The temporal lobe was sometimes

*The distribution of etiologies reported here is generally consistent with that reported by Wertz, Rosenbek, and Deal's (1970) analysis of etiologies in a group of 176 adults with AOS.

involved but never alone. When only a single lobe was implicated, it was most often the frontal but occasionally the parietal. The lesion was confined to subcortical structures in some cases.

Somewhat surprisingly, 16% of the cases were associated with degenerative disease. Most of these conditions were not precisely specified, but some of the patients had probable Alzheimer's disease or a similar dementing condition. The few remaining patients had diagnoses of PPA, CJD, or leukoencephalopathy. In some of these cases, AOS was the only or the initial sign of disease or was among the most significant deficits at the time of diagnosis. They illustrate that some degenerative neurologic diseases can present as focal disturbances. They also demonstrate that AOS can be the first sign of a slowly progressive degenerative neurologic disease.

Surgical trauma was the etiology in 13% of the cases. In all but one of them, surgery involved the left hemisphere, most often the frontal lobe. One left-handed patient had a right frontal lobe tumor resection and was also aphasic postoperatively; he likely had right hemisphere dominance for speech and language. A few patients had sustained a closed head injury (CHI), further establishing that focal motor speech disturbances can result from such trauma.

Six percent of the patients had a left hemisphere tumor, all of which included the frontal lobe. In three of these patients, AOS was among the initial neurologic signs. In one patient, AOS was the only clinically apparent evidence of neurologic disease, the tumor being identified on subsequent CT scan.

In the category "other," one patient had AOS in association with a seizure disorder. Of interest, 4% of patients had acquired AOS (or "expressive aphasia") as the only evidence of neurologic disease, leaving the etiologic diagnosis undetermined.

How often was nonverbal oral apraxia (to be discussed shortly) present? In patients for whom observations about it were made (60% of the sample), 63% had evidence of it. Therefore, consistent with the literature, there was a frequent but not invariable co-occurrence of AOS and nonverbal oral apraxia.

How often was aphasia present? In patients for whom observations about aphasia were made (99% of the sample), 78% had evidence of aphasia. Thus, it appears that for individuals in whom AOS is the most prominent speech or language disturbance, an accompanying aphasia is very often, but not always, present. This is in agreement with reports that AOS can occur independent of language disturbance. It is not appropriate to conclude from these observations, however, that 22% of people with AOS have no aphasia; that is, the sample did not include patients in whom aphasia was the primary speech-language disturbance. If all patients with AOS as the primary *or* secondary speech-language disturbance were included, the percentage of patients with AOS but without evidence of accompanying aphasia would be considerably less than 22%.

How often was dysarthria present? In patients for whom observations about dysarthria were made (99% of the sample), dysarthria was present in 29%. When dysarthria type was specified, it was most often unilateral UMN or spastic. The fairly frequent co-occurrence of AOS and dysarthria is consistent with the proximity of crucial speech motor programming structures and pathways to cortical and subcortical components of the direct and indirect activation pathways that execute speech motor programs. Unilateral UMN dysarthria is the expected dysarthria on this basis, with spastic dysarthria occurring in patients with lesions in more than just the left hemisphere.

In 70% of the patients, AOS was among the initial symptoms of neurologic disease. This fact is not surprising because of the high proportion of vascular etiologies in which speech-language and motor and sensory deficits usually are present together at onset. More illuminating, however, is the fact that AOS was the only problem at onset or the only clinical evidence of neurologic disease at the time of neurologic and speech evaluation, for 23% of the patients. This fact establishes that AOS can be an isolated, presenting sign of neurologic disease and that its accurate diagnosis can contribute to neurologic localization and diagnosis.

Patient perceptions and complaints

Patients with AOS may offer complaints that are quite different from those with dysarthria or aphasia. When AOS occurs without dysarthria or aphasia, individuals often say something like "my speech won't come out right. I know the words I want to say but they won't come out the right way." Phrases such as "not as fluent as before" and words like *mispronounce* are common descriptors. Complaints nearly always center on articulation and rarely on breathing, phonation, or resonance. When AOS is not severe, patients sometimes note being surprised by errors that intrude into an otherwise fluent narrative. Others report having to speak slowly or carefully in order to prevent errors. Some predict errors on difficult-to-pronounce multisyllabic words, and many recognize errors when they occur and attempt to correct them. The word *stutter* is occasionally used to describe associated dysfluencies, effortful groping for articulatory postures, and attempts at error correction. Patients admit that the problem may be more obvious under conditions of stress or fatigue.

Those with isolated AOS do not complain of chewing, swallowing, or drooling difficulties. If such problems are present, they should raise concerns about neuromuscular deficits and the possibility of an accompanying dysarthria. Patients also deny difficulties with verbal comprehension, reading comprehension, or the linguistic aspects of writing. Because AOS so frequently co-occurs with aphasia, however, all patients with suspected AOS should be considered aphasic until comprehensive language assessment proves otherwise.

Clinical findings

Nonverbal oral mechanism. In spite of left hemisphere damage, there may be no evidence of right lingual or central facial weakness. Similarly, the gag reflex and chewing and swallowing functions may be entirely normal, and there may be no pathologic oral reflexes.

Although the oral mechanism may be normal, it is more often the case that the causative lesion is large enough to have damaged corticobulbar pathways. It is thus common to find a right central facial weakness and sometimes right lingual weakness. A unilateral UMN dysarthria may be present as a result of such weakness. Any speech deficits attributed to unilateral face or tongue weakness are part of the dysarthria and not the AOS, however.

Because motor programming and control is a *sensori*motor process, it is reasonable to ask if oral sensation (for example, oral form identification, two-point oral discrimination, and mandibular kinesthetic abilities) is impaired. A few studies have addressed this issue, some finding evidence of deficits and a relationship to severity of AOS (for example, Rosenbek, Wertz, and Darley, 1973) and others failing to find such deficits or relationships (for example, Deutsch, 1981). Wertz, LaPointe, and Rosenbek (1984) concluded from their review of such studies that some patients with AOS have oral sensory deficits that may or may not be related to AOS severity. In general, the available data do not support a primary causative role of oral sensory deficits in AOS or the necessity for testing for such deficits in order to diagnose AOS.

Nonverbal oral apraxia. A substantial proportion of patients with AOS will exhibit a *nonverbal oral apraxia (NVOA),** which is characterized by an inability to imitate or follow commands to

perform volitional movements of speech structures; the inability cannot be attributed to poor task comprehension or to sensory or neuromuscular deficits. The lesions leading to it tend to include the frontal and central (rolandic) opercula, adjacent portions of the first temporal convolution, and the anterior portion of the insula (Tognola and Vignolo, 1980).

Although the co-occurrence of AOS and NVOA is quite high, there is no one-to-one correspondence between the two, and either one can exist in the absence of the other. For example, De Renzi, Pieczuro, and Vignolo (1966) found a strong correlation between the presence of NVOA and articulatory disturbances that probably represented AOS in a large group of patients with left hemisphere lesions. They noted that NVOA and speech errors were dissociated in some patients, however. Nonverbal oral apraxia was much more frequent in patients with Broca's aphasia than in those with Wernicke's or nonclassifiable aphasia types. Limb apraxia and NVOA also tended to co-occur, but the relationship between them was not as strong as that between NVOA and AOS. The fact that AOS and NVOA can occur independently argues against the notion that AOS is simply a reflection of a more fundamental disturbance of nonverbal oral movement (Wertz, LaPointe, and Rosenbek, 1984).

Commonly used sensitive tasks for detecting NVOA include imitating or following commands to cough, click the tongue, smack the lips, blow, or whistle (see Table 3–2 for a list of tasks and suggestions for evaluating NVOA).* Patients with the disorder invariably attempt to respond but do so awkwardly or with off-target responses, effortful groping for correct movements, or inconsistent trial-and-error attempts. Sometimes they try to perform the act but simultaneously say the command. For example, when asked to cough a patient may say "cough" and simultaneously attempt to cough. Patients usually are perplexed, frustrated, amused, or embarrassed by these off-target responses and often try to correct themselves, usually with inconsistent success. It is common to observe at a later time accurate reflexive performance of the failed voluntary act; patients may

---

*Nonverbal oral apraxia is also referred to by terms such as *oral nonverbal apraxia, buccofacial apraxia, lingual apraxia, oral apraxia,* and *facial apraxia.*

---

*Johns and LaPointe (1976) suggested that volitional coughing, blowing, and whistling were among the most difficult items for their patients because they require coordination of the breath stream, laryngeal activity, and oral movements. LaPointe and Wertz (1974) and Mateer and Kimura (1977) suggest that sequences of nonverbal oral motor movements (for example, click teeth together and then pucker the lips) are more difficult for aphasic patients than single discrete movements. Performance on such tasks can be confounded by verbal comprehension deficits (on commanded tasks) or by short-term retention difficulties (on imitation tasks), however.

cough reflexively, lick their lips, or blow out air in an exhausted sigh after failing to perform the same act on imitation or command. Patients with suspected AOS should always be assessed for NVOA because its presence is a sign of left hemisphere pathology.

Limb, nonverbal oral, other speech-language deficits, and patient complaints that may accompany AOS are summarized in Table 11–1.

Auditory processing skills. Central to discussions about whether AOS might actually reflect a language disturbance are questions about auditory processing skills. Auditory comprehension deficits are present in most patients with aphasia, and their severity is usually correlated with verbal output deficits. Such auditory deficits in pure AOS would raise suspicions about language deficits and might even suggest a causal role for auditory deficits in AOS errors.

Today, there seems to be a general consensus that auditory deficits are not present in patients with pure AOS and that when they are present in those with AOS and aphasia they do not explain speech errors that are considered apraxic in nature. These conclusions are based on a number of studies of apraxic speakers that have demonstrated adequate perception of stimuli to be produced and, at the least, auditory skills that were superior to speech production skills. The most convincing and thorough investigation of this issue was reported by Square-Storer, Darley, and Sommers (1988). They tested 4 individuals with pure AOS, 10 with aphasia, 10 with aphasia and AOS, and 11 control subjects on an extensive battery of auditory pro-

cessing and metalinguistic perceptual skills. Tasks included judgments of tone sequences and the phonemic accuracy of word productions, same-different judgments of real and nonsense word pairs, identification of target syllables and their location within trisyllabic words, and identification of objects whose labels began with the same sounds. The AOS patients performed as well as controls on all tasks. The aphasic and aphasic-apraxic groups were deficient but similar to each other. The investigators concluded that auditory processing abilities can be normal in AOS and that AOS and aphasia are distinguishable deficits from both motor speech and auditory processing perspectives.

It does appear that apraxic speakers are susceptible to the effects of disrupted auditory feedback, however. Chapin and others (1981) found that delayed auditory feedback (DAF) severely disrupted speech in those with Broca's aphasia, more so than in speakers with any other aphasia type. This effect does not necessarily argue for a causal role for disrupted auditory feedback in AOS, however. Chapin and others argued, for example, that it may be that the output deficit (in AOS) "is so fragile that any perturbation of the articulatory system ... seriously affects the quality of their output" (p. 112). It might be argued that apraxic speakers are particularly reliant on adequate auditory feedback to speak as well as they do.

It is reasonable to conclude that AOS can exist in the absence of auditory processing difficulties, but, because AOS usually occurs with aphasia, auditory processing deficits are often present in

Table 11–1 Common limb, nonverbal oral, other speech-language deficits, and patient complaints associated with AOS.

Limb	Right hemiparesis and/or associated sensory deficits
	Babinski sign
	Hyperactive stretch reflexes
	Limb apraxia, usually bilateral
Nonverbal oral	Right lower face weakness
	Right lingual weakness
	Nonverbal oral apraxia
	Oral sensory deficits
Language and other speech deficits	Aphasia, most often Broca's aphasia when language deficit can be categorized by type, but may be present in other types as well
	Unilateral UMN dysarthria
Patient complaints	"Speech doesn't come out right"
	Mispronunciation
	Stuttering
	Must speak slowly to prevent errors

None of these deficits and complaints is invariably present in AOS.
AOS, apraxia of speech; *UMN,* upper motor neuron.

apraxic speakers. Their presence, however, is not likely to be causally related to their motor speech disorder, although such deficits might serve to exacerbate it.

Speech. Tasks placing demands on the volitional sequencing of a variety of sounds and syllables are most likely to elicit the salient and distinguishing features of AOS. Conversational and narrative speech and reading can be revealing for this purpose, particularly if language and reading skills are good and the patient can give more than brief and unelaborated conversational or narrative responses.

Imitative tasks assist the clinical "hunt" for AOS because they can contain stimuli that challenge speech programming abilities and because they circumvent demands on word retrieval and other aspects of language formulation. This is important because the aphasia can make assessment of motor speech difficult. Aphasia also can mask or be difficult to distinguish from AOS.

Among the tasks most sensitive to AOS are *speech sequential motion rates (SMRs)* and *imitation of complex multisyllabic words and sentences.* It is not unusual for a vague suspicion of AOS generated during conversation and responses to simple language tasks to blossom into an unequivocal diagnosis after observing attempts to sequence SMRs and repeat words and sentences like "catastrophe," "statistical analysis," and "the municipal judge sentenced the criminal." Patients' repeated attempts at such tasks not only demonstrate apraxic errors but also highlight the inconsistency and variety of errors that are characteristic of many apraxic speakers.

The challenging tasks just described are not always useful for patients with marked or severe AOS. For such patients it is more valuable to discover what they are able to do and to contrast that with the nature of the tasks in which performance breaks down. Thus, it may be discovered that a patient who cannot converse intelligibly and cannot perform SMRs or even attempt to imitate multisyllabic words is able to count, imitate simple consonant-vowel-consonant (CVC) syllables, sing a familiar tune, and produce speech alternating motion rates (AMRs) because they are highly overlearned, can be produced "automatically," or place minimal demands on sequencing abilities. From this standpoint, examination reflects a search for the threshold at which patients succeed and fail on tasks reflecting a continuum of speech programming demands. For some, the threshold is high and tasks should be difficult; for others the threshold is low and tasks should be simple. For a few, AOS is so severe that a search for a stimulus that can elicit just a trace of phonation is most appropriate.

Table 3–6 provides a list of tasks and scoring notations that are useful for assessing AOS. Published tasks for the diagnosis of AOS—namely, the *Apraxia Battery for Adults* (Dabul, 1979) and the *Comprehensive Apraxia Test* (DiSimoni, 1989)—were discussed in Chapter 3.

Wertz, LaPointe, and Rosenbek (1984) point out that our modern descriptions of the perceptual characteristics of AOS have evolved over a number of years, beginning perhaps with Darley's clinical observations in the late 1960s (1968, 1969) and an important published study by Johns and Darley (1970) and then evolving to the present through a substantial number of perceptual and acoustic and physiologic studies.*

Descriptions of the articulatory and prosodic characteristics of AOS have been influenced by the results of acoustic and physiologic studies (to be reviewed in the next section) and the results of perceptual studies employing narrow phonetic transcription. Narrow transcription studies have highlighted the presence of vowel errors and the relative pervasiveness of distortions in AOS and established that what we perceive as substitutions in AOS (because of our "desire" as listeners to perceive meaningful units and because of many prior investigations' use of broad transcription and linguistic phonologic process analyses) may be the result of motor or phonetic level distortions. For example, Odell and others (1990) found that apraxic speakers produced more consonant distortions than substitutions and that half of their perceived substitutions were also perceived as distortions. This suggests that a significant proportion of the substitution characteristics described in the next box, when encountered clinically, will probably also be associated with distortions.

In spite of the separation of articulation from rate, prosody, and fluency characteristics as delineated in the boxes on page 270, it should be kept in mind that they usually co-occur in AOS. Rate and prosodic abnormalities are particularly pervasive problems that may be even more important to

---

*Clinical overviews and data-based studies that have contributed to the summary of perceptual speech characteristics offered here include Darley (1969, 1982); Darley, Aronson, and Brown (1975); Deal and Darley (1972); Dunlop and Marquardt (1977); Johns and Darley (1970); Keller (1978); LaPointe and Johns (1975); McNeil and Kent (1990); McNeil and others (1990b); Odell and others (1990); Rosenbek (1985); Rosenbek, Kent, and LaPointe (1984); Sasanuma (1971); Shankweiler and Harris (1966); Square, Darley, and Sommers (1981, 1982); Trost and Canter (1974); and Wertz, LaPointe, and Rosenbek (1984). Particularly valuable comprehensive historic, theoretical, or clinical overviews of AOS can be found in Buckingham (1981); McNeil and Kent (1990); Rosenbek, Kent, and LaPointe (1984); Wertz, LaPointe, and Rosenbek (1984); and Odell and others (1990).

clinical diagnosis than articulatory characteristics. It is of interest in this regard that Wertz, LaPointe, and Rosenbek (1984) consider trial-and-error groping, dysprosody without extended periods of normal stress and rhythm, difficulty initiating utter-

ances, and articulatory inconsistency to be the most salient features of AOS; three of these four characteristics can be considered prosodic abnormalities.

The meaning of rate and prosodic abnormalities in AOS is uncertain. Three possibilities exist: (1) they could represent a fundamental feature of AOS, as important as the disorder's articulatory deficits, (2) they could be a simple by-product of a fundamental problem with articulation (for example, how could rate and prosody possibly be normal in the context of the disorder's characteristic articulatory deficits?), or (3) they could reflect efforts at compensation for a fundamental deficit in articulation. It may be that all three explanations are valid, but today's definitions of the disorder usually consider prosodic disturbances to be among the defining features of AOS, and some acoustic and physiologic studies suggest that some prosodic characteristics in some apraxic speakers are not simply compensatory in character.

The boxes on this page summarize common articulatory, rate, prosody, and fluency characteristics of AOS. Not all patients with AOS display all of these characteristics, and some may actually run counter to them. The reasons for this are not entirely clear, but they may be related to the

---

ARTICULATORY CHARACTERISTICS OF APRAXIA OF SPEECH.

Perceived substitutions, distortions, omissions, additions, and repetitions. Substitutions more frequently perceived than other error types, but many substitutions may actually reflect or include distortions if narrow transcription is employed

Perceived substitutions tend to rank from highest to lowest frequency as follows: place > manner > voicing > oral/nasal

Bilabials and lingual-alveolar consonants less frequently in error than other places of articulation

Affricates and fricatives more frequently in error than other manners of production

Some but not many perceived substitutions are anticipatory or regressive ("nanana"/ banana), some are reiterative/perseverative ("popado"/potato), and some metathetic ("Dofter Ducky"/Doctor Duffy)

Consonant clusters more frequently in error than singletons

Vowel errors/distortions occur; when consonants and vowels differ in error frequency, consonant errors generally more frequent

Consonant substitutions sometimes perceived as complications rather than simplifications of target sounds; distortions and perceived substitutions tend to be close to target features

Sound position within words may not influence error frequency; when it does, initial position is most difficult, especially if delays in initiation and groping for articulatory positions are included as error characteristics

Error rates higher for infrequently occurring sounds

Error rates higher for nonsense syllables and words than for meaningful words

Error rates increase with increased word length; error rates increase as distances between successive points of articulation increase (for example, SMRs are more difficult than AMRs)

Error rates higher for volitional/purposive versus automatic/reactive utterances

Inconsistent errors; same sounds not always in error; error types not always the same in specific utterances

Errors occur on both imitative and spontaneous speech tasks; imitation errors generally do not exceed spontaneous speech errors on comparable productions

Speakers often aware of articulatory errors, can sometimes predict them, and often attempt to correct them

---

AMR, alternating motion rate; *SMR,* sequential motion rate.

PERCEIVED ABNORMALITIES IN RATE, PROSODY, AND FLUENCY IN APRAXIA OF SPEECH.

Rate and prosody

Rate for utterances more than one syllable in length is usually slow

Prolonged consonants and vowels

Silent pauses preceding initiation of speech; pauses between syllables or words give them a segregated character

Dysprosody very common

Equalized stress across syllables and words

Difficulty varying propositional stress in spontaneous and imitated sentences

Restricted or altered pitch, durational, and loudness contours within utterances

Altered prosody occasionally leads to the perception of a foreign accent in monolingual speakers

Fluency

False articulatory starts and restarts and repetitive attempts to produce words

Effortful visible and audible trial-and-error groping for articulatory postures ("conduite d'approche"), especially at the beginning of utterances; facial grimacing may accompany such efforts

Sound and syllable repetitions

Initiation of utterances particularly difficult

CHARACTERISTICS OF SEVERE AOS

Limited repertoire of speech sounds.
Speech may be limited to a few meaningful or unintelligible utterances.
Imitation of isolated sounds may be in error, and errors may be limited in variety.
Errors may be highly predictable.
Automatic speech may not be better than volitional speech.
Error responses may approximate target if stimuli are chosen carefully.
Muteness may be present, but rarely persists for more than 1 or 2 weeks if other speech, language, or cognitive deficits are not present.
Usually accompanied by severe aphasia, but can occur in the absence of aphasia.
Usually accompanied by NVOA.

AOS, apraxia of speech; *NVOA,* nonverbal oral apraxia.

possible existence of subtypes of AOS, to various contaminating effects of concomitant aphasia, or to variability associated with AOS severity. For example, variability of errors, although common in patients with mild to moderate AOS, may not be characteristic of those with severe AOS.

Severe apraxia of speech. Patients with mild to moderate (and perhaps marked) AOS represent the data base from which much of our understanding of the characteristics of the disorder is based. Unfortunately, there has been very little systematic study of severe AOS. This is probably because people with severe AOS tend to have significant and often severe aphasia that contaminates the study of AOS. This is unfortunate because marked or severe (hereafter called *severe*) AOS probably occurs much more frequently than generally milder, pure AOS. It is additionally unfortunate because the characteristics of severe AOS may not simply reflect a greater magnitude of the characteristics that define milder forms, especially the disorder's articulatory characteristics.

The box above summarizes the speech characteristics of many patients with severe AOS whose speech characteristics depart from those described for less severe forms. The features that distinguish severe AOS from less severe forms are primarily related to *reduced variability of articulatory characteristics.* This difference is important because variability of errors has traditionally been thought of as a hallmark of AOS.

Rosenbek (1985) has provided a helpful description of severe AOS. He points out that speech in severe AOS may be limited to a few meaningful or meaningless utterances on imitation, reading, and spontaneous speech tasks. Even attempts to imitate isolated sounds may be in error, and the types of error responses limited (less severely impaired patients may also make errors on isolated sounds, but their errors may vary across stimuli or repeated trials). Because their verbal repertoire is limited, errors may not approximate the target unless the target happens to resemble sounds or syllables in their repertoire. Although prosody and the expected number of syllables may be adequate, automatic speech may not be noticeably better than volitional speech (for example, a severely impaired patient might produce "dun, do, dee, daw, digh" when attempting to count from one to five); singing of a familiar tune may contain the correct number of syllables, with correct stress and tune, but contain only a single consonant and a few vowels (for example, "hatee turtee too too"/ "Happy birthday to you"). When only a few different sounds can be produced, errors may be highly predictable, sometimes giving the impression that the patient has actually "lost" sounds from the motor repertoire.

The severity continuum for AOS extends to muteness. Most clinicians agree that muteness (or apraxia of phonation) in pure AOS is an early and transient problem, usually resolving within a few days, at least when the lesion is confined to Broca's area (Mohr, 1980). It is very rare for muteness due to AOS alone to last for more than one to two weeks. In fact, a gratifying aspect of clinical practice is eliciting the first utterances in mute apraxic patients a few days following their strokes by having them count or sing a familiar tune with cuing from the clinician. Persistence of AOS mutism for more than a few weeks should raise suspicions about a different diagnosis or an additional problem, such as severe aphasia, anarthria, akinetic mutism, or psychogenic mutism. The distinctions among AOS and other forms of mutism will be addressed in Chapter 12.

Mute apraxic patients nearly always make attempts to speak on request, with attempts characterized by silent groping attempts to move the jaw, lips, and tongue to articulate and by gestural and facial expressions of frustration. A severe NVOA is usually present. It is rare that articulation ability significantly exceeds the patient's inability to phonate; that is, apraxia of phonation is nearly always accompanied by severe articulation difficulties.*

---

*A case study by Marshall, Gandour, and Windsor (1988) represents a dramatic exception. Their patient had a selective impairment of phonation (a laryngeal apraxia) for an extended period of time and was able to speak normally when using an electrolarynx.

Acoustic and physiologic findings

Acoustic and physiologic studies have provided confirmation for many of the disorder's clinical perceptual characteristics and have identified additional features that have shaped what clinicians should attend to perceptually. Equally important, they have provided a substantial body of data that supports a conclusion that many features of AOS probably do reflect a phonetic disorder of motor programming rather than deficits that are fundamentally linguistic in character. The following somewhat arbitrary subsections summarize the results of a number of representative acoustic and physiologic studies that have helped to characterize further the disorder's clinical features and clarify its general underlying nature. These acoustic and physiologic findings are summarized in Table 11–2.

Voice onset time. Voice onset time (VOT) is the duration between the articulatory release of a consonant and the onset of voicing for a following vowel. It is measured acoustically from the onset of the noise burst reflecting stop release to the onset of periodicity in the waveform reflecting the onset of glottal pulsing. Voiced stops are characterized by voicing lead (the onset of voicing before

Table 11–2 Summary of acoustic and physiologic findings in studies of AOS. Many of these observations are based on studies of only one or a few speakers, and not all apraxic speakers exhibit these features. Also, these characteristics may not be unique to AOS; some may also be found in dysarthrias or nonneurologic conditions.

Voice onset time	Overlap of VOT values for voiced and voiceless stops and fricatives VOT values in the range between voiced and voiceless values for normal speakers Increased variability and abnormal distribution of VOT values, even when perceived as phonemically accurate
Rate	Slow overall rate Excessive lengthening of consonants and vowels in multisyllabic words, word strings, and sentences Increased interword intervals and verbal response times Reduced ability to adjust speech rate on request, especially to produce faster rates, even in presence of demonstrated ability to produce some normally fast rates Delayed onset and inconsistency of coarticulation Slowed formant trajectories, with steady-state components in diphthongs Longer lower lip plus jaw movement and more velocity changes and movement variability during word repetition, in spite of normal peak velocity
Prosody and stress	Flattening of intensity envelope (syllable-to-syllable intensity variability) in phrases and sentences Reduced f_o decline over the course of lengthy sentences Reduced final word lengthening, relative to nonfinal words, in sentences Increased intersyllabic pauses and pause duration within utterances Uniform syllable durations within utterances, regardless of stress or position within sentences Acoustic evidence of equal stress on stressed and unstressed syllables within utterances
Precision and fluency	Failure to achive complete vocal tract closure for stops Abnormal F1 and F2 for vowel production with bite block in place Misdirected, exaggerated, and "perseverative" formant trajectories Acoustic or EMG evidence of reduplicated, aborted, or "stuttered" attempts, especially for initial segments of utterances
Variability and inconsistency	Greater than normal acoustic variability in onset of coarticulation, formant trajectories, attainment of vowel targets, and vowel duration Greater than normal variability in the direction, duration, velocity, and relationships between amplitude and velocity of jaw, lip, tongue, and velar movements

AOS, apraxia of speech; *EMG,* electromyography; f_o, fundamental frequency; *F1, F2,* formants; *VOT,* voice onset time.

the release of the stop), simultaneous voice onset and stop release, or voice lag (onset of voicing within about 20 ms after the stop release). Voiceless stops are characterized by voice lag of 40 ms or more.

Voice onset time has been a popular acoustic measure of coordination in studies of AOS because it reflects relative timing between supralaryngeal articulators (for example, the lips and tongue) and laryngeal events* that are essential to signaling phonologic distinctions. The VOT measures have provided valuable insights about motor programming versus phonologic deficits in patients with AOS.

Several studies indicate that the distribution of VOT values for voiced and voiceless stops overlap considerably in people with AOS, that their VOT values may fall in a range between normal voiced and voiceless values (that is, between 25 and 40 ms), and that they have greater than normal variability in VOT values, even when stop productions are perceived as accurate. These abnormalities have also been documented for initial voiced and voiceless fricatives (Baum and others, 1990). Although AOS patients sometimes produce VOT values that suggest a phonologic error (for example, a VOT value for a /b/ that clearly falls in the normal range for /p/), the general trend in the data is indicative of a pervasive phonetic rather than phonologic disorder (Blumstein and others, 1980). In fact, VOT values for productions perceived as substitutions are not always distributed in a manner consistent with normal productions of the perceived substituted phoneme.

In general, this overlap of VOT values and their greater than normal variability has been interpreted as reflecting a phonetic level deficit, an interpretation more consistent with poor motor programming than incorrect phoneme selection; that is, they suggest the correct phoneme (voiced or voiceless) has been selected but that the timing of articulatory and laryngeal activity is poorly regulated (for example, Blumstein and others, 1977, 1980; Freeman, Sands, and Harris, 1978; Hardcastle, Barry, and Clark, 1985; Itoh and others, 1982; Itoh and Sasanuma, 1984; Tuller, 1984). The pervasiveness of VOT abnormalities has led to a conclusion that AOS is particularly susceptible to phonetic parameters requiring the integration of activities of more than one articulator (Baum and others, 1990).

Rate. Slow rate is a common perceived abnormality in AOS. Studies of its acoustic and physiologic correlates generally support and refine these

clinical perceptions. Some of them provide insight into whether slowed rate is a primary feature of AOS or reflects compensatory efforts to maintain articulatory control.

A number of acoustic studies have quantified slow rate in AOS (for example, Gandour, Petty, and Dardarananda, 1989; Kent and Rosenbek, 1983; Pellat and others, 1991; Skenes, 1987; Square-Storer and Apeldorn, 1991). Several have documented excessive lengthening of consonants (for example, McNeil and Kent, 1990; Weismer and Liss, 1991) as well as increased vowel duration in multisyllabic words, word strings, and phrases (for example, Collins, Rosenbek, and Wertz, 1983; Caligiuri and Till, 1983; Kent and Rosenbek, 1982; McNeil and Kent, 1990; Ryalls, 1981).

Because vowel duration does not carry specific linguistic meaning in many contexts, it is difficult to argue that increased vowel durations reflect an underlying linguistic disorder, especially when some findings also indicate that AOS speakers do follow certain rules for vowel duration. For example, Collins, Rosenbek, and Wertz (1983) demonstrated that AOS speakers, like normal speakers, reduced vowel duration in segments as the number of segments in an utterance increased (for example, the vowel in the syllable *cat* in the word *catapult* was shortened relative to the vowel in the syllable *cat* produced in isolation). In addition, AOS speakers obey the "vowel shortening rule" to signal the voicing feature for syllable final consonants (that is, vowels preceding voiceless final consonants are shorter than vowels preceding the voiced cognate) (Baum and others, 1990; Caligiuri and Till, 1983; Duffy and Gawle, 1984). Thus, like normal speakers, apraxic speakers vary vowel duration to signal linguistic contrasts, even though their vowel durations tend to be longer than those of normal speakers.

Acoustic analyses also demonstrate increased interword intervals in AOS, a finding that supports the perception of syllable segregation. This suggests that apraxic speakers engage in independent (syllable-by-syllable) programming of syllables to a greater extent than normal speakers (Gandour, Petty, and Dardarananda, 1989; Kent and Rosenbek, 1983; McNeil and Kent, 1990; Mercaitis, 1983; Ziegler and Von Cramon, 1986). Strand and McNeil (1987) have shown that apraxic speakers, similar to normal speakers, decrease interword intervals in sentences relative to interword intervals in word strings but that they are less consistent in doing so. They interpreted this as reflecting an impaired mechanism for activating and executing motor plans. Findings of increased verbal response times in apraxic speakers (Mercaitis, 1983; Strand, 1987; Towne and Crary, 1988) also support this conclusion.

It has been difficult to establish if slow rate in AOS is compensatory (that is, articulatory accuracy may

---

*Laryngeal events associated with timing for VOT may be more accurately described as laryngeal-respiratory events based on recent findings of Hoit, Solomon, and Hixon (1993) that VOT tends to be longer at high lung volumes and shorter at low lung volumes.

be achieved if rate is "intentionally" slowed) or a reflection of a primary part of the disorder. Addressing this issue, McNeil and others (1990a) acoustically analyzed durations under controlled, slowed, and fast speech rates. They (as well as Robin, Bean, and Folkins, 1989) found that apraxic speakers were less efficient in adjusting rates, especially increasing rate, even though they were able to produce some normally fast rates. This was interpreted as reflecting a problem with motor control and as evidence against the notion that all slowed rate in AOS is compensatory. Skenes (1987) also found that AOS speakers had difficulty changing rate when instructed to speak rapidly, again arguing against explanations of slowed rate in AOS as reflecting only compensatory efforts. Finally, McNeil and Kent (1990) suggest that certain temporal parameters in AOS may be an artifact of slow rate because even normal speakers show some evidence of decomposition or increased variability of relative timing patterns at slow rates when compared to average or fast rates.

Studies of coarticulation also provide evidence of delayed (or deficient) onset of coarticulation. Ziegler and Von Cramon (1986), examining acoustic evidence of coarticulation in unstressed vowels and stop noise bursts in trisyllabic utterances, found inconsistency and a relative lack of evidence of coarticulation that made prediction of upcoming articulatory events difficult (Ziegler and Von Cramon, 1985). This finding was interpreted as reflecting a disturbance in phase relationships of individual articulatory gestures. The authors noted that this mistiming was generally in the direction of delays of anticipatory coarticulation. Weismer and Liss (1991) also found acoustic evidence of slowed formant trajectories in diphthongs of apraxic speakers. Their apraxic speakers displayed some long steady-state portions within diphthongs, something not observed in normal speakers.

McNeil, Caligiuri, and Rosenbek (1989) used movement transducers to measure lower lip plus jaw movements in apraxic and normal speakers during a word repetition task. Average movement durations were longer and more variable in apraxic speakers, but peak velocity (the maximum speed attained) did not differ. Apraxic speakers also had a greater number of velocity changes and greater velocity variability during movement. These results suggest that lip movements are not fundamentally slower than normal, even though lip gestures take longer to achieve.* The authors speculated that

movements took longer because some were larger (involved greater displacement) or because movements had a greater number of movement aberrations over the course of movement (dysmetrias). Of interest, they noted that such dysmetrias are not dissimilar to those observed in ataxic dysarthria associated with cerebellocortical programming problems. They pointed out, however, that the dysmetrias may reflect an artifact of slow speaking rate because some normal speakers can look dysmetric when speaking at slow rates.

In summary, speech rate in AOS is generally slower and more variable than normal. Acoustic and physiologic findings generally support a conclusion that these rate aberrations reflect motor or phonetic level deficits rather than linguistic deficits, especially because apraxic speakers appear generally capable of signaling linguistic distinctions that are dependent upon rate modifications. Although such studies tend to argue against linguistic explanations for rate deficits, they do raise questions about distinctions between AOS and abnormalities found in certain types of dysarthria, particularly ataxic dysarthria.

Prosody and stress. Prosodic abnormalities are considered by some to be a universal and defining feature of AOS. Although some investigators argue that prosodic disturbances may not be present in all patients or at least may not be present within all utterances (Square-Storer and Apeldoorn, 1991), acoustic data documenting rate and variability abnormalities are strongly predictive and supportive of perceived prosodic abnormalities in many apraxic speakers. A number of additional acoustic studies have addressed prosody and stress abnormalities in AOS directly. They also are supportive of perceived abnormalities.

Apraxic speakers tend to show a reduction of intensity variation from syllable to syllable within phrase or sentence utterances (Gandour, Petty, and Dardarananda, 1989; Kent and Rosenbek, 1983). This generally means that unstressed syllables are produced with relatively greater intensity than normal, making them less distinguishable from stressed syllables. This tendency toward temporal and amplitude uniformity seems to be correlated with neutralization of stress and dysprosody (McNeil and Kent, 1990).

Abnormalities in regulation of fundamental frequency (f_o) may also be apparent in AOS. In normally spoken declarative sentences, f_o tends to decline in a linear fashion over the course of an utterance, with the greatest and most rapid decline occurring at the end of the utterance. In addition, the terminal words of declarative sentences tend to be lengthened, signaling the end of the utterance. Danly and Shapiro (1982) have shown that Broca's aphasics, while demonstrating a decline in f_o

---

*Similarly, Robin, Bean, and Folkins (1989) found that apraxic speakers were able to generate high peak lip velocities when asked to speak rapidly and when a bite block was in place. They also found no differences in peak lip velocities between perceived accurate and inaccurate word productions.

at the end of simple sentences, may not do so over longer utterances. They also found that final words were not clearly longer in duration than initial or medial words and that, in some instances, final words were actually shorter; this lack of durational distinction may be due to an increase in the length of nonfinal words rather than a shortening of final words. This occurrence could be characterized by the patient's effortful articulation or difficulty with syntax, reflecting a smaller scope of linguistic planning, motor planning, or both. McNeil and Kent (1990) also suggest that f_o may be used in a compensatory fashion, such as when a speaker increases f_o within a sentence to signal an intent to continue talking.

Acoustic studies have also documented increased intersyllabic pauses within utterances (Ziegler and von Cramon, 1986), suggesting that each syllable is being programmed independently. Acoustic findings of longer pause time, increased number of pauses within utterances, greater pause duration, stress on each syllable including non-stressed syllables, slower overall rate, shorter phrases, and uniform syllable durations regardless of stress or sentence position (Gandour, Petty, and Dardarananda, 1989; Kent and Rosenbek, 1983) all provide support for the frequent perception of prosodic and stress abnormalities in AOS. Taken together, these findings imply a simplification of motor programming in AOS; that is, the perception that each syllable is stressed or produced as a single unit, rather than merged with other syllables and words in a phrase, suggests that some speakers must approach the programming of speech in a syllable-by-syllable manner and that normal stress and prosodic flow are lost in the process.

Articulatory precision and fluency. Many of the acoustic and physiologic findings already discussed carry an implication that articulation is imprecise, if not inaccurate, in place, manner, and voicing. A few additional findings add to such evidence and also provide support for perceived dysfluencies in AOS.

Regarding articulatory imprecision, there is acoustic evidence that Broca's aphasic or AOS speakers may fail to achieve complete vocal tract closure for stops (Shinn and Blumstein, 1983; Weismer and Liss, 1991). The resulting noise (spirantization), instead of silence reflecting closure, suggests distortion rather than a true fricative for stop substitution.

Imprecision extends to vowels. With a bite block in place, normal speakers are able to achieve normal formant positions for targeted vowels, often at the first glottal pulse of their initial effort. In contrast, Sussman and others (1986) found that speakers with Broca's aphasia (and, presumably, AOS), attempting to produce /i/ with a bite block

in place, had higher than normal F1 and lower F2 values, indicative of undershooting of tongue elevation and fronting. At the least, this finding suggests that AOS is associated with difficulties in making on-line adjustments for compensatory articulation, including vowels.

Weismer and Liss (1991) found evidence of misdirected formant trajectories in the connected speech of apraxic speakers; for example, rather than formants following a normal monotonic course, they would sometimes initially rise and then fall. They also found evidence of exaggerated formant trajectories (by inference, exaggerated extent of movement), in which the frequency change in a formant transition was greater than normal. Finally, they observed perseverative trajectories, in which formant transitions sometimes resembled those in preceding syllables. Each of these observations implies imprecision or inaccuracy of articulatory movements during speech. Of interest, Weismer and Liss noted that some of these characteristics are ataxic-like in character, whereas others might reflect effort at compensation.

A few studies have documented the occurrence of events that support the perception of dysfluencies or aborted articulatory attempts in AOS. For example, Towne and Crary (1988) found EMG evidence of reduplicated attempts during the initial segments of words, Weismer and Liss (1991) commented on acoustic evidence of aborted articulatory attempts, Katz and others (1990) found evidence of "stuttered" initial consonant segments, and Fromm and others (1982) reported kinematic and EMG data suggestive of added movements and groping.

Variability and inconsistency. Inconsistency is considered by many to be a hallmark of AOS, at least at less than severe degrees of impairment. McNeil and Kent (1990) point out that variability in AOS tends to argue for a speech mechanism that is linguistically and biomechanically sound but characterized by a phonetic level defect.

Acoustic studies have provided considerable evidence of greater than normal variability in AOS. These studies are theoretically important because measures of variability often have been computed on productions perceived as accurate on broad phonetic transcription. Abnormal variability in phonologically accurate productions makes it difficult to argue that such disturbances are linguistically based.

Several studies have examined vowel formant trajectories for evidence of coarticulation, rate of change, and attainment of proper vowel targets, with task demands sometimes requiring speech rate or stress adjustments. In addition to documenting reduced rate and evidence of less than adequate coarticulation, these studies usually document greater than normal variability (McNeil and others, 1990; Ryalls, 1981, 1986; Weismer and Liss, 1991; Zeigler and von Cramon, 1986). Similarly, studies of vowel duration in single syllable, multisyllabic, and phrase productions have generally documented greater than normal variability in vowel duration (for example, Caligiuri and Till, 1983; Duffy and Gawle, 1984; Shankweiler, Harris, and Taylor, 1968; Weismer and Liss, 1991).

Physiologic measures of jaw, lip, tongue, and velar movements during speech have also documented greater than normal variability. For example, Itoh and Sasanuma (1984) and Itoh, Sasanuma, and Ushijima (1979); found marked variability in the height and segmental duration of velar movements across repetitions of the same stimuli, in spite of the fact that a fairly normal pattern of velar movement was maintained. Highly variable coarticulatory patterns for labial and velar movements during speech, especially for measures of spatial displacement, were identified by Katz and others (1990). Similarly, studies of lip and jaw movements have identified greater than normal variability in peak velocity, velocity changes, and relationships between movement amplitude and velocity (Forrest and others, 1991; McNeil, Caliguiri, and Rosenbek, 1989). Finally, McNeil and others (1990), examining nonspeech isometric force and static position control of the lips, tongue, and jaw, found greater than normal force and position instability in individuals with AOS (and in subjects with ataxic dysarthria). They noted, however, that the pattern of instability was not consistent across all structures tested and that not all AOS subjects demonstrated instability.

Although it is not included in this review, some speakers with conduction aphasia and Wernicke's aphasia have displayed acoustic and physiologic abnormalities similar to those found in AOS. Such abnormalities are usually of lesser magnitude than those found in AOS, and they do not argue for linguistic explanations of AOS. They do suggest, however, that some degree of motor programming and control difficulty may be present in patients who do not display perceptual evidence of AOS.

CASES

Case 11.1

A 68-year-old woman awoke one morning unable to speak and with mild right-sided weakness. Emergency room examination revealed a right central facial weakness, mild right hemiparesis, and inability to speak.

Speech evaluation the following day demonstrated normal oral movements with the exception of limited tongue excursion to the right, but she produced only off-target groping movements of her jaw and lips when asked to clear her throat, click her tongue, blow, or whistle. Her reflexive cough was normal. She produced only awkward, groping, off-target jaw and lip movements when asked to count, sing a familiar tune, or imitate simple sounds or syllables. She could awkwardly produce the vowel "ah" and with effort imitated the vowels /ou/ and /u/. She was able to produce /m/ in isolation but could imitate no other isolated sounds. She achieved correct articulatory place for /f/ but could not simultaneously move air to produce frication.

Verbal comprehension was normal, even for the most difficult portion of the Token Test (DeRenzi and Vignolo, 1962). Reading comprehension was normal. Writing with her preferred right hand was awkward because of hemiparesis, but spelling, word choice, and sentence structure were normal.

A CT scan five days postonset identified a lesion in the left hemisphere at the junction of the posterior frontal and parietal lobes. The neurologic diagnosis was left hemisphere stroke.

Speech therapy was undertaken. At the time of discharge six weeks later, she was producing most sounds within single syllables, although very slowly and with excess and equal stress when she attempted to string syllables together. When reassessed two months later, she was speaking laboriously in sentences, with moderately slowed rate and excess and equal stress, very careful articulation, and pervasive mild articulatory distortions. When reassessed two years later, speech was functional but characterized by moderately slowed rate and occasional perceived articulatory substitutions, especially on multisyllabic words. She had consistent difficulty with /s/, /z/, /l/, and all consonant clusters.

Commentary. *(1) Stroke is the most common cause of AOS, and AOS may be the only or most prominent manifestation of stroke; (2) AOS may be characterized by muteness at onset, although patients mute from AOS usually attempt to speak; (3) although AOS usually occurs with aphasia, it can exist without any evidence of language impairment, sometimes even when severe, (4) AOS is frequently accompanied by an NVOA; and (5) when caused by stroke, AOS tends to improve over time, sometimes dramatically. The gains may be greatest when there is no or minimal language impairment.*

Case 11.2

A 63-year-old man was hospitalized following a left carotid endarterectomy at another institution six weeks previously. Postoperative difficulties included speech problems and right hemiparesis. Neurologic examination noted a mild right hemiparesis, "dysarthria from facial weakness and a nonfluent aphasia."

Speech-language evaluation revealed mild difficulty with verbal and reading comprehension and inability to write intelligibly because of right hemiparesis. Speech was telegraphic and characterized by numerous articulatory revisions, hesitancy, and repetitions, as well as reduced loudness, mild hoarseness, and consistent mild articulatory distortions. A right central facial weakness was present.

The clinician concluded that the patient had "an AOS which is the major variable contributing to his commu-

nication disorder, a nonfluent (Broca's-like) aphasia, and a unilateral UMN dysarthria." Speech-language therapy was recommended.

A CT scan and cerebral angiogram the following day identified the presence of a mass in the left frontoparietal region. He underwent surgery for gross total removal of a meningioma. Reassessment two days postoperatively indicated that the aphasia had resolved. Mild AOS and unilateral UMN dysarthria remained but were improved. He received therapy for one week prior to his discharge. At the time of discharge, he was able to carry on a conversation without significant difficulty. He still had a mild AOS, which was most apparent when he was anxious or attempting to speak at normal rate. Reassessment by his neurologist several months later suggested that he had continued to improve but that residual speech difficulty remained.

Commentary: (1) Apraxia of speech often occurs with aphasia and unilateral UMN dysarthria. In this case, all three disorders were present initially, with the AOS being the most evident deficit. (2) Etiology of AOS may include vascular disturbances, as well as tumor. In this case, stroke initially appeared to be the etiology, although subsequent identification of a tumor raised the possibility that it was causing the AOS. (3) AOS is associated with a range of severity. In this case, it was relatively mild, and improvement was good but not complete.

Case 11.3

A 51-year-old woman was admitted to the hospital after several hours of progressive speech and writing difficulty, difficulty counting change, and not knowing how to start her car. Emergency room evaluation revealed a right central facial weakness, disorientation, limb apraxia, and difficulty with verbal expression. Comprehension appeared normal. A cerebral angiogram conducted four days postonset identified occlusion of two of the ascending frontal parietal branches of the left middle cerebral artery. A CT scan was negative. A diagnosis of left frontoparietal stroke was made.

Speech-language examination a few days later revealed AOS as her most prominent communication deficit, although there was an accompanying aphasia. The AOS was characterized by articulatory substitutions, omissions, and distortions; groping for articulatory postures; slow rate; and altered prosody. Articulatory difficulties increased with increasing word or utterance length. Speech AMRs were slow, and she had difficulty sequencing SMRs. She had a right central facial weakness and equivocal tongue weakness. The clinician felt she might also have had a unilateral UMN dysarthria.

She had good comprehension for single and two-step commands, but she performed poorly on the more difficult portions of the Token Test. Linguistically, verbal expression was quite good. She was a bit telegraphic, but the clinician wondered if it reflected compensation for the AOS. She had no difficulty with picture naming, but rapid word retrieval abilities fell outside the normal range. Reading comprehension for sentences and short paragraphs was adequate. Writing was linguistically adequate, but she had some difficulty with letter forma-

tion, suggestive of limb apraxia. There was no evidence of NVOA.

The clinician concluded that the patient had a moderately severe AOS and a mild accompanying aphasia. She improved significantly by the time of her discharge a few days later. For example, during a 10-minute conversation, she exhibited only three perceived substitutions and one episode of groping for articulatory posture. Slowing of speech rate facilitated articulation. She was minimally frustrated by her speech difficulty and confident that she would continue to improve. She decided not to pursue speech therapy after discharge.

Commentary: (1) Apraxia of speech and aphasia are frequently the initial manifestations of left hemisphere stroke. (2) AOS can be the prominent communication deficit in patients with AOS and aphasia. When it is relatively mild at onset, significant recovery can be expected. (3) Frequently AOS and NVOA co-occur, but AOS can be present without evidence of NVOA.

Case 11.4

An 81-year-old man was admitted to the rehabilitation unit because of speech and limb control difficulties of 2 years' duration, presumably the result of a left hemisphere stroke. A CT scan revealed mild cerebral atrophy but was otherwise normal. An electoencephalogram was suggestive of a left hemisphere lesion. He was referred for speech-language assessment and recommendations.

During the initial interview, the patient reported that his speech had been slowly deteriorating. Oral mechanism examination revealed a mild right central facial weakness and an NVOA characterized by difficulty voluntarily clicking his tongue and coughing, with associated groping, off-target movements.

He had moderate difficulties comprehending complex spoken sentences and mild difficulties with similar reading tasks. On confrontation picture naming, he made several semantic paraphasic errors, which he self-corrected. Conversational speech was slow and characterized by short phrases, which were occasionally telegraphic, and infrequent semantic errors, which he usually corrected. He made numerous spelling errors when writing to dictation. His self-generated written sentences were telegraphic, with self-corrected grammatic errors and some uncorrected spelling errors.

Motor speech evaluation revealed reduced rate (−2); irregular articulatory breakdowns (1,2); articulatory substitutions, distortions, and sequential errors, with associated groping for articulatory postures; and dysprosody (2,3). Speech AMRs were slow (−1), and SMRs were inadequately sequenced. He had considerable difficulty repeating multisyllabic words. Intelligibility was very mildly impaired.

The clinician concluded that the patient had a "moderately severe AOS, perhaps with accompanying unilateral UMN dysarthria, both suggestive of left hemisphere posterior frontal dysfunction." He also had a "mild-moderate aphasia affecting all language modalities, although expressive functions were more impaired than receptive. This is also suggestive of left perisylvian, predominantly pre-rolandic dysfunction." The clinician expressed concerns about the patient's report of slow *progression of symptoms and raised the possibility of a slowly progressive degenerative condition rather than stroke as the etiology for his problems. Subsequently, behavioral neurology consultation concluded that the patient might have an asymmetric cortical degenerative disease, such as primary progressive aphasia.*

The patient made some equivocal functional gains in speech during his hospital stay. When seen six months later for follow-up, he reported that his speech had worsened and said, "I can't read very much . . . words run together." He was unable to write and had significant difficulty coordinating movements of his right arm. He had had a brief period of speech therapy following his hospital discharge but did not feel it helped. Exam again revealed a significant NVOA. His AOS was similar in character but clearly worse than during initial evaluation. There was little evidence of worsening of his aphasia.

The clinician concluded that he, "continues to exhibit a marked AOS which is worse than six months ago. He also has a significant NVOA (and upper limb apraxia). His behavior during examination is quite characteristic of patients with significant AOS and mild-moderate aphasia. I observed no evidence of behavior which is more typical of patients with generalized cognitive impairment."

Because the patient felt strongly that he would not benefit from speech therapy and because he had benefited minimally from therapy in the past, continued therapy was not recommended. He was advised, however, that therapy might be beneficial if his speech deteriorated to a point where functional verbal communication was difficult. Augmentative means of communication were discussed.

Neuropsychological assessment revealed little evidence of difficulty beyond the speech and language realm. A single photon emission computed tomography scan was conducted and showed diffusely decreased uptake in the left parietal region and somewhat less decreased uptake in the left frontal region. It was concluded that the patient had an asymmetric degenerative process, with the left parietal and left frontal regions being predominantly affected. The patient was not seen again for follow-up, but a phone call to the patient's wife two years later established that he was mute and had no functional use of his right upper extremity. His wife believed his verbal comprehension and use of his left upper extremity were good.

Commentary. *(1) Apraxia of speech and aphasia can be among the most prominent signs of an asymmetric cortical degenerative process. The nature of the AOS and language disturbance may be indistinguishable from that seen in stroke. (2) Apraxia of speech sometimes cooccurs with significant LA, which can make assessment of the linguistic aspects of writing and nonverbal intellectual abilities very difficult. (3) Apraxia of speech (and aphasia) can represent for a considerable length of time the prominent or only manifestations of degenerative neurologic disease. (4) Issues related to the management of AOS in patients with degenerative disease differ from those for nondegenerative etiologies. They are discussed in the chapters on management.*

SUMMARY

1. Apraxia of speech is a motor speech disorder resulting from impairment of the capacity to program sensorimotor commands for the positioning and movements of muscles for the volitional production of speech. It can occur without significant weakness or neuromuscular slowness, and in the absence of disturbances of thought or language.

2. It is nearly always the result of pathology in the left (dominant) cerebral hemisphere. It occurs as the primary speech pathology diagnosis at a rate comparable to that for several of the major single dysarthria types. It is also very frequently a secondary speech pathology diagnosis in people with left hemisphere pathology and is clinically distinguishable from dysarthrias, aphasia, and other neurologic disorders that may affect communication.

3. Apraxia of speech frequently occurs with other motor and sensory signs of left hemisphere damage, but it can occur as the only evidence of neuropathology. Some patients with AOS also have limb apraxia, although limb apraxia and AOS can occur independent of one another.

4. It is usually caused by vascular disturbances and sometimes by tumor or trauma. It occasionally is the presenting sign of a degenerative CNS disease.

5. There is debate about whether AOS is a linguistic as opposed to a motor speech disorder. At this time, the weight of perceptual, acoustic, and physiologic evidence supports motor speech disorder explanations of AOS, in spite of the fact that AOS usually occurs in association with aphasia. Whether there are subtypes of AOS has not been clearly established.

6. It may occur in association with dysarthria, most often unilateral UMN dysarthria or spastic dysarthria. Many but not all patients with AOS have an accompanying nonverbal oral apraxia that is also a sign of left hemisphere pathology. Oral sensation may be impaired in AOS, but such impairments do not have a clear causal relationship with AOS. People with AOS but no evidence of aphasia generally have normal auditory processing skills.

7. Deviant speech characteristics associated with AOS include a number of abnormalities of articulation, rate, prosody, and fluency. The most distinctive of these characteristics include trial-and-error groping, dysprosody, difficulty initiating utterances, and articulatory inconsistency. Unlike patients with milder degrees of

impairment, patients with severe AOS may have a limited phonetic repertoire, little difference between voluntary and automatic speech utterances, and a highly consistent pattern of perceived speech errors.

8. A number of acoustic and physiologic studies have provided confirmation for the clinical perceptual characteristics of AOS and have documented a number of additional acoustic and movement traits that characterize the disorder. In general, they provide strong support for the notion that AOS is a motor speech disorder rather than a linguistic disorder.

REFERENCES

Adams RD and Victor M: Principles of neurology, New York, 1991, McGraw-Hill.

Baum SR and others: Temporal dimensions of consonant and vowel production: an acoustic and CT scan analysis of aphasic speech, Brain Lang 39:33, 1990.

Blumstein SE and others: The perception and production of voice onset time in aphasia, Neuropsychologia 15:371, 1977.

Blumstein SE and others: Production deficits in aphasia: a voice-onset time analysis, Brain Lang 9:153, 1980.

Brookshire RH: An introduction to neurogenic communication disorders, ed 4, St Louis, 1992, Mosby–Year Book.

Buckingham HW: Explanation in apraxia with consequences for the concept of apraxia of speech, Brain Lang 8:202, 1979.

Caligiuri MP and Till JA: Acoustical analysis of vowel duration in apraxia of speech: a case study, Folia Phoniatr Logop 35:226, 1983.

Caselli RJ and Jack CR: Asymmetric cortical degeneration syndromes: a proposed clinical classification, Arch Neurol 49:770, 1992.

Caselli RJ and others: Asymmetric cortical degenerative syndromes: clinical and radiologic correlations, Neurology 42:1462, 1992.

Chapin C, Blumstein SE, and Meissner B: Speech production mechanisms in aphasia: a delayed auditory feedback study, Brain Lang 14:106, 1981.

Collins M, Rosenbek JC, and Wertz RT: Spectrographic analysis of vowel and word duration in apraxia of speech, J Speech Hear Res 26:224, 1983.

Dabul B: Apraxia battery for adults. Tigard, 1979, CC Publications.

Danly M and Shapiro B: Speech prosody in Broca's aphasia, Brain Lang 16:171, 1982.

Darley FL: Apraxia of speech: 107 years of terminological confusion. Paper presented to the American Speech and Hearing Association, Denver, CO, 1968 (unpublished).

Darley FL: Aphasia: input and output disturbances in speech and language processing. Paper presented to the American Speech and Hearing Association, Chicago, 1969 (unpublished).

Darley FL: Aphasia, Philadelphia, 1982, WB Saunders.

Darley FL, Aronson AE, and Brown JR: Motor speech disorders, Philadelphia, 1975, WB Saunders.

Deal JL and Darley FL: The influence of linguistic and situational variables on phonemic accuracy in apraxia of speech, J Speech Hear Res 15:639, 1972.

De Renzi E: Methods of limb apraxia examination and their bearing on the interpretation of the disorder. In Roy EA, editor: Neuropsychological studies of apraxia and related disorders, New York, 1985, North Holland.

De Renzi E, Pieczuro A, and Vignolo LA: Oral apraxia and aphasia, Cortex 2:50, 1966.

De Renzi E and Vignolo LA: The Token Test: a sensitive test to detect receptive disturbances in aphasics, Brain 85:665, 1962.

Deutsch SE: Oral form identification as a measure of cortical sensory dysfunction in apraxia of speech and aphasia, J Commun Disord 14:65, 1981.

Deutsch SE: Prediction of site of lesion from speech apraxic error patterns. In Rosenbek JC and others, editors: Apraxia of speech: physiology, acoustics, linguistics, and management, San Diego, 1984, College Hill.

DiSimoni FG: Comprehensive apraxia test (CAT), Dalton, PA, 1989, Praxis House.

Dronkers NF, Redfern B, and Shapiro JK: Neuroanatomic correlates of production deficits in severe Broca's aphasia, J Clin Exp Neuropsychol 15:59, 1993.

Duffy JR: Slowly progressive aphasia. In Brookshire RH, editor: Clinical aphasiology, Minneapolis, 1987, BRK Publishers.

Duffy JR and Duffy RJ: The limb apraxia test: an imitative measure of upper limb apraxia. In TE Prescott, editor: Clinical aphasiology, vol 18, Boston, 1989, College-Hill.

Duffy JR and Duffy RJ: The assessment of limb apraxia: The limb apraxia test. In GE Hammond, editor: Cerebral control of speech and limb movements, New York, 1990a, Elsevier Science.

Duffy JR and Gawle CA: Apraxic speakers' vowel duration in consonant-vowel-consonant syllables. In Rosenbek C, McNeil MR, and Aronson AE, editors: Apraxia of speech: physiology, acoustics, linguistics, management, San Diego, 1984, College-Hill.

Duffy JR and Petersen RC: Primary progressive aphasia, Aphasiology 6:1, 1992.

Duffy JR, Watt JR, and Duffy RJ: Path analysis: a strategy for investigating the multivariate causal relationships in communication disorders, J Speech Hear Res 24:474, 1981.

Duffy RJ and Duffy JR: Three studies of deficits in pantomime expression and pantomime recognition in aphasia, J Speech Hear Res 24:70, 1981.

Duffy RJ and Duffy JR: The relationship between pantomime expression and recognition in aphasia: the search for causes. In Hammond GE, editor: Cerebral control of speech and limb movements, New York, 1990b, Elsevier Science.

Dunlop JM and Marquardt TP: Linguistic and articulatory aspects of single word production in apraxia of speech, Cortex 13:17, 1977.

Forrest K and others: Kinematic, electromyographic, and perceptual evaluation of speech apraxia, conduction aphasia, ataxic dysarthria, and normal speech production. In Moore CA, Yorkston KM, and Beukelman DR, editors: Dysarthria and apraxia of speech: perspectives on management, Baltimore, 1991, Paul H Brookes Publishing.

Freeman FJ, Sands ES, and Harris KS: Temporal coordination of phonation and articulation in a case of verbal apraxia: a voice onset time study, Brain Lang 6:106, 1978.

Fromm D and others: Simultaneous perceptual-physiological method for studying speech apraxia. In Brookshire RH, editor: Clinical aphasiology: conference proceedings, Minneapolis, 1982, BRK Publishers.

Gandour J, Petty SH, and Dardarananda R: Dysprosody in Broca's aphasia: a case study, Brain Lang 37:232, 1989.

Goodglass H and Kaplan E: The Boston diagnostic aphasia examination, Malvern, PA, 1983, Lea and Febiger.

Hardcastle WJ, Morgan Barry RA, and Clark CJ: Articulatory and voicing characteristics of adult dysarthric and verbal dyspraxic speakers: an instrumental study, Br J Disord Commun, 20:249, 1985.

Heilman KM: Apraxia. In Heilman KM and Valenstine E, editors: Clinical neuropsychology, Oxford, 1979, Oxford University Press.

Hoit JD, Solomon NP, and Hixon TJ: Effect of lung volume on voice onset time (VOT), J Speech Hear Res 36:516, 1993.

Itoh M and others: Voice onset time characteristics in apraxia of speech, Brain Lang 17:193, 1982.

Itoh M and Sasanuma S: Articulatory movements in apraxia of speech. In Rosenbek C, McNeil MR, and Aronson AE, editors: Apraxia of speech: physiology, acoustics, linguistics, management, San Diego, 1984, College-Hill.

Itoh M, Sasanuma S, and Ushijima T: Velar movements during speech in a patient with apraxia of speech, Brain Lang 7:227, 1979.

Johns DF and Darley FL: Phonemic variability in apraxia of speech, J Speech Hear Res 13:556, 1970.

Johns DF and LaPointe LL: Neurogenic disorders of output processing: apraxia of speech. In Whitaker H and Whitaker HA, editors: Studies in neurolinguistics 1, New York, 1976, Academic Press.

Katz W and others: A kinematic analysis of anticipatory coarticulation in the speech of anterior aphasic subjects using electromagnetic articulography, Brain Lang 38:555, 1990.

Keller E: Parameters for vowel substitutions in Broca's aphasia, Brain Lang 5:265, 1978.

Kent RD and Rosenbek JC: Acoustic patterns of apraxia of speech, J Speech Hear Res 26:231, 1983.

Kertesz A: Western aphasia battery, San Antonio, 1982, The Psychological Corporation.

Kertesz A: Subcortical lesions and verbal apraxia. In Rosenbek JC, McNeil MR, and Aronson AE, editors: Apraxia of speech: physiology, acoustics, linguistics, management, San Diego, 1984, College-Hill.

LaPointe LL and Johns DF: Some phonemic characteristics in apraxia of speech, J Commun Disord 8:259, 1975.

LaPointe LL and Wertz RT: Oral-movement abilities and articulatory characteristics of brain-injured adults, Percept Mot Skills 39:39, 1974.

Liepman H: Das Krankheitsbild der apraxie (moterischen asymbolie) auf grund eines falles von einseitiger apraxie, Monatsschrift für Psychiatrie und Neurologie 8:15, 1900.

Luria AR: Higher cortical functions in man, New York, 1980, Basic Books.

Mandell AM, Alexander MP, and Carpenter S: Creutzfeldt-Jakob disease presenting as isolated aphasia, Neurology 39:55, 1989.

Marshall RC, Gandour J, and Windsor, J: Selective impairmnet of phonation: a case study, Brain Lang 35:313, 1988.

Mateer C and Kimura D: Impairment of nonverbal oral movements in aphasia. Brain Lang 4:262, 1977.

McNeil MR and Kent RD: Motoric characteristics of adult apraxic and aphasic speakers. In GR Hammond, editor: Cerebral control of speech and limb movements, New York, 1990, North Holland.

McNeil MR and others: Effects of speech rate on the absolute and relative timing of apraxic and conduction aphasic sentence production, Brain Lang 38:135, 1990a.

McNeil MR and others: Oral structure nonspeech motor control in normal, dysarthric, aphasic and apraxic speakers: Isometric force and static position control, J Speech Hear Res 33:255, 1990b.

McNeil MR, Calguiri M, and Rosenbek JC: A comparison of labiomandibular kinematic durations, displacements, velocities, and dysmetrias in apraxic and normal adults. In Prescott TE, editor: Clinical aphasiology, vol 18, Boston, 1989, College-Hill.

Mercaitis PA: Some temporal characteristics of imititative speech in non-brain-injured, aphasic, and apraxic adults (unpublished doctoral dissertation) University of Massachusetts, Amherst, 1983.

Mesulam MM: Principles of behavioral neurology, Philadelphia, 1985, FA Davis.

Mohr JP: Revision of Broca's aphasia and the syndrome of Broca's area infarction and its implications for aphasia therapy. In Brookshire RH, editor: Proceedings of the conference on clinical aphasiology, Minneapolis, 1980, BRK Publishers.

Mumenthaler M: Neurology, ed 3, New York, 1990, Thieme Medical.

Odell K and others: Perceptual characteristics of consonant production by apraxic speakers, J Speech Hear Disord 55:345, 1990.

Odell K and others: Perceptual comparison of prosodic features in apraxia of speech and conduction aphasia. In Prescott TE, editor: Clinical aphasiology, vol 19, Austin, TX, 1991, Pro-Ed.

Pellat J and others: Aphemia after a penetrating brain wound: a case study, Brain Lang 40:459, 1991.

Robin DA, Bean C, and Folkins JW: Lip movement in apraxia of speech. J Speech Hear Res 32:512, 1989.

Rosenbek JC: Treating apraxia of speech. In Johns DF, editor: Clinical management of neurogenic communicative disorders, Boston, 1985, Little, Brown.

Rosenbek JC, Kent RD, and LaPointe LL: Apraxia of speech: an overview and some perspectives. In Rosenbek JC, McNeil MR, and Aronson AE, editors: Apraxia of speech: physiology, acoustics, linguistics, management, San Diego, 1984, College-Hill.

Rosenbek JC, Wertz RT, and Darley FL: Oral sensation and perception in apraxia of speech and aphasia, J Speech Hear Disord 16:22, 1973.

Rosenfield DB and others: Speech apraxia in cortical-basal ganglionic degeneration, Ann Neurol 30:296, 1991.

Rosenfield DB and others: Speech apraxia in cortical-basal ganglionic degeneration (abstract), Ann Neurol 30:296, 1991.

Roy EA and Square-Storer PA: Evidence for common expressions of apraxia. In Hammond GE, editor: Cerebral control of speech and limb movements, New York, 1990, Elsevier Science.

Ryalls JH: Motor aphasia: acoustic correlates of phonetic disintegration in vowels, Neuropsychologia 19:365, 1981.

Ryalls JH: An acoustic study of vowel production in aphasia, Brain Lang 29:48, 1986.

Sasanuma S: Speech characteristics of a patient with apraxia of speech, Annual Bulletin, Research Institute of Logapedics and Phoniatrics, University of Tokyo, 5:85, 1971.

Shankweiler D and Harris KS: An experimental approach to the problem of articulation in aphasia, Cortex 2:277, 1966.

Shankweiler D, Harris KS, and Taylor ML: Electromyographic studies of articulation in aphasia, Arch Phys Med Rehabil 49:1, 1968.

Shinn P and Blumstein SE: Phonetic disintegration in aphasia: Acoustic analysis of spectral characteristics for place of articulation, Brain Lang 20:90, 1983.

Shuttleworth EC, Yates AJ, and Paltan-Ortiz J: Creutzfeldt-Jakob disease presenting as progressive aphasia, J Natl Med Assoc 77:649, 1985.

Skenes LL: Durational changes of apraxic speakers, J Commun Dis 20:61, 1987.

Square PA, Darley FL, and Sommers RK: Speech perception among patients demonstrating apraxia of speech, aphasia, and both disorders. In Brookshire RH, editor: Clinical aphasiology: conference proceedings, Minneapolis, 1981, BRK Publishers.

Square PA, Darley FL, and Sommers RK: An analysis of the productive errors made by pure apractic speakers with differing loci of lesions. In Brookshire R, editor: Clinical aphasiology conference proceedings, Minneapolis, 1982, BRK Publishers.

Square-Storer PA and Apeldoorn S: An acoustic study of apraxia of speech in patients with different lesion loci. In Moore CA, Yorkston KM, and Beukelman DR, editors: Dysarthria and apraxia of speech: perspectives on management, Baltimore, 1991, Paul H Brookes Publishing.

Square-Storer P, Darley FL, and Sommers RK: Nonspeech and speech processing skills in patients with aphasia and apraxia of speech, Brain Lang 33:65, 1988.

Square-Storer PA and Roy EA: The apraxias: commonalities and distinctions. In Square-Storer PA, editor: Acquired apraxia of speech in aphasia adults, New York, 1989, Taylor and Francis.

Strand EA: Acoustic and response time measures in utterance production: a comparison of apraxic and normal speakers (unpublished doctoral dissertation), University of Wisconsin–Madison, 1987.

Strand EA and McNeil MR: Evidence for a motor performance deficit versus a misapplied rule system in the temporal organization of utterances in apraxia of speech. In Brookshire RH, editor: Clinical aphasiology, vol 17, Minneapolis, 1987, BRK Publishers.

Sussman H and others: Compensatory articulation in Broca's aphasia, Brain Lang 27:56, 1986.

Tognola G and Vignolo LA: Brain lesions associated with oral apraxia in stroke patients: a clinico-neuroradiological investigation with the CT scan, Neuropsychologia, p 257, 1980.

Towne RL and Crary MA: Verbal reaction time patterns in aphasic adults: consideration for apraxia of speech, Brain Lang 35:138, 1988.

Trost JE and Canter GJ: Apraxia of speech in patients with Broca's aphasia: a study of phoneme production accuracy and error patterns, Brain Lang 1:63, 1974.

Tuller B: On categorizing aphasic speech errors, Neuropsychologia 22:547, 1984.

Weismer G and Liss JM: Acoustic/perceptual taxonomies of speech production deficits in motor speech disorders. In Moore CA, Yorkston KM, and Beukelman DR, editors: Dysarthria and apraxia of speech: perspectives on management, Baltimore, 1991, Paul H Brookes Publishing.

Wertz RT, LaPointe LL, and Rosenbek JC: Apraxia of speech in adults: the disorder and its management, New York, 1984, Grune and Stratton.

Wertz RT, Rosenbek JC, and Deal JL: A review of 228 cases of apraxia of speech: classification, etiology, and localization. Presentation at the American Speech and Hearing Association, New York, 1970.

Yamanouchi H, Budka H, and Vass K: Unilateral Creutzfeld-Jakob disease, Neurology 36:1517, 1986.

Ziegler W and von Cramon D: Anticipatory coarticulation in a patient with apraxia of speech, Brain Lang 26:117, 1985.

Ziegler W and von Cramon D: Disturbed coarticulation in apraxia of speech: acoustic evidence, Brain Lang 29:34, 1986.

12 Neurogenic Mutism

*MUTISM IS LIKE A SPHINX—IT IS BOTH
CAPTIVATING AND DISQUIETING. IT STARES
AT US DEFIANTLY, AND WE FIND IT
DIFFICULT TO SOLVE ITS SILENT RIDDLE.*
(LEBRUN, 1990, P 106)

Disease can leave its victims conscious, alert, and able to comprehend their environment, but without speech. Sometimes this condition is accompanied by cognitive deficits that make speechlessness an accurate reflection of the person's inner state. Sometimes the motor system is so damaged that a normally formulated message cannot be spoken. In the cruelest of circumstances, a cognitively intact person may be "locked in," unable to convey basic thoughts in any conventional way.

Mutism is the absence of speech. Unlike motor speech disorders, which by definition are neurologic in origin, mutism may have multiple origins. It may be deliberate (elected or chosen) or a product of subconscious psychiatric disturbances. It may also be organic but nonneurologic, as in some people with profound congenital hearing loss or peripheral structural loss, such as laryngectomy.

Mutism also can be neurogenic. Neurogenic mutism may be congenital or acquired, and it can result from peripheral nervous system (PNS) or central nervous system (CNS) pathology. *Acquired neurogenic mutism* will be addressed in this chapter. Congenital neurogenic mutism will not be addressed here, nor will muteness associated with deafness or musculoskeletal deficits. Psychogenic mutism will be addressed in Chapter 14; it is of special interest because it is often difficult to distinguish from, or is intertwined with, neurogenic mutism.

Neurogenic mutism can take several forms. It can result from severe dysarthria, apraxia of speech (AOS), aphasia, and a variety of nonaphasic cognitive and affective conditions. It may also occur under specific medical circumstances (for example, in association with seizures or after surgical sectioning of the corpus callosum), even though the underlying nature of the mutism may be uncertain. Distinctions among these forms of neurogenic mutism can be quite important to differential diagnosis, localization, and management. The definition and clinical manifestations, neurologic substrate, and common etiologies of each of several forms of neurogenic mutism will be addressed in the remainder of this chapter. Table 12–1 summarizes types of neurogenic mutism, their neurologic substrates, and common clinical characteristics.

MOTOR SPEECH DISORDERS AND MUTISM

Several single dysarthria types or combinations of them, as well as AOS, can be severe enough to cause mutism. In this section, several subcategories of dysarthria associated with mutism will be discussed, including the generic disorder anarthria, which captures all forms of dysarthric mutism, but also locked-in syndrome, the bi-opercular syndrome, and cerebellar mutism. These latter subcat-

Table 12–1 Types of neurogenic mutism and their neurologic substrates and distinguishing clinical features

Type	Localization	Primary clinical manifestations
Motor speech disorders		
Anarthria		
Spastic (including locked-in syndrome)	Bilateral UMN	Oromotor spasticity and weakness, severe dysphagia, pathologic reflexes; quadriplegia if locked-in, but preserved eye movements
Flaccid	LMN	Oromotor and/or respiratory weakness/paralysis, dysphagia, absent reflexes, atrophy, fasciculations
Hypokinetic or hyperkinetic	Basal ganglia control circuit	Oromotor & respiratory rigidity & hypokinesia, or hyperkinetic movement disorder
Cerebellar mutism	Cerebellar control circuit	Ataxia (& other neuromuscular or programming deficits?)
Bi-opercular syndrome	Lower precentral & postcentral gyri	Minimal voluntary orofacial mobility, hypotonic & weak orofacial muscles, dysphagia, absent gag reflex, relatively preserved cough, yawn & emotional orofacial responses, ? AOS, ? NVOA
Apraxia of speech	Left hemisphere	Groping efforts to speak, aphonic, normal swallowing & automatic oral movements, NVOA
Aphasia	Left hemisphere	Severe multimodality impairments of language, accompanying AOS & NVOA
Diffuse cognitive/affective deficits		
Arousal	Reticular activating system	Coma, unresponsive or responding only to vigorous stimulation; disturbed sleep-wake cycle
Persistent vegetative state	Cerebral cortex, diffuse	Preserved wake-sleep cycle, no visual tracking or response to stimulation
Apallic state	Cerebral cortex, diffuse	Preserved wake-sleep cycle, may respond to painful stimuli, alterations in tone & posture
Frontal/limbic system		
Akinetic mutism	Frontal lobes	Preserved motor & sensory ability; seemingly alert but abulic, unresponsive, & apathetic; delayed responses; grasp & snout reflexes
Etiology specific		
Commissurotomy	Corpus callosum (frontal lobes, SMA?)	Uncertain mechanism (AOS, aphasia, akinetic mutism possible)
Seizure-related speech arrests	Right or left SMA, dominant language cortex	Variable explanations (AOS, aphasia, akinetic mutism, others)

AOS, apraxia of speech; *LMN,* lower motor neuron; *NVOA,* nonverbal oral apraxia; *SMA,* supplementary motor area; *UMN,* upper motor neuron.

egories are given explicit recognition because they are rare and represent special challenges to differential diagnosis and management or because the nature of the dysarthria (or other underlying deficits) is poorly understood. Mutism associated with AOS will also be discussed.

Anarthria

Definition and clinical characteristics. The term anarthria refers to *speechlessness due to a severe loss of neuromuscular control over the speech musculature.* Although the term has sometimes been used to refer to AOS, its use today by speech pathologists and most neurologists is reserved for dysarthria in its most severe form.

The language and cognitive abilities of anarthric patients may be intact, as may be their emotional drive or desire to communicate, but their neuromuscular system does not permit speech. Thus, anarthric individuals do not speak because they cannot speak.

The specific types of dysarthria underlying anarthric muteness can be very difficult to establish or technically impossible if differential diagnosis is restricted to distinctions among deviant speech characteristics. Type of dysarthria can be presumed in those with progressive disorders when evaluation prior to the loss of speech was able to establish dysarthria type. Inferences about the types of dysarthria also can be made on the basis of confirmatory features and information about etiology and lesion localization. In addition, in many cases the use of the term anarthria is not absolute; the label often is used to mean that "for all practical purposes" the patient is mute. Many anarthric individuals can make some visible attempts to speak; some can produce a few sounds or some voice and even approximate some syllables. These efforts, combined with observations of movement and reflexes during oral mechanism examination and other physical examination findings (limb strength, tone, reflexes, etc.), permit judgments about the compatibility of the inferred dysarthria type with known etiology and localization. If etiology and localization are unknown, the clinical observations may help to establish them.

In general, flaccid dysarthria alone seldom leads to anarthria because it is unusual for multiple cranial nerves supplying the speech muscles to be involved bilaterally (a near requirement for anarthria to develop from lower motor neuron [LMN] weakness alone). Flaccid dysarthria associated with myasthenia gravis, Guillain-Barré syndrome, and brainstem tumors affecting multiple cranial nerves bilaterally can lead to mutism, however. It is also unusual for ataxic dysarthria to be so severe that anarthria is the result, although "cerebellar mutism" (discussed in a subsequent section) may represent an exception. Similarly, hyperkinetic dysarthria, although capable of producing devastating effects on speech intelligibility, only infrequently results in anarthria.

Spastic and hypokinetic dysarthria are the most likely culprits when a single dysarthria type leads to anarthria, with spastic dysarthria probably representing the most frequent cause in vascular etiologies. As might be expected, mixed dysarthrias probably account for more cases of anarthria than single types, although this has not been studied systematically. Based on the distribution of types of mixed dysarthrias reviewed in Chapter 10 (Table 10–4), it is likely that mixed spastic-flaccid, spastic-ataxic, and spastic-hypokinetic dysarthrias account for many cases of anarthria.

Neurologic substrates and etiologies. Bilateral final common pathway lower motor neuron involvement of speech cranial and respiratory nerves, bilateral direct and indirect activation pathway involvement, and bilateral control circuit pathology may, separately or in combination, lead to anarthria. Combined direct and indirect pathway involvement (as in spastic dysarthria) or basal ganglia control circuit pathology (as in hypokinetic or hyperkinetic dysarthria) are probably more frequently implicated in anarthria than are other components of the motor system.

Table 12–2 summarizes the etiologies and primary speech diagnoses for 24 cases with anarthria, including locked-in syndrome. The cases illustrate but do not exhaust what the literature suggests

Table 12–2 Etiology and type of motor speech disorder for 24 quasirandomly selected cases seen at the Mayo Clinic with a primary speech pathology diagnosis of anarthria, including locked-in syndrome.

Etiology	Speech diagnosis
Brainstem stroke (7)	LiS, unspecified dysarthria type (4)
	Anarthria, unspecified dysarthria type (2)
	LiS, spastic (1)
Multiple, bilateral strokes (5)	Anarthria, unspecified dysarthria type (3)
	Anarthria, spastic (1)
	Anarthria, spastic + AOS (1)
Closed head injury (5)	Anarthria, unspecified dysarthria type (3)
	Anarthria, spastic (2)
Undetermined CNS degenerative disease (2)	Anarthria, spastic (1)
	Anarthria, unspecified dysarthria + AOS (1)
ALS (1)	Anarthria, spastic-flaccid
PSP (1)	Anarthria, spastic-hypokinetic
Brainstem tumor, post-surgical (1)	LiS, flaccid
Anoxic encephalopathy (1)	Anarthria, spastic
MS + multiple strokes (1)	Anarthria, unspecified dysarthria type

ALS, amyotrophic lateral sclerosis; *AOS,* apraxia of speech; *CNS,* central nervous system; *LiS,* locked-in syndrome; *MS,* multiple sclerosis; *PSP,* progressive supranuclear palsy.

regarding etiology. Vascular events were the most frequent etiology. A majority of the strokes were in the brain stem, and a single brainstem stroke was sufficient to cause anarthria (and locked-in syndrome) in a number of cases. Multiple strokes leading to anarthria were more widely dispersed, often including cortical or subcortical hemispheric events, but always bilateral; multiple strokes sometimes also included a lesion in the brain stem. Closed head injury (CHI) was also a frequent cause, often associated with multifocal and diffuse injuries, frequently including or largely limited to the brain stem. Degenerative disease, including amyotrophic lateral sclerosis (ALS), progressive supranuclear palsy (PSP), and multiple sclerosis (MS) led to anarthria in some cases. Anoxic encephalopathy, as well as multiple cranial nerve injuries associated with a brainstem tumor and subsequent neurosurgery, represented other causes. One individual had MS plus multiple strokes.

Anarthria may also result from severe extrapyramidal diseases (for example, Parkinson's and Wilson's diseases, dystonia musculorum deformans). A number of other diseases may be associated with mutism that may reflect anarthria, but the severe cognitive impairments typically associated with them in their later stages make it difficult to determine if muteness is motor or cognitive in origin (for example, Alzheimer's disease, Creutzfeldt-Jakob disease, Huntington's chorea, normal pressure hydrocephalus, Pick's disease, progressive multifocal leukoencephalopathy).

Vogel and von Cramon (von Cramon, 1981; Vogel and von Cramon, 1982, 1983) have studied mutism and dysarthria in a number of individuals with traumatic midbrain injuries. Their patients were mute for several days-to-months after they regained consciousness and had evidence of hemiparesis or quadriparesis and limb spasticity and/or ataxia. They demonstrated severe limitations of jaw, lip, and tongue mobility. Phonation was apparent only during coughing or gagging. Speech reemerged slowly and was initially characterized by a poorly modulated sound that conveyed affective information such as pain, followed by emergence of a breathy-whispered dysphonia, often high in pitch and poorly modulated, with poor articulation and respiratory control. The dysarthria of these patients was described as mixed spastic and hypokinetic in form.

Locked-in syndrome

Definition and clinical characteristics. When anarthria is accompanied by total immobility of the body except for vertical eye movements and blinking, but the individual is sufficiently intact cognitively to communicate with eye movements, the condition is referred to as locked-in syndrome (LiS) (Plum and Posner, 1966). It is also sometimes referred to as the *de-efferentiated state* (Ruff and others, 1987), *ventral pontine syndrome,* or *bilateral brain pyramidal system syndrome* (Chia, 1991). Its distinction from coma is made on the basis of the LiS patient's ability to communicate with eyeblinks or, in rare cases, by electroencephalogram (EEG) demonstrating normal cortical electrical activity (Bauer, Gerstenbrand, and Rumpl, 1979; Patterson and Grabois, 1986). Therefore, LiS is a special and dramatic manifestation of anarthria, one that presents special challenges to diagnosis and management.

Patients with "classical" LiS are mute and usually have a spastic quadriplegia and no craniofacial movements except for upper eyelid and vertical eye movements. Respiratory difficulties are common (Morariu, 1979a). Locked-in syndrome is occasionally "incomplete," with remnants of additional voluntary movements (most often horizontal gaze or face movement, according to Patterson and Grabois, 1986). Rarely, "total" LiS occurs, in which even eye movements are absent. A review of 139 cases by Patterson and Grabois (1986) found 64% to have classical manifestations, 33% to have incomplete manifestations, and only 2% to have total LiS.

The anarthria of LiS most often reflects severe spastic or mixed spastic-flaccid dysarthria. Typically, the patient cannot move the jaw, face, tongue, palate, or vocal cords voluntarily. Dysphagia is severe. Sometimes stereotyped chewing and sucking movements or a facial grimace can be elicited by perioral or noxious stimuli. People with incomplete LiS may produce some face, tongue, jaw, head, or forehead movements (McGann and Paslawski, 1991; Patterson and Grabois, 1986).

The outlook for locked-in patients is generally poor. Patterson and Grabois (1986) reported an overall 87% mortality within the first four months postonset. The most common cause of death within the first week postonset was extension of the brainstem lesion, but pulmonary complications were the most common cause of death overall. Many patients required mechanical ventilatory support and assisted secretion management, and a number needed tracheostomy and intubation.

Long-term survival with LiS is unusual but possible. Survivors tend to remain locked in (McCusker and others, 1982). People with nonvascular etiologies tend to show earlier and more complete recovery than those with vascular etiology, and functional recovery in vascular cases is generally quite limited in the first four months (Patterson and Grabois, 1986). Functional improvement in communication is possible in LiS of vascular etiology, however. Haig, Katz, and Sahgal (1986), for example, conducted a long-term study of 27 LiS patients who were locked in for from one to more than 12 years. About 40% were able to point, type, or trigger a switch to communicate. Over half could be fed orally.

There are case reports of dramatic improvement in LiS, sometimes over the course of several years (McCusker and others, 1982; Ruff and others, 1987). In such cases, speech tends to improve later than limb movement, but functional communication, sometimes including intelligible (but dysarthric) speech, as well as ability to eat orally, can occur. Youth and an absence of hypertension or previous stroke may be favorable prognostic signs for such recovery (McCusker and others, 1982). McGann and Paslawski (1991) documented the cases of two highly motivated individuals with LiS from basilar artery strokes who progressed from an eye blink form of communication to the use of computerized communication devices. Importantly, they noted that neither patient was entirely intact cognitively, consistent with what little is known about the cognitive status in people with LiS. They stress the importance of cognitive and language assessment in such patients and provide a valuable overview of issues relevant to managing communication problems in LiS. All of these studies emphasize the need for vigorous physical, dysphagia, and speech-communication therapy for their cases.

Neurologic substrate and etiologies. In the vast majority of cases, LiS is caused by vascular occlusion of the basilar artery, affecting the ventral aspect of the pons and severing descending motor pathways to the spinal cord and lower cranial nerves (Lebrun, 1990; Segarra and Angelo, 1970). Much less commonly, infarction is in the ventral midbrain or the internal capsule, bilaterally (Chia, 1984, 1991). Other etiologies include trauma, central pontine myelinolysis, tumor, encephalitis, MS, and drug toxicity or abuse (Patterson and Grabois, 1986).

The preservation of consciousness, eye movements, and the ability to communicate in LiS are accounted for by sparing of supranuclear oculomotor pathways and the reticular formation of the pons and midbrain, as well as their connections with the relatively intact functions of the cerebral cortex (Bauer, Gerstenbrand, and Rumpl, 1979; Chia, 1991).

Bi-opercular syndrome

Definition and clinical characteristics. The bi-opercular syndrome is a rare disorder that is often associated with mutism. It has also been called *flaccid facial diplegia, facio-labio-linguopharyngeal palsy of cortical-subcortical origin,* the *Foix-Chavany-Marie syndrome,* and the *opercular syndrome* (Lebrun, 1990). It is caused by bilateral damage to the rolandic operculum (lower part of the precentral and postcentral convolutions of the cerebral hemispheres).

The syndrome's defining clinical features (Cappa and others, 1987; Lebrun, 1990; Mariani and others, 1980; Weller, 1993) are

1. Severely reduced voluntary orofacial mobility. Lip, tongue, jaw, and palatal movements are hypotonic, weak, and restricted. The upper face is also often affected, with inability to voluntarily close the eyes or frown. Hypotonicity gives the face a void appearance.
2. Preserved reflexive cough and yawning, and preserved automatic and emotional facial and jaw movements, laughing and crying.
3. The patient is mute or capable only of minimal, distorted, low-volume speech.
4. Severe dysphagia. Chewing ability is severely limited, and food must often be pushed to the back of the mouth to trigger the pharyngeal phase of swallowing, which may be normal. The gag reflex is usually absent. There is a high risk of aspiration pneumonia. Percutaneous endoscopic gastrostomy may be required.
5. Limb movements may be preserved. There may be no significant aphasia, and communication through writing may be normal. When the etiology is vascular, the severe dysarthria and dysphagia tend to persist, although facial movement and chewing may show some improvement.

A number of the syndrome's features resemble those encountered in pseudobulbar palsy and muteness resulting from the anarthria of spastic dysarthria. In fact, it has been called an extreme form of pseudobulbar palsy (Cappa and others, 1987; Weller, 1993). However, in the bi-opercular syndrome the speech muscles appear hypotonic rather than spastic, pseudobulbar laughter and crying are atypical, and the pharyngeal phase of swallowing may be normal (Lebrun, 1990). Of special interest is the apparent dissociation of voluntary and automatic movements. For example, Cappa and others (1987) noted "normal" but stereotypic laughter and crying in appropriate situations in their patient, even though swallowing was severely impaired and an undifferentiated moan was the only "speech" than could be produced.

Neurologic substrate and etiologies. Bilateral damage to the lower part of the precentral and postcentral convolutions are the apparent cause of the syndrome (Lebrun, 1990; Mariani and others, 1980).* Stroke is nearly always the etiology. The

---

*Starkstein, Berthier, and Leiguarda (1988) reported an unusual case in which a right-hander developed bilateral lower face and tongue weakness, muteness, and inability to chew and swallow, but with preserved automatic oral function and language following a unilateral stroke in the right insula and no other identifiable lesion. They interpreted the findings as representing a "bilateral opercular syndrome" due to unilateral lesion and "crossed aphemia."

syndrome frequently occurs after a unilateral opercular lesion, from which there may be good recovery, followed by a second stroke on the other side, after which the syndrome emerges. Traumatic, neoplastic, and infectious etiologies are also possible. The syndrome also may emerge as a variant of primary lateral sclerosis or other focal degenerative central nervous system (CNS) disease (Lang and others, 1989; Weller, 1993; Weller, Poremba, and Dichgans, 1990).

The categorization of the bi-opercular syndrome into a category of motor speech disorder is difficult. On the one hand, it almost certainly reflects a severe dysarthria that resembles spastic dysarthria, but the absence of pseudobulbar affect, gag reflex, and pathologic oral reflexes, as well as "preserved" emotional laughter and crying, are atypical for people with spastic dysarthria. The voluntary-automatic dissociation is consistent with a degree of anatomic separation of corticobulbar pathways for voluntary and automatic control of orofacial structures, and it suggests that the lower precentral gyrus is not essential for driving involuntary facial movements (Weller, 1993). The voluntary-automatic dissociation raises the possibility that the condition is complicated by a nonverbal oral apraxia (NVOA) and, perhaps, AOS. This author has followed a few individuals who *may* have had the syndrome as the result of degenerative disease. Their speech deficit began as an AOS (with an accompanying NVOA) with an accompanying dysarthria that was difficult to characterize but resembled spastic dysarthria because of slow rate, effortful and strained voice quality, and prosodic excess.

It seems reasonable to conclude that the muteness associated with the syndrome represents an anarthria in which the underlying dysarthria type is unclear but perhaps spastic and in which NVOA and AOS may complicate the clinical picture. Recognition of the syndrome is important because of its localizing value, its clinical distinction from more typical manifestations of anarthria, and the apparently poor prognosis for recovery of functional speech, at least when the etiology is vascular or degenerative.

Cerebellar mutism

Definition and clinical characteristics. Cerebellar lesions acquired in adulthood seldom cause mutism. Although rare, a number of cases have been reported in which children undergoing surgery for cerebellar or posterior fossa tumors (or, in a few cases, arteriovascular malformations [AVMs]) have developed mutism postoperatively. Its development has been perplexing and its mechanism poorly understood. The condition is often referred to as *mutism of cerebellar origin*.

A review of reported cases by Dietze and Mickle (1990–91) and examination of some of the more adequately described case reports permit the following summary of the primary features of the disorder:

1. Most cases have large midline posterior fossa tumors and preoperative cerebellar deficits. Preoperatively, mutism is not present, and dysarthria generally is not mentioned.

2. Mutism usually does not develop until one-to-three days after surgery, with adequate speech noted before that. The mutism persists for an average of three months but ranges from several weeks to seven months or longer. Cranial nerve deficits are not apparent, and patients are cognitively alert and without any obvious aphasia.

3. When speech reemerges, severe dysarthria is apparent. When type has been specified, it has been called ataxic (Hudson, Murdoch, and Ozanne, 1989). Some recover completely whereas others remain dysarthric.

4. All but one reported case have been children. The only adult was a 20-year-old man who had a tumor removed from the cerebellar vermis (Salvati and others, 1991). His pre- and postoperative characteristics and recovery were not obviously different from reported childhood cases. Muteness developed 46 hours after surgery and persisted for four weeks, after which dysarthria (unspecified as to type) was apparent. By seven weeks he was mildly dysarthric.

Neurologic substrate and etiology. Dietze and Mickle (1990–91) concluded that the mutism results from acute injury to the midportion of the cerebellum, with a higher risk of mutism with widespread injury to the midportion and the dentate nuclei. Ferrante and others (1990) noted that mutism may develop after a "generous resection" of a cerebellar lobe or part or all of the vermis.

The physiologic mechanism for the muteness is unclear, but it may not be just the result of cerebellar injury. Ferrante and others (1990) noted a fairly high frequency of postoperative meningitis or hydrocephalus (treated with shunting) as possible contributing factors; they also noted the possible contributions of vascular disturbances or edema. Nagatani, Waga, and Nakagawa (1991) point out that bilateral stereotactic ablation of the dentate nuclei can cause mutism, as can bilateral thalamotomy (damaging cerebellocortical projections). This raises the possibility of a contribution of the superior cerebellar peduncles, which connect the dentate nuclei to the thalamus. Finally, there is a tendency to label some of these cases as psychogenic in origin. Psychological mechanisms are certainly possible (Ferrante and others, 1990), although they do not explain the dysarthria that becomes apparent when speech emerges.

Assuming that muteness is due to a motor speech disorder, it is possible that it represents more than severe ataxic dysarthria in some cases. One of the six cases of Rekate and others (1985) was unable to imitate limb and tongue movements during the period of mutism, and phonation emerged during laughter and crying. Another of their cases could only "whine" when attempting to speak (this author has also observed these characteristics in two cases of cerebellar mutism). These behaviors are apraxic-like in character and could implicate motor programming deficits as a mechanism in the muteness. It is clear that careful preoperative and postoperative examination and follow-up of a series of cases undergoing surgery for posterior fossa lesions, with special attention to their specific postoperative speech and oral mechanism characteristics, are essential for a better understanding of this unusual and interesting problem.

Apraxia of speech and mutism

It is not unusual for AOS to be associated with mutism, but it seldom lasts for more than a few days. Sometimes, however, the mutism persists beyond the acute stage, even in the absence of aphasia or significant dysarthria. There is no clear evidence that the lesions associated with prolonged muteness in AOS, particularly pure AOS, are situated differently than lesions associated with more rapid emergence of speech.

Several case studies have documented persistent mutism in association with left hemisphere surgery or stroke (Bone, 1984; Jürgens, Kirzinger, and von Cramon, 1982; Marshall, Gandour, and Windsor, 1988; Ruff and Arbit, 1981), with emergence from mutism usually occurring between three and ten weeks postonset. These patients tended to have an accompanying NVOA. Some were unable to phonate, whisper, hum, or articulate under any circumstance, but some were observed to hum or articulate without phonation during the otherwise mute period. These cases suggest that prolonged muteness in AOS is at least sometimes associated with a *disproportionate degree of apraxia of phonation.* In fact, when speech first emerges in some apraxic patients, phonation may be whispered.

Levin and others (1983) reported that about 3% of 350 consecutive cases with traumatic brain injury (TBI) were mute even though they were not in a persistent vegetative state, locked in, or akinetically mute. Several of the cases had evidence of focal left basal ganglia lesions and tended to have more rapid recovery of consciousness and better overall language and communication outcomes than those with severe diffuse injuries. It is quite possible that the mutism in some of the patients with focal basal ganglia lesions was primarily due to AOS. This is im-

portant to recognize because TBI mutism can also be associated with much more severe cognitive, affective, and neuromuscular disorders.

Lebrun (1990) discusses what he calls mutism associated with a "pyramidal hemisyndrome." It is associated with a unilateral cerebral hemisphere lesion, hemiplegia, and facial weakness. If this occurred only with lesions in the left hemisphere, it could be assumed that the mutism reflected AOS or aphasia. However, he also refers to reported cases with muteness associated with right hemisphere lesions in the third frontal and first temporal convolutions and the insula, the inner surface of the operculum, and part of the corona radiata (and one case with a lesion in the supplementary motor area). He indicates that such mutism generally remits after a few days but with residual "dysarthria." Although speculative, it is possible that these cases reflect AOS in individuals with crossed or mixed dominance for motor speech programming (and, very possibly, language). Thus, what Lebrun calls mutism associated with a pyramidal hemisyndrome may actually be mutism associated with AOS, even in patients with right hemisphere lesions.

Prolonged mutism in individuals presumed to have AOS should raise suspicions about the influence of dysarthria, aphasia, or psychological factors on the mutism. For example, Groswasser and others (1988) discussed three nonaphasic patients for whom "buccofacial apraxia" was presumed to be the source of their prolonged mutism. However, although the patients had NVOA and, very possibly, AOS, the description of their limited speech, the presence of significant dysphagia, and the presence of bilateral frontal lobe lesions suggest they also had significant dysarthria (?spastic). The mutism may thus have been due to dysarthria rather than AOS or to a combination of the two disorders. In general, however, it is important to bear in mind that mutism can persist beyond the acute stage in AOS, even when it is the only manifestation of neurologic disease.

APHASIA AND MUTISM

Mutism in the acute period following the onset of aphasia in adulthood is not unusual. However, persisting mutism, even in patients with global aphasia, is uncommon.* Mutism associated with subcortical lesions leading to aphasia may be more common than aphasia caused by cortical lesions,

---

*Aphasia acquired in childhood (from stroke or trauma, for example) is often associated with a period of mutism (see, for example, Alajouanine and Lhermitte, 1965; Cooper and Flowers, 1987; Hecaen, 1976; Miller and others, 1984).

but it is possible that the mutism in such cases is contributed to by, or due to, AOS and dysarthria.

Acute lesions in the dominant hemisphere superior premotor area may produce complete muteness for several days and then evolve into so-called *transcortical motor aphasia* in which spontaneous speech is limited in amount and complexity, but repetition, naming, and reading aloud may be preserved (Mesulam, 1985). Emergence from mutism in such cases may be characterized by slowly initiated, brief, unelaborated, and sometimes perseverative verbal responses. The patient may mouth or whisper words before normal phonation emerges, and their prosody may be flat, consistent with their overall affect. Alexander, Benson, and Stuss (1989) suggest that these patients have difficulty activating speech and communication that reflects damage to frontal lobe activation mechanisms. It is questionable whether the mutism in such cases is due to a language deficit (aphasia) per se. Nonaphasic cognitive deficits associated with frontal lobe pathology, such as akinetic mutism (discussed later in this chapter), may be a better explanation (and label) for these deficits than transcortical motor aphasia. Of course, some individuals may have aphasia and nonaphasic cognitive communication deficits simultaneously.

In general, persisting mutism in aphasia should raise suspicions about the accuracy of the aphasia diagnosis or the presence of additional problems such as motor speech disorders or nonaphasic cognitive deficits.

NONAPHASIC COGNITIVE AND AFFECTIVE DEFICITS ASSOCIATED WITH MUTISM

Thus far we have discussed mutism secondary to disorders of execution (dysarthrias), a disorder of programming (AOS), and a disorder specifically affecting language (aphasia). In this section, mutism secondary to defects in arousal, affect and drive, cognition, and motor planning and initiation will be addressed. There is considerable clinical overlap among such disorders. For example, many patients with mutism associated with defects in affect or drive have significant cognitive deficits, and many with deficits in motor initiation have defects in affect and drive as well as cognition.

Disorders of arousal

The reticular activating system (RAS) in the pons, midbrain, and diencephalon is crucial to arousal. When severely damaged, all voluntary behavior is diminished or absent. If damage is widespread, the individual may be in a *coma,* a state of complete unresponsiveness often accompanied by disrupted vegetative functions such as respiration and heart rate. The unresponsiveness reflects a failure to activate (arouse) functions above the brainstem level. In a sense, the mutism of coma is hardly thought of as a variety of mutism because speechlessness is expected when a person is neither aroused nor arousable.

Some patients with severe midbrain RAS involvement, although technically not comatose, are in a state of *hypersomnolent mutism* (Turkstra and Bayles, 1992). Although generally unconscious, they may respond to repeated vigorous stimulation. These responses may include vocalization and even speech. This state is sometimes considered a variant of *akinetic mutism,* which will be discussed in a subsequent section.

Mutism resulting from RAS involvement and decreased arousal can have multiple causes, but TBI and vascular events are probably the most common etiologies encountered in speech pathology practices.

Diffuse impairments of cortical functions (persistent vegetative state, apallic state, coma vigil)

Persistent vegetative state. Patients in a persistent vegetative state fail to show evidence of viable higher level cerebral function. Unlike those in true coma, their wake-sleep cycles are relatively preserved. However, when awake they do not visually track or respond to external stimulation, and EEG, computed tomography (CT) and magnetic resonance imaging (MRI) scan, and measures of cerebral metabolic activity are consistent with gross abnormalities or absence of cortical functioning. Their muteness is therefore consistent with their severely reduced level of arousal and cognition (Turkstra and Bayles, 1992; Yorkston and Beukelman, 1991). Severe TBI, anoxia, drug toxicity, and Wernicke's encephalopathy exemplify etiologies capable of producing the widespread cortical damage leading to a persistent vegetative state.

Apallic state (coma vigil). Apallism refers to the absence of the pallium or gray matter of the cortex. Patients in an *apallic state* or *coma vigil* can appear very similar to those in a persistent vegetative state, and the difference between the two conditions may be only one of degree. They may also resemble but are more impaired than patients with akinetic mutism.

Individuals in an apallic state are unresponsive, make few spontaneous movements, and do not generally make reflexive defensive or protective movements, although they do respond to painful stimuli. They occasionally move or shout spontaneously, demonstrating some capacity for movement (Lebrun, 1990). They may lie with their eyes open and occasionally visually follow the examiner, but eye movements are usually random (Segarra and Angelo, 1970). They tend to remain in any position in which they are placed, may have prominent sucking and grasping reflexes, and may develop marked alterations in tone and posture, such as rigidity and extrapyramidal hyperkinesia (Mumenthaler, 1990). Their behavior suggests that the bases for feeling, thought, and motivation to act are absent.

The apallic state is distinguished from akinetic mutism by its victims' prompt responses to painful stimuli, their occasional spontaneous movements, and their tendency to develop marked alterations in muscle tone and posture (Lebrun, 1990; Segarra and Angelo, 1970).

The apallic state is associated with widespread destruction of cortical gray matter. Etiologies include anoxia, carbon monoxide poisoning, degenerative disease (for example, Creutzfeldt-Jakob disease), meningovascular syphilis, chronic viral encephalitis, and severe TBI (Morariu, 1979; Segarra and Angelo, 1970).

Akinetic mutism (frontal lobe–limbic system pathology)

Definition and clinical characteristics. Pathology in the anterior or mesial portions of the frontal lobes may lead to *abulia,* or a lack of initiative. Abulia can be pronounced enough to cause mutism. This form of mutism, therefore, reflects a lack of drive or motivation to speak, difficulty initiating and sustaining the cognitive and motor effort required for speech, or an apparent "absence" of content or information to be communicated. The term we will use for this abulic state is *akinetic mutism.* Other terms with anatomic references that refer to a constellation of deficits that include akinetic mutism are the *prefrontal syndrome,* the *anterior cerebral artery syndrome,* and the *SMA syndrome* (Turkstra and Bayles, 1992).

Akinetic mutism (AM) is *a state of muteness and general unresponsiveness and reluctance to perform even simple motor activities, in spite of preservation of alertness, basic motor and sensory abilities, and at least some fundamental cognitive abilities.* It may be difficult to distinguish from what have been called "pseudoakinetic states" (Segarra and Angelo, 1970) of LiS and basal ganglia diseases associated with severe hypokinesia and rigidity (that is, anarthria). It is important to do so because AM is not due to neuromuscular difficulties.

Akinetically mute patients typically sit with their eyes open, seemingly alert and on the verge of responding to simple requests and questions, but basically unresponsive and apathetic. They may follow movement but not truly react to it and may respond only to painful stimuli. Their apathy and indifference often leads to incontinence (Trimble, 1990). They may have a grasp and snout reflex and vegetative jaw and face movements, and they may swallow food after it is placed in the mouth but often only after a significant delay (Lebrun, 1990).

There may be gradations of severity. When emerging from the mute state, as in recovery after infarct or trauma, a patient may respond with movement or speech when stimuli are powerful and persistent. Movements are simple, brief, and delayed, sometimes delayed for as long as two minutes (Lebrun, 1990). Speech is *brief, aphonic, whispered or reduced in loudness, and monotonic,* with articulation and intelligibility appearing more intact than phonation. Content is *unelaborated*—but not truly telegraphic—and *concrete* and *literal* (Aronson, 1990; Lebrun, 1990; Morariu, 1979; Trimble, 1990). For example, asked if they can tell the examiner the time, the patient may simply respond, "yes." Patients may also seem to be stubbornly refusing to cooperate and sometimes appear to resist the examiner's attempt to open the mouth. The overall impression given is one of indifference, apathy, lethargy, and sometimes somnolence.

The clinical characteristics of patients with AM have been interpreted as reflecting deficits in affect, personality, and emotion. The disturbed functions that produce them are related to a damaged drive mechanism for action and emotion that translates into reduced or absent movement, insight, and affective expression (Sapir and Aronson, 1985).

Neurologic substrate and etiologies. Two general lesion loci are associated with AM. The first is the mesial surface of one or both frontal lobes, including the SMA. Involvement of the anterior cingulate region, which is the frontal surface of the limbic system, may be quite important for the syndrome's emergence (Segarra and Angelo, 1970). Stuss and Benson (1984), however, point out that whereas an "apathetico-akinetico-abulic syndrome" tends to reflect damage to the prefrontal convexity it is most characteristic of massive frontal lobe damage.

The SMA, its connections to the cingulate gyrus, and its projections to dorsolateral frontal cortex (including Broca's area), the motor cortex, and the striatum are important to the activation of motor responses. Damage to the left SMA reduces the drive to speak, sometimes enough to induce mutism. In general, damage to the right SMA also reduces output but does not generally lead to mutism (Alexander, Benson, and Stuss, 1989).

Small lesions in the SMA may cause transient muteness, after which articulation may be normal but verbal output is delayed in initiation and sparse. With small lesions, improvement to sentence length utterances may occur within a few weeks (Alexander, Benson, and Stuss, 1989). Larger lesions tend to be associated with longer periods of mutism, and with noticeable apathy, disconcern, and slowness in initiating responses. In such cases, there seems to be an impairment in cingulate cortex and SMA activities that play a role in response activation, as well as in more anterior frontal areas that are involved in organization and executive control (Alexander, Benson, and Stuss, 1989).

Patients with so-called transcortical motor aphasia are often mute at onset. The mutism usually clears within a few days but is sometimes prolonged. Although repetition may be good, when nonimitative speech does return, it is often sparse, slow to emerge, flat in its prosodic features, and perseverative. Lesions are usually in the left dorsolateral area. As noted previously, at least in some cases, transcortical motor aphasia may not reflect a disorder of language per se.

Akinetic mutism may also result from lesions in the mesencephalic-diencephalic region, a location where disconnection of thalamic nuclei from ascending RAS impulses is possible. The anatomic distance between the frontal and deeper sites of damage that can lead to AM is explained by Stuss and Benson (1984), who point out that the brainstem-frontal system is an integrated system, with the brainstem RAS influencing states of alertness. Thus, severe brainstem pathology may lead to coma or a somnolent akinetic state. Frontal lobe pathology may not be associated with marked somnolence because the RAS is intact, but abulia and lack of drive limit responsiveness and initiative.

Akinetic mutism may have multiple etiologies. Infarction of the anterior cerebral arteries or perforating branches of the posterior cerebral artery can cause the frontal lobe and mesencephalic variants of AM, respectively (Damasio, 1979; Segarra and Angelo, 1970). Tumor, TBI, encephalitis, vascular malformations, ruptured aneurysms, obstructive hydrocephalus, cerebral hypoxia, and thalamotomy are additional possible causes (Aronson, 1990; Morariu, 1979; Mumenthaler, 1990; Trimble, 1990).

ETIOLOGY-SPECIFIC NEUROGENIC MUTISM

Neurogenic mutism is sometimes associated with very specific events or characteristics, even though the mechanism underlying the mutism is not always clear. Mutism following commissurotomy and speech arrests are examples of such conditions.

Mutism following commissurotomy

Surgical transection of the corpus callosum is sometimes undertaken to control severe, unlocalized epilepsy that is refractory to medical management. Sectioning of the anterior portion of the corpus callosum can result in mutism or decreased spontaneity of speech for several days to months postoperatively (Gazzaniga and others, 1984; Polkey, 1989; Reeves, 1992). In one reported case, a nearly complete mutism persisted for 16 months (Sussman and others, 1983). Comprehension and ability to communicate by writing can be spared. During recovery, patients tend to go through a period of whispering or hoarseness, and an NVOA may be present (Bogen and Vogel, 1975; Sussman and others, 1983).

The mechanism for the muteness is unclear. It is generally not considered the result of the transection per se, however. Mechanical trauma from operative traction or diaschisis or ischemia affecting the parasaggital cortex, including the SMA, may be significant (Reeves, 1992; Sussman and others, 1983). Because the brains of individuals with epilepsy are not normal, it has been speculated that preoperative dominance for speech is bilateral in some individuals. As a result, speech cannot be supported postoperatively because the two hemispheres are disconnected, and a single hemisphere cannot immediately control speech without the help of the other.

The behavioral basis for the mutism is also unclear. Some suggest that "aphemia" (AOS) is the explanation in some cases (Sussman and others, 1983), but aphasia and psychological explanations have also been mentioned (Benes, 1990). If malfunction of the SMA is the source of difficulty, then difficulty with initiation of speech from motor or cognitive drive mechanism deficits would be implicated.

Callosotomy is also undertaken in individuals undergoing surgical removal of tumors in the third ventricle and pineal region. Sectioning of the anterior, middle, or posterior third of the corpus callosum is undertaken as the chosen route of the surgical approach to such tumors. Benes (1990) notes that mutism is one of the most serious side effects of the procedure, although only rarely does it last more than several weeks. Children under the age of 10 years have fewer postoperative deficits, apparently including mutism, than older individuals. Similar to callosotomy for seizure control, the mechanism for the mutism is often undetermined.

Speech arrests

One of the most common events associated with partial seizures is speech arrest (Brown, 1972), commonly called *ictal speech arrest,* in which speech in progress at the onset of a seizure is halted, even though consciousness is maintained. Efforts to speak on such occasions may result only in indistinct sounds (Lebrun, 1990). Cascino and others (1991) note that arrests can occur with frontal seizures, especially when the SMA or the dominant hemisphere inferior rolandic area are involved. Speech arrest or aphasia may be the only behavioral evidence of seizure activity in some cases (Cascino and others, 1991; Jonas, 1981).

Although speech arrests are often labelled as "aphasic," Rosenbaum and others (1986) point out that the arrest of speech is really not proof of aphasia. The fact that arrests can originate in the right or left hemisphere SMA suggests that they may be more strongly tied to interference with mechanisms involved in the initiation of motor activity or its programming or organization (AOS).

Speech arrest has been observed in electrical stimulation studies of individuals with seizures. Penfield and Roberts (1959) induced it with stimulation of the temporal-parietal area, Broca's area, and the SMAs of both hemispheres. Stimulation of the ventrolateral thalamus during stereotactic procedures can also arrest speech (Botez and Barbeau, 1971). Lesions, including tumors, in the SMA can produce sudden speech arrests or uncontrolled vocalization (Jonas, 1981). Speech arrest accompanied by right leg weakness but preserved writing and comprehension has also been observed during migrainous episodes (Jenkyn and Reeves, 1979).

CASES

Case 12.1

A 65-year-old woman was admitted to the hospital for evaluation of episodes of unsteady gait, facial weakness, and speech difficulty. Following admission, she had several transient ischemic attacks (TIAs) and two weeks later a stroke. A CT scan revealed infarcts in the temporal and occipital lobes, basal ganglia, and cerebellum.

She was seen for speech evaluation two weeks after her stroke. She was mute but attempted to speak, producing only a grunt with minimal articulatory movements. Her face and tongue were weak, and, on request, she protruded her tongue slowly and with limited range of movement. The palate moved minimally on attempts at phonation and during a gag. Responses on language tasks were noticeably delayed, and verbal and reading comprehension were significantly impaired; responses often were perseverative. These deficits appeared more related to general cognitive impairments than a focal impairment of language.

An attempt was made to establish an augmentative means of communication, but the patient's cognitive impairments prevented success. She was discharged to a nursing home but readmitted two months later for rehabilitation. She was still mute but was more responsive nonverbally, answering yes-no questions with head nods or eye blinks, without perseveration. Oral mechanism examination was unchanged. Because of marked visual impairments and inability to use her limbs for pointing or other gestural responses, head nods and simple eye blinks remained the most viable means of communication.

The clinician concluded that the patient's muteness was primarily due to anarthria resulting from bilateral UMN involvement.

Commentary: *(1) Multiple strokes can lead to mutism. (2) Cognitive deficits frequently accompany anarthric mutism. In combination with visual and limb motor deficits, they may place limits on the sophistication of the augmentative means of communication that are possible.*

Case 12.2

A 71-year-old woman presented to neurology with a two-year history of decline in gait, speech, and bowel and bladder control. Examination revealed weakness and spasticity in all limbs and the face, with a generalized increase in reflexes and positive snout, suck, and jaw jerk reflexes. She was unable to speak and had significant difficulty with chewing and swallowing.

A CT scan revealed generalized cerebral atrophy but provided no evidence of stroke or tumor. Her neurologist concluded that she probably had a primary degenerative CNS disease that could not be further specified.

During speech evaluation she confirmed being unable to speak for the last three months, following a nearly two-year gradual decline in speech ability. She answered yes-no questions by raising one or two fingers (she was unable to write secondary to bilateral upper extremity weakness). Her verbal comprehension for simple and complex commands and yes-no questions was quite good, as was sentence-level reading comprehension.

Jaw, face, and tongue movements were markedly slowed and restricted in range. The gag reflex was normal. She was unable to cough or clear her throat with normal sharpness. She did produce a very brief nonvolitional sigh and yawn. She was otherwise completely mute. There was no evidence of nonverbal oral apraxia or apraxic-like groping during attempts at speech. It was concluded that her muteness was due to anarthria stemming from severe spastic dysarthria. She did not remain at the clinic and was referred to a speech pathologist near her home for consideration of alternative communication devices.

Commentary: *(1) Anarthria can be the product of degenerative CNS disease. (2) Anarthria can be present without significant cognitive or sensory impairments.*

Case 12.3

A 22-year-old man was admitted to the rehabilitation unit for management of deficits stemming from a motor vehicle accident 2.5 years earlier. He had made only minimal progress during previous rehabilitation efforts.

A CT scan at the time of admission revealed significant generalized cerebral atrophy as well as low attenuation changes in the centrum semiovale bilaterally. An EEG showed marked diffuse nonspecific abnormalities with a potentially epileptogenic focus in the left occipital-parietal region. The patient did have occasional seizures.

During speech evaluation, he demonstrated a nearly total disregard for auditory or visual stimuli and showed no evidence of comprehension of any verbal statement made to him. He did not attempt to vocalize or generate any sound volitionally or reflexively. He occasionally grimaced, made some sucking motions with his mouth, ground his teeth, and lifted his head toward the left, all for no obvious reason. He did not respond to persistent strong auditory, visual, or tactile stimulation during several periods of observation, nor was he observed to do so by any other staff.

The clinician concluded that the patient's muteness was due to his severely reduced level of arousal and cognition. Neuromotor impairments could not be ruled out as an additional contributor to his muteness.

During neurologic evaluation, the patient appeared alert but did not make any meaningful responses to any stimuli. Some dystonic posturing of the arms and legs was apparent. He did not clearly blink in response to visual threat. He groaned for no apparent reason on a few occasions. The neurologist concluded the patient had a severe encephalopathy and was in a persistent vegetative state.

Efforts to increase responsiveness over several weeks were unsuccessful. The patient was discharged to a nursing home.

Commentary: (1) Mutism may be associated with diffuse impairment of cortical function, leading to a persistent vegetative or apallic state. (2) A common cause of this form of mutism is CHI.

Case 12.4

A 5-year-old right-handed boy underwent neurosurgery for removal of a large fourth ventricle medulloblastoma. Preoperatively, he had had a history of headaches and ataxic gait, but no speech or language difficulty.

On the first postoperative day, he made a few normal-sounding utterances. On the second postoperative day, he became mute.

He was referred for speech assessment 10 days postoperatively because of continued mutism. He was awake, somewhat restless, and agitated, but not clearly oppositional. Several times per minute he cried for 1 to 3 seconds, without tears, and for no apparent reason, although it most often followed a verbal request or comment directed to him. He made no attempt to communicate verbally or gesturally, and he made no purposeful movements with his upper extremities, except to scratch his nose and eyes with his right hand. He did not respond to verbal requests to point, answer yes-no questions, or look at objects. Observation a few hours later was similar, although when asked to close his eyes he made some upper face–forehead movements without closing his eyes. They were closed by the examiner and

maintained by him, but he did not then open his eyes on command, although he appeared to try. He responded similarly when asked to open and close his mouth, and these activities triggered crying. His jaw and lower face were not obviously weak. His cry sounded normal. He did not protrude his tongue under any voluntary or involuntary circumstances but did retract it during eating and crying. Sucking was adequate. He had no difficulty swallowing solids or liquids but did occasionally lose liquids and solids out of his mouth, as if their oral handling was uncoordinated. On one occasion, he laughed briefly at a humorous comment by the clinician.

Five days later, he was able to protrude his tongue to lick a lollipop; he did this on several trials but with some apparent groping for movement before protrusion. Intermittent crying was still present. He achieved and maintained eye contact more consistently and laughed appropriately on two occasions.

Although the patient's neurologists were suspicious of elective (psychogenic) mutism, the speech pathologist concluded that he had "muteness of undetermined origin. There are several possibilities. Elective mutism is unlikely; it doesn't explain his lack of response to nonspeech demands and electively mute individuals often communicate adequately nonverbally. It also does not explain the paucity of purposeful limb activity. Conversion mutism is also a possibility, but the same arguments against it apply. If psychogenic explanations are active, strongly suspect there is an additional neurogenic component. Normal chewing and swallowing and normal cry argue against a severe spastic or flaccid dysarthria. Could this be a variant of akinetic mutism? (Crying, restlessness/agitation, and relatively rapid feeding would be unusual, however.) Perhaps more likely is a severe loss of cerebellar control for speech movements or an apraxia of speech. Cases of mutism following posterior fossa surgery in children have been reported in the literature."

The patient was discharged from the hospital shortly thereafter. Follow-up phone conversation with his mother indicated that he began to speak 23 days postoperatively. At that time his articulation was reasonably good, but his mother noted that his "accent" was not appropriate and that he was occasionally excessively loud. The excessive loudness had resolved, but his mother felt the melody of his speech remained impaired.

The patient was seen four years later as part of a learning disorders assessment. His receptive and expressive language abilities fell in the low-average range. Speech rate was moderately slowed. Excess and equal stress, a voice tremor, and subtle irregular articulatory breakdowns were noted. Speech AMRs were irregular (2,3). The clinician concluded that he had a mild-moderate ataxic dysarthria that did not impair speech intelligibility.

Commentary. (1) Mutism sometimes develops after neurosurgery for cerebellar–fourth ventricle tumors in children. (2) The etiology of "cerebellar mutism" is not always clear, but psychogenic factors, anarthria, and motor programming (AOS) deficits often need to be considered. (3) In this case, psychogenic etiology was *considered unlikely, and severe dysarthria or apraxic-like deficits were considered likely during the period of mutism. The emergence of an ataxic dysarthria following the period of mutism suggests that anarthria was, at the least, a significant contributor to mutism in this case.*

Case 12.5

A 45-year-old man was admitted to the hospital with a two-month history of bilateral frontal headaches and recently developed left hemiplegia and diffuse neurologic deficits. A CT scan demonstrated bilateral basal ganglia infarcts. A multitude of additional neurologic tests led to a suspicion that he had a CNS vasculitis.

During initial speech-language evaluation, the patient was unresponsive to any commands for oral volitional movement, with the exception that he slowly protruded his tongue on request, after a significant delay. He followed some one-step commands and identified some large print letters accurately, but after significant delays. There was no spontaneous speech and he did not respond to attempts to have him count or sing. He made a few unintelligible sounds when attempting to imitate some single-syllable words. He wrote his first name after a significant delay. He wrote a few single words to dictation, with significant spelling errors (he had only a seventh-grade education).

The clinician stated, "The most impressive features of this exam are: consistent, markedly latent responses; frequently, no responses; nearly all "errors" are of omission, not commission; reduced amplitude of response; absence of groping or off-target attempts at speech and absence of speech except for a few sounds; drowsy/obtunded appearance, often with failure to achieve eye contact. His general behavior resembles that of abulic or akinetically mute patients, but is complicated by his drowsiness/obtundation. There is no convincing evidence of aphasia or apraxia of speech, although they could be masked by his other deficits." Therapy was not recommended at the time.

Examination one month later was similar. He was mute but did phonate while yawning. He did not respond to any requests for nonverbal oral movements. He identified a few body parts, pictures, and letters on request after lengthy delays. Again, the clinician concluded that the patient was akinetically mute but was unable to rule out dysarthria or AOS. By the time of his discharge, the patient was more alert and able to follow some commands, although with delays. He was not seen for futher follow-up.

Commentary. (1) Diagnosis of the underlying nature of mutism is often difficult. (2) The patient's marked response latencies to simple concrete tasks and frequent complete unresponsiveness supported the impression of akinetic mutism. The absence of speech or production of very limited speech, particularly in the presence of bilateral basal ganglia infarcts, left open the possibility that the patient was also dysarthric and had an AOS.

Case 12.6

A 51-year-old man was admitted to the rehabilitation unit two months following a pontine infarction that left him mute and quadriplegic. He was tracheostomized and fed through a nasogastric tube.

On initial speech evaluation, the patient was alert and responsive, and there was no evidence of aphasia or confusion. His jaw was weak bilaterally, but he was able to partially open, close, and lateralize it. He had a moderate degree of facial weakness but was able to approximate his lips and retract and purse them slowly. He had minimal ability to protrude, retract, lateralize, and elevate his tongue. The palate was immobile, and a gag reflex could not be elicited. The patient was mute, although he did attempt to mouth some words and had fairly good jaw and lower face and lip movement during speech attempts.

He was able to answer yes-no questions correctly with head nods or eye blinks. He correctly identified large-print words, letters, and numbers by closing his eyes to stop the examiner's scanning of choices. He was able to spell words using a combination of head movements and eye blinks as an alphabet board was scanned.

The clinician concluded that the patient was "anarthric, with an incomplete LiS, with some limited ability to move his articulators. Speech would be nonfunctional even if he were not trached." He was considered an excellent candidate for an augmentative system of communication.

For the next month, the patient communicated with an eye gaze communication system with letters or pictures representing choices. This was slow but an effective means of communication, particularly between the patient and his wife. He next proceeded to be able to use his right index finger to activate a switch that triggered an electronic scanner on a large alphabet board. It also contained some common phrases. He gradually became able to make some lip and tongue movements and to produce weak stops.

Two weeks later he received a speaking trach and was able to phonate quite well, although he tired quickly. Over the next several weeks, he became able to produce some sounds and syllables, although with considerable difficulty synchronizing exhalation and articulation. His trach tube was removed shortly thereafter. Voice quality was breathy and somewhat hypernasal. Bilateral vocal cord weakness was apparent on laryngeal examination.

Over the next two months, his speech improved to a point where he was considered 100% intelligible in quiet speaking situations. He was discharged from the hospital shortly thereafter but returned five months later for reassessment. His speech at that time was characterized by a breathy-strained voice quality (3); hypernasality (2); slow rate (−2); there was clear-cut left-sided weakness of the palate and left-sided vocal cord weakness. Speech intelligibility was generally good but considered reduced in noise.

The patient was seen two years later for follow-up. Speech was relatively unchanged, and he was considered to have a mixed spastic-flaccid dysarthria and *speech characteristics attributable to respiratory, laryngeal, velopharyngeal, and articulatory impairments. There was also a significant respiratory contribution to his speech difficulties; he clearly exhibited a clavicular pattern of breathing.*

Commentary. *(1) Incomplete LiS frequently results from brainstem infarction causing quadriplegia, spasticity of cranial nerves supplying bulbar muscles, and cranial nerve LMN impairment. (2) A mixed flaccid-spastic dysarthria is not infrequently the underlying cause of the anarthria in LiS. (3) Substantial recovery from LiS, while unusual, is possible. (4) Patients who recover from LiS frequently progress from increasingly sophisticated means of alternative communication, to the emergence of some functional speech, to the development of intelligible speech and the discarding of augmentative means of communication. (5) Patients with LiS present special challenges to management and, particularly when considerable recovery occurs, require a number of approaches to treatment.*

SUMMARY

1. Mutism, the absence of speech, may have multiple origins, including neurologic disease. When it results from acquired neurologic disease, it may reflect severe dysarthria (anarthria), AOS, aphasia, and a variety of nonaphasic cognitive and affective conditions.

2. Anarthric mutism may result from a variety of different dysarthria types, lesion loci, and a number of different neurologic diseases. Anarthria most commonly results from bilateral or diffuse neurologic damage, however. When a single vascular event causes anarthria, its locus is usually in the brain stem.

3. Locked-in syndrome is characterized by anarthria plus immobility of the body except for vertical eye movements and blinking, which allow communication through eye movements. It is usually caused by occlusion of the basilar artery, which affects the ventral aspect of the pons.

4. Anarthria occasionally results from bilateral damage to the lower part of the precentral and postcentral convolutions (a bi-opercular syndrome) and may leave limb movements, language, and cognitive abilities relatively intact. "Cerebellar mutism" is a rare form of mutism that may occur in children following neurosurgery for large midline posterior fossa tumors. The mechanism for the mutism is unclear, although significant dysarthria is usually present when the mutism begins to clear.

5. Mutism associated with AOS is not unusual in the first few days postonset. Rarely, it persists for several months and is often charac-

terized by a disproportionately severe apraxia of phonation.

6. Mutism in the acute period following the onset of aphasia is not unusual, but it usually does not persist. When it does, suspicion should be raised about an accompanying AOS, dysarthria, or nonaphasic cognitive deficits.

7. Mutism may result from cognitive and affective deficits that are distinct from motor speech disorders and aphasia. Severe disorders of arousal stemming from reticular activating system involvement and diffuse impairments of cortical functions can be associated with mutism. Damage to frontal lobe–limbic system structures may lead to akinetic mutism that is usually associated with general unresponsiveness or reluctance to perform simple motor activities in spite of preserved alertness and basic motor and sensory abilities. Akinetic mutism is strongly associated with deficits reflecting a lack of initiative, as well as impairments in affect, personality, and emotion.

8. Neurogenic mutism may also result from specific neurologic events. For example, mutism following transection of the corpus callosum for control of epilepsy or removal of tumors in deep midline structures is not unusual. Speech arrests during partial seizures are common, typically reflecting involvement of the supplementary motor area or dominant hemisphere language areas.

9. The distinction among different forms of neurogenic mutism can contribute to the localization of neurologic disease, an understanding of the underlying nature of the mutism, and an appreciation of factors that must be considered in its management.

REFERENCES

Alajouanine TH and Lhermitte F: Acquired aphasia in children, Brain 88:653, 1965.

Alexander MP, Benson DF, and Stuss DT: Frontal lobes and language, Brain Lang 37:656, 1989.

Aronson AE: Clinical voice disorders, ed 3, New York, 1990, Thieme.

Bauer G, Gerstenbrand F, and Rumpl E: Varieties of the locked-in syndrome, J Neurol 221:77, 1979.

Benes V: Advantages and disadvantages of the transcallosal approach to the III ventricle, Childs Nerv Syst 6:437, 1990.

Bogen J and Vogel P: Neurological status in the longterm following complete cerebral commissurotomy. In Michel F and Schott B, editors: Les syndromes de disconnexion calleuse chez l'homme, Lyon, France: Hôpital Neurogique, 227, 1975.

Bone DI: Mutism following left hemisphere infarction, J Neurol Neurosurg Psychiatry 47:1342, 1984.

Botez MI and Barbeau A: Role of subcortical structures, and particularly of the thalamus, in the mechanisms of speech and language, Int J Neurol 8:300, 1971.

Brown JW: Aphasia, apraxia, and agnosia, Springfield, IL, 1972, Charles C Thomas.

Cappa SF and others: Speechlessness with occasional vocalizations after bilateral opercular lesions: a case study, Aphasiology 1:35, 1987.

Cascino GD and others: Seizure-associated speech arrest in elderly patients, Mayo Clin Proc 66:254, 1991.

Chia LG: Locked-in state with bilateral internal capsule infarcts, Neurology 34:1365, 1984.

Chia LG: Locked-in syndrome with bilateral ventral midbrain infarcts, Neurology 41:445, 1991.

Cooper JA and Flowers CR: Children with a history of acquired aphasia: residual language and academic impairments, J Speech Hear Disord 52:251, 1987.

Damasio A: The frontal lobes. In Heilman KM and Valenstein E, editors: Clinical neuropsychology, New York, 1979, Oxford University Press.

Dietze DD and Mickle JP: Cerebellar mutism after posterior fossa surgery, Pediatr Neurosurg 16:25, 1990–91.

Ferrante L and others: Mutism after posterior fossa surgery in children, report of three cases, J Neurosurg 72:959, 1990.

Gazzaniga MS and others: Neurologic perspectives on right hemisphere language following surgical section of the corpus callosum, Semin Neurol 4:126, 1984.

Groswasser Z and others: Mutism associated with buccofacial apraxia and bihemispheric lesions, Brain Lang 34:157, 1988.

Groswasser Z, Groswasser-Reider I, and Korn C: Bioopercular lesions and acquired mutism in a young patient, Brain Inj 5:331, 1991.

Haig AJ, Katz RT, and Sahgal V: Mortality and complications of the locked-in syndrome, Arch Phys Med Rehabil 68:24, 1987.

Hecaen H: Acquired aphasia in children and the ontogenesis of hemispheric functional specialization, Brain Lang 13:114, 1976.

Hudson LJ, Murdoch BE, and Ozanne AE: Posterior fossa tumours in childhood: associated speech and language disorders post-surgery, Aphasiology 3:1, 1989.

Jenkyn L and Reeves A: Aphemia with hemiplegic migraine, Neurology 29:1317, 1979.

Jonas S: The supplementary motor region and speech emission, J Commun Dis 14:349, 1981.

Jürgens U, Kirzinger A, and von Cramon D: The effects of deep-reaching lesions in the cortical face area on phonation, a combined case report and experimental monkey study, Cortex 18:125, 1982.

Lang C and others: Foix-Chavany-Marie syndrome—neurological, neuro-psychological, CT, MRI, and SPECT findings in a case progressive for more than 10 years, Eur Arch Psychiatry Neurol Sci 239:188, 1989.

Lebrun Y: Mutism, London, 1990, Whurr Publishers.

Levin HS and others: Mutism after closed head injury, Arch Neurol 40:601, 1983.

Mariani C and others: Bilateral perisylvian softenings: bilateral anterior opercular syndrome (Foix-Chavany-Marie syndrome), J Neurol 223:269, 1980.

Marshall RC, Gandour J and Windsor J: Selective impairment of Phonation: a case study, Brain Lang 35:313, 1988.

McCusker EA and others: Recovery from the "locked-in" syndrome, Arch Neurol 39:145, 1982.

McGann WM and Paslawski TM: Incompleted locked-in syndrome: two cases with successful communication outcomes, Am J Speech-Language Pathol 1:32, 1991.

Mesulam M-M: Principles of behavioral neurology, Philadelphia, 1985, FA Davis.

Miller JF and others: Language behavior in acquired childhood aphasia. In Holland AL, editor: Language disorders in children: recent advances, San Diego, 1984, College-Hill.

Morariu MA: Locked-in syndrome. In Major neurological syndromes, Springfield, IL, 1979a, Charles C Thomas.

Morariu MA: Akinetic mutism (coma vigil). In Major neurological syndromes, Springfield, IL, 1979b, Charles C. Thomas.

Mumenthaler M: Neurology, ed 3, New York, 1990, Thieme Medical.

Nagatani K, Waga S, and Nakagawa Y: Mutism after removal of a vermian medullobastoma: cerebellar mutism, Surg Neurol 36:307, 1991.

Patterson JR and Grabois M: Locked-in syndrome: a review of 139 cases, Stroke 17:758, 1986.

Penfield W and Roberts L: Speech and brain-mechanisms, Princeton, 1959, Princeton University Press.

Plum F and Posner J: Diagnosis of stupor and coma, Philadelphia, 1966, FA Davis.

Polkey CE: Surgical treatment of chronic epilepsy. In Trimble MR, editor: Chronic epilepsy, its prognosis and management, New York, 1989, John Wiley and Sons.

Reeves AG: Corpus callosotomy. In Resor SR and Kutt H, editors: The medical treatment of epilepsy, New York, 1992, Marcel Decker.

Rekate HL and others: Muteness of cerebellar origin, Arch Neurol 42:697, 1985.

Rosenbaum DH and others: Epileptic aphasia, Neurology 36:822, 1986.

Ruff RL and Arbit E: Aphemia resulting from a left frontal hematoma, Neurology 31:353, 1981.

Ruff and others: Long-term survivors of the "locked-in" syndrome: patterns of recovery and potential for rehabilitation, J Neuro Rehabil 1:31, 1987.

Salvati M and others: Transient cerebellar mutism after posterior cranial fossa surgery in an adult, Clin Neurol Neurosurg 93:313, 1991.

Sapir S and Aronson AE: Aphonia after closed head injury: aetiologic considerations, Br J Disord Commun 20:289, 1985.

Segarra JM and Angelo JN: Anatomical determinants of behavioral change. In Benton AL, editor: Behavioral change in cerebrovascular disease, New York, 1970, Harper and Row.

Starkstein SE, Berthier M, and Leiguarda R: Bilateral opercular syndrome and crossed aphemia due to a right insular lesion: a clinicopathological study, Brain Lang 34:253, 1988.

Stuss DT and Benson DF: Neuropsychological studies of the frontal lobes, Psychol Bull, 95:3, 1984.

Sussman NM and others: Mutism as a consequence of callosotomy, J Neurosurg 59:514, 1983.

Trimble MR: Psychopathology of frontal lobe syndromes, Semin Neurol 10:287, 1990.

Turkstra LS and Bayles KA: Acquired mutism: physiopathy and assessment, Arch Phys Med Rehabil 73:138, 1992.

Vogel M and von Cramon D: Dysphonia after traumatic midbrain damage: a follow-up study, Folia Phoniatr Logop 34:150, 1982.

Vogel M and von Cramon D: Articulatory recovery after traumatic mutism, Folia Phoniatr Logop 35:294, 1983.

Von Cramon D: Traumatic mutism and the subsequent reorganization of speech functions, Neuropsychologia 19:801, 1981.

Weller M: Anterior opercular cortex lesions cause dissociated lower cranial nerve palsies and anarthria but no aphasia: Foix-Chavany-Marie syndrome and "automatic voluntary dissociation" revisited, J Neurol 240:199, 1993.

Weller M, Poremba M, and Dichgans J: Opercular syndrome without opercular lesions: Foix-Chavany-Marie syndrome in progressive supranuclear motor system degeneration, Eur Arch Psychiatry Neurol Sci 239:370, 1990.

Yorkston KM and Beukelman DR: Motor speech disorders. In Yorkston KM and Beukelman DR, editors: Communication disorders following traumatic brain injury: management of cognitive, language, and motor impairments, Austin, TX, 1991, Pro-Ed.

Not all neurogenic disturbances of speech are captured under the heading of motor speech disorders. This was implied in the previous chapter in which it was made clear that neurogenic mutism can reflect disturbances in arousal, drive, motivation, and affect, as well as specific motor speech disorders. Similarly, speaking individuals' verbal output may be aberrant for reasons other than dysarthria and apraxia of speech (AOS). The recognition of these "other" problems as distinct from motor speech disorders is important to understanding the organization of speech, language, and communication in the brain, and it has implications for localization and management. These problems are the focus of this chapter.

The speech disorders discussed here represent a heterogeneous collection of problems that have a variety of close and distant relationships to motor speech disorders. Some are clearly distinct from the dysarthrias and AOS and fall in the realm of cognitive, affective, or linguistic disturbances. Others might be motor speech disorders in their own right but have not been considered so by convention or because their nature is poorly understood. Still others may represent an unusual prominence of a characteristic that is part of an identifiable motor speech disorder.

There is no generally accepted way for categorizing these diverse speech disorders. For organizational purposes, in this chapter they will be grouped under three broad anatomic headings: (1) those that are associated with bilateral, diffuse, or multifocal central nervous system (CNS) lesion sites; (2) those usually associated with left hemisphere (LH) lesions; and (3) those usually associated with right hemisphere (RH) lesions. These headings and the deficits to be discussed under them are summarized in Table 13–1.

OTHER SPEECH DISTURBANCES ASSOCIATED WITH BILATERAL, DIFFUSE, OR MULTIFOCAL CENTRAL NERVOUS SYSTEM LESION SITES
Acquired neurogenic dysfluency or stuttering-like behavior (neurogenic stuttering)

Central nervous system (CNS) disease occasionally is associated with disrupted speech fluency that is characterized by sound or syllable repetition, prolongation, or hesitation. Sometimes these dysfluencies are the only evident speech abnormality. Sometimes they are embedded within a constellation of symptoms that represent dysarthria, AOS, or aphasia. Sometimes they represent a psychological response to neurologic disease, a condition that will be discussed in the next chapter, which addresses psychogenic speech disturbances. Dysfluent speech acquired as a direct result of neurologic disease has been given a variety of labels, including *acquired stuttering, cortical stuttering,* and *neurogenic stuttering.*

The heading used for this section obviously reflects some reservations about the label "stuttering." These reservations stem from a desire to

Table 13–1 Designation, lesion loci, and nature of deficits associated with neurogenic speech disturbances that may or may not be explained by dysarthria or apraxia of speech

Designation	Anatomic locus	Nature of deficit
Bilateral, diffuse, or multifocal lesion sites		
Neurogenic stuttering	Left hemisphere	Aphasia
		Apraxia of speech
	Basal ganglia	Hypokinetic dysarthria
	Multiple lesion sites	Other dysarthria types
		Unknown: ? dysequilibrium of a bilateral innervated system
Palilalia	Basal ganglia ? frontal lobes	? Damaged inhibitory motor circuits
Echolalia	Left hemisphere, diffuse, multifocal	Preserved input/output, lowered threshold for responding to external stimulation, poor propositional language
Attenuated speech/hypophonia	Frontal lobe/limbic, thalamic Basal ganglia	Cognitive-affective Hypokinetic dysarthria
Disinhibited vocalization	Diffuse, multifocal ? Basal ganglia control circuit	Cognitive-affective Hyperkinesia (e.g., Tourette's)
Left hemisphere		
Aphasia		Nonfluency
		Word retrieval deficits
		Phonologic errors
Pseudoforeign accent		? Motor programming (apraxia of speech)
		? Syntactic deficits (aphasia)
Right hemisphere		
Aprosodia		? Dysarthria
		? Motor programming
		? Cognitive-affective
		? Other

avoid (1) confusing this disorder with behavioral, etiologic, and theoretic issues associated with developmental stuttering, or suggesting that acquired neurogenic dysfluencies represent strong evidence for a neurogenic basis for developmental stuttering; (2) implying that all dysfluencies associated with acquired CNS damage reflect the same underlying disturbance; and (3) implying that all acquired stuttering-like behavior is neurogenic—it can be psychogenic in origin, even in people with neurologic disease.

With these reservations stated, the designation *neurogenic stuttering (NS)* will be adopted here in an effort to maintain consistency with its frequent use in the literature and because it makes explicit the presumed neurogenic etiology of the problem. The designation "stuttering," it should be understood, represents a shorthand for "stuttering-like behavior," which is not identical in a number of respects to developmental stuttering, the disorder

for which the label "stuttering" traditionally has been reserved.

Clinical characteristics. Whether NS in aphasic, apraxic, and dysarthric speakers represents a symptom of those problems or a concomitant but separate speech disorder may be very difficult to determine in individual cases. However, there have been a sufficient number of reported cases without aphasia, AOS, or significant dysarthria to suggest that NS can be "isolated." The characteristics and common associated deficits and etiologies of NS are summarized in the box on page 299.

Neurogenic stuttering is characterized by repetition, prolongation, or blocking on sounds or syllables in a manner that interrupts the normal rhythm and flow of speech (Helm, Butler, and Benson, 1978). Rosenbek and others (1978) suggested that sound-syllable repetitions are the most frequent type of dysfluency, with a majority occurring in the initial position. Ludlow and others

NEUROGENIC STUTTERING— CHARACTERISTICS AND COMMON ASSOCIATED DEFICITS AND ETIOLOGIES

Characteristics

Sound/syllable repetitions, prolongations, and blocking
May not be restricted to initial syllables
May include content and function words
Awareness of dysfluencies but without significant anxiety or secondary struggle behavior
May not show adaptation effect or improvement with choral reading or singing

Associated deficits

Aphasia
Apraxia of speech
Dysarthrias (perhaps hypokinetic more than other types)

Common etiologies

Multiple, but stroke and closed head injury most common
Also in Parkinson's disease, progressive supranuclear palsy, dementia, seizure disorders, dialysis dementia, tumors, anoxia, bilateral thalamotomy, drug toxicity or abuse

(1987) described the dysfluencies of individuals with penetrating head injuries as "like it was 'shot from a gun,'" with intermittent and unpredictable bursts of rapid and unintelligible speech, uncontrolled repetitions or prolongations, and long silences without struggle" (p. 62). These patients were aware of their dysfluencies but felt that they could not control them.

Many descriptions of NS are framed in comparison to those associated with developmental stuttering. They address the locus of dysfluencies within words and phrases, the kinds of tasks in which dysfluencies are exacerbated or reduced, whether there is an adaptation effect (a reduction of dysfluencies with repeated readings), and whether there is evidence of anxiety, avoidance, or secondary struggle associated with the dysfluencies. In this context, people with NS have been reported to (1) not necessarily adapt on repeated readings, (2) have dysfluencies that are not restricted to initial syllables, (3) be dysfluent on function words as well as content words, (4) have no consistent differences between spontaneous speech and imitation, and (5) demonstrate annoyance and awareness of dysfluencies but generally not significant anxiety or secondary struggle behavior beyond mild facial grimacing (Ardila and Lopez, 1986; Helm, Butler, and Benson, 1978; Peach, 1984; Rosenbek, 1984; Rosenbek and oth-

ers, 1978). Helm-Estabrooks (1986) anecdotally suggests that an adaptation effect and secondary motor behaviors may be more likely when the etiology is closed head injury. Some have noted that there may be no significant reduction of dysfluency with choral reading or singing (Miller, 1985; Rentschler, Driver, and Callaway, 1984).

Varieties of neurogenic stuttering. Neurogenic stuttering is not a homogeneous disorder. It is associated with a number of etiologies and may be transient or persistent. It may be the predominant or only deficit affecting speech or may occur in association with aphasia, AOS, or dysarthria. Market and others (1990), in a survey study that identified 81 cases of acquired stuttering, reported that 32% of the cases were aphasic, 12% had dysarthria, and 11% had aphasia and dysarthria (they apparently did not inquire about AOS). It is this possible association with other speech and language deficits that represents the most logical way to think of "types" of neurogenic dysfluencies at this time.

Dysfluencies may occur with aphasia, often as a manifestation of word retrieval difficulties or efforts to organize verbal expression or to correct errors. Farmer (1975) found stuttering-like repetitions in people with Wernicke's, conduction, Broca's and anomic aphasia, indicating that NS is not associated with any specific type of aphasia. She suggested that LH damage that causes inefficiencies in language can also lead to temporal disorganization in the form of stuttering repetitions.

Rosenbek (1984) argued that when dysfluencies are embedded within the numerous manifestations of aphasia, they should not be labeled as stuttering because aphasia is not a necessary condition for NS. In contrast, Lebrun and others (1983) concluded from their literature review that although NS occurs in the context of aphasia in about two thirds of cases, the relationship between the dysfluencies and aphasia may not be causal. Sometimes dysfluencies may be "remarkable" and deserving of special mention as an unusually prominent deficit in aphasia. Consider, for example, the dysfluencies—in the form of word repetitions and "fillers"—during the following 33-second sample of an aphasic man's attempt to describe people's efforts to help him with word retrieval:

and uh, and uh, and, and uh, the, the first, the uh nurse, uh um, the nurse, uh would just . . . wait awhile and then and uh sometimes she she would, she would fill in uh, for the the word, and uh and uh and uh and uh and uh, it it got to be uh, to be more and more and more uh more, helpful to get somebody to, to come up with the right word.

Similarly, prominent dysfluencies may be present in people with AOS (Johns and Darley,

1970; Schuell, Jenkins, and Jiminez-Pabon, 1964). Such dysfluencies may reflect efforts to establish or correct articulatory postures for sound or syllable production. Rosenbek (1984) suggests that it may be inappropriate to label as stuttering the sound and syllable repetitions and prolongations that reflect attempts to correct articulatory or speech movement errors but also notes that some apraxic speakers may be dysfluent on correctly produced sounds and syllables. Consider the following 30-second sample of a patient's description of his speech and reading difficulties; the sample reflects a combination of his AOS and aphasia:

> Well, I thing gits uh, git the . . . the words to come, together, the right uhhh, in a sen sen . . . ss . . . ss . . . I yuh . . . wellll . . . I juh juh, hard hard hard time uh make makin' a sen, sens, sentence . . . greading, puh poor uh hard, I have a hard time, rea reading. [Note that several transcribed substitutions are actually distortions, and that distortions are present in some words transcribed as accurate.]

Dysfluencies may also be prominent in dysarthria, especially hypokinetic dysarthria, and may be a relatively early manifestation of hypokinetic dysarthria in parkinsonism or progressive supranuclear palsy (PSP) (Helm-Estabrooks, 1986). Consider the following relatively rapidly spoken, but broken with pauses, 8-second sample from a man with hypokinetic dysarthria who is describing his work: "i i i it's dea dealing wi wi with a lo lot of people [2-second pause] . . . wh who [2-second pause] . . . ha have a lot of needs."

Etiologies. Neurogenic stuttering may have multiple etiologies. In their survey study of acquired stuttering, Market and others (1990) reported an association with TBI in 38%, stroke in 37%, drugs in 6%, and neurosurgery in 4%. These data confirm impressions from the literature that stroke and TBI are probably the most frequent causes of NS.

Other documented causes of NS include degenerative diseases such as Parkinson's disease, PSP, and dementia; seizure disorders; dialysis dementia; metastatic brain tumors; anoxia; and bilateral thalamotomy (Helm-Estabrooks, 1986; Helm, Butler, and Canter, 1980; Janati, 1986; Madison and others, 1977; Manders and Bastijns, 1989; Quinn and Andrews, 1977; Rosenbek and others, 1978). Of interest, acquired dysfluencies have also been associated with use of drugs such as tricyclic antidepressants, benzodiazepine derivatives (such as Tranxene and Librium), phenothiazines, phenytoin (Dilantin), and theophylline for the treatment of disorders such as depression, anxiety, schizophrenia, seizures, and asthma (McCarthy, 1981; Mclean and McClean, 1985; Nurnberg and Green-wald, 1981; Quader, 1977; Rentschler, Driver, and Callaway, 1984). Stuttering symptoms have remitted in some cases after drug withdrawal or a change in drugs. It should be noted that the onset of NS may be delayed following stroke or TBI (Fleet and Heilman, 1985; Meyers, Hall, and Aram, 1990), although Market and others (1990) reported that most of their survey cases developed dysfluencies within one month postonset.

Of interest are cases in which developmental stuttering has remitted or reemerged with the onset or progression of neurologic disease. For example, the remission of lifelong developmental stuttering has been reported in adults during the course of multiple sclerosis with cerebellar lesions (Miller, 1985), following closed head injury (CHI) (Helm-Estabrooks and others, 1986), and following neurosurgery for tumor or vascular disturbances in the right or left hemisphere in people with amytal test-confirmed bilateral language representation (Jones, 1966). Manders and Bastijns (1989) described a child whose developmental stuttering emerged, escalated in severity, and then remitted following a seizure. Conversely, the reemergence of developmental stuttering has been reported following LH stroke (for example, Helm-Estabrooks and others, 1986; Rosenbek and others, 1978), as an initial complaint in probable Alzheimer's disease (Quinn and Andrews, 1977), and as an initial symptom in olivopontocerebellar atrophy (Hartman and O'Neill, 1989). Caution must be exercised in these latter cases, however, because they do not necessarily represent reemergence of developmental stuttering. The adult onset dysfluencies may have been only coincidentally related to the resolved developmental problem; that is, they might have developed in the absence of the developmental problem.

Anatomic correlates. The survey study of acquired stuttering by Market and others (1990) reported that 38% of the cases had left hemisphere damage (LHD), 9% right hemisphere damage (RHD), 11% subcortical lesions, and 10% bilateral lesions; lesions were not identified in 32% of the cases. These data confirm impressions that when NS develops in association with a unilateral lesion, it is most often in the LH (Lebrun and others, 1983), and they are consistent with observations of a frequent association of NS with aphasia and AOS.

The natural occurrence of dysfluencies in unselected patients does appear to be considerably higher in LHD than RHD. Yairi, Gintautas, and Avent (1981) found three times as many dysfluencies during spontaneous speech in a group with Broca's aphasia and LHD than in a non-brain-injured control group and a group of people with

RHD. The control and RHD groups did not differ significantly in the frequency of dysfluencies.

It is noteworthy that NS also has been reported in several cases with single RH lesions without evidence of aphasia or AOS (Ardila and Lopez, 1986; Fleet and Heilman, 1985; Horner and Massey, 1983; Rosenbek and others, 1978). Fleet and Heilman (1985) have suggested that because women may have a greater tendency than men to have bilateral representation of language would predict a higher incidence of RHD in women and LHD in men who acquire NS. Data are insufficient to assess the accuracy of this prediction, however.

The frontal, temporal, and parietal lobes may be involved in people with NS. This is consistent with the cortical stimulation findings of Penfield and Roberts (1959), who reported being able to elicit sound and word repetitions from all cortical areas except the occipital lobes. The association of NS with parkinsonian syndromes and PSP also implicates the basal ganglia control circuit in the disorder (Helm-Estabrooks, 1986; Janati, 1986). In an examination of NS in Vietnam veterans with penetrating head injuries, Ludlow and others (1987) found that lesions in the internal and external capsules, frontal white matter, and striatum were present more often in those with NS than in those without NS. They also reported that cortical speech regions such as Broca's area and the primary motor area were involved in 80% of NS patients but that the frequency of such lesions was not significantly greater than that for nonstuttering individuals.

Single lesions seem less likely to produce lasting NS than multifocal or diffuse lesions. Helm, Butler, and Benson (1978) found that multifocal lesions were most common in their group of 10 NS patients. Patients with persisting NS had bilateral lesions and those with unilateral lesions tended to have their dysfluencies resolve. Neurogenic stuttering can be persistent in some patients with unilateral lesions, however (Lebrun and others, 1983).

It is also of interest to examine the site of lesion or neural activity that may be associated with a cessation of dysfluencies. Bhatnagar and Andy (1989), for example, reported a case of an adult whose acquired dysfluencies developed in association with intractable pain. The dysfluencies were relieved by self-stimulation through an electrode placed in the left centromedian nucleus of the thalamus in an effort to relieve the pain. Cooper (1983) reported the case of an adult with developmental stuttering whose dysfluencies remitted for six weeks following a brainstem contusion (see additional references to cases with remission under the discussion of etiologies).

To summarize, NS may occur in the aftermath of lesions in the brain stem, cerebellum, right or left cerebral hemispheres, and frontal white matter of both cerebral hemispheres. The only innocent structures seem to be the occipital lobes and the cranial nerves (Rosenbek, 1984). Neurogenic stuttering tends to be more persistent with multifocal or bilateral lesions, but it can occur with single, unilateral lesions. Not infrequently, it may develop in individuals without identifiable lesions, as in certain degenerative diseases, CHI, and drug-related etiologies.

Nature of the problem. Why does NS develop? There are a number of possible explanations. As already discussed, when associated with aphasia, dysfluencies may simply be secondary to efforts at word retrieval, verbal formulation, and attempts to revise or correct linguistic errors. When associated with AOS, they may reflect attempts to achieve or correct articulatory movements or perceptual goals. When part of hypokinetic dysarthria, they may represent difficulties with initiation of movements, freezing, or festination, problems analogous to other movement deficits associated with rigidity, bradykinesia, and akinesia.

An explanation is more difficult to come by when dysfluencies are disproportionate to those usually encountered in aphasia, AOS, or dysarthria or when they occur in the absence of those deficits. In such cases, it may be that the offending pathology—which varies considerably in etiology and localization—disrupts the equilibrium in a bilaterally innervated system (Rosenbek and others, 1978) that existed before the lesion. The multiplicity of lesion sites associated with NS—and the fact that it can emerge when the dominant perisylvian language and motor speech programming apparatus is spared—suggests that "speech rhythm and rate control are not dependent on the left cortical regions traditionally associated with speech and language" (Ludlow and others, 1987, p. 65).

Some alternative explanations do not invoke a direct neurologic cause; that is, some patients may become dysfluent in response to the psychological trauma of their other speech or language deficits, or their other neurologic deficits, or in response to the general impact of suffering an injury to the brain. In such cases, the stuttering-like behavior can be considered psychogenic in origin and must be separated diagnostically from the communication deficits that are direct consequences of brain injury; they may also be managed quite differently. Acquired psychogenic stuttering-like behavior will be discussed in the next chapter.

Palilalia

Clinical characteristics. Another variety of dysfluency that may be associated with CNS disease, but that is quite different from NS, is *palilalia.* Palilalia, sometimes referred to as *autoecholalia* or *pathologic reiterative utterances,* is the *compulsive repetition of utterances, often in a context of increasing rate and decreasing loudness* (LaPointe and Horner, 1981). Repetitions generally involve words and phrases. Sound and syllable repetitions are usually excluded from definitions of palilalia, although sound and syllable repetitions may be present in palilalic speakers. The characteristics and common associated deficits and etiologies of palilalia are summarized in the box below.

The clinical characteristics of palilalia can be summarized as follows:

1. *Word and phrase repetitions,* with *stereotypic prosody,* but often with *progressively reduced loudness and increased rate,* very much like the acceleration and reduced loudness associated with hypokinetic dysarthria. Some observers suggest, however, that palilalia may be present in the absence of dysarthria (Boller and others, 1973) and that increasing rate and reduced loudness over the course of repetitions are not invariably present

(Kent and LaPointe, 1982). Repetitions may be numerous; a case study by LaPointe and Horner (1981) documented up to 52 repetitions in a single occurrence!

2. Reiterations occur most often *during conversation, narratives, and elicited speech* and least often during reading, repetition, and automatic responses such as counting (Boller and others, 1973; Brown, 1972; LaPointe and Horner, 1981).

3. Reiterations may occur *anywhere within an utterance* (Horner and Massey, 1983), although clinical reports suggest they occur more often at the end of utterances. Some cases have had more reiterations in the beginning than in middle or final sentence segments (LaPointe and Horner, 1981).

4. Based on LaPointe and Horner's (1981) case study, it seems that the *locus of reiterations may be inconsistent* across repeated readings and that *adaptation (reduced reiteration) does not occur* during repeated readings of the same material.

5. Palilalic *speakers tend to be aware* of their reiterations and are agitated by them (Marie and Levy, 1925). There is *no obvious struggle* or effort to inhibit them during their course, but they may be able to *inhibit reiterations* temporarily with effort and encouragement (Brown, 1972; Wallesch, 1990).

Etiologies. Palilalia has been reported in people with postencephalitic parkinsonism, Parkinson's disease, Alzheimer's disease, Pick's disease, progressive supranuclear palsy, posttraumatic encephalopathy, multiple sclerosis, Tourette's syndrome, traumatic basal ganglia lesions, and bilateral cerebral calcinosis (Ackerman, Ziegler, and Oertel, 1989; Boller and others, 1973; Brown, 1972; Wallesch, 1990). Horner and Massey (1983) reported a case in which palilalia emerged two years after a large RH middle cerebral artery stroke; they concluded that its emergence was related to degeneration of the subcortical projection system. Brown (1972) noted that "palilalic-like" symptoms may occur in association with parasaggital meningiomas in the region of the secondary motor area.

Anatomic and physiologic correlates. As a number of the possible etiologies of palilalia suggest, the disturbance is generally considered to reflect *bilateral basal ganglia pathology.* This is also consistent with the association of palilalia with hypokinetic dysarthria. The only case reported with unilateral pathology is that of Horner and Massey (see previous section), and they nonetheless attributed the disorder to degeneration of subcortical structures. Bilateral frontal lobe involvement has also occasionally been associated with palilalia (for example, Valenstein, 1975), but Brown (1972) has questioned the justification for this association.

PALILALIA—CHARACTERISTICS AND COMMON ASSOCIATED DEFICITS AND ETIOLOGIES

Characteristics

Repetitions of words or phrases

Increased rate and decreased loudness with successive repetitions (not invariable)

Most prominent during spontaneous and elicited speech; reduced during reading, repetition, and automatic speech tasks

Most common toward end of utterances, but may occur anywhere

Adaptation effect uncommon

Awareness of deficit but no anxiety or secondary struggle

Reiterations can be inhibited temporarily, with effort

Associated deficits

Hypokinetic dysarthria frequent but not invariably present

Variety of deficits that may occur with bilateral basal ganglia pathology

Common etiologies

Parkinson's disease, Alzheimer's disease and other dementias, progressive supranuclear palsy, closed head injury, stroke, tumor, multiple sclerosis, Tourette's syndrome

---

It has been suggested that palilalia reflects damage to inhibitory motor circuits (Boller and others, 1973). Wallesch (1990) notes that it bears some resemblance to the acceleration of gait with progressively smaller steps and the difficulty with terminating movement that may occur in Parkinson's disease. Ackerman, Ziegler, and Oertel (1989) reported a case with Parkinson's disease in which palilalia occurred during peak dose levels of L-dopa with associated hyperkinesias. They suggested that palilalia may not be related to dopamine depletion but rather to abnormal properties or distributions of dopaminergic receptors in the basal ganglia.

Echolalia

Definition and clinical characteristics. Echolalia is the *motorically normal unsolicited repetition of another's utterances.* In its full-blown form, it may be automatic, compulsive, and parrotlike in quality, without comprehension of meaning. In its less complete form, it may be characterized by repetition of all or part of what apparently has been understood. Sometimes a reply may contain only some of the words in a question or statement, with appropriate grammatical alterations, as if the repetition is serving as an aid to comprehension (Brown, 1972; Wallesch, 1990); for example, a patient may respond, "Something I like to do is golf" in response to the inquiry, "Tell me something you like to do."

Echolalia may not be restricted to speech explicitly directed to the patient. Fisher (1988) described the occurrence of *ambient echolalia* in demented patients, in which portions of speech from television programs or conversations going on around them are echoed.

Variations of echolalia may also be observed in the form of appropriate pronoun changes or spontaneous correction of syntactic errors; a patient may echo "Where am I going?" in response to "Where am you going?" These occurrences are sometimes called *mitigated echolalia.* Thus, echolalia does not always occur in the complete absence of linguistic processing. The box at the right summarizes the characteristics and common associated deficits and etiologies of echolalia.

Etiologies. Echolalia has been reported in stroke, Pick's disease, Alzheimer's disease and other dementing conditions, schizophrenia, mental retardation, Tourette's syndrome, carbon monoxide poisoning, and when consciousness emerges after coma (Brown, 1972; Rubens and Kertesz, 1983; Wallesch, 1990).

Anatomic and physiologic correlates. Echolalia usually occurs with diffuse or multifocal cortical pathology, as implied by many of its etiologies.

It is not an uncommon symptom in stroke(s) that leads to transcortical sensory aphasia or, more dramatically, mixed transcortical aphasia ("isolation of the speech area"). In this latter syndrome, the perisylvian language area is relatively spared but surrounded by widespread areas of infarction or degeneration of the anterior and posterior association cortex, as may occur in widespread border zone strokes, medial frontoparietal infarction in the area of the anterior cerebral artery, carbon monoxide poisoning, or dementia (Alexander, Benson, and Stuss, 1989; Albert and others, 1981; Brown, 1972; Gonzalez Rothi, 1990; Rubens and Kertesz, 1983). Such lesions relatively preserve basic input and output circuits for spoken language, permitting repetition, but isolate input and output channels from cognitive processes necessary for comprehension and language formulation. Wallesch (1990) suggests that the mechanism for echolalia may reflect an inability to propositionize, in combination with a lowered threshold to react to external stimuli. In contrast to palilalia, in which lower-level motor mechanisms appear disinhibited, echolalia seems more strongly tied to higher-level cognitive deficits.

Cognitive and affective disturbances

There are a few conditions whose speech characteristics are not easily captured under the other headings in this chapter. Disturbance of nonlinguistic cognitive and affective functions most likely underlie their clinical manifestations. Behaviorally, they can be divided crudely into disorders that attenuate speech and those that reflect apparent disinhibition of vocalization. The box

---

ECHOLALIA—CHARACTERISTICS AND COMMON ASSOCIATED DEFICITS AND ETIOLOGIES

Characteristics

Unsolicited repetition of others' utterances
Compulsive, parrotlike quality
Repetition may be complete or partial, sometimes with
spontaneous correction of syntax

Associated deficits

Aphasia
Diffuse deficits of cognition

Common etiologies

Stroke, carbon monoxide poisoning, Alzheimer's
disease, Pick's disease, other dementias,
schizophrenia, mental retardation, autism, and
pervasive developmental disorders

below summarizes the characteristics and common associated deficits and etiologies of these disorders.

Attenuation of speech. Neurogenic mutism (discussed in Chapter 12) represents attenuation of speech in the extreme. It can reflect anarthria, AOS, and aphasia but can also be the result of disorders that are not confined to speech or language. Among the cognitive and affective deficits associated with mutism, frontal lobe–limbic system pathology leading to abulia and akinetic mutism is of greatest interest here.

Individuals with frontal lobe–limbic system pathology associated with abulia and akinetic mutism tend to have extensive frontal lobe damage, although the anterior or mesial portions of the frontal lobes, including the supplementary motor area (SMA), may be most commonly involved (the common etiologies of these lesions were reviewed in Chapter 12). The deficits that derive from these lesions appear to reflect reduced drive, initiative, motivation, and ability to sustain cognitive and motor effort. These translate into apathy, listlessness, unconcern, and slowness in responding, with associated decreased verbal output, facial expression, and gesture (Alexander, Benson, and Stuss, 1989; Stuss and Benson, 1984).

When damage to frontal activating mechanisms is not so severe as to produce mutism, there often is a constellation of distinctive speech, voice, and language characteristics that seem to reflect an attenuation rather than alteration of normal speech output. The term *attenuation* in this context refers to *reduced speed of verbal responding, reduced linguistic and cognitive complexity of content, reduced vocal loudness and completeness of phonation, and flattened prosody.* To be more explicit, the patient may be very slow to initiate verbal responses and show little or no behavioral evidence of effort during the delay. When responses emerge, they often are *brief, unelaborated,* and *literal.* Rather than inadequacies or errors in language per se, content reflects limited thought, with indifference to its lack of detail or impact on the listener.

It should be noted that reduced loudness (often called *hypophonia*) and flattened prosody also may be associated with damage to subcortical structures that have important connections to cortical frontal and limbic structures. Therefore, for example, patients with hypokinetic dysarthria due to basal ganglia pathology (discussed in Chapter 7) may have attenuated loudness and prosody as prominent speech characteristics. Additional speech abnormalities and the general clinical milieu in which these attenuations occur tie them to motor rather than cognitive deficits. Taken as isolated symptoms, however, they may be very similar to the decreased loudness and prosody associated with the abulic and cognitive deficits associated with cortical frontal-limbic pathology. Similarly, hypophonia and flattened prosody (as well as variable alertness and attention, decreased insight, flat affect, and lack of initiative) are frequently associated with thalamic lesions* (for example, see Graff-Radford and Damasio, 1984; Graff-Radford and others, 1984; Mohr, Watters, and Duncan, 1975; Jonas, 1982). Ignoring other

---

COGNITIVE AND AFFECTIVE DISTURBANCES ASSOCIATED WITH ATTENUATED OR DISINHIBITED SPEECH: CHARACTERISTICS AND COMMON ASSOCIATED DEFICITS AND ETIOLOGIES

Attenuation of speech

Characteristics

Reduced loudness and hypophonia
Flattened prosody
Reduced speed of responding
Brief, unelaborated responses with reduced complexity of content

Associated deficits

Cognitive and affective impairments
Dysphonia/aphonia associated with postintubation, psychogenic, and "inertial" factors

Common etiologies

Closed head injury common, but includes anything that may damage frontal lobes, limbic system, basal ganglia, or thalamus

Disinhibited vocalization

Characteristics

Involuntary speech or phonation
Inappropriate shouting or laughter
Grunting noises
Verbal and vocal tics
? palilalia, echolalia

Associated deficits

Diffuse cognitive deficits

Common etiologies

Alzheimer's disease and other dementing conditions, Tourette's syndrome

---

*Recall that certain thalamic nuclei have important connections to the frontal lobes, including the supplementary motor area.

behaviors that may distinguish thalamic from cortical pathology, this constellation of symptoms is very similar to the cortical frontal-limbic deficits previously described.

The phonatory characteristics of these attenuations of speech deserve further mention because the reasons for them can be in doubt. For example, patients with TBI who have emerged from an akinetic mute state and are abulic and aphonic or dysphonic could be so because of vocal cord edema resulting from intubation or extubation (Lesser, Williams, and Hoddinott, 1986; Scholefield, 1987; Woo, Kelly, and Kirsner, 1989). It is certainly the case that many patients with TBI have been intubated for varying durations after their injury and that dysphonia can occur after removal of endotracheal tubes in patients without brain injury (Beckford and others, 1990; Colice, Stukel, and Dain, 1989; Jones and others, 1992; Yonick and others, 1990). Therefore, the effects of intubation and extubation must be considered as a source of phonatory abnormality, especially when cognitive abilities and overall affect seem less affected than phonation.

Sapir and Aronson (1985) present a cogent discussion of the aphonia that may be associated with closed head injury. This was an outgrowth of their experience with two patients with posttraumatic aphonia and no evidence of vocal cord weakness, dysarthria, or AOS, who regained their voices after one session of symptomatic therapy. Although there was no provable cause of the aphonia, they suggested that "damage or disturbance of the frontal lobes, limbic system, and other subcortical structures, as well as to interconnections among these systems, seems to produce a disorder of affect and cognition that, in turn, influences a patient's vocal behavior" (p. 293). They discussed two additional possible explanations for their patients' aphonia. First, especially given their rapid response to symptomatic therapy, the aphonia may have represented an acute emotional reaction to the trauma or its physical and psychological consequences. Second, there may have been an initial vocal cord paralysis (or weakness, or edema from intubation) or an apraxia of phonation, with persistence of aphonia after those disorders cleared. They indicate that such "inertial aphonia" can occur in patients who are placed on voice rest following thyroidectomy and that such patients respond well to symptomatic therapy. A similar mechanism may have been at work in their patients.

Disinhibited vocalization. Sometimes neurologic disease can lead to apparently involuntary vocalization, a phenomenon that may reflect disinhibition of vocal mechanisms. For example, Jonas (1981) has noted that SMA lesions may disinhibit speech, leading to involuntary automatic speech and paroxysmal involuntary phonation. This may happen more frequently with LH than RH lesions.

Other examples of disinhibited vocalization include (1) the shouting and inappropriate laughter that sometimes emerges in severely impaired individuals with Alzheimer's disease (Appell, Kertesz, and Fisman, 1982) (sometimes cognitively impaired patients with diffuse or multifocal involvement also make apparently involuntary, brief grunting noises of which they are unaware); and (2) the verbal and vocal tics associated with Tourette's syndrome (see Chapter 8).

Finally, inhibitory mechanisms may be implicated in echolalia and perhaps palilalia, as well as some of the dysfluencies that may occur in some forms of neurogenic stuttering. These deficits have been discussed under other headings in this chapter.

OTHER SPEECH DISTURBANCES ASSOCIATED WITH LEFT HEMISPHERE LESIONS
Aphasia—language-related speech disturbances

Aphasia is a *CNS disturbance of the capacity to interpret and formulate symbols for communicative purposes. It generally affects all modalities of language use (speech, verbal comprehension, reading, writing, and nonverbal propositional communication) but cannot be attributed to global impairments of cognitive functions, confusion, or sensory or motor deficits.* Although it has prominent effects on spoken language expression, it is not a motor speech disorder.

Aphasia is nearly always the result of damage to the LH perisylvian language zone, which includes posterior frontal and temporal and parietal cortex. Damage to subcortical structures in the LH, including the basal ganglia and thalamus, may also be associated with aphasia. This LH dominance for language exists for about 98% of right-handers and 60% to 70% of left-handers. Among left-handers who are not LH-dominant for language are individuals who are either RH-dominant or have mixed language dominance. Stroke is the most common cause of aphasia.

The manifestations of aphasia usually are most evident in spoken language. In many instances, it is clear that the ability to formulate messages has gone awry, and there is little to suggest that the motor aspects of speech are deficient. However, when AOS is also present—which it often is—separating the language problem from the motor speech deficit can be difficult. It is appropriate, therefore, to summarize some of the common verbal output characteristics of aphasia that may affect the phonemic accuracy and prosodic features of speech. The box below summarizes the characteristics of aphasia that affect the fluency and flow of verbal output, as well as common associated deficits and etiologies.

Nonfluency. Aphasia may affect grammar and syntax. Such deficits are most evident in the agrammatic or telegraphic speech of some patients with so-called *Broca's or nonfluent aphasia,* who, for example, may say "the fork ... eat, meat, potatoes" to describe what one does with a fork. Nonfluent patients' utterances tend to be reduced in length, often with simplified grammar and a relative absence of function words. They are often *produced slowly* with an *abnormal prosodic pattern* that sounds more like a listing of words than the "melodic line" of normally structured sentences. The content of nonfluent utterances reflects the underlying language deficit in many patients, and the abnormal prosody is a natural consequence of the structure of the utterance; that is, prosodic flow is disturbed by the absence of parts of speech that receive varying stress (sentences containing only nouns and verbs naturally have a pattern of excess and equal stress). In addition, because most patients with Broca's aphasia have an accompanying AOS, it is possible that reduced utterance length and telegraphic content represent an attempt to economize on speech programming demands.

APHASIA—SPEECH CHARACTERISTICS AND COMMON ASSOCIATED DEFICITS AND ETIOLOGIES

Characteristics

Nonfluency: slow rate; altered prosody with tendency to excess and equalized stress; simplified grammar and telegraphic structure
Word retrieval deficits: slow overall rate; interrupted prosodic flow
Phonologic errors: phonemic paraphasias and neologisms, usually in context of normal prosody

Associated deficits

Apraxia of speech
Unilateral upper motor neuron dysarthria

Common etiologies

Stroke most common, but can include any process capable of damaging dominant hemisphere language areas

---

The characteristics summarized here include only those aphasic deficits that alter the fluency and flow of speech.

Word retrieval deficits. Nearly all aphasic persons have difficulty with word retrieval. This is often characterized by hesitancy and delays that are sometimes silent but that may also be loaded with fillers such as "um" and "uh" or asides about the problem ("it's a ... oh I know what it is ... it's a, a, fork"). Patients may make semantic errors that may or may not be recognized by the patient ("It's a knife, no it's not a knife, it's a, oh, it's a fork"). Delays for word retrieval efforts, filled or unfilled, result in a *slowed overall rate* of expression and *interrupted prosodic flow,* giving speech a *halting, hesitant* character. In the absence of AOS, this reduced rate and aborted prosodic flow reflect the underlying linguistic disturbances and not a motor speech problem.

In some patients, word retrieval and other language formulation and expression difficulties are associated with dysfluencies that may have a stuttering-like character. These were discussed earlier in the chapter in the section on neurogenic dysfluency.

Phonologic errors. Some aphasic patients make phonologic errors, called *phonemic or literal paraphasias,* which are substitutions, omissions, additions, or transpositions of phonemes in correctly retrieved lexical units ("religerator" for "refrigerator"). Such errors are most often made by patients who speak fluently and grammatically and with relatively normal motor effort and prosody (they are often said to have Wernicke's or conduction aphasia).

Relatively severely affected patients who nonetheless have fluent and prosodically normal speech may produce *neologisms,* or words with no currency in the language ("grundel" for "cigarette," "taidillion" for "pencil"). These phonologically aberrant productions may superficially suggest AOS, but their fluent and effortless production, usually without recognition or efforts at self-correction, are usually not confused with apraxic errors. The distinction between apraxic and phonologic errors on semantically interpretable words, especially when the patient shows awareness of errors and attempts to self-correct, can be much more difficult (this issue is addressed in Chapters 11 and 15).

To summarize, when aphasia is the only communication disorder, phonation, resonance, and the rate at which individual words and many portions of utterances are produced are usually normal. However, there may be abnormalities in prosodic flow that are by-products of the language formulation problem, with slowed rate and hesitancy associated with delays during word retrieval efforts, correction of semantic errors, and revisions of statements that fail to convey semantic intent.

Prosody also may be altered by grammatic and syntactic deficits that remove usually unstressed words (the, a, of) and disturb prosodic flow. Phonologic errors may suggest articulatory deficits, but distortions of sounds usually are not evident, errors may not be recognized by the speaker, and they occur in utterances that may be produced effortlessly.

Pseudoforeign accent

Neurologic disease occasionally produces an unusual disorder whose articulatory and prosodic characteristics are perceived as a foreign accent. Because the etiology is neurogenic and because the accents are not entirely consistent with those of nonnative speakers of specific languages, this disorder is referred to as *pseudoforeign accent.**

Pseudoforeign accent is rare. Aronson (1990) identified 12 published cases from 1907 to 1978 and added 13 cases from Mayo Clinic files. Only a handful of cases have been reported since.

Clinical characteristics. The clinical characteristics of pseudoforeign accent can be summarized as follows:

1. *The disorder is not language-specific.* The literature contains reports of native speakers of British and American English, Czech, French, Norwegian, and Spanish who developed a pseudoforeign accent. The accents perceived have included Alsatian, American English, Chinese, Dutch, French, German, Hungarian, Irish, Italian, Norwegian, Polish, Scandinavian, Scottish, Slavic, Spanish, Swedish, and Welsh. Of importance, the type of accent perceived often differs among listeners or cannot be classified. True speakers of the perceived language report that the accent is not really that of their language (Ardila, Rosselli, and Ardila, 1988).

2. *There is considerable heterogeneity among the specific speech characteristics* that have been reported. In general, however, they include consonant and vowel changes and, most notably, alterations of linguistic prosodic patterns relative to premorbid patterns. These abnormalities can be summarized as follows (based primarily on reports from Aronson, 1990; Ardila, Rosselli, and Ardila, 1988; Blumstein and others, 1987; and Graff-Radford and others, 1986).

Vowel changes. These may include diphthongization; distortions and prolongations of vowels; omission of unstressed vowels; inser-

tion of epenthetic vowels between words or at the end of CVC syllables (for example, "dis *uh* boy" for "this boy," "nice*uh*" for "nice"); equalization of vowel duration; vowel shifts (for example, "feet" for "fit," "soam" for "some," "bock" for "back").

Consonant changes. These may include alterations in voicing, place, and manner features, leading to perception of substitutions; poor control of voice onset time (VOT), such as long prevoicing of initial stops; slightly off-target consonants (allophonic variations), such as fronting of alveolar consonants; anomalous consonant production, such as voicing assimilation ("yez I know"); and production of full alveolar stops instead of flapping in the medial position, as in "butter" for "budder."

Prosodic changes. These may include generally altered prosody, failure to reduce unstressed syllables within words, equalized syllabic stress, prolonged intervals, inappropriate pitch patterns, prosody characterized by large f_o (fundamental frequency) excursions, abnormal melodic line such as uncharacteristic rising pitch contours at the end of simple declaratives, slow rate, reduced fluency, initial consonant blocking, and poor transitions across word boundaries. Some of these features could occur independently of abnormalities or differences in segmental or articulatory aspects of speech; others could be secondary to such abnormalities or differences.

Nonspecific changes. Some changes may cross vowel, consonant, and prosodic dimensions, including sound substitutions, nonelided word boundaries, nonnative phonemes, broadening of phonemic boundaries, inconsistency of deviant characteristics, hesitancy, and word searching.

3. *Other motor and speech and language deficits frequently accompany pseudoforeign accent.* Many affected patients have a right hemiparesis and right central facial weakness. More relevant, many are or have been mildly aphasic, usually with relatively mild nonfluent verbal output characteristics (Broca's aphasia). Aronson's (1990) review observed that 68% of affected cases had their accent embedded in or following dysarthria, aphasia, or AOS. Among Aronson's 13 Mayo Clinic patients, 62% had AOS as an antecedent to the perception of an accent.

Etiologies and anatomic correlates. Stroke and closed head injury are the most common etiologies of pseudoforeign accent. For example, Aronson's (1990) review of 25 cases reported etiology as stroke in 56% and as closed head injury in 25% of the cases. Twenty percent had otherwise negative

*The problem has also been referred to as "dysprosody of pseudoforeign dialect" (Aronson, 1990), "foreign accent syndrome" (Berthier and others, 1991; Blumstein and others, 1987), and "unlearned foreign accent" (Graff-Radford and others, 1986).

neurologic exams or equivocal neurologic diagnoses. This suggests that lesions may be very small in some cases and illustrates one of the reasons why the disorder is often diagnosed as psychogenic in origin.

When lesion site can be determined, it has almost always been in the *left hemisphere,* very often in the premotor area (Broca's area) or frontotemporoparietal cortex. Lesions have also been reported in the subcortical white matter of the prerolandic and postrolandic gyri. Berthier and others (1991), studying four patients with the disorder, reported good recovery of accent in two patients with premotor cortex lesions and sparing of primary motor cortex, but persistence of accent in two patients with lesions of the primary motor and adjacent sensory cortex.

The following box summarizes the characteristics and common associated deficits and etiologies of pseudoforeign accent.

Nature of the problem. The underlying nature of this disorder is unclear. However, because of its association with LH pathology, its frequent localization to areas involved in motor programming, and its frequent association with Broca's aphasia, it is reasonable to speculate that it represents a type of motor speech disorder. Aronson (1990), noting the frequent occurrence of vowel distortions, allophonic consonant variations, sound substitutions, initial consonant blocking, equalized stress, prolonged intervals, inappropriate pitch variability, and inconsistency of speech characteristics, concluded that the problem most closely resembles AOS. It does seem possible that the accent reflects a variant of AOS in which prosodic abnormalities predominate and in which articulatory deficits are relatively confined to distortions of vowels and consonants, with a minimum of perceived frank consonant substitutions and groping for articulatory postures. The addition of syntactic and morphologic errors that may characterize relatively mild Broca's aphasia may also contribute to the perception that the speaker is influenced by a foreign language ("broken English") (Ardila, Rosselli, and Ardila, 1988). Why the disorder is so rare is unclear, although isolated AOS (the "typical variety") is rare in itself.

What leads to the perception of accent? It may be that the loss of verbal fluency, a broadening of phonemic boundaries, inadequate suprasegmental features, and agrammatism combine to convey the impression (Ardila, Rosselli, and Ardila, 1988). Blumstein and others (1987) suggest that listeners may categorize the speech as an accent because, even though the abnormalities are not part of the native language phonetic repertoire, they do reflect "stereotypical features which are part of the universal properties found in natural language" (p. 243). Unlike the deviations of articulation and prosody that characterize many of the dysarthrias and AOS, many of the speech abnormalities in patients with accent may not cross universal boundaries of speech production, even though they may cross phonetic and prosodic boundaries for their native language. For example, Blumstein and others point out that characteristics such as syllable timed speech rhythm, CVCV syllable structure, and intonational patterns with rising final contours may be pathologic for English but are nonetheless characteristic of natural languages. This would also explain why the perceived accent cannot be identified reliably; the accent is a generic one, not tied to a particular language. The categorical perception of this speech disorder as an accent, therefore, may be similar to the tendency of clinicians to perceive distorted consonants as substitutions in speakers with AOS.

PSEUDOFOREIGN ACCENT: CHARACTERISTICS AND COMMON ASSOCIATED DEFICITS AND ETIOLOGIES

Characteristics

Unreliability among listeners about accent perceived

Vowels: diphthongization, distortions, prolongations, insertions

Consonants: voice, place, and manner distortions, substitutions, and allophonic variations

Prosody: equalized or altered stress, prolonged intervals, inappropriate pitch contours, slow rate, reduced fluency, blocking

Other: substitutions, nonnative phonemes, broadening of phonemic boundaries, hesitancy and word searching, grammatic and syntactic errors

Associated deficits

Aphasia

Apraxia of speech

Nonverbal oral apraxia

Common etiologies

Stroke and closed head injury most common

OTHER SPEECH DISTURBANCES ASSOCIATED WITH RIGHT HEMISPHERE LESIONS—APROSODIA

The limbic system plays a crucial role in emotional experience and internal feelings of emotion, but it appears that the RH plays a dominant role in recognizing the emotional aspects of information and in producing the affective components of behavior. It also seems to make an important contribution to the perception, comprehension and production of the prosodic components of speech, especially those tied to the expression of attitudes, emotion, and emphasis (Joanette, Goulet, and Hannequin, 1990; Myers, 1994).

In recent years, increasing attention has been given to the processing and production of prosody in people with RH lesions. This has contributed to clinical descriptions of deficits associated with RHD and to our understanding of the role of the RH in the comprehension and production of verbal messages.

Some claim that the RH is specialized for the processing of prosody in the same way that the LH is specialized for the processing of language. Ross (1981), who coined the term "aprosodia" for prosodic deficits associated with RHD, has proposed a model that predicts forms of disordered prosody that mirror the major classically defined types of aphasia. Thus, for example, he discusses motor aprosodia, sensory aprosodia, transcortical motor and sensory aprosodia, global aprosodia, and so on. This model has received criticism (Cancelliere and Kertesz, 1990; Joanette, Goulet, and Hannequin, 1990), much of it related to uncertain reliability and validity of assessment protocols and judgments of aprosodia, weaknesses in the classical notions of aphasia types upon which the model of aprosodia is based, and the small number of patients thus far systematically examined. Nonetheless, clinical observations and some formal studies do suggest that a subgroup of patients with RHD have difficulty with the prosodic aspects of spoken language.

Aprosodia can be defined as *a deficit in the interpretation or production of distinctions in the durational, amplitude, or fundamental frequency (f_o) variations in speech that convey emotional tone, emphasis, and certain linguistic information.* In the context of this chapter, the term *aprosodia* refers to deficits specifically associated with RHD, but it should be recognized that the production of prosody is complex and not localizable to any single area of the brain. Attenuation of prosodic distinctions in speech production can occur in motor speech disorders (for example, hypokinetic dysarthria). Other disturbances of prosody (dysprosody) can occur in virtually every type of dysarthria. Neurogenic cognitive-affective disorders (for example, abulia) and psychiatric conditions (for example, depression) can also be associated with attenuation of prosodic features.

The term *dysprosody* is sometimes preferred to the term *aprosodia* in reference to RHD-related

prosodic deficits (Bryan, 1989; Ryalls and Behrens, 1988) because the prosodic disturbances do not seem to be characterized by a total absence of prosodic variations. The term *aprosodia* will be retained here as a way of identifying a problem that *may* be uniquely associated with RHD.

In keeping with the purposes of this book, we will focus on prosodic *production* deficits associated with RHD. The reader should keep in mind, however, that patients with RHD may also have deficits in the comprehension of prosodic variations. These problems include difficulty identifying and discriminating emotions conveyed by prosody, as well as problems with linguistic prosody that may alter meaning, provide emphatic stress, and convey information about sentence type (Heilman and others, 1984; Tompkins and Flowers, 1985; Tucker, Watson, and Heilman, 1977). The nature of these difficulties is unclear, but some suggest that they may be tied to deficits at an early stage of perceptual decoding rather than to the emotional nature of the prosody (Joanette, Goulet, and Hannequin, 1990). The relationship between these prosodic input difficulties and prosodic production difficulties in patients with RHD has not been clearly established.

It should also be kept in mind that RHD patients may have a variety of additional cognitive and perceptual impairments that affect communication and that such deficits may be more prevalent and handicapping than difficulties with the production of prosody. These problems have been categorized by Myers (1994) as nonlinguistic and extralinguistic in character.* Nonlinguistic impairments may, for example, include left-sided neglect, visuoperceptual problems, and attentional deficits. Extralinguistic impairments that, according to Myers, are at the heart of RHD communication problems interfere with the ability to understand and convey intentions, implied meanings, and emotional tone, especially in situations in which verbal and nonverbal cues must be used to assess and convey communicative intents that go beyond the explicit meaning of utterances. As a result, patients with RHD may seem indifferent or flat in affect and may have difficulty interpreting emotions conveyed by facial expression and speech. Problems with the interpretation and production of prosody,

---

*Not all patients with RHD have the nonlinguistic, extralinguistic, or prosodic deficits that are described here; the incidence of such deficits in the RHD population is unknown. Also, some people with LHD and aphasia are not entirely free of nonlinguistic and extralinguistic deficits; for example, aphasic patients sometimes have difficulty with the comprehension and production of prosody (Cancelliere and Kertesz, 1990; Joanette, Goulet, and Hannequin, 1990).

therefore, may be just one of their extralinguistic deficits. Unfortunately, the relationship between prosodic deficits—especially prosodic production deficits—and the nonlinguistic and other extralinguistic impairments is unclear. In general, however, it is possible for prosodic production deficits to be dissociated from other nonlinguistic and extralinguistic deficits; that is, some patients with significant nonlinguistic and extralinguistic deficits have no apparent deficits in prosodic expression (that are not explainable by the dysarthria that may be present), and some with significant aprosodia may have little or no clinical evidence of other nonlinguistic and extralinguistic deficits.

Assessing prosodic production

It may help at this point to establish the types of tasks that commonly have been used to study prosodic production deficits. Some of these tasks go beyond those commonly used in the assessment of the dysarthrias and AOS.

The most essential observations for the diagnosis of aprosodia are made during conversational and narrative speech, particularly when the patient addresses topics likely to generate a range of affective feelings (for example, likes and dislikes, description of family members and relationships, and the impact of their illness on life-style). It is during these responses that the characteristics of aprosodia may be most evident. It can be argued that if prosodic abnormalities are not apparent during extended spontaneous conversational interaction the diagnosis of "aprosodic" speech cannot be made with confidence.

Beyond conversational speech, many studies have examined *linguistic and affective prosody* at the word, phrase, and sentence levels.* Such tasks may include imitation, reading, and answers to questions in which response content is controlled by picture stimuli or the nature of the questions.

Linguistic or *lexical stress* may be examined by contrasting production of compound words (for example, *greenhouse, whitecaps*) with phonetically identical noun phrases (for example, *green house, white caps*). *Emphatic stress* may be examined by inducing target stress patterns in responses to questions with prescribed answers (for example, the word "John" should receive stress in the sentence "John loves Mary" in response to the question "*Who* loves Mary?"). Production of vari-

ous sentence forms (for example, declaratives, interrogatives, imperatives) is another way to examine sentence-level linguistic stress. The examination of *emotional prosody* may employ tasks that require the imitation, reading, or spontaneous production of linguistically neutral or emotional sentences with requested emotions such as happiness, sadness, and anger.

Studies of prosodic production have used perceptual ratings and a variety of acoustic measures. Acoustic studies have examined the f_o, amplitude, and durational components of syllables, words, phrases, and sentences that define prosody. Considerable emphasis has been placed on measures of f_o because it has tended to yield the greatest differences between RHD patients and neurologically normal speakers.*

Speech characteristics of patients with right hemisphere damage

What are the salient perceptual features of aprosodia? Answering this question on the basis of empiric data is difficult because of the highly variable methods and patient selection criteria in studies of patients with RHD. General clinical descriptions provide a starting point, however. The box on page 311 summarizes common complaints, perceptual and acoustic characteristics, and accompanying deficits of RHD patients who have prosodic abnormalities.

Clinical observations. The speech of RHD patients who are said to be aprosodic has been described as *flat; indifferent; computer-like or robotlike; devoid of expression and emotion; monotonous in pitch, loudness, and duration; poorly intoned and lacking in emphasis.* Patients have been described as having *little spontaneous prosody, trouble with question forms,* and an *inability to modulate the voice* to convey emotions or express the subtleties of irony and sarcasm.

In spite of the denial of deficits by some people with RHD, it is interesting that some aprosodic patients spontaneously complain that their voices do not convey the emotions they feel and wish to

---

*A comprehensive protocol for the assessment of prosodic production has been summarized by Robin, Klouda, and Hug (1991). It includes examples of tasks and stimuli, procedures for making perceptual ratings of prosodic adequacy, and a discussion of the acoustic features that can be analyzed to quantify and further characterize prosodic productions.

*Frequently used f_o and durational measures have included f_o and duration of stressed versus unstressed words (f_o and duration increase in stressed words); f_o pattern over the course of a sentence (it tends to drop over the course of a neutral, declarative sentence); f_o and duration in question forms (f_o tends to rise and duration increases on the last word relative to neutral declarative sentences); f_o during "happy" versus "sad" expressions (happiness has higher mean f_o and greater variability than affectively neutral sentences, whereas sadness has a lower mean f_o and flatter contour; sadness is associated with increased sentence duration, and happiness with reduced duration but increased durational variability) (Robin, Klouda, and Hug, 1991).

COMMON PATIENT COMPLAINTS, PERCEPTUAL AND ACOUSTIC CHARACTERISTICS, AND ACCOMPANYING CLINICAL CHARACTERISTICS OF RHD PATIENTS WHO HAVE DIFFICULTY WITH THE PROSODIC ASPECTS OF SPEECH PRODUCTION. NOTE THAT NOT ALL RHD PATIENTS WILL DISPLAY ALL OF THESE CHARACTERISTICS, EVEN IF THEY ARE JUDGED AS APROSODIC.

Patient complaints

Voice does not convey felt emotions
Altered pitch, either lower or higher
Reduced pitch range
Reduced loudness
Hoarseness

Perceptual characteristics

Flattened spontaneous prosody
Robotlike
Monotonous
Reduced affect, expression, and emotion; indifferent
Reduced pitch and loudness variation
Reduced or abnormal intonational range
Tendency to equalize stress
Poor expression of irony and sarcasm
Poorly projected
Lack of emphasis
Abnormal quality to emotional crying and laughter

Acoustic characteristics

Less salient and fewer acoustic cues for linguistic stress in narratives
Abnormal amplitude variations in emphasized and nonemphasized sentence final nouns
Reduced linearity and flatter f_o decline in declarative sentences
Poor f_o modulation to distinguish yes-no sentences from other sentence forms
Abnormally high mean f_o in sentences
Restricted f_o modulation for emotional expression during reading
Rapid rate for some speech segments
Reduced acoustic energy in middle and high frequency range
Evidence of nasalization
Reduced acoustic contrast in sentences
Failure to achieve stop closure
"Fused" (flat, indistinct syllable chain) prosodic pattern, similar to hypokinetic dysarthria

Accompanying deficits

Paucity of spontaneous emotional and propositional gestures
Left central facial weakness
Dysarthria, unilateral UMN
Left hemiparesis
Left-sided neglect
Visuoperceptual disturbances
Cognitive-communication deficits

f_o, fundamental frequency; *RHD*, right hemisphere damage.

express. Some complain of altered pitch, reduced pitch range, reduced loudness, hoarseness, or even a strangled feeling (Ryalls, Joanette, Feldman, 1987).* They may report professional, social, and

emotional problems because of these difficulties (Ross and Mesulam, 1979). These complaints are captured in the following self-description by a man who had an RH stroke and aprosodic speech:

I lack dynamics in my voice, I lack inflection in my voice ... it doesn't have the dynamicism that I had before my stroke, nor do I have any measurable amount of inflection to make my voice more interesting and

*It is of potential significance that some of these specific complaints are often heard from dysarthric patients.

more ... motivating when I talk to people ... and motivate them to my way of thinking which of course is the way I used my voice my whole career at work.

Findings and issues raised by the results of representative studies that have specifically examined the perceptual characteristics of prosody in people with RHD can be summarized as follows:

1. Based on the work of Benke and Kertesz (1989), RHD patients, as a group, are more impaired in prosody (reduced affective inflection, monotony and tendency to equal stress, and a lack of emphasis and effort), whereas LHD patients have more prominent articulation deficits and reduced rate.* Both RHD and LHD groups had all of these problems, however. These findings indicate that dysprosody may be relatively more prominent or apparent in RHD than in LHD, but it is not clear if it reflects dysarthria or a distinctive disorder of prosody; although some studies of prosodic production in people with RHD have excluded those with dysarthria, others have included them or have failed to note whether dysarthria was present. Because many RHD patients with aprosodic speech are dysarthric early postonset (Mesulam, 1985), it is possible that dysarthria has been a significant contributor to the perceived prosodic abnormalities in some studies.[†] It is crucial that any study of prosodic deficits in patients with RH (or LH) lesions take into account the possible contribution of dysarthria to prosodic abnormalities.

2. People with RHD may have trouble producing emphatic and lexical stress, imitating emphatic stress, and imitating or reading interrogative and declarative sentences with appropriate intonation contours. Their prosody during narrative discourse may be abnormal (Bryan, 1989; Shapiro and Danly, 1985; Weintraub, Mesulam,

and Kramer, 1981). They may also have less pitch variation and restricted intonational range when reading or imitating sentences expressing specified emotions (Shapiro and Danly, 1985; Tucker, Watson, and Heilman, 1977).* Some of these deficits may be present in patients with LHD but they are generally discounted as attributable to aphasia (Bryan, 1989).

These results suggest that aprosodia may affect linguistic and propositional prosody as well as affective and emotional prosody. This implies that the flat affective prosody of some patients with RHD may not reflect their mood and that aprosodia is not necessarily indicative of depression or unconcern (Ross, 1981). They also suggest that aprosodic patients may have a specific deficit in the modulation of prosody that is independent of affective disturbances that may occur with RHD (Bryan, 1989; Shapiro and Danly, 1985; Weintraub, Mesulam, and Kramer, 1981).

3. Clinical impression suggests that prosodic disturbances caused by stroke are usually most evident in the first few days postonset (Joanette, Goulet, and Hannequin, 1990) and that they frequently resolve over time, although not always (Mesulam, 1985; Ross and Mesulam, 1979). However, recovery from aprosodic speech has not been studied systematically.

Acoustic findings. Findings and associated issues raised by acoustic studies can be summarized as follows:

1. People with RHD produce acoustic cues to linguistic prosody in a manner similar to normal speakers but generally use fewer and less salient cues than normal. Their ability to convey stress at the phrase level (for example, compound nouns versus noun phrases) and for emphatic stress at the sentence level seems preserved (Behrens, 1988; Emmorey, 1987; Hird and Kirsner, 1993). This suggests that production of linguistic prosody may be spared at the word and noun phrase level.

2. People with RHD may also produce sentence intonational contours that are normal in overall direction and rate of f_o decline for imperatives and interrogatives. Their f_o contours on sentence intonation tasks tend to be less linear and flatter in f_o decline in declarative sentences, and

---

*Cancelliere and Kertesz (1990), however, found no significant difference in the frequency of prosodic deficits (receptive or expressive) between groups of patients with RH and LH damage.

[†]For example, Ross and others (1981) reported a case of "motor aprosodia" in which the RH lesion was in the posterior two thirds of the anterior limb, the entire genu, and the anterior third of the rostral internal capsule. There was also a smaller, similarly located lesion in the LH that was considered "silent" because the patient had no prior history of right-sided deficits. A moderate left-central facial weakness was present. Because unilateral UMN dysarthria often occurs with lesions of the internal capsule (see Chapter 9), and because the patient was reportedly "mildly dysarthric," many, most, or all of the deviant prosodic characteristics could have been due to a unilateral UMN dysarthria or even a spastic dysarthria in which the effects of the left hemisphere lesion were unmasked by the RH lesion.

---

*On repetition tasks, adequate perception of stimuli is required for adequate performance. Thus, poor performance on prosodic repetition tasks could reflect indifference, neglect, or comprehension and discrimination problems (Joanette, Goulet, and Hannequin, 1990) rather than a deficit in prosodic production per se.

they may have difficulty using f_o to distinguish yes-no sentences from other sentence forms (Behrens, 1989). Behrens suggests that this may reflect problems with the modulation of f_o at the sentence level and that such difficulties may contribute to the impression of speech that is devoid of emotion.

3. Some people with RHD produce greater amplitude for unemphasized than emphasized sentence final nouns, a pattern that is the opposite of that observed in normal speakers (Behrens, 1988).

4. During Wada testing in the RH, patients may lose the ability to convey happiness, boredom, anger, and surprise during repetition of semantically neutral sentences. Their spontaneous speech may be flat relative to pre-Wada speech. Statistical analysis suggests that the flattening of prosody is primarily through f_o, not loudness or duration (Ross and others, 1988).

5. Some people with RHD may have a basic abnormality in mean pitch level. In their acoustic analysis of f_o mean and variability in read sentences expressing happiness, sadness, anger, and questioning, Colsher, Cooper, and Graff-Radford (1987) found that two RHD patients had higher mean f_o and f_o variability relative to controls, but when the data were normalized to control for mean f_o differences the control speakers had greater variability for most utterances.

6. Some speakers with RHD may have a rapid rate of speech, at least for some speech segments. For example, Hird and Kirsner (1993) found that speakers with RHD had shorter than normal durations for both noun phrases and compound nouns, even though they were able to vary duration to distinguish noun phrases from compound nouns.

7. Kent and Rosenbek's (1982) acoustic analysis of three RHD patients with prosodic deficits found reduced acoustic energy in the middle and high frequency range for vocalic segments, and strong low-frequency (below 500 Hz) energy, probably reflecting nasalization and perhaps inadequate articulation. Perceptually, these features translate to monotone, hypernasality, and imprecise articulation. Speakers also occasionally failed to achieve stop closure, accompanied or characterized by continuous voicing. The overall prosodic pattern was described as "fused," in which the relief of the syllable chain was flattened or indistinct, and consecutive syllables were blurred together into a continuous vocalization, sometimes with a reduction of syllables. Of interest, the prosodic pattern is very similar to that encountered in hypokinetic dysarthria, the dysarthria type most likely to be characterized by a reduction of prosodic contrast (aprosodia). This highlights the possible influence of dysarthria in prosodic disturbances; at the least, it suggests that the clinical distinction between aprosodia and hypokinetic dysarthria may be difficult. Relatedly, Ryalls, Joanette, and Feldman (1987) questioned whether their patients with RHD had a dysphonia that might have contributed to prosodic difficulties.

8. There is great variability among acoustic parameters within groups of RHD and neurologically normal speakers (Behrens, 1988) and considerable overlap between the two groups. For example, some studies have found no differences on sentence repetition between RHD and control speakers in average f_o, f_o range, contour shape, and sentence duration, as well as no differences between anterior or posterior lesions (Ryalls, Joanette, and Feldman, 1987).

Associated clinical characteristics and supporting data

Clinical characteristics that may occur in patients with aprosodia, as well as some clinical findings in brain-injured people that support a role for the RH in prosodic production disorders, can be summarized as follows:

1. Aprosodic patients often have flat nonverbal affect and a paucity of spontaneous emotional and extralinguistic gesturing (for example, Blonder and others, 1993; Ross, 1981). In spite of this, some RHD patients with aprosodic speech may cry in an all-or-none fashion, suggesting that extremes of emotional expression may rely on motor systems that are not identical to RH mechanisms involved in prosody. Observations that the emotional cry and smiling and laughing may seem stilted or feigned in aprosodic patients (Ross and Mesulam, 1979) suggest some overlap in such mechanisms, however.

2. Patients undergoing callosal section may have difficulty repeating different sentence types and sentences expressing different emotions. Some findings suggest that the modulation of f_o may be more disturbed than durational prosodic distinctions (Klouda and others, 1988). In addition, patients with LHD and mixed transcortical aphasia, while able to repeat propositional speech, may have trouble imitating affective prosody (Speedie, Coslett, and Heilman, 1984). It is possible in such cases that the left perisylvian area is disconnected from RH structures that mediate affective prosody.

3. The presence of dysarthria and facial weakness in aprosodic patients has already been noted. Dysarthria represents a potential confounding variable in any study of aprosodia in people with RHD.

Anatomic correlates

The localization of RH lesions that lead to aprosodia has not been well delineated. As might be expected, however, some evidence suggests that frontal lobe (or frontoparietal) lesions are most likely to lead to prosodic production deficits (Shapiro and Danly, 1985; Edmonson and others, 1987; Ross, 1981; Ross and Mesulam, 1979). Prosodic difficulties have also been reported in patients with RH subcortical lesions (Ross and others, 1988; Benke and Kertesz, 1989; Cancelliere and Kertesz, 1990). Ross and Mesulam (1979) have suggested that permanent aprosodia is associated with subcortical lesions.

Nature of the problem

The underlying nature of aprosodia is not understood. Explanations generally focus on the role of motor programming and execution disturbances and on affective and cognitive impairments.

Although some investigations suggest that dysarthria may explain prosodic deficits of some patients (Kent and Rosenbek, 1982; Ryalls, Joanette, and Feldman, 1987), some people with RHD have no discernible dysarthria. Even when unilateral UMN dysarthria is present, some patients' prominent prosodic abnormalities do not seem explainable by their neuromuscular deficits. If, as some studies suggest, the primary acoustic features of aprosodia stem from problems in the modulation of f_o, it would indeed be an unusual "focal" form of dysarthria, unlike any other CNS dysarthria yet described.

The possible role of underlying affective disturbances is central to the understanding of aprosodic speech. At a very basic level, for example, it could be that aprosodic speech reflects decreased arousal or responsiveness or an inattention to extralinguistic cues (Myers, 1994). As an emotional disturbance, it could reflect depression, although Ross and Rush (1981) have reported the persistence of aprosodia after depression was effectively treated.

Although the emotional or affective aspects of prosody seem to be more pervasively affected than linguistic prosody, findings that some aspects of linguistic prosody are sometimes impaired suggest that prosodic production deficits may exist independent of affective disturbances. The nature of such independence is unclear, however. For example, it may be that limbic system functions that drive the expression of affective prosody are disconnected from speech programming and motor control, effectively leaving speech "emotionless" (Ryalls and Behrens, 1988), or the motor programming of affective and some aspects of linguistic prosody, for which the RH may play a dominant role, may be disturbed, resulting in prosodic production errors that may be a variant of AOS (Myers, 1994). Myers has suggested that prosodic production deficits may be analogous to constructional apraxia, in which features are produced without integration; that is, aprosodia may reflect an impaired ability to synthesize or integrate features into a normal prosodic melody, but with preservation of linguistic stress and articulation because they reflect segmental (LH) processing. Relatedly, Ryalls, Joanette, and Feldman (1987) imply an analogy between efforts to understand prosodic deficits and efforts to distinguish the phonologic and phonetic errors that separate aphasia from AOS when they state, "We cannot be sure whether the patient's problem is one of organizing an emotionally appropriate prosodic contour or one of motor realization of an appropriately organized response" (p. 685). Thus, aprosodia could reflect a higher-level cognitive deficit in which an appropriate prosodic pattern cannot be "retrieved" and organized or a problem in the motor programming of adequately identified patterns.

It is apparent from studies of prosodic production deficits associated with RHD that results are inconsistent and that clinical impressions of impaired prosody have been difficult to quantify. Some studies find no acoustic evidence of prosodic disturbance at all, even when perceptual judgments suggest abnormalities (Ryalls, Joanette, and Feldman, 1987). Others have found evidence of deficits in affective but not linguistic prosody, and others have found abnormalities in both. To some extent, the inconsistent findings may be attributed to different methods of speech elicitation, differences in perceptual and acoustic measures,* and variability in the time afteronset of patients studied (Ryalls and Behrens, 1988). Another possibility is that aprosodia simply has not been present in many of the patients studied; that

---

*Perceptual and acoustic measures have focused largely on prosody at the word, phrase, and sentence level. Is it possible that the impression of monotonous and colorless speech in aprosodia derives from the gestalt provided by *discourse extending over a number of sentences,* giving evidence of a prosodic pattern that is relatively fixed, repetitive, and stereotypic and lacking the variations in pause, rhythm, and inflection that reflect the ebb and flow of emotions and emphasis that emerge over time during communicative interaction?

is, group studies have generally tested patients unselected for the presence of aprosodia, perhaps because there is no good operational definition of the disorder. However, assuming that aprosodic speech is not universally present in RHD and may not be very common beyond the acute phase after stroke, group studies probably contain a number of patients without prosodic deficit or whose prosodic deficits are attributable to unilateral UMN dysarthria. If true, the effect would be to wash out the influence of individuals with "true" aprosodia in group statistical comparisons. It may be more productive in developing a full description and understanding of the characteristics and underpinnings of aprosodia to study only patients who meet some predefined operational clinical criteria for the diagnosis of the disorder.

CASES

Case 13.1

A 63-year-old woman presented with a seven-month history of progressive speech and gait difficulty. Neurologic examination revealed a gait disturbance and speech difficulty. Magnetic resonance imaging (MRI) showed evidence of subcortical demyelinization.

During speech evaluation, she complained that her speech was rapid, with words run together, and that she occasionally repeated words. Oral mechanism examination was normal, although she had difficulty maintaining a steady tongue posture on protrusion, suggesting either motor impersistence or dyskinesia. Her speech was characterized by rapid rate with acceleration. Articulation was imprecise during periods of rapid speech, and monopitch and monoloudness were present. She also frequently repeated words or short phrases, usually with accelerating rate and decreasing loudness. These repetitions rarely exceeded three times per event. There was no evidence of aphasia. She was somewhat uninhibited, occasionally impulsively interrupting the examiner and frequently laughing for no apparent reason.

The clinician concluded that the patient had a "marked hypokinetic dysarthria with palilalia. Conversational intelligibility is approximately 70% to 80%." Speech therapy was recommended, and the patient elected to pursue it closer to her home.

The neurologist concluded that the patient had a subcortical encephalopathy associated with apraxia of gait, ataxia, and an extrapyramidal speech disorder. The cause was undetermined.

Commentary. *(1) Palilalia may occur in bilateral subcortical disease affecting the basal ganglia control circuit. When present, it is often associated with hypokinetic dysarthria. (2) In spite of its frequent association with hypokinetic dysarthria, etiologies of palilalia are not limited to Parkinson's disease. In this case, it was associated with a degenerative subcortical process of undetermined etiology.*

Case 13.2

A 72-year-old right-handed man presented with a six-week history of imbalance, slurred speech, and hearing loss. Neurologic examination revealed adequate mental status, marked hearing difficulty, slow speech that did not sound dysarthric, and gait imbalance. Strength was good. The neurologist thought the patient may have had a vascular event and that his hearing loss might have been related to a medication he was taking for poor circulation. A computed tomography (CT) scan was normal. Audiometric evaluation shortly before his initial neurologic assessment showed a moderate bilateral sensorineural hearing loss.

The patient returned three weeks later, complaining of loss of appetite, increased dizziness, confusion, and imbalance. On examination, gait had clearly worsened, and some jerking in the extremities was apparent. He had bilateral Babinski signs. He appeared unable to hear, but he read adequately.

Speech examination four days later found the patient unable to comprehend any spoken language, as if he were deaf. Examination was carried out through written instructions. Speech was noticeably slowed in rate, primarily secondary to prolonged vowels that altered prosody in a manner suggestive of a pseudoforeign accent. He had irregular articulatory breakdowns and some difficulty with correct articulatory sequencing for multisyllabic words. He also had fairly frequent sound, syllable, word, and, occasionally, phrase repetitions without obvious overt struggle. Speech alternating motion rates were equivocally slowed but regular. There was no evidence of aphasia in any language modality.

The clinician concluded, "This is a very unusual speech problem which, I think, reflects multifocal or diffuse impairment. His drawn out speech rate, pseudoforeign accent, and occasional articulatory sequencing difficulties probably reflect an apraxia of speech, suggesting dominant hemisphere involvement. He also exhibits a number of stuttering-like behaviors, some of which may be secondary to his apraxia of speech, but others which appear almost palilalic in nature, although without hypokinetic elements. Finally, some of his irregular articulatory breakdowns are suggestive of ataxic dysarthria, although these may also be secondary to apraxia of speech. There is no evidence of aphasia, nor is he obviously confused or demented. His rapidly progressive hearing loss is very unusual; I don't believe his speech abnormalities can be attributed to his hearing loss, however. Finally, it should be noted that the patient occasionally became oppositional and agitated." Therapy was not recommended because of the rapidly progressive nature of the problem and the undetermined diagnosis.

The patient's condition continued to deteriorate. An electroencephalogram (EEG) one week later was abnormal in a manner strongly suggestive of Creutzfeldt-Jakob disease. An MRI was negative.

The patient continued to deteriorate and died six weeks later. Autopsy was consistent with the diagnosis of Creutzfeldt-Jakob disease with predominant involvement of the cerebral cortex.

Commentary. *(1) Pseudoforeign accent may be perceived in patients with identifiable apraxia of speech. (2) Stuttering-like behavior can be associated with apraxia of speech, but the nature of the relationship is not always clear. (3) Palilalia may occur in patients with stuttering-like behavior and without clear evidence of hypokinetic dysarthria. (4) Identification of ataxic dysarthria in the presence of AOS may be difficult. (5) Pseudoforeign accent, neurogenic stuttering, palilalia, and apraxia of speech may co-occur, and they may be associated with degenerative neurologic disease. It is likely that their co-occurrence reflects diffuse or multifocal pathology. (6) Degenerative neurologic disease may produce multiple, co-occurring motor speech and related speech disorders. (7) Changes in speech may be the first or among the first signs of degenerative neurologic disease, including Creutzfeldt-Jakob disease.*

Case 13.3

A 59-year-old right-handed woman was seen for evaluation two months following the relatively acute onset of what outside records described as "aphasia." Neurologic exam was normal with the exception of her speech. A CT scan was normal. She was referred for speech assessment.

She reported that, at onset, "The words just wouldn't come out." She believed she was greatly improved. She noted some mild difficulty following conversations in noise or with groups of people. She had no complaints about reading or writing.

Oral mechanism exam was normal. Conversational speech and reading aloud were characterized by numerous brief sound prolongations and repetitions, occasional hesitations, and slight delays before word initiation. These dysfluencies were the only evidence of speech abnormality. Performance on a variety of taxing language tasks assessing verbal comprehension and expression, reading, and writing was normal.

The clinician concluded that the patient had "stuttering-like behavior associated with CNS disease. There are no objective signs of a focal aphasic language impairment, although the patient's history and current complaints suggest that aphasia was present and may continue to be present at a subclinical level. Given her history and current speech dysfluencies, her dysfluencies may reflect left hemisphere pathology. It should be noted, however, that stuttering following brain damage has been reported with right or left hemisphere lesions, bilateral lesions, and subcortical lesions." The patient had been receiving speech therapy for her dysfluencies. It was recommended that she continue with therapy.

Commentary. *(1) Neurogenic stuttering can develop in association with acute neurologic events, such as stroke. Although neurologic exam and CT were normal, by history the patient had been aphasic. (2) Stuttering-like behavior can occur in association with aphasia. In some cases, dysfluencies persist after resolution of clinically apparent language difficulties.*

Case 13.4

A 55-year-old man was referred for speech-language assessment following surgery for removal of a recurrent bifrontal, biparietal parasaggital meningioma. Preoperatively, he had had seizures, progressive "mental slowing," and mild right and left lower extremity weakness.

During evaluation, the patient offered no spontaneous speech and was minimally responsive during social interaction. His wife noted that his responses to questions and commands, if he responded, were accurate. During formal testing, he followed nearly all simple commands but failed to respond at all to two-step commands. He read words correctly, named pictures accurately, defined a few words, and answered some questions. All responses were produced with long latencies, and some required prompting. For example, the patient initially failed to respond within 30 seconds to a request to define the word "island." After being asked, "Is it a kind of building?" he stated, after another 10-second delay, "It's a land mass." His verbal responses were relatively reduced in loudness and flat prosodically. Content was consistently brief and unelaborated. He did not write anything on request or spontaneously, even though he adequately grasped a pencil.

The clinician concluded that the patient's behavior was very similar to that of patients who are emerging from akinetic mutism and that his difficulties with speech could not be attributed to aphasia, apraxia of speech, or dysarthria, but were more likely a manifestation of cognitive and affective disturbances. When discharged from the hospital three weeks later, the patient was more verbal and responded more rapidly but continued to have abnormal response latency.

Commentary. *(1) Attenuation of speech can occur with bifrontal damage. (2) The speech characteristics of this patient appeared to reflect reduced drive, motivation, initiative, and affect. (3) A clue to the distinction between reduced output secondary to cognitive and affective disturbances versus aphasia is that all of this patient's errors were those of omission rather than commission and that accurate responses emerged if sufficient time was permitted.*

Case 13.5

A 24-year-old man was seen for speech-language assessment 12 days following a motorcycle accident. An MRI demonstrated an area of hemorrhage in the right frontal lobe, with surrounding edema. Neuropsychological assessment demonstrated evidence of moderate, diffuse cognitive impairment.

Language evaluation revealed no evidence of aphasia. He was, however, slow to respond to all tasks and did not initiate any verbal interaction with the examiner. His performance on more abstract tasks (word definitions and proverb explanations) was adequate linguistically but slowly formulated. His affect was flat.

Speech was characterized by moderately reduced loudness, moderately reduced pitch and loudness variability, and mild-moderate breathiness. Speech AMRs and SMRs were normal, and articulation was precise.

Intelligibility was normal in the quiet setting but reduced in noise because of his reduced loudness. His reduced loudness and flat prosody, as well as slowness to initiate speech, were considered his primary communication deficits.

The clinician concluded that the patient's reduced loudness and flat prosody were consistent with frontal and/or subcortical injury associated with CHI and that he had no obvious dysarthria. There was evidence of reduced short-term memory for verbally presented materials and slowness in processing and producing complex language, consistent with a nonaphasic, cognitively based communication deficit. There was no evidence of aphasia. His speech normalized within the next month, but his cognitive deficits remained evident, mostly in the form of slowed processing. He was discharged to another facility for continued rehabilitation.

Commentary. (1) Reduced loudness and prosody and delayed initiation of speech are not uncommon in closed head injury. Such difficulties are consistent with reduced drive, motivation, affect, and general cognitive functioning, and they often reflect impairments in frontal lobe–limbic system function. (2) The patient's right frontal hemorrhage raises the possibility that his reduced prosody reflected an aprosodia associated with right hemisphere lesion, although he did not have any other lateralizing motor or cognitive deficits. The distinction between right hemisphere aprosodia and flattened prosody associated with more widespread neurologic involvement can be difficult.

Case 13.6

An 81-year-old woman was seen in neurology for evaluation of mental status changes and speech difficulty of two years' duration. She had a history of a stroke 4 to 5 years previously, after which her speech was "slurred, repetitive, stuttering, and fast." Her speech seemed to have been stable after her stroke, but in the last two years she had had reduced memory abilities and increased confusion. Examination noted disorientation, difficulty following commands, reduced mental status, and bilateral Babinski signs and hyperreflexia. A CT scan showed diffuse cerebral atrophy as well as areas of low attenuation within the centrum semiovale bilaterally, suggestive of demyelinization or multiple infarcts.

During speech assessment, her husband reported that her speech problem had worsened in the last two years and that she was talking a great deal more than she had in the past. During language assessment there was no clear evidence of aphasia. However, she spoke compulsively and made numerous comments that ranged from marginally appropriate to frankly inappropriate. Her speech was characterized by frequent rapid initial phoneme and word and short phrase repetitions. Articulatory precision was good, as was prosody. Intelligibility was frequently poor secondary to her dysfluencies and rapid speech rate.

The speech diagnosis was "(1) Palilalila characterized by rapid word-phrase repetitions; she also has a number of stuttering-like behaviors, including rapid phoneme repetitions. (2) Hypokinetic- like dysarthria, although this is not a full-blown hypokinetic dysarthria and may be secondary to her palilalia. (3) Cognitive impairments and apparent confusion, but no evidence of focal aphasic language impairment. It should be noted that palilalia is almost always associated with bilateral and/or diffuse dysfunction." The clinician did not believe the patient would benefit from speech therapy because of her cognitive difficulties. It was suggested that, if her cognitive difficulties improved, speech therapy should be reconsidered.

Commentary. (1) Palilalia and stuttering-like behavior can co-occur, particularly in the presence of hypokinetic dysarthria. Lesions leading to palilalia (and hypokinetic dysarthria with stuttering-like dysfluencies) are almost always bilateral and subcortical in origin. (2) By history, the patient's "stuttering-like" behavior was present since her stroke but had worsened significantly in recent years. The mechanism for this worsening was unclear in this case, but it is unlikely that her palilalia could be explained by a single unilateral stroke. The neurologist ultimately concluded that the patient had a degenerative CNS disease of undetermined origin.

Case 13.7

A 48-year-old woman was referred for speech-language assessment after admission to the rehabilitation unit three weeks following surgery for a right frontotemporal arteriovenous malformation, with subsequent evacuation of an intracerebral hematoma that developed postoperatively. Afterward, she had a marked left hemiparesis and left-sided neglect.

Examination failed to reveal evidence of aphasia. She had considerable difficulty reading, most often reading only the right half of printed materials on a page, with accompanying statements that the material did not make sense. When presented with pictured scenes, she consistently ignored information on the left and frequently misinterpreted depicted information. She had a tendency to talk excessively about pictured scenes, frequently labeling objects rather than stating conclusions or interpretations about pictured activities.

Most impressive was the prosodic pattern of her speech. There was no evidence of dysarthria or apraxia of speech, and voice quality, resonance, rate, and articulatory precision were normal. Although there was evidence of pitch and loudness variability in her speech, the overall affect conveyed was one of lack of emotion, even when she was discussing emotion-laden information. During the course of a narrative, for example, the intonational pattern of many of her sentences was stereotypic, with little variation as a function of emotional content or salience of information. She was able to place emphatic stress on appropriate words in sentences when answering questions and imitating sentences, but her manner of doing so seemed somewhat artificial and "conscious," almost robotlike. She tended not to reduce pitch and loudness at the end of declarative sentences, often ending them with rising inflection, a pattern that was striking for its frequent occurrence *during extended narratives. Finally, the emotions conveyed during a narrative about things that made her happy versus angry was readily apparent in linguistic content but indistinguishable prosodically.*

Commentary. *(1) Alterations in prosody can occur following RH lesions and in the absence of any recognizable dysarthria or apraxia of speech. (2) The "aprosodia" associated with RH pathology is often associated with cognitive impairments and neglect. (3) Aprosodia is not necessarily a complete "flattening" of the prosodic features of speech, as might be heard in hypokinetic dysarthria or the prosody of patients with frontal lobe–limbic system impairments. Rather, it may have a robotlike rhythm and stress pattern, with a recurring repetitive prosodic pattern across many utterances. (4) The aprosodia associated with RHD is not clearly associated with depression. In this patient, the emotions expressed prosodically were much less apparent than those conveyed by the content of her language.*

SUMMARY

1. Neurologic disease can alter speech in ways that are not attributable to commonly described dysarthrias or apraxia of speech. It is possible that some of these disturbances represent motor speech disorders in their own right or an unusual prominence of a characteristic that may logically be related to a known motor speech disorder. Other alterations in speech can be attributed to cognitive, affective, or linguistic disturbances. These heterogeneous problems are sometimes associated with lesions confined to the left or the right hemisphere; others may be associated with bilateral, diffuse, or multifocal CNS lesions.

2. Neurogenic stuttering is characterized by various patterns of dysfluency that may occur with or without accompanying aphasia, apraxia of speech, or dysarthria. When associated with aphasia, apraxia of speech, or dysarthria, the dysfluencies may be part of the language or motor speech disturbance, a response to the language or motor speech disturbance, or relatively independent of the language or motor speech disturbance. Lesion sites associated with neurogenic stuttering are multiple and sometimes not readily apparent, as when dysfluencies develop in response to drugs, metabolic disturbances, and closed head injury.

3. Palilalia is the compulsive repetition of words and phrases, often in a context of increasing rate and decreasing loudness. It generally reflects bilateral basal ganglia pathology and is frequently but not always associated with hypokinetic dysarthria.

4. Echolalia is the motorically normal, unsolicited repetition of another's utterances. The repetition may be exact or modified in a way that demonstrates some degree of linguistic processing. It usually occurs with diffuse or multifocal cortical pathology in which there is relative sparing of the perisylvian language area, permitting adequate input and output of speech but with limited linguistic processing for meaning.

5. Cognitive and affective disturbances can alter the character of speech. Frontal lobe–limbic system pathology may reduce speed of verbal responding, reduce linguistic and cognitive complexity of content, and reduce vocal loudness, completeness of phonation, and prosody. These changes in speech appear to reflect a reduction in drive, initiative, motivation, and sustained cognitive and motor effort. Other cognitive and affective disturbances can lead to disinhibited vocalization and involuntary phonation, inappropriate shouting or laughter or other noises, and verbal and vocal tics.

6. Aphasia, a disturbance of language, can alter the character of speech. Grammatic and syntactic deficits, word retrieval deficits, and phonologic errors are the primary manifestations of aphasia that alter the rate, fluency, and prosodic flow of verbal expression.

7. A pseudoforeign accent occasionally develops in patients with neurologic disease. The perception of accent seems to reflect an articulatory and prosodic disturbance that is associated with left hemisphere pathology and frequently with aphasia or apraxia of speech. Pseudoforeign accent may represent a variant of apraxia of speech.

8. Aprosodia is a disturbance that has been associated with right hemisphere dysfunction. Although prosodic disturbances may be associated with a variety of lesion sites, motor speech disorders, and cognitive and affective deficits, there is some evidence to suggest that distinctive deficits in prosody may occur with right hemisphere lesions. This aprosodic speech pattern is often described as flat, indifferent, devoid of expression and emotion, and computerlike or robotlike. Studies of aprosodia have produced heterogeneous results. Neither the defining characteristics of the problem nor the nature of the disturbance underlying aprosodia is well understood.

REFERENCES

Ackerman H, Ziegler W, and Oertel W: Palilalia as a symptom of L-DOPA induced hyperkinesia, J Neurol Neurosurg Psychiatry 52:805, 1989.

Albert ML and others: Clinical aspects of dysphasia, New York, 1981, Springer-Verlag.

Alexander MP, Benson DF, and Stuss DT: Frontal lobes and language, Brain Lang 37:656, 1989.

Appell J, Kertesz A, and Fisman M: A study of language functioning in Alzheimer patients, Brain Lang 17:73, 1982.

Ardila A and Lopez MV: Severe stuttering associated with right hemisphere lesion, Brain Lang 27:239, 1986.

Ardila A, Rosselli M, and Ardila O: Foreign accent: an aphasic epiphenomenon? Aphasiology 2:493, 1988.

Aronson AE: Clinical voice disorders, ed 3, New York, 1991, Thieme.

Beckford NS and others: Effects of short-term intubation on vocal function, Laryngoscope 100:331, 1990.

Behrens SJ: The role of the right hemisphere in the production of linguistic stress, Brain Lang 33:104, 1988.

Behrens SJ: Characterizing sentence intonation in a right hemisphere–damaged population, Brain Lang 37:181, 1989.

Benke T and Kertesz A: Hemispheric mechanisms of motor speech, Aphasiology 3:627, 1989.

Berthier ML and others: Foreign accent syndrome: behavioral and anatomic findings in recovered and non-recovered patients, Aphasiology 5:129, 1991.

Bhatnagar S and Andy OJ: Alleviation of acquired stuttering with human centremedian thalamic stimulation, J Neurol Neurosurg Psychiatry 52:1182, 1989.

Blonder L and others: Right hemisphere facial expressivity during natural conversation, Brain Cogn 21:44, 1993.

Blumstein SE and others: On the nature of the foreign accent syndrome: a case study, Brain Lang 31:215, 1987.

Boller F, Albert M, and Denes F: Palilalia, Br J Disord Commun 10:92, 1975.

Boller F and others: Familial palilalia, Neurology 23:1117, 1973.

Brown JW: Aphasia, apraxia and agnosia, Springfield, IL 1972, Charles C Thomas.

Bryan KL: Language prosody and the right hemisphere, Aphasiology 3:285, 1989.

Cancelliere AEB and Kertesz A: Lesion localization in acquired deficits of emotional expression and comprehension, Brain Cogn 13:133, 1990.

Colice GL, Stukel TA, and Dain B: Laryngeal complications of prolonged intubation, 96:877, 1989.

Colsher PL, Cooper WE, and Graff-Radford N: Intonational variability in the speech of right-hemisphere damaged patients, Brain Lang 32:379, 1987.

Cooper E: A brain stem contusion and fluency: Vicky's story, J Fluency Disord 8:269, 1983.

Edmondson JA and others: The effect of right-brain damage on acoustical measures of affective prosody in Taiwanese patients, J of Phonetics 15:219, 1987.

Emmorey KD: The neurological substrates for prosodic aspects of speech, Brain Lang 30:305, 1987.

Farmer A: Stuttering repetitions in aphasic and nonaphasic brain-damaged adults, Cortex 11:391, 1975.

Fisher CM: Neurologic fragments. I. Clinical observations in demented patients, Neurology 38:1868, 1988.

Fleet WS and Heilman KM: Acquired stuttering from a right hemisphere lesion in a right-hander, Neurology 35:1343, 1985.

Gonzalez Rothi LJ: Transcortical aphasias. In LaPointe LL, editor: Aphasia and related neurogenic language disorders, New York, 1990, Thieme Medical.

Graff-Radford NR and others: An unlearned foreign "accent" in a patient with aphasia, Brain Lang 23:86, 1986.

Graff-Radford NR and Damasio AR: Disturbances of speech and language associated with thalamic dysfunction, Semin Neurol 4:162, 1984.

Graff-Radford NR and others: Nonhemorrhagic infarction of the thalamus: behavioral, anatomic, and physiologic correlates, Neurology 34:14, 1984.

Hartman DE and O'Neill BP: Progressive dysfluency, dysphagia, dysarthria: a case of olivopontocerebellar atrophy. In

Yorkston KM and Beukelman DR, editors: Recent advances in clinical dysarthria, Boston, 1989, College-Hill.

Heilman K and others: Comprehension of affective and nonaffective prosody, Neurology 34:917, 1984.

Helm NA, Butler RB, and Benson DF: Acquired stuttering, Neurology 28:1159, 1978.

Helm NA, Butler RB, and Canter GJ: Neurogenic acquired stuttering, J Fluency Disord 5:267, 1980.

Helm-Estabrooks N: Diagnosis and management of neurogenic stuttering in adults. In The atpyical stutterer: principles and practices of rehabilitation, St Louis, 1986, Academic Press.

Helm-Estabrooks N and others: Stuttering: disappearance and reappearance with acquired brain lesions, Neurology 36:1109, 1986.

Hird K and Kirsner K: Dysprosody following acquired neurogenic impairment, Brain Lang 45:46, 1993.

Horner J and Massey EW: Progressive dysfluency associated with right hemisphere disease, Brain Lang 18:71, 1983.

Janati A: Case report: progressive supranuclear palsy: report of a case with torticollis, blepharospasm, and dysfluency, Am J Med Sci 292:391, 1986.

Joanette Y, Goulet P, and Hannequin D, Right hemisphere and verbal communication, New York, 1990, Springer-Verlag.

Johns DF and Darley FL: Phonemic variability in apraxia of speech, J Speech Hear Res 13:556, 1970.

Jonas S: The supplementary motor region and speech emission, J Commun Disord 14:349, 1981.

Jonas S: The thalamus and aphasia, including transcortical aphasia: a review, J Commun Disord 15:31, 1982.

Jones MW and others: Hoarseness after tracheal intubation, Anaesthesia 47:213, 1992.

Jones RK: Observations on stammering after localized cerebral injury, J Neurol Neurosurg Psychiatry 29:192, 1966.

Kent RD and LaPointe LL: Acoustic properties of pathologic reiterative utterances: a case study of palilalia, J Speech Hear Res 25:95, 1982.

Kent RD and Rosenbek JC: Prosodic disturbance and neurologic lesion, Brain Lang 15:259, 1982.

Klouda GV and others: The role of callosal connections in speech prosody, Brain Lang 35:154, 1988.

LaPointe LL and Horner J: Palilalia: a descriptive study of pathological reiterative utterances, J Speech Hear Res 46:34, 1981.

Lebrun Y and others: Acquired stuttering, J Fluency Disord 8:323, 1983.

Lesser THJ, Williams RG, and Hoddinott C: Laryngographic changes following endotracheal intubation in adults, Br J Disord Commun 21:239, 1986.

Ludlow CL and others: Site of penetrating brain lesions causing chronic acquired stuttering, Ann Neurol 22:60, 1987.

Madison DP and others: Communicative and cognitive deterioration in dialysis dementia: two case studies, J Speech Hear Disord 42:238, 1977.

Manders E and Bastijns P: Sudden recovery from stuttering after an epileptic attack: a case report, J Fluency Disord 13:421, 1989.

Marie P and Levy G: A singular trouble with speech: palilalia (dissociation of voluntary speech and of automatic speech), Le Monde Medical 64:329-344, 1925.

Market KE and others: Acquired stuttering: descriptive data and treatment outcome, J Fluency Disord 15:21, 1990.

Mazzuchi H and others: Clinical observations on acquired stuttering, Br J Disord Commun 16:19, 1981.

McCarthy MM: Speech effect of theophylline (letter to the editors), Pediatrics 68:5, 1981.

McClean MD and McLean A: Case report of stuttering acquired in association with phenytoin use for post-head-injury seizures, J Fluency Disord 10:241, 1985.

Mesulam M-M: Principles of behavioral neurology, Philadelphia, 1985, FA Davis.

Meyers SC, Hall NE, and Aram DM: Fluency and language recovery in a child with a left hemisphere lesion, J Fluency Disord 15:159, 1990.

Miller AE: Cessation of stuttering with progressive multiple sclerosis, Neurology 35:1341, 1985.

Mohr JP, Watters WC, and Duncan GW: Thalamic hemorrhage and aphasia, Brain Lang 2:3, 1975.

Myers PS: Communication disorders associated with right hemisphere brain damage. In Chapey R, editor: Language intervention strategies in adult aphasia, ed 3, Baltimore, 1994, Williams and Wilkins.

Nurnberg HG and Greenwald B: Stuttering: an unusual side effect of phenothiazines, *Amer J of Psychiatry* 138:386, 1981.

Peach RK: Acquired neurogenic stuttering, Grand Rounds Communic Disord 9:177, 1984.

Penfield W and Roberts L: Speech and brain mechanisms, Princeton, 1959, Princeton University Press.

Quader S: Dysarthria: an unusual side effect of tricyclic antidepressants, *British Medical J* 2:97, 1977.

Quinn PT and Andrews G: Neurological stuttering—a clinical entity? J Neurol Neurosurg Psychiatry 40:699, 1977.

Rentschler GJ, Driver LE, and Callaway EA: The onset of stuttering following drug overdose, J Fluency Disord 9:265, 1984.

Robin DA, Klouda GV, and Hug LN: Neurogenic disorders of prosody. In Vogel D and Cannito MP, editors: Treating disordered speech motor control, Austin, TX, 1991, Pro-Ed.

Rosenbek JC: Stuttering secondary to nervous system damage. In Curlee RF and Perkins WH, editors: Nature and treatment of stuttering: new directions, San Diego, 1984, College-Hill.

Rosenbek J and others: Stuttering following brain damage, Brain Lang 6:82, 1978.

Ross ED: The aprosodias: functional-anatomic organization of the affective components of language in the right hemisphere, Arch Neurol 38:561, 1981.

Ross ED: Right-hemisphere lesions in disorders of affective language. In Kertesz A, editor: Localization in neuropsychology, New York, 1983, Academic Press.

Ross ED and Mesulam M-M: Dominant language functions of the right hemisphere? Prosody and emotional gesturing, Arch Neurol 36:144, 1979.

Ross ED and others: How the brain integrates affective and propositional language into a unified behavioral function: hypothesis based on clinicoanatomic evidence, Arch Neurol 38:745, 1981.

Ross ED and others: Acoustic analysis of affective prosody during right-sided Wada test: a within-subjects verification of the right hemisphere's role in language, Brain Lang 33:128, 1988.

Ross ED and Rush AJ: Diagnosis and neuroanatomical correlates of depression in brain-damaged patients: implications for a neurology of depression, Arch Gen Neurol 38:1344, 1981.

Rubens AB and Kertesz A: The localization of lesions in transcortical aphasias. In Kertesz A, editor: Localization in neuropsychology, New York, 1983, Academic Press.

Ryalls J, Joanette Y, and Feldman L: An acoustic comparison of normal and right-hemisphere-damaged speech prosody, Cortex 23:685, 1987.

Ryalls JH and Behrens SJ: Review: an overview of changes in fundamental frequency associated with cortical insult, Aphasiology 2:107, 1988.

Sapir S and Aronson AE: Aphonia after closed head injury: aetiologic considerations, Br J Disord Commun 20:289, 1985.

Scholefield JA: Aetiologies of aphonia following closed head injury, Br J Disord Commun 22:167, 1987.

Schuell HM, Jenkins JJ, and Jiminez-Pabon E: Aphasia in adults, New York, 1964, Harper and Row.

Shapiro BE and Danley M: The role of the right hemisphere in the control of speech prosody in propositional and affective contexts, Brain Lang 25:19, 1985.

Speedie LJ, Coslett HB, and Heilman KM: Repetition of affective prosody in mixed transcortical aphasia, *Arch Neurol* 41:268, 1984.

Stuss DT and Benson DF: Neuropsychological studies of the frontal lobes, Psychol Bull 95:3, 1984.

Tompkins CA and Flowers CR: Perception of emotional intonation by brain-damaged adults: the influence of task processing levels, J Speech Hear Res 28:527, 1985.

Tucker DM, Watson RT, and Heilman KM: Discrimination and evocation of affectively intoned speech in patients with right parietal disease, Neurology 27:947, 1977.

Valenstein E: Nonlanguage disorders of speech reflect complex neurologic apparatus, Geriatrics 30:117, 1975.

Wallesch C-W: Repetitive verbal behaviour: functional and neurological considerations, Aphasiology 4:133, 1990.

Weintraub S, Mesulam M-M, and Kramer L: Disturbances in prosody: a right-hemisphere contribution to language, Arch Neurol 38:742, 1981.

Woo P, Kelly G, and Kirsner P: Airway complications in the head injured, Laryngoscope 99:725, 1989.

Yairi E, Gintautas J, and Avent JR: Disfluent speech associated with brain damage, Brain Lang 14:49, 1981.

Yonick TA and others: Acoustical effects of endotracheal intubation, J Speech Hear Disord 55:427, 1990.

14 Acquired Psychogenic Speech Disorders

Speech is a mirror of personality and emotional state in healthy and ill individuals. It is particularly sensitive to intrinsic psychological abnormalities and to the routine, catastrophic, or tragic physical and emotional traumas that can attach themselves to our lives. Alterations and abnormalities of speech that are acquired by adults as a result of these psychological states or events, particularly those that may be difficult to distinguish from neurologically based speech disorders, are the focus of this chapter.

The following definition, adapted from Aronson's (1990) description of psychogenic voice disorders, will help to establish the boundaries of the disturbances that will be discussed here. *Acquired psychogenic speech disorders represent a wide variety of speech disturbances that result from one or more types of psychological dysequilibrium, such as anxiety, depression, conversion reaction, or personality disorders that interfere with volitional control over any component of speech production.*

Psychogenic speech disorders are not unusual within a large multidisciplinary medical practice. They accounted for 4.5% of all acquired communication disorders seen in the section of Speech Pathology at the Mayo Clinic between 1987 and 1990 (Figure 1–1). Of relevance to this chapter, many of these patients were referred for speech evaluation as part of a medical workup to determine the cause of their symptoms.

This chapter will address psychologically based problems that most often may be difficult to distinguish from neurologic disease, or that may

co-occur with neurologic disease. In this context, a few general principles are worth keeping in mind.

1. Neurologic and psychiatric diseases can and do co-occur.
2. Speech disorders in people with neurologic disease may be psychological in origin.
3. Speech disorders in people with psychiatric disease may be neurological in origin.
4. It may be very difficult to distinguish neurogenic from psychogenic speech disturbances in some cases.
5. Psychogenic speech disorders are most often manifest as voice, fluency, or prosodic disturbances, but any component of speech production can be affected.

ETIOLOGIES

Some of the most common etiologies of psychogenic speech disorders will be discussed in this section. In general, depression, manic depression, and schizophrenia tend to lead to logically predictable speech disturbances; in fact, the character of speech may help to define the psychopathology. In contrast, responses to life stress, conversion disorders, somatization disorders, and factitious disorders and malingering have much less predictable effects on speech and are more challenging to the diagnostic and management efforts of speech pathologists.

Depression

Description. Depression is an affective disorder of mood. Primary or major depression can exist without any nonaffective psychiatric disorder or any serious organic disorder, whereas secondary or minor depression is associated with preexisting organic or psychiatric illness. The lifetime prevalence in the general population for major depression may be as high as 9% in women and 4% in men (Hirschfeld and Goodwin, 1988). It may occur throughout the adult years. There is a presumed precipitating event (emotional loss, chronic stress) in about 25% of cases (Tomb, 1981).

Depression may be accompanied by mania in some people, a condition known as *manic depression*. Mania is a near emotional mirror image of depression, with characteristic symptoms including excited mood, euphoria, low frustration tolerance, elevated self-esteem, poor judgment, disorganization, paranoia, little need for sleep, and boundless energy (Tomb, 1981).

Depressed mood, characterized by sadness and feeling low, hopeless, and gloomy, is the most common characteristic of depression (Nicholi, 1988; Tomb, 1981). It, or loss of interest or pleasure, must be present for a diagnosis of major depression, according to the *Diagnostic and Statistical Manual of Mental Disorders (DSM-III-R)* of the American Psychiatric Association (APA, 1987).* Other symptoms may include increased or decreased appetite, insomnia or hypersomnia, loss of energy, feelings of worthlessness or guilt, and difficulty with thinking, memory, concentration, or decision making. Depressed people may also exhibit *psychomotor retardation* which may be characterized by reduced speech and facial expression, fixed gaze and reduced eye scanning, stooped posture, and slow movement.

Neurologic disease and depression. As many as one third of patients with neurologic disease may have severe depression or anxiety (Sapir and Aronson, 1990). Depression is one of the most common emotional sequelae after traumatic brain injury (Uomoto, 1991). Major or minor depression seems to occur in almost half of unselected stroke patients and may persist for one to two years (Starkstein and Robinson, 1990). It tends to last longer with cortical lesions than when lesions are elsewhere, but it can be associated with basal ganglia, thalamic, and limbic system lesions (Sapir and Aronson, 1990; Starkstein and Robinson, 1990). It is more likely to occur with lesions of the left than the right hemisphere and is more likely with frontal lesions, especially in the left hemi-

sphere (Robinson and others, 1984a & b; Robinson, Lipsey, and Price, 1985).

Most stroke patients with significant depression have left frontal or basal ganglia lesions (Starkstein and Robinson, 1990). This has obvious implications for patients with aphasia and apraxia of speech and, in fact, depression is more common in nonfluent aphasic patients than those with global or fluent aphasia (Robinson and Benson, 1981). Starkstein and Robinson (1988) have suggested that depression in aphasic people is not necessarily a reaction to the aphasia but that depression and aphasia can be separate, coexisting outcomes of brain injury. Poststroke depression may be effectively treated with tricyclic antidepressants (Starkstein and Robinson, 1990).

Depression can occur in numerous other neurologic diseases and is common in Parkinson's disease, epilepsy, Alzheimer's disease, multiple sclerosis, systemic lupus erythematosis, and Huntington's disease. There is a 40% to 50% risk of depression in Parkinson's disease, and depression may precede the onset of motor deficits, suggesting that it may have a neurophysiologic basis (Schiffer, 1990). This notion receives support from observations that basal ganglia lesions may be associated with a range of psychiatric disorders, including depression, mania, and obsessive-compulsive and schizophrenia-like disorders (Rogers, 1990).

In the elderly, depression may be mistaken for progressive dementia, and depression is the most common alternative diagnosis in dementia. Of interest, it has been suggested that cognitive impairments associated with depression may not be due to psychological factors but rather to reversible neurologic impairment associated with neurochemical changes (Freeman and others, 1985).

Schizophrenia

Schizophrenia is the most common psychotic disorder, affecting over 2 million people in the United States (Tomb, 1981). It usually begins in adolescence or early adulthood. It has no pathognomonic features, and its exact nature is unclear. The *DSM-III-R* criteria for its diagnosis describe symptoms during the active phase of the illness that include bizarre, somatic, grandiose, religious, nihilistic, and other delusions; auditory hallucinations; incoherence; illogical thinking; and poverty of speech content. Symptoms present prior to or following active phases of the illness may include social isolation or withdrawal; peculiar behavior (talking to self in public); reduced or inappropriate affect; digressive, vague, overelaborate, or metaphorical speech; and odd or bizarre thinking or perceptual experiences. Depression and mania may develop after the onset of psychotic symptoms.

---

*The *DSM-III-R* (APA, 1987) contains criteria for the diagnosis of more than 150 categories of mental disorders. It is currently accepted as the standard language of communication for mental health professionals in the United States and is widely used in clinical practice, research, and training programs (Williams, 1988).

Many neurologic disorders can produce schizophrenia-like symptoms. Schizophrenia-like psychoses have been associated with diffuse cerebral injuries, with some association of them with temporal lobe lesions. Examples of etiologies associated with such symptoms include closed head injury, encephalitis, temporal lobe epilepsy, Huntington's chorea, Wilson's disease, and demyelinating disease. The distinction between the psychotic features of schizophrenia and mental disorders induced by substance abuse also can be very difficult (Nicholi, 1988).

Stress and stress reactions

Stress is a state of bodily or mental tension resulting from factors that tend to alter equilibrium. It is a normal part of life that may be necessary and invigorating to our sense of well-being and accomplishment. Stress comes from many sources, such as working conditions and family and social relationships and events.

Reactions to stress are determined by the degree and chronicity of stress but also by intrinsic personality traits such as flexibility, perfectionism, compulsivity, and ambition. When the tension generated by psychological stress is not appropriately released, it may build to a point at which abnormal functioning develops. Excessive tension may occur in individuals with or without serious psychiatric disease.

People may be predisposed by personality or physiologic makeup to hyperreact to stress through a particular neuromuscular or visceral system (Aronson, 1990). An especially relevant example is the susceptibility of the laryngeal muscles to emotional stress, perhaps because of the voice's prominent role in conveying emotional information and its strong links to limbic system influences. Thus, the larynx can be a site of neuromuscular tension arising from stress associated with fear, anger, anxiety, and depression.

Stress and other psychological factors sometimes seem to play a causal role in organic disease. When this happens, the resulting disorder may be called psychosomatic. *Psychosomatic disorders,* therefore, are related to the effects of psychological and sociocultural stresses on the "predisposition, onset, course, and response to treatment of some physiological changes and biochemical disorders" (Thompson, 1988, p. 493). This notion of psychological factors that can affect physical conditions depends on the co-occurrence of factors that include (1) a biologic predisposition to a particular organic disorder, (2) a personality vulnerability or a type or degree of stress that a person cannot manage, and (3) the presence of significant chronic psychosocial stress in the sus-

ceptible personality area (Thompson, 1988; Tomb, 1981).

There are a number of organic diseases in which psychological factors may play a role. They include, but are not limited to, cardiovascular (coronary artery disease, hypertension), respiratory (bronchial asthma), gastrointestinal (peptic ulcer, ulcerative colitis), and musculoskeletal (tension headache, low back pain) functions. Some laryngeal pathologies, including vocal cord nodules, polyps, and contact ulcer, may also be linked to such factors (Aronson, 1990). It thus appears that the relationship between stress and organic disease can be bidirectional. Not only can organic pathologies (for example, neurologic disease) lead to stress and other psychological sequelae but also stress and other psychological reactions may play a causal role in the onset and course of organic disease.

Conversion disorders

Description. Conversion disorder is a subtype of *somatoform disorders* that involves physical symptoms "for which there are no demonstrable organic findings or known pathophysiologic mechanism to account for the disturbance and for which there is positive evidence, or a strong presumption, of a link between the somatic symptoms and psychologic factors or conflicts" (Williams, 1988, p. 219). In conversion disorders there is an actual loss or alteration of volitional muscle control or sensation that represents an unconscious simulation of illness. It appears that the conversion symptoms, or the *conversion reaction,* enables the patient to prevent conscious awareness of emotional conflict or stress that would be intolerable if faced directly. In some cases, the symptom may have a symbolic relationship to the underlying event or conflict. For example, a person may become aphonic because of conflict over verbally expressing anger at someone who has hurt them emotionally. Symptom "choice" may also relate to the person's experience with or conception of illness (Ziegler and Imboden, 1962). In addition to the *primary gain* of avoiding or displacing mental conflict, conversion reactions may be associated with *secondary gain* such as sympathy, preventing a court appearance, or necessitating a leave of absence from a hated job. Patients are generally unaware of these gains or the relationship of them to their physical symptoms, and they tend to resist psychological explanations (Sapir and Aronson, 1990).

Conversion disorder is sometimes called "hysteria" or "hysterical neurosis, conversion type," although hysteria refers to a personality type rather than a conversion response. The hysterical personality is characterized by immaturity and egocentricity, and sometimes by flirtatious, hostile, manipulative, dramatic, and emotionally labile behavior. A tendency to develop subjective physical complaints may be present in people with hysterical personalities, but they do not necessarily develop conversion reactions, and conversion reactions may occur in any personality type (Aronson, 1990; Carden and Schramel, 1966).

Characteristics of affected individuals. Conversion disorder can occur in the presence or absence of other psychiatric or organic disorders. It may occur in people with average or better than average psychological stability who find themselves in unusually stressful situations. Depression, schizophrenia, dependent, histrionic, or antisocial personalities, or passive-aggressive personality disorders are present in a high percentage of cases, however (Lazare, 1981). Affected people may be immature or shallow, and there is a tendency toward lower intelligence or lower socioeconomic status. In better educated people, symptoms tend to resemble known organic disease more closely (Ford and Folks, 1985). A history of disturbed sexuality, including sexual abuse, seduction, and incest, may be present (Lazare, 1981), and it is not uncommonly associated with drug abuse and alcoholism (Ford and Folks, 1985). Ford and Folks (1985) note that conversion disorder may be "facilitated in some patients by a brain predisposed by hereditary influences or injury" (p. 381).

Although unusual in the general population, conversion disorders are common in a general hospital population. Psychiatric consultations in a general hospital may be associated with conversion diagnoses in 5% to 16% of cases, and 20% to 25% of patients admitted to a general hospital may have had a conversion reaction at one time in their lives (Folks, Ford, and Regan, 1984; Lazare, 1981). Most agree that conversion responses are diagnosed more often in women, although they are frequent in men in combat situations and seem to have been higher in U.S. soldiers in the Vietnam War than in other wars (Carden and Schramel, 1966).

Course. Conversion symptoms tend to be abrupt in onset and sometimes remit rapidly. They often emerge on the heels of acute stress or trauma, but they may follow the "true" cause by a prolonged time, suggesting that there may be a latent period until a suitable "face-saving event" permits the conversion to occur (Carden and Schramel, 1966). The history may raise suspicions about previous conversion reactions, with first episodes emerging in adolescence or early adult-

hood. Patients are generally cooperative with examination but may be indifferent (*la belle indifference*) to their symptoms, although it has been noted that indifference is an unreliable indicator of conversion reactions and that some people with a conversion disorder are very interested and concerned about their problems (Ford and Folks, 1985; Lazare, 1981).

Many conversion symptoms are transient. Persisting symptoms tend to be seen more often in tertiary care settings (Ford and Folks, 1985). The patients with the best prognoses for recovery are those whose conversion symptoms developed recently and abruptly and who have an identifiable precipitating event, good premorbid health, and an absence of major psychiatric or organic illness (Ford and Folks, 1985; Lazare, 1981).

Relationship to neurologic disease. Conversion symptoms are very often neurologic in character and often present first to neurologists or neurosurgeons (Ford and Folks, 1985). Symptoms may include tremor, paresthesia, paraplegia, hemiplegia, lingual weakness, torsion dystonia, seizures (Baker and Silver, 1987; Fahn and Williams, 1988; Keane, 1986; Koller and others, 1989; Tomb, 1981), and a wide variety of speech disturbances, just to name a few. The high incidence of conversion symptoms in patients with a history of closed head injury or other organic injury suggests possible biologic mechanisms for some patients with conversion reactions. There also seems to be a predisposition in families and various ethnic and social groups, indicating hereditary and sociocultural mechanisms as well (Lazare, 1981).

It is important to remember that diagnosis of conversion disorder is not one of exclusion and that a link between symptoms and psychological factors must be apparent for a confident diagnosis. This is particularly important because conversion diagnoses are common in people with neurologic disease and often accompany depression, anxiety, or other psychological disturbances (Merskey, 1990; Sapir and Aronson, 1990). Based on follow-up studies, 15% to 30% of patients with conversion reaction diagnoses actually have organic disease, often neurologic disease. It may be that some neurologic diseases predispose people to conversion reactions or that neurologic disease can be sufficiently subtle, nonspecific, or unusual in its presentation to be mistaken for nonorganic disease. Neurologic conditions frequently misdiagnosed as conversion disorders include epilepsy, multiple sclerosis, frontal lobe lesions, postconcussion syndrome, encephalitis, dementia, tumor, stroke, and myasthenia gravis (Lazare, 1981; Tomb, 1981). There is a high incidence of conversion disorders in people with severe behavior disorders following diffuse brain injury (Eames, 1992).

Complicating the differential diagnosis between conversion disorder and organic disease is the factor of *somatic compliance,* which is the tendency for conversion symptoms to develop in an organ affected by organic disease, such as psychogenic seizures in people with neurologic seizures, or psychogenic aphonia in people with vocal cord weakness (Sapir & Aronson, 1987; 1990).

Somatization disorder

Somatization disorder, also known as *Briquet's syndrome,* is a subcategory of somatoform disorder. It is a chronic illness characterized by recurrent, multiple physical complaints and a belief that one is ill (Williams, 1988). It may be accompanied by conversion symptoms.

People with the disorder tend to have numerous, dramatic complaints involving multiple organs. They usually insist on and receive multiple tests and treatment and generally fail to be reassured when told there is no evidence of organic disease. They are at risk for drug dependence and complications from unnecessary medications and invasive procedures.

The disorder usually develops before the age of 30 and is more common in women of lower intelligence and socioeconomic status who have interpersonal problems. It tends to run in families and may be accompanied by significant sexual dysfunction and hysterical or antisocial personality traits (Nicholi, 1988; Teitelbaum and McHugh, 1990).

Unlike conversion disorders, somatization disorder is not frequently associated with organic illness (Tomb, 1981). It is also distinguished from conversion disorders by the wide variety of complaints within affected individuals and a lack of evidence that symptoms reflect subconscious repression of underlying acute conflict, stress, or anxiety. Patients are rarely indifferent to their symptoms and tend to be highly demanding and manipulative in their efforts to get help. Like conversion disorders, complaints may raise suspicion of neurologic disease, and patients are frequently suspected of having multiple sclerosis, myasthenia gravis, or seizures (Teitelbaum and McHugh, 1990).

Volitional disorders

Some psychogenic disturbances are under volitional control. They can be very difficult to distinguish from neurologic disease and psychiatric disturbances that are not volitional. They can be divided into factitious disorders and malingering.

Factitious disorders. Individuals with a factitious disorder *consciously and deliberately feign physical or psychological symptoms of disease but do so for uncontrolled, unconscious psychological reasons that lead them to seek out the role of the patient or sick person* (Stoudemire, 1988; Tomb, 1981; Williams, 1988). They are generally loners with personality disorders, often with a history of abuse, trauma, or deprivation. They may give a dramatic history with complaints that may, for example, be neurologic (seizures, headache, loss of consciousness), abdominal, or dermatologic. They submit to recommended medical tests and procedures, and they are at risk for drug addiction and complications from multiple surgeries (Stoudemire, 1988; Tomb, 1981).

The best-known factitious disorder is *Munchausen's syndrome,* named after a Russian army calvary officer who wandered from town to town telling outlandish war stories. The syndrome is characterized by pathological lying and extensive wandering among cities and hospitals, presenting with a wide variety of factitious illnesses. Factitious disorders can also occur in people whose general behavior is more socially acceptable but who may feign or induce illness by techniques that may include injection or insertion of contaminated substances, self-induced bruises, thermometer manipulation and urinary tract manipulation (Stoudemire, 1988).

Malingering. Malingering involves *the deliberate, voluntary feigning of physical or psychological symptoms for consciously motivated external purposes* (to avoid work or combat, for financial gain, to evade prosecution). To achieve their goals, malingerers may stage events (getting hit by a slow-moving car), alter medical tests, take advantage of natural events (use an accident or injury to maximize compensation), self-inflict injury (a minor gunshot wound to avoid combat), or invent symptoms that may be neurologic in nature.

Malingering is not considered a mental disorder, but it can be very difficult to distinguish from organic disease and factitious disorders. Among the clinical markers that are useful to its detection are examination and diagnostic test data incompatible with history and complaints, ill-defined and vague symptoms, overdramatized complaints, uncooperativeness with workup, resistance to a favorable prognosis, history of recurrent accidents or injury, potential for financial compensation, potential to avoid legal proceedings, requests for addictive drugs, and antisocial personality traits (Stoudemire, 1988). It is clear that such traits may belong to many people with organic disease and mental disorders, so their diagnostic usefulness is as circumstantial evidence rather than proof. The most important aspect of the workup of such patients is careful and objective assessment and documentation of examination findings, including their degree of correspondence with known patterns of disease.

SPEECH PATHOLOGY
Distribution of psychogenic speech disorders in clinical practice

The incidence and prevalence of psychogenic speech disorders in the general population and in medical practice are unknown. Similarly, little is known about the distribution of specific types of psychogenic speech disorders, although some sense of it may be gained by examining their distribution within a speech pathology practice in a large multidisciplinary medical setting. Table 14–1 summarizes the distribution of types of speech disturbance within the group of 215 individuals with psychogenic speech disorders who were seen over a 4-year period in the section of speech pathology at the Mayo Clinic.

About 80% of the cases had some type of voice disorder. This high proportion seems consistent

Table 14–1 Distribution of psychogenic speech disorders in 215 cases seen for speech pathology evaluation at the Mayo Clinic from 1987 to 1990

Diagnosis	Percent of cases
Psychogenic voice disorders	80
Aphonia	30
Hoarseness	22
Spasmodic dysphonia	
Adductor	13
Abductor	1
High pitch	6
Ventricular dysphonia	4
Miscellaneous voice problems	3
Inappropriate loudness	<1
Falsetto (excluding mutational falsetto)	<1
Psychogenic fluency, prosodic, and other speech disorders	20
Stuttering	11
Articulation deficits	3
Dysprosody	3
Infantile speech	2
Mutism	<1
Psychotic language	<1

with the attention paid to such deficits in the medical and speech pathology literature. About 65% of the voice disorders were characterized by aphonia, hoarseness, or adductor spasmodic dysphonia; aphonia was the most frequent diagnosis in the entire group of 215 cases. A variety of other problems were also present, including high pitch, ventricular dysphonia, abductor spasmodic dysphonia, inappropriate loudness, and falsetto. About 3% had voice abnormalities that did not fit into any other category, probably because of their atypical characteristics.

Twenty percent of the cases had problems with fluency, prosody, articulation, or some other aspect of speech that was not isolated to laryngeal function. Stuttering-like behavior represented more than half of the cases in this category. Psychogenic articulation deficits, prosodic abnormalities, and patterns of infantile speech were also encountered. Mutism and psychotic language were rarely diagnosed, perhaps because such cases infrequently were difficult to distinguish from neurologic disorders or did not require language or speech therapy. A high proportion of these disorders appeared to reflect conversion disorders or responses to life stresses.

Examination

The assessment of speech disorders that may be psychogenic in origin usually should include all components of the motor speech disorders examination. When a stress-induced speech disorder, conversion disorder, somatization disorder, factitious disorder, or malingering is suspected, several components of the assessment deserve special attention because of their value to differential diagnosis, particularly the distinction between organic and psychogenic etiology. These relate to the patient's history and to observations of speech during examination.

History. The conditions under which psychogenic speech problems first emerge can differ from those usually associated with neurologic disease. For example, there may have been an associated cold or similar nonneurologic illness shortly before, during or after onset. The problem may have developed at the time of or shortly after a physically or psychologically traumatic event; with physical trauma, there may not have been any loss of consciousness or injury to the head, face, or neck. When an organic or psychologically significant event cannot be associated with the onset of the speech problem, it is important to review the more distant history for similar evidence. The current deficit may reflect an ongoing pattern of psychological disturbance or a delayed response to a temporally distant traumatic event.

The history following onset is also important because the disorder sometimes develops in anticipation of a difficult encounter or illness, such as an anticipated emotional confrontation with a boss or family member or fear of a life-threatening disease. When a psychologically significant event is discovered and considered causally related to the speech disorder, it is important to explore if the stress or conflict is currently active or has dissipated. When the triggering event is no longer active, the prognosis for resolution of the speech disorder is usually better than when stress and conflict, or primary or secondary gain issues, remain active.

It is also important to establish if the problem has been constant since onset or if there have been periods of remission, even if brief. Transient problems certainly may be neurogenic, so the conditions under which exacerbations and remissions occur are also important. Close ties between symptom fluctuation and stressful events or encounters with particular individuals should raise suspicions about psychogenic etiology. Reports of sudden, dramatic deterioration of speech immediately after brief exposure to nonregulated fumes, odors, or environments should raise similar suspicions. The possibility of secondary gain should also be considered (for example, litigation related to the speech disturbance or its alleged cause, or inability to work because of the speech problem, especially if work is described as dissatisfying or stressful).

The clinician should keep in mind that evidence of significant life stress, by itself, does not establish that a speech deficit is psychogenic. Heavy reliance on such evidence can blind one to signs of neurologic or other organic explanations, especially if the patient also believes his or her difficulty is psychological. In general, patients who spontaneously express a belief that their problem is psychological should heighten suspicions about organic etiology, whereas those who insist on an organic explanation or deny the possibility of a psychological explanation should heighten suspicions about psychogenic etiology. Although such suspicions may be unfounded, they help to maintain diagnostic vigilance.

Important observations. Several questions should be addressed as the clinician conducts and evaluates the results of examination:

1. *Can the speech disorder be classified neurologically?* Do the speech deficits fit lawful patterns associated with the dysarthrias, apraxia of speech, or other neurogenic speech disturbances? Departures from these lawful patterns may reflect psychogenic etiology or a significant psychogenic contribution to the speech disorder. In people with confirmed neurologic disease, speech symptoms that are incongruent or inconsistent with the localization, character, and severity of the disease should raise suspicions about psychogenic etiology.

2. *Is the oral mechanism examination consistent with the speech disorder and patterns of abnormalities found in neurologic disease?* In neurologic disease, speech and oral mechanism findings generally have a predictable relationship. Incongruities may occur in psychogenic disorders. For example, strength testing may reveal weakness that is grossly disproportionate to the severity of the speech deficit. The patient may exhibit "give-way" weakness or no ability to resist movement on strength testing, and their efforts may be accompanied by dramatic posturing of oral structures or complaints that the exam is too difficult or uncomfortable to permit compliance.

3. *Is the speech deficit consistent?* Most neurogenic and other organic speech disorders are constant and consistent during examination. Significant fluctuations—especially from normal to grossly abnormal speech—as a function of speech task (for example, casual conversation versus reading or repetition) or emotional content (for example, reading versus discussion of personal relationships) are uncommon when etiology is neurologic. In contrast, some patients with psychogenic speech disorders may speak much more adequately during conversation than during formal assessment tasks, and others may regress significantly when sensitive psychosocial issues are addressed. Some patients have grossly irregular speech alternating motion rates (AMRs) in the absence of any irregular articulatory breakdowns during contextual speech or any other evidence of ataxic or hyperkinetic dysarthria, a very unusual finding in neurogenic speech disorders.

4. *Is the speech deficit suggestible?* Is there anything the clinician can do to dramatically improve or worsen the deficit? For example, some patients with psychogenic speech disorders dramatically worsen if it is suggested that a task is likely to be difficult.

5. *Is the speech deficit susceptible to distractibility?* Neurologic disease rarely is. Psychogenic speech disorders may improve noticeably if the clinician breaks out of the formal examination mode to speak casually with the patient or to clarify points in the history.

6. *Does speech fatigue in a lawful manner?* With the exception of the flaccid dysarthria associated with myasthenia gravis, motor speech disorders do not fatigue dramatically over the course of examination, even when continuous

speaking is required. Some people with psychogenic speech disorders deteriorate dramatically during speech stress testing, especially if myasthenia gravis is a possibility. However, the character of such "fatigue" may be inconsistent with progressive weakness and may actually reflect an increase in musculoskeletal tension. For example, instead of increasing breathiness, short phrases, and hypernasality that lawfully reflect increasing weakness, a patient may develop a strained voice quality with associated orofacial struggle and exaggerated articulation, behaviors associated with increased rather than decreased muscular contraction.

7. *Is the speech deficit reversible?* Unfortunately, motor speech and other neurologic speech disturbances do not completely remit with symptomatic speech therapy. In contrast, it is not unusual for people with psychogenic speech disorders, particularly those with dysphonia, aphonia, or dysfluencies reflecting a conversion disorder or response to life stresses, to respond dramatically to symptomatic treatment during the examination. Also, the catharsis of confronting the psychological dynamic underlying the development of the speech disorder during review of the history is sometimes associated with dramatic improvement or resolution of the speech problem. Symptom reversibility rules out neurologic causes for the speech deficit observed during evaluation and confirms the diagnosis as psychogenic.

Answers to the preceding questions are valuable to diagnostic decision making and to decisions about management and referrals to other medical subspecialists (neurology, psychiatry). In general, when examination results are incongruent with expectations for neurogenic or other organic speech deficits, and when the history provides evidence of psychological factors that are logically related to the disorder, the probability that the speech disorder is psychogenic can be considered high.

Speech characteristics associated with specific psychiatric conditions

Depression and manic-depression. The speech characteristics of depressed people often lead to a perception of depression, so there seems to be a close match between underlying mood and speech in the disorder. In general, depressed people have reduced loudness, pitch, and inflectional range, giving speech a dead or listless quality (Aronson, 1990; Darby, Simmons, and Berger, 1984) that seems consistent with the cognitive, vegetative, and general clinical features of the disorder.

In a study of depressed men before they were treated with antidepressants, Darby, Simmons, and Berger (1984) found a predominance of reduced loudness and loudness variability, with a tendency to trail off at the end of utterances, as well as a repetitious, singsong pattern of stress and inflection. The typical triad of patients' characteristics included *reduced stress, monopitch,* and *monoloudness.* The authors noted that reduced loudness and monoloudness conveyed an impression of reduced respiratory drive and effort and that the flat prosody seemed to reflect overall reduced vitality. There were no differences from control subjects in rate or periods of silence during speech, although reduced rate has been noted by others (Darby and Hollien, 1977). Darby, Simmons, and Berger also noted that the relatively consistent speech patterns of their patients seemed to represent an index of depression in that the patients' depression and speech pattern both improved with antidepressant medication.

Of special interest, Darby, Simmons, and Berger noted that a number of speech characteristics of depression are *hypokinetic-like* in character and suggestive of extrapyramidal system disturbance, an association made more interesting by the common occurrence of depression in Parkinson's disease. This raises questions about the neurology of depression and highlights the fact that the speech of depression may sometimes be difficult to distinguish from the speech of hypokinetic dysarthria. Relatedly, the common occurrence of stroke-related depression, especially in people with left hemisphere lesions, suggests that some prosodic abnormalities associated with nonfluent aphasia, apraxia of speech, and perhaps unilateral upper motor neuron (UMN) dysarthria may reflect the influence of depression as well as the primary speech or language disturbance in some patients.

In people with manic depression there may be a dramatic change in speech during the manic phase of the illness. Speech may become *loud* and *pressured* (rapid, as if the drive to speak cannot be controlled) with *vigorous articulation,* a *lively and vital voice, frequent emphasis,* and occasional *word rhyming (clanging).* Ideas may flow freely and be incoherent (Aronson, 1990; Tomb, 1981). Manic speech tends not to be confused with dysarthrias or apraxia of speech, but sometimes may resemble fluent, Wernicke's aphasia.

Schizophrenia. Schizophrenic speech is not usually mistaken for a motor speech disorder. Schizophrenia does not have a single pathognomonic speech pattern, but it does have variations in content and manner of expression that distinguish it from normal speech. Experienced psychologists and psychiatrists, for example, can distinguish schizophrenic from nonschizophrenic speakers during reading, apparently because they can perceive schizophrenic speakers' slowed rate, dependence, inefficiency, and moodiness (Todt and Howell, 1980).

Schizophrenia may have exaggerated as well as attenuated speech characteristics that reflect different phases or varieties of the illness. The active phases of the disorder can be associated with *rapidly altering melody and pitch,* with *inappropriate stress patterns* that do not have a clear relationship to ideational content (Aronson, 1990). Speech may contain *verbigeration,* the stereotypic and seemingly meaningless repetition of words and sentences. Content may contain *loose associations,* in which ideas have no apparent relation to one another, and *word salad,* in which words have no apparent relationship to one another. In general, content may be *incoherent, illogical, digressive, vague,* or *excessively detailed.* Some patients have a tendency to *pun* and *rhyme words,* and *verbal paraphasias, neologisms,* and *perseveration* may be present. These characteristics may be accompanied by inappropriate affect, such as giggling and smiling, that may be incongruent with verbal content (Gerson, Benson, and Frazier, 1977; Nicholi, 1988).

A number of these "active" speech characteristics are similar to the verbal behaviors associated with Wernicke's aphasia. The similarities can be so striking that the term "schizophasia" has been used to describe the language of some schizophrenic patients (Lecours and Vanier-Clement, 1976). Distinctions between the disorders can be made, however. Comparisons between schizophrenic and aphasic speech by Gerson, Benson, and Frazier (1977) and DiSimoni, Darley, and Aronson (1977) suggest that schizophrenic speakers (1) have fewer dysfluencies than aphasic speakers; (2) tend to reiterate themes, whereas aphasic speakers reiterate words and phrases; (3) comprehend, read, and write adequately if they attend to the task, whereas aphasic speakers do poorly; (4) make fewer semantic and phonemic errors than aphasic speakers; (5) have good naming and syntax compared to aphasic speakers; (6) tend to be irrelevant, whereas aphasic responses are usually relevant; and (7) show little awareness of deficits, whereas aphasic speakers show some awareness and frustration. These contrasts are consistent with general notions of aphasia as a language disorder and schizophrenia as a thought disorder, and they are useful to differential diagnosis. In addition, the typical gradual emergence at a relatively young age without evidence of a focal neurologic lesion in schizophrenia, versus the common sudden emergence at a relatively older age with evidence of focal left hemisphere pathology in aphasia, usually helps to distinguish between the two disorders.

During the more chronic phases of schizophrenia, speech and language characteristics may be "negative" or passive, with a general *decrease in expressiveness and responsiveness.* Patients' speech may be *monotonous, weak, flat, colorless,* and *gloomy* in character (Aronson, 1990). Some patients may exhibit a *poverty of speech, mutism, increased response latency,* with *reduced gestures and spontaneous movement* and *poor eye contact* (Nicholi, 1988). Such characteristics have the potential to be confused with motor speech disorders (hypokinetic dysarthria) or frontal lobe–limbic system cognitive and affective deficits. Again, dissimilarities in onset, course, and neurologic findings between schizophrenia and these other disorders help to clarify the diagnosis in many cases.

Psychogenic voice disorders

Voice abnormalities probably represent the largest proportion of symptoms of psychogenic speech disturbances. As suggested earlier, this dominance of voice disorders probably reflects the voice's prominent role in the expression of emotion, the links between laryngeal control mechanisms and the limbic system, and the voice's subsequent susceptibility to the effects of stress.

Aronson (1990) suggests that some people may be "laryngoresponders," predisposed by personality or physiologic makeup to react through muscular hypercontraction of the laryngeal muscles to emotional stress, such as fear, anxiety, anger, frustration, and depression. Aronson, Peterson, and Litin (1966) found frequent evidence of acute or chronic stress, marital discord, poor sex identification, anger, immature-dependent personality, neurotic life adjustment, or depression in 27 people with psychogenic voice disorders.

In some cases, vocal hyperfunction can lead to organic laryngeal pathology such as nodules, polyps, and contact ulcer. Such structural pathologies will not be discussed here, however, because they are rarely confused with neurologic disease. Of greater interest are voice disturbances that are not associated with structural laryngeal changes. Such disorders often lead patients on a pilgrimage for diagnosis and treatment, frequently with misdirected efforts to establish an organic explanation. These voice problems include dysphonias associated with excessive musculoskeletal tension in response to life stress, conversion aphonia or dysphonia, some spasmodic dysphonias, iatrogenic and inertial voice disorders, and voice disorders that may develop as secondary responses to other psychogenic symptoms.

Musculoskeletal tension disorders. Prolonged hypercontraction of laryngeal muscles in response to psychological stress is often associated with elevation of the larynx and hyoid bone and with pain and discomfort in response to digital palpation in the area because of muscular soreness.* *Hoarseness, strained-breathiness, alterations in pitch,* and *aphonia* may result in spite of an absence of laryngeal lesions. Such difficulties can develop without serious psychopathology in people under considerable psychological stress, particularly those who also must talk under demanding or stressful situations. These dysphonias usually are not mistaken for neurologic disease, and patients are often most concerned about structural laryngeal pathology. Ruling out structural pathology and identifying the presence of musculoskeletal tension and the underlying sources of psychological stress usually lead to accurate diagnosis and recommendations for management.

Conversion aphonia. Aphonia is listed in many psychiatric texts as a common conversion symptom. Conversion aphonia can occur in the absence of laryngeal pathology; is usually linked to stress, anxiety, depression, or conflict; and serves as a vehicle for avoiding underlying psychological conflict (Aronson, Peterson, and Litin, 1966). It may also have symbolic significance, such as reflecting an inability to confront verbally a person who has hurt the patient in some way (Aronson, 1990).

Patients with conversion aphonia involuntarily whisper. The whisper may be *pure, harsh, or sharp,* sometimes with *high-pitched squeaky* traces of phonation, and sometimes with *traces of normal phonation.* The sharpness of the whisper and its strained and high-pitched components are very different from the weak, breathy, and hoarse quality associated with vocal cord weakness or paralysis. The *cough is usually sharp,* another clue to the capacity for vocal cord adduction. Excessive musculoskeletal tension can be detected as a narrowing of the thyrohyoid space during digital examination, as well as patients' frequent pain or discomfort response during that examination.

The onset of the aphonia is often sudden and may seem to have been triggered by a cold or flu in which the aphonia persists after the physical illness subsides. The patient may complain of pain in the neck, throat, and chest. The history often reveals acute or chronic emotional stress, as well as evidence of primary or secondary gain from the symptom. A history of previous episodes of voice loss or other possible conversion symptoms may be present. Some patients are indifferent to the aphonia and unimpressed by the rapid return of their voices with symptomatic treatment. Others are very concerned and then pleased when the voice returns with symptomatic treatment. Still others may not focus much on their improved voice when it returns because they are focused on their discovery during discussion with the clinician of the underlying psychological reason for the conversion reaction.

Conversion aphonia is commonly investigated as a manifestation of neurologic disease. Myasthenia gravis and multiple sclerosis seem to be among the most common neurologic diseases being investigated in patients referred to speech pathologists for assessment of conversion aphonia.

Conversion dysphonia. Conversion disorder can also be manifested as dysphonia, which may be characterized by *hoarseness with or without a strained component, high-pitched falsetto pitch breaks, breathiness, intermittent whispering,* and a wide variety of other abnormal voice characteristics (Aronson, 1990). Aronson, Peterson, and Litin (1966) established that patients with conversion dysphonias are not fundamentally different from those with conversion aphonia or muteness in history, personality, or clinical criteria for conversion disorder diagnosis. Aronson (1990) also notes that, among such patients, "few have incapacitating psychiatric disturbances. In many ways, they have adjusted to their anxiety and depression" (p. 134).

Psychogenic spasmodic dysphonia. Neurogenic spasmodic dysphonia and general demographic characteristics associated with all forms of spasmodic dysphonia were discussed in Chapter 8. In spite of the growing tendency for higher proportions of spasmodic dysphonias to be diagnosed as neurogenic, some are clearly psychogenic in origin, sometimes reflecting conversion disorder or a response to life stresses that is not necessarily conversion in nature.

The diagnosis of psychogenic spasmodic dysphonia may be very difficult in many cases. Symptom reversibility in some patients confirms the diagnosis as psychogenic. The common emergence of tremor and dystonia as the basis for spasmodic dysphonia in some patients with histories of prominent acute or chronic psychologic stress raises questions about spasmodic dysphonia as a psychosomatic disorder in some patients with neurogenic or idiopathic spasmodic dysphonia.

Psychogenic spasmodic dysphonia can be adductor or abductor in form. The *adductor form* is characterized by a *continuous or intermittent strained, jerky, grunting, squeezed, groaning, and*

---

*Aronson (1990) very clearly describes the examination of laryngeal musculoskeletal tension, as well as methods for relieving such tension during diagnostic assessment and management of psychogenic voice disorders.

effortful quality. The *abductor form* has *continuous or intermittent breathy or aphonic segments.* Their vocal characteristics can be highly similar to those of neurogenic or idiopathic etiology, although underlying voice tremor or evidence of laryngeal dystonia should not be encountered in psychogenic etiologies unless a combination of causes is present. Careful history and examination can help to identify a probable etiology, although it is not unusual for the etiology to remain uncertain. It should be noted that the prolonged persistence (years) of spasmodic dysphonia is expected when etiology is neurogenic but is less common when conversion response or reaction to life stresses is responsible, especially when the psychogenic triggers have ceased to exist or vary in their presence or intensity. The specific history and personality traits associated with psychogenic spasmodic dysphonia may be quite similar to those of patients with psychogenic aphonia, dysphonia, and muteness, according to Aronson (1990).

Iatrogenic voice disorders. An iatrogenic disorder is one *induced by the actions of the clinician and dependent on suggestibility and other psychological characteristics of affected patients.* For example, carotid endarterectomy carries some risk for vocal cord paralysis, and patients are typically informed of this risk when they must decide whether to consent to surgery; a suggestible patient may develop a postoperative psychogenic dysphonia in response to the "suggestion" that it might occur. On a deeper psychological level, a psychogenic voice disorder may represent unconscious hostility toward the surgeon following laryngeal surgery (Aronson, 1990). Finally, patients who are placed on voice rest—very often unnecessarily or inappropriately as a treatment for vocal abuse, musculoskeletal tension dysphonia, or other psychogenic dysphonia—may develop a fear of speaking, with subsequent dysphonia or aphonia, because of the suggestion that to speak would be harmful.

Inertial aphonia or dysphonia. Some patients with voice disorders of neurogenic origin, secondary to laryngeal pathology, or in response to psychological factors or a recommendation for voice rest may develop an *inertial aphonia or dysphonia.** In these cases, patients "seem to lose

their sense or feel for volitional phonation . . . some sort of loss of recall, memory, or even praxis for normal voice production" (Aronson, 1990, p. 142). Sapir and Aronson (1985) have suggested that inertial factors may explain the persistence of aphonia in some head-injured patients. This notion may also explain the persistence of conversion or nonconversion psychogenic voice disorders that persist after triggering psychological events have subsided or resolved.

Dysphonias as secondary responses to other psychogenic symptoms. Certain physical manifestations of psychological difficulties, particularly those that involve the airway, can have indirect effects on the voice. For example, chronic coughing or throat clearing linked to psychological factors may result in dysphonia secondary to vocal cord trauma.

Dysphonia may also develop in association with "paradoxical vocal cord function" or "functional stridor" in which there is stridor or high-pitched wheezing caused by abnormal vocal cord adduction without identifiable cause. Affected individuals tend to be females in their teens to thirties. The problem may represent a conversion disorder in some cases, but a variety of psychiatric disorders may be responsible (George, O'Connell and Batch, 1991; Kellman and Leopold, 1982; Pannbacker, 1990).*

Psychogenic stuttering-like dysfluency of adult onset (psychogenic stuttering)

That stuttering can emerge in adulthood as a manifestation of psychological difficulties has been recognized for many years. In 1922, for example, Henry Head observed that stuttering was one of the possible manifestations of hysteria. Only in recent years has the disorder received much attention in the speech pathology literature, however.

Acquired neurogenic stuttering was discussed in Chapter 13. The reservations expressed there about using the term *stuttering* to refer to dysfluencies acquired in adults hold here, but the term also will be retained here to maintain consistency with much of the literature and to highlight the difficulties that may arise when attempting to establish etiology of acquired stuttering as neurogenic or psychogenic. The designation, *psychogenic stuttering (PS),* will be used to refer to

---

*The influence of somatic compliance may be important in such cases. For example, Hartman, Daily, and Morin (1989) discussed a case with a psychogenic voice disorder that co-occurred or evolved along with signs of a unilateral superior laryngeal nerve paresis in which the psychogenic component reflected either a conversion reaction or a musculoskeletal tension disorder. Voice therapy relieved the psychogenic component of the problem.

---

*Wheezing and stridor have also been reported in a person with a posterior fossa subarachnoid cyst, which presumably caused the symptoms by compressing the brain stem. The symptoms resolved following surgical treatment (Patton and others, 1987).

stuttering-like behavior that emerges in adulthood and is psychogenic in origin.

Psychogenic stuttering is not nearly as common as are psychogenic voice disorders, but it is probably more frequently mistaken as a sign of CNS disease than are psychogenic voice disorders. Although uncommon, a number of cases of PS have been reported. Most illustrate the need to establish etiology as neurogenic or psychogenic because many have occurred in the presence of confirmed central nervous system (CNS) disease or symptoms that raised the possibility of CNS disease.

Baumgartner and Duffy (1986), in an unpublished retrospective study, summarized the characteristics of 49 people with PS in the absence of neurologic disease and of 20 people with PS in the presence of neurologic disease. Because their series is the largest reported to date, their findings will serve as a vehicle for summarizing the features of PS. Relevant demographic characteristics of the two groups are summarized in Table 14–2.

There were no substantial differences between the two groups in education or age at onset. About as many men as women were affected, a noticeable difference from the predominance of women in those with psychogenic aphonia. Educational level approximated the national average. Age at onset was younger than the average age of many adult-onset neurologic disorders. Some patients were seen soon after onset of their PS, but about half in each group had the problem for more than three months, indicating that PS often was of more than brief duration.

For those who had formal psychiatric assessment, the most common diagnosis was conversion disorder, followed by depression, anxiety neurosis, and hysterical neurosis. Some patients had personality or adjustment disorders, and some were dealing with drug dependence or posttraumatic difficulties. There were no clear differences in the distribution of psychiatric diagnoses between those with or without neurologic disease. These diagnoses, plus combat neurosis, are consistent with those reported in the literature (Brookshire, 1989; Deal, 1982; Duffy, 1989; Mahr and Leith,

Table 14–2 Characteristics of individuals with psychogenic stuttering with or without evidence of neurologic disease

	Without neurologic disease (n = 49)	With neurologic disease (n = 20)
Male:female	26:23	9:11
Education (M & SD)	12.6 (3.7)	12.6 (2.6)
Age at onset		
M	46.2	44.4
SD	8.5	10.1
Range	21–68	26–69
Duration of disorder at time of assessment		
1–90 days	50%	53%
91–365 days	24%	16%
> 1 year	26%	32%
Psychiatric diagnoses	Conversion	Conversion
	Anxiety neurosis	Hysterical neurosis
	Depression	Depression
	Personality disorder	Personality disorder
	Reactive depression	
	Posttraumatic disorder	
	Adjustment disorder	
	Drug dependence	
Response to sx therapy*		
Normal	47%	45%
Near normal	28%	18%
Some improvement	19%	18%
No change	4%	18%

*Provided in one or two sessions, often including initial diagnostic encounter. Results of treatment are based on responses of the 43% of patients without neurologic disease and the 55% of patients with neurologic disease who were treated.
Based on data from Baumgartner and Duffy, 1986. *M*, mean; *SD*, standard deviation; *sx*, symptomatic.

1992; Roth, Aronson, and Davis, 1989; Wallen, 1961).

The specific chronic or acute life stresses that emerge in the histories of patients with PS include marital discord or divorce; coping with family tragedies, illnesses, or deaths; inability to manage work responsibilities; anger and loss of self esteem from unemployment; physical disability; accumulation of psychologically traumatic childhood experiences; dissatisfaction with work but conflict over change; unjust accusations of wrongdoing; religious differences with offspring; and emotional shock from an accident (Attanasio, 1987; Duffy, 1989; Roth, Aronson, and Davis, 1989).

Roth, Aronson, and Davis (1989) reported that their patients with PS were similar to those with psychogenic mutism, aphonia, or dysphonia. They displayed a tendency to emotional immaturity and neurotic life adjustments, and some had a history of multiple conversion symptoms. A common theme for their patients was struggle over expressing anger, fear, or remorse in conventional ways or a breakdown in communication with an important person. The authors observed that voice problems are rarely switched for stuttering and that stuttering, unlike voice problems, rarely develops in the aftermath of an upper respiratory infection. They also noted that both PS and psychogenic voice disorders tend to be highly responsive to symptomatic therapy and disclosure of conflict.

More than 80% of Baumgartner and Duffy's cases without neurologic disease had nonspeech complaints of a neurologic nature, including weakness or incoordination, fatigue, sensory difficulties, seizures, and cognitive difficulties, but none had neurologic disease confirmed. Those with neurologic disease most often had degenerative disease, convulsive disorder, or traumatic brain injury.* Their lesions included the right and left cerebral hemispheres and the brain stem and cerebellum. About three quarters of the patients with neurologic disease had no associated dysarthria, apraxia of speech, or aphasia. Twenty percent had a dysarthria, and a few had equivocal evidence of aphasia or apraxia of speech.

More than half of the patients in both of Baumgartner and Duffy's groups who received brief periods of symptomatic therapy improved to normal or near normal within one or two sessions, change dramatic and lasting enough to rule out neurologic etiology.* This observation highlights the diagnostic value of attempts to modify dysfluencies (and other speech disturbances) within the diagnostic setting when psychogenic etiology is suspected.

The box on page 334 summarizes the characteristics of dysfluencies and other speech-related behaviors that were present in Baumgartner and Duffy's (1986) cases. They are representative of those described in the literature. The dysfluencies themselves are similar to those described for developmental stuttering, with *sound and syllable repetitions* occurring most frequently. *Struggle behavior* in the form of facial grimacing or bizarre face, neck, or limb shaking or tremorous movements was quite common. *Rate abnormalities* during periods of fluency were present in some patients. In addition, 10% of the cases had *telegraphic syntax/grammar* that superficially resembled that encountered in nonfluent or Broca's aphasia, a characteristic that could fuel suspicions of neurologic etiology; in most instances, however, such telegraphic language had an infantile structure and prosody that should not be mistaken for aphasia or apraxia of speech.

In their review of PS, Deal and Cannito (1991) suggested that PS dysfluencies, in contrast to those associated with developmental stuttering, are not generally reduced by choral reading, masking, delayed auditory feedback, singing, or mimed speaking. They noted that these traits of PS are not universally reported in the literature, however. They also concluded that evidence of secondary struggle behavior or concern about stuttering is often absent in people with PS. However, Baumgartner and Duffy noted some form of struggle in more than half of their patients, and many of them expressed distress over their speech disorder. Baumgartner and Duffy also observed that variables that influenced the presence and severity of PS had highly variable effects across patients within their groups. For example, some had speech that was unvarying under any observed circumstance, including adaptation, whereas others varied according to task, environment, or time of day. In some patients, the near absence of any variability in dysfluency was considered incompatible with neurologic etiology (see Case 14.3 for such an example); in others the situational specificity or seemingly random presence or absence of dysfluencies was considered incompatible with

---

*Several case studies help confirm that PS may be associated with neurologic disease, including epilepsy (Attanasio, 1887; Deal and Doro, 1987; Tippett and Siebens, 1991), stroke (Brookshire, 1989), and anoxic encephalopathy (Tippett and Siebens, 1991).

---

*Some patients seem to require a longer period of treatment to make major gains. For example, Brookshire (1989) reported marked improvement after 21 therapy sessions in a patient whose probable PS developed after a stroke that produced speech and language problems and dyskinesias.

CHARACTERISTICS OF DYSFLUENCIES ASSOCIATED WITH PSYCHOGENIC STUTTERING IN PEOPLE WITHOUT EVIDENCE OF NEUROLOGIC DISEASE. PERCENTAGE OF CASES IN WHICH CHARACTERISTICS WERE OBSERVED ARE GIVEN IN PARENTHESES.

Dysfluencies

Sound or syllable repetitions (80%)
Prolongations (27%)
Hesitations (27%)
Word repetitions (20%)

Blocking (18%)
Tense pauses (14%)
Phrase repetitions (8%)
Interjections (2%)

Associated behaviors

Secondary struggle (e.g., facial grimacing) (49%)
"Bizarre" struggle (12%)
Telegraphic speech (10%)
Slow rate (10%)
Fast rate (4%)

Factors influencing dysfluencies

Unvarying (27%)
Intermittent/unpredictably present (27%)
Situationally specific (22%)
Conversation more fluent than reading (10%)
No adaptation effect (8%)
Adaptation effect (2%)
Reading more fluent than conversation (2%)
Fluctuation by time of day (2%)

Based on data from Baumgartner and Duffy, 1986.

neurologic etiology. It seems that too little is known at this time to establish a single diagnostic rule about adaptation, choral speaking, singing, responses to masking, and the like in PS. It may be that such variables actually have no consistent relationships with PS.

Other manifestations of psychogenic speech disorders

The data in Table 14–1 suggest that most psychogenic speech disturbances are reflected in abnormalities of voice or fluency. Although rarely reported in the literature, they also can be manifested as disturbances in articulation, resonance, and prosody. It is also noteworthy that psychogenic speech disturbances can also have multiple effects on speech, in which voice, fluency, articulation, resonance, and prosody may all be affected in the same individual.

It is not always clear why some psychogenic speech disorders take these less conventional routes of expression. The existence of varieties of psychogenic speech disorders raises questions about the symbolic differences among voice abnormalities versus stuttering versus disorders of resonance, articulation, or prosody. In cases of physical trauma, somatic compliance may be im-

portant; for example, a neck injury may lead to dysphonia, whereas oral surgery may lead to an articulation problem (malingering or true organic explanations deserve serious consideration in such cases). In other cases, the symptom may reflect the affected individual's experiences or ideas about the effects of illness on speech.

Psychogenic articulation, resonance, and prosodic abnormalities seem most often to be associated with conversion or somatization disorders, rather than a "simple" response to life stress. In some cases, malingering may be suspected, especially if litigation is pending.

Articulation disorders. Acquired articulation disturbances can have a psychogenic basis. Most psychogenic articulation difficulties raise questions about oral structure abnormalities or about flaccid or hyperkinetic dysarthria.

The problems may develop following traumatic injury to oral structures, such as occurs during oral surgery. When that is the case, they may also be associated with oral sensory complaints. When they represent a conversion disorder, the articulation problem is not usually subtle. The errors may be quite consistent and isolated to specific sounds, not infrequently the most difficult to produce consonants (/r/, /l/, /s/). Sometimes the errors are bizarre and associated with unusual tongue posturing, such as speaking with the tongue consistently elevated and retracted. The consistency of errors can seem to reflect lingual weakness and raise suspicions about flaccid dysarthria; however, when the deficit is dramatic but limited to only a few sounds, and especially when there are no associated chewing or drooling difficulties, true weakness can be ruled out. When problems are subtle, differential diagnosis can be very difficult.

When abnormal posturing of articulators is responsible for the articulation problem, a movement disorder (hyperkinetic dysarthria) must be considered. An "atypical dysarthria" has been reported in a person with Munchausen's syndrome who was initially suspected of having multiple sclerosis, partly because of a speech pattern that contained pervasive glottal stop substitutions (Kallen, Marshall, and Casey, 1986).

Resonance disorders. Although rarely the case, acquired hypernasality may be psychogenic in origin. Psychogenic hypernasality may be a symptom of conversion reaction or may reflect the effects of speech lacking in vigor as the result of poor self-image (Aronson, 1990). Oral or sinus surgery may serve as a trigger for a conversion reaction or a somatic compliance function in some cases. Malingering must be considered if litigation is involved.

Psychogenic hypernasality can be difficult to distinguish from oral or nasal structural defects or from flaccid dysarthria. Psychogenic hyponasality is very rare but should be given consideration in cases without evidence of nasal obstruction.*

Prosodic disturbances. Prosody may be disturbed on a psychogenic basis in ways that are quite different from the prosodic attenuations or exaggerations that are associated with depression, mania, and schizophrenia, and in ways that are not simply secondary to psychogenic voice or stuttering disorders. Such disturbances may be accompanied by abnormal resonance and articulation. In most instances they appear associated with conversion or somatization disorders; in some cases, malingering may be suspected. The abnormal prosody can be highly variable. It may have a *deaflike quality* or convey the impression of accent, not dissimilar to the *pseudoforeign accent* that may be associated with neurologic disease. These disturbances of prosody are often associated with suspicions about neurologic rather than peripheral structural disease.

Infantile speech. Speech sometimes appears to regress to an infantile level. The perception of infantile speech is created by a combination of prosodic, voice, resonance, and articulatory alterations that usually include an *increase in pitch, exaggerated inflectional patterns,* and production of common *developmental articulation errors* (for example, lisping, w/r or w/l substitutions). These are usually accompanied by nonvocal affective behaviors that convey an impression of childlike behavior (for example, demure gestures and wide-eyed, childish smiling). Infantile speech sometimes develops in adults suspected of having neurologic disease, especially when it is accompanied by other deficits in volitional motor control (walking, dressing). It seems to serve the purpose of avoiding interactions on the adult plane (Aronson, 1990). It may reflect a conversion disorder, hysterical personality disorder, or other psychopathology.

Psychogenic mutism

Mutism can be psychogenic or neurogenic in origin (see Chapter 12). It may occur in schizophrenia, severe depression, and other severe psychiatric conditions (Nicholi, 1988). Mutism may also be a symptom of a conversion disorder and may often be mistaken for neurologic disease when it is. People with conversion mutism are quite similar to those with conversion aphonia and dysphonia in their personality traits, their histories, and the fact that they meet criteria for conversion disorder diagnosis (Aronson, Peterson, and Litin, 1966).

Patients with psychogenic mutism either make *no attempt to speak* or they *mouth words without voice or whispering.* They usually have no chewing, swallowing, or drooling difficulties Their cough is normal, establishing the capacity for vocal cord adduction. They often initiate writing to communicate their thoughts and answer questions and may show no distress at their inability to speak. They may exhibit other psychogenic speech disturbances as they emerge from their mute state. For example, Aronson (1990) discussed a case in which telegraphic speech and stuttering-like blocking was present as the transition during symptomatic therapy was made from mutism to normal speech. Finally, it is important to remem-

---

*An unusual problem, known as *patulous eustachian tube,* can lead to hyponasality that is misinterpreted as psychogenic in origin. This syndrome is characterized by a roaring sound and sense of fullness in the ears; hyponasality; depression, anxiety, and preoccupation with the problem; and disappearance of the problem when lying down. The cause of the symptoms is patency of the eustachian tube because of loss of tissue mass around its orifice or a change in velopharyngeal muscle tone. Causes include significant weight or tissue fluid loss, nasopharyngeal radiation, and estrogen hormones. The reason for hyponasality is probably protective; palatal closure prevents voice and other airway noise from reaching the open eustachian tube and producing excessive loudness. The symptom disappears when reclining because of venous engorgement of the area around the opening of the tube, helping to close it off (Aronson, 1990).

ber that organic mutism following an acute neurologic insult, such as closed head injury, may persist on a psychogenic basis after the neurologic barriers to speech have resolved (Lebrun, 1990).

CASES

Case 14.1

A 31-year-old woman came to the clinic with a four-month history of voice difficulty, pharyngitis, and pain with swallowing. Her physical examination by an internist was normal with the exception that her voice was a "barely audible whisper." Subsequent examinations of thyroid function were normal, as were all other tests during a complete physical examination. She was referred for Ear, Nose, and Throat (ENT) and neurologic evaluations, both of which were normal. The ENT exam raised suspicions about spasmodic dysphonia.

During speech evaluation, the patient reported losing her voice following an upper respiratory infection. She had seen six different physicians about the problem and had been placed on antibiotics, given flu shots, and provided with several thyroid investigations, all failing to explain or remediate her aphonia.

Psychosocial history revealed that she had been working for a large department store for about a year. Three months prior to the onset of her voice problem, she was transferred from a personnel office to an automotive department, at which time she lost her voice for about a week. She was unhappy with the new job and was promised that she could eventually return to personnel. She subsequently discovered that this would not be the case, but was not told so directly by her supervisor. Shortly after this, she lost her voice again. She had been out of work since that time because of her inability to speak. She planned to go back to work when her voice returned.

The patient lived with her parents and a younger brother. She had a relationship with a man but felt he was pushing her too hard toward marriage. Her parents thought she could do better than her current boyfriend. She admitted to uncertainty about whether to continue the relationship.

Her voice was completely aphonic, but her whisper was strong. All other aspects of speech and oral mechanism exam were normal. She experienced pain with minimal digital pressure in the thyrohyoid space. Symptomatic voice therapy was undertaken. Within 40 minutes her voice returned to normal. She was able to speak without effort for the next hour, including in the presence of her mother and uncle, who had accompanied her to the clinic.

The clinician subsequently told the patient that there was no current physical restriction to her speaking normally, even though her initial aphonia might have been triggered by organic illness. The roles of stress, conflict, and other emotional factors in the maintenance of her aphonia were discussed, as was the importance of confronting issues that could be producing conflict. At this time, the patient admitted that she did not like her job and wanted to quit and strike out on her own. She admitted that she had never confronted her employer about being "double crossed" regarding her transfer to a more acceptable job. She declined to pursue psychiatric assessment. She was asked to write to the clinician about her voice in one month, and she agreed.

The clinician concluded that the patient had a "psychogenic aphonia, resolved with symptomatic therapy. The exact mechanism for her aphonia is not entirely clear, but work-related and perhaps family and personal relationship issues are probably involved."

A month later the clinician received a letter from the patient stating that her voice had remained normal. She also stated, "I took care of the important things we discussed. I went back to my place of employment to confront my boss in personnel. I was asked to stay on but I made my final decision and said no. Now I'm looking for another job. Also, I ended a relationship that I thought was causing a lot of stress. I feel I'm more capable of handling stress now, due to your interest in me. Thank you for your encouragement in dealing with my symptoms. It was a great help and opened my eyes."

Commentary. (1) Psychogenic aphonia often develops on the heels of an upper respiratory infection or cold. (2) The psychosocial history frequently reveals significant stress, anxiety, or conflict and is essential to understanding the mechanism underlying the speech disorder. (3) Psychogenic aphonia often leads to multiple medical examinations and recommendations for the treatment of a presumed organic cause, which often serve to reinforce the notion that the problem is organic. (4) Symptomatic therapy, combined with discussion of psychosocial issues, often results in rapid return of normal voice. (5) Psychiatric assessment may be declined by patients with psychogenic voice disorders and, in some cases, is not essential. This patient appears to have done quite well after her voice returned to normal, but the long-term outcome for her was uncertain. (6) Effective management of psychogenic voice disorders usually must be multidisciplinary. Speech evaluation and management proved crucial in this case, but it was not likely to have been successful if the patient had not been reassured by other medical subspecialists about the absence of serious organic illness.

Case 14.2

A 50-year-old woman came to the clinic with a 10-month history of fatigue and an 8-month history of severe pain in her right shoulder and the fingers of her right hand. Local evaluation suggested a brachial plexus neuropathy of unknown cause. Three months after onset of her initial symptoms, she developed a voice problem following a flulike illness. Neurologic evaluation suggested a spasmodic dysphonia or "neurologic amyotrophy" of undetermined etiology. An immunologist suspected a viral infection and told her it would take a long time for her nerves to regenerate. One month prior to coming to the clinic, she developed increasing shortness of breath, a tremorlike disorder of breathing, and an unsteady gait. The internist who first saw her at the clinic noted the striking dysphonia and "tremorous loss of organized muscle activity in the muscles of breathing." There was no evidence of airway compromise. His impression was that the patient had a neurologic disorder, most likely on a degenerative or inflammatory basis.

Neurologic examination suggested mild residual weakness in her right arm and shoulder and evidence of an old right radiculopathy. There was no evidence of a peripheral neuropathy or defect in neuromuscular transmission. Magnetic resonance imaging (MRI) of the head and cervical spine and additional x-rays and laboratory studies were negative. The neurologist noted her voice difficulty and irregularities in breathing and felt the patient had an indeterminate CNS disease as their cause. A second neurologist evaluated the patient and felt there was evidence of laryngeal myoclonus or dystonia and maybe respiratory myoclonus, perhaps on an autoimmune basis. Multiple laboratory tests failed to reveal evidence of autoimmune disease. Botox injection for her voice problem was recommended.

Prior to Botox injection, the patient was seen for speech evaluation. She stated that her voice difficulty was accompanied by shortness of breath, a rushing sound in her ears, and a need to maintain conscious awareness of swallowing because her throat felt full. Her voice worsened under conditions of stress and fatigue.

During speech and occasionally at rest, there were coarse, somewhat jerky, side-to-side, tremorlike movements of her head and occasional myoclonic-like jerking of her arms. Her breathing was paradoxic and jerky, and inspiratory and expiratory cycles tended to be short, especially during speech. There was considerable neck tension during speaking. She engaged in some effortful and dramatic groping when attempting to puff her cheeks. The thyrohyoid space was markedly narrowed, and she experienced considerable pain with minimal pressure in that area. Her speech was characterized by a continuous marked strained, tight, spasmodic voice quality with mildly reduced loudness. Phrase length was variable secondary to the dysphonia and abnormal breathing. She could not sustain a vowel for more than 4 seconds. Her attempts to produce speech AMRs were accompanied by significant orofacial struggle.

The clinician suspected a psychogenic component to the voice problem, and symptomatic therapy was undertaken. The patient's voice returned to normal within about 15 minutes and was maintained for the next 45 minutes without noticeable effort on her part. As her voice improved, her breathing pattern normalized, and her coarse head tremor and shakiness subsided. The myoclonic jerking of her arms and torso persisted but were reduced in frequency. The patient was extremely pleased with the improvement of her voice. The scheduled Botox injection was canceled.

The patient was a medical science writer and was perplexed at her dramatic improvement. Her psychosocial history was discussed, and she revealed that she had been under considerable stress because of a difficult-to-manage adolescent son who had problems with the law and drug abuse. She was urged to complete her medical workup and return in several days to evaluate her progress. Five days later, she reported that her voice had remained normal. She was also reevaluated by her neurologist, who stated, "I am left to conclude that her movement disorder(s) were not due to primary organic etiology. Her response to voice therapy is obviously very gratifying." The final neurologic diagnosis was that she had had a brachial plexus injury but that there was no evidence of other neurologic disease. Follow-up assessment was recommended.

The patient returned six months later. She had had no recurrence of her voice difficulty but did have some ongoing problems with shoulder pain. Family stresses persisted, but she, her husband, and her son were receiving counseling. The possible causes of her spastic dysphonia were discussed and the meaning of the "nonorganic" or "psychological" origins of her problem clarified. She was told that her problem might best be viewed as a learned response to her neck-shoulder pain and to a viral illness that was present at the time her voice difficulty began. It was suggested that her physical response to her organic illnesses became habituated and that therapy was effective because it helped put her physical manner of speaking into a more normal mode. The role of psychological stress in producing her disorder was also discussed. She was urged to contact the clinician if she had any further questions or difficulties. Nine months later the patient called the clinician to indicate that she maintained her normal voice in spite of an occasional sensation of tightness in her neck, often associated with stress. Her mother had died recently, and she was grieving and had become responsible for her father's care. Her son continued to have difficulty. She had not developed any breathing difficulty or abnormal movements in her torso or arms.

Commentary. (1) Adductor spasmodic dysphonia can be psychogenic in origin. (2) Psychogenic voice disorders can develop in association with neurologic disease (brachial plexus injury in this case) as well as respiratory or upper respiratory functions. (3) Psychogenic voice disorders can be misinterpreted as neurologic in origin. The voice problem may be associated with other nonorganic disorders of movement, such as the abnormal patterns of breathing and jerkiness in the limbs noted in this patient. (4) Symptomatic therapy can lead to the rapid resolution of psychogenic voice disorders, with obvious benefits to the patient and with clear implications for diagnosis. (5) Successful treatment of psychogenic voice disorders can put an end to treatment recommendations based on an assumption of organic illness. (Botox injection was planned in this case.) This eliminates the risks and expense associated with an invasive procedure, as well as reinforcement of the patient's belief that the symptoms are organic. (6) The exact mechanism for psychogenic voice disorders is not always apparent. In this case, the patient's brachial plexus injury, the suggestion to her about the possible serious nature of her voice and breathing difficulty, and perhaps issues related to family stress may have combined to set the stage for her nonorganic movement disorders.

Case 14.3

A 38-year-old man presented to the emergency room with swelling and pain on the left side of his face of three days' duration. He had also been "stuttering" since his discharge from a local hospital three months earlier when he was first worked up for pain, headache, and right extremity tremor. The admitting resident was suspicious of primary CNS disease. Neurologic consultation identified the presence of speech abnormality, right extremity tremor, and gait difficulty but raised suspicions that at least some of his problems might be nonorganic.

Subsequent neurologic tests were negative with the exception that an electromyogram demonstrated a mild right ulnar neuropathy at the elbow. An electroencephalogram showed mild generalized irregularities that were nonspecific. He had periauricular and facial cellulitis, which responded rapidly to treatment with antibiotics. Speech and psychiatric evaluations were requested.

During speech evaluation, the patient reported some fluctuation of his stuttering since onset but no return to normal. He had had some speech therapy at his local hospital but without improvement. The oral mechanism was normal with the exception of what appeared to be give-way weakness during testing of lower face strength. His conversational speech, reading, and repetition were characterized by a remarkable degree of dysfluency in which he repeated each phoneme of each word 4 to 6 times. Repetitions were accompanied by mild facial grimacing, eye closing, and neck extension. He did not adapt during repeated readings of the same material. Prolonged vowel was produced in a staccato or repetitive manner consistent with the speech repetitions. Speech AMRs were irregular and slow but followed the same pattern as his conversational dysfluencies. His conversational speech was telegraphic and often characterized by omissions of articles, pronouns, prepositions, and the like. He admitted to doing this intentionally in order to economize physical effort.

During 40 minutes of symptomatic speech therapy, he became able to prolong a vowel normally and could initiate some simple single words without repeating. During one hour of therapy the following day, the clinician was able to alter the patient's abnormal pattern from one of multiple sound and syllable repetitions to one of exaggerated prolongation of all syllables produced. He returned to his presenting speech pattern whenever he stopped concentrating on the new pattern of speech, however. The extreme length of time it took the patient to produce any utterances precluded a review of psychosocial history, and it was assumed this would be addressed during his scheduled psychiatric consultation.

The clinician concluded that the patient had "stuttering-like behavior of adult onset, almost certainly psychogenic in origin. His repetitions do not reflect a palilalia, nor are they consistent with typical manifestations of neurogenic stuttering. His repetitions are remarkably consistent; this is highly unusual, even in developmental stuttering, and would be very rare in neurogenic stuttering." The clinician told the patient that his current speech difficulty was not likely organic in nature. He was reassured that his problem might improve spontaneously or with therapy. The patient did not argue with this explanation but self-mockingly referred to the problem as being "all in my head." He was somewhat indifferent to the severity of his speech difficulty, the efforts made to help him improve, and the explanation given to him about the nature of his deficit.

Psychiatric evaluation the following day noted his bizarre speech. The psychiatrist found no evidence of prior psychiatric disease. The psychiatrist stated, "The only finding of note is his consistency of denial of ever experiencing or knowing distressful emotions such as fear, anxiety, anger, or sadness, and constantly minimizing the effects of trying to keep up with three jobs and raising three children." (The patient was divorced.) The patient admitted to chronic tiredness but denied any awareness or need to give in to it or change his patterns. His affect was described as inappropriately indifferent. The psychiatrist felt the findings supported a diagnosis of conversion disorder. Psychotherapy was not recommended because the patient had so little awareness of his emotions. Continued speech and physical therapy were suggested. The patient chose to return home to pursue such therapies. He was not heard from again.

Commentary. (1) Stuttering-like behaviors can develop in adulthood. They can be psychogenic in origin but may present in a milieu suggestive of neurologic disease. (2) The nature of the patient's dysfluencies and their remarkable consistency seemed incompatible with dysfluencies encountered in neurogenic stuttering. Although symptomatic therapy did not really improve speech, it did alter it. These observations led to a conclusion that the stuttering was psychogenic. (3) Psychogenic speech disorders often develop at about the same time as other physical deficits that may appear to represent organic disease. (4) The diagnosis of conversion disorder, in the absence of rapid resolution of symptoms, is often based on circumstantial evidence. Multidisciplinary evaluations can increase confidence in the diagnosis, however.

Case 14.4

A 44-year-old man came to the clinic with a fifteen-month history of tremors in his arms and hands, severe headaches, and speech difficulty, problems for which his local physicians were unable to establish a cause.

Neurologic history indicated that he developed the sudden onset of numbness and weakness on the left side of his body 15 months ago. This was accompanied by sudden hearing impairment on the left and speech difficulty described as "stuttering and slurring." Angiogram and MRI scan were normal at the time of onset. These problems resolved over several days, with some persistence of mild numbness in the left hand and arm. A week later a tremor developed in his left upper extremity, and he was unable to return to work as an insurance agent. He had been out of work for a year. For several months he had had some visual spells and headaches, and three months ago he developed "halting speech." The neurologic exam revealed the presence of tremor but noted that there were "few hard findings" and raised suspicion about nonorganic causes. Subsequent MRI scan, however, showed evidence of an old small hemorrhage in the right brain stem that might have been responsible for his initial deficits.

During speech evaluation the patient described his speech as "stuttering" with slow rate and poor enunciation. He denied difficulty with language. He denied a childhood history of speech or language problems, although he had a brother who stuttered as a child.

The AMRs of the tongue, lip, and jaw were produced with hesitation and struggle, but not like that encountered in ataxia or neurologic movement disorders. His speech was characterized by frequent repetition and prolongation of initial phonemes and sometimes the initial phoneme of the second syllable of a multisyllabic word. These dysfluencies were accompanied by some orofacial tension and eye closing. He was slow to initiate speech, and overall rate was moderately reduced. Prosody was flat, as was his overall affect, with the exception of an occasional sudden smile or laugh. His head nodding in response to yes-no questions was also hesitant and somewhat jerky. Dysfluencies during reading were similar to contextual speech. Speech AMRs were markedly irregular and hesitant but not in a manner consistent with ataxia or hyperkinetic dysarthria. His conversational language was telegraphic but not like that typically heard in Broca's aphasia.

During 30 minutes of symptomatic therapy that focused on adoption of a prolonged and somewhat sing-song prosody, fluency improved markedly, and by the end of the session speech was approximately 90% normal, with only infrequent hesitancies or repetitions. As fluency improved, facial animation also improved. The patient was seen again the following day. He had maintained his speech improvement and described it as "97% normal." The clinician agreed.

The clinician concluded, "His speech difficulty is best characterized as stuttering of psychogenic origin. Its presentation was inconsistent with neurogenic stuttering and its resolution during a brief period of behavior modification does not occur in neurogenic stuttering. We did not explore the possible origin of this problem but I explained to the patient that whatever event tipped him into his speech problem was no longer active. I also explained that his speech gains could be maintained and that further improvement could be expected, perhaps in a short period of time." The patient accepted this explanation, although somewhat blandly, and expressed confidence that his speech gains would be maintained.

When he was seen for psychiatric consultation four days later, his speech was normal. The psychiatrist established that a number of his symptoms had developed shortly after he became extremely angry during a confrontation with a claims adjuster at the insurance company where he worked. History also established a difficult childhood, an early failed marriage to a repeatedly unfaithful woman, rejection by a church of his attempts to become a minister, remarriage to a person with significant visual and hearing deficits necessitating fairly constant assistance from him, and frustrations in his and his spouse's attempts to adopt a disabled child. The psychiatrist described the patient as intense and tense, rigid, and only superficially insightful. Affect was generally flat. He hesitated to call the patient's problems a conversion reaction but did feel he was amplifying his symptoms. He offered the patient inpatient treatment that would include physical and speech therapy, if necessary, as well as psychotherapy. The patient opted to return home, however.

Commentary. (1) Psychogenic speech disorders can occur in individuals with neurologic disease. This patient's brainstem hemorrhage probably explained some of his early symptoms but did not explain his speech deficit. (2) Symptomatic therapy for psychogenic stuttering can result in rapid improvement of speech, help confirm the diagnosis as psychogenic, and faciliate psychiatric evaluation. (3) Patients who develop psychogenic speech disorders may have what appears to be a single triggering event, but their histories often contain evidence of multiple stress factors. (4) Psychogenic stuttering is sometimes accompanied by a nonfluent pattern of speech that may superficially resemble Broca's aphasia. Of interest, the patient's telegraphic speech resolved as his dysfluencies resolved.

Case 14.5

A 45-year-old woman was seen at the clinic for evaluation of a two-year history of leg weakness and speech difficulty. She initially had used a wheelchair but had graduated to a walker and then a cane. An MRI of the head and spine was normal.

Neurologic evaluation revealed a bizarre flailing and lurching gait. She would not stand alone and would not stand without touching something with both hands. There was no evidence that her ability to control her center of gravity was impaired, and her ability to remain upright despite her bizarre movements suggested excellent balance. She gave way during muscle testing, but there was no evidence of loss of muscle bulk. The neurologist felt that her gait disorder was hysterical in nature. The remainder of the neurologic workup was normal.

During speech evaluation, the patient denied any change or difficulty with speech but admitted that her husband felt her pitch was higher. She admitted that when she answered the phone people would ask if they could talk to her mother. There was marked give-way weakness on strength testing of the jaw, face, and tongue and bizarre, strugglelike behavior when she was asked to perform oral volitional movements. There was no evidence of weakness, spasticity, incoordination, or movement disorder during physical exam.

Speech was high in pitch; infantile in prosody, grammar, and content; and frequently accompanied by dysfluencies that included hesitancies and some phrase and word repetitions, with accompanying facial grimacing and eye closing. Eye contact was nearly nonexistent, and her nonverbal behavior was floridly infantile. A brief attempt was made to modify her voice and speech pattern. No change occurred.

The clinician concluded that she had a "psychogenic infantile speech pattern characterized by elevated pitch, immature prosody, and some grammatical variations which are infantile. I hear no evidence to suggest the presence of a dysarthria or apraxia of speech or other neurogenic motor speech disturbance." The clinician felt that the patient's denial of speech change or difficulty precluded the likelihood that she would benefit from therapy at that time.

Psychiatric examination failed to find evidence of a depressive, psychotic, or chemical dependency disorder. Her father had died when she was three months old, and the patient had always been sickly. She had lost two infants between her living children's births. Her mother had been neurotically overprotective, and it appeared that her husband was the same. She appeared to the psychiatrist to be "totally regressed," unable to walk and speaking in a childlike manner. A probable conversion disorder was diagnosed, and inpatient psychiatric therapy was recommended. The patient refused, returned home, and was lost to follow-up.

Commentary. *(1) Infantile speech can develop as a symptom of conversion disorder. (2) Conversion disorder can occur in a context suggestive of neurologic disease. (3) Symptomatic therapy for psychogenic speech disorders is not always recommended. At the least, the patient must be aware of and express some concern about speech difficulty, an attitude not present in this case. (4) Oral mechanism examination is often helpful for diagnosis of psychogenic speech disorders. In this case, the deficits observed were disproportionate to anything that would be predicted by her speech pattern.*

Case 14.6

A 26-year-old man was seen at the clinic for evaluation of low back pain, leg numbness, and dysarthria. His problem began two months prior to evaluation, following a fall while leaving a restaurant. There was no loss of consciousness, but he had immediate onset of severe low back pain, which required hospitalization for several weeks. His pain improved, but one week after hospital discharge he became unable to walk because of cramps in his legs. He also developed markedly slurred speech that could not be understood. He stated, "The tongue would curl up inside my mouth and I couldn't control it." This problem had improved somewhat. After a complete neurologic examination and appropriate laboratory tests, the neurologist concluded, "Neither the story nor the examination would support a diagnosis of a radiculopathy, peripheral nerve lesion, or spinal cord lesion. The distribution of his pain did not conform to any known organic neurologic condition." The neurologist referred the patient for speech evaluation.

During speech evaluation the patient revealed that he had two children through an earlier marriage, was divorced two years ago, remarried a year ago, and recently had another child about one month after the onset of his speech problem. He had owned a used car dealership for about six months but had to close it down since his illness. Of interest, he reported that his father once ran a used car dealership but had to close his business 13 years ago after suffering "crushed vertebrae" in an automobile accident. His father fully recovered and was able to begin another business.

During oral mechanism examination, the tongue was held in an elevated posture with some spontaneous variable movements at rest, usually characterized by further retraction or lateralized movements. With prodding he was able to move his tongue forward and protrude it. He was also able to lateralize, elevate, and point the tongue toward his chin. Tongue strength was grossly normal. He was able to swallow water without difficulty.

His speech was characterized by numerous articulatory distortions secondary to his retracted and elevated tongue posture. Anterior lingual fricatives and affricates were fairly consistently omitted or slighted, and lingual alveolar stops and nasals were palatized. Oral resonance was noticeably altered by his abnormal tongue posturing. Speech AMRs were normal. During conversation there were secondary struggle behaviors in the form of eye closing, mild facial grimacing, and neck extension.

An attempt was made to modify his tongue posture. With great effort he was able to produce some anterior lingual stops and nasals and reduce some of his secondary struggle behaviors. He was unimpressed with his ability to change these behaviors but did admit that they represented improvement. He stated that he felt his speech had been improving and that he did not feel a need for speech therapy.

The clinician concluded that the patient had a "probable psychogenic articulation disorder which, at this point in time, seems resistant to symptomatic therapy. Although there is a possibility that his abnormal tongue posturing represents a hyperkinetic-like dysarthria (lingual dyskinesia), I have never seen it take this specific form. The absence of chewing or swallowing difficulty in the presence of lingual retraction and elevation is quite unusual in organic disturbance." The patient was told that his speech problem might represent a psychological reaction to his recent medical difficulties or other undefined problems. He was told that his speech problem did not fit any commonly recognized neurologic speech deficit and was also told that his pattern of slow, steady improvement was reason for optimism about continued recovery. He was told that he might benefit from symptomatic speech therapy if improvement ceased or regression occurred.

The speech pathologist and the patient's neurologist recommended psychiatric consultation, but the patient declined. He was lost to follow-up, but two years later the neurologist and speech pathologist were called to give depositions related to a suit the patient had initiated against the owner of the restaurant where he had fallen.

Commentary. *(1) Psychogenic speech disorders can affect articulation. (2) Psychogenic speech disturbances often begin following a physical injury. (3) Psychosocial history occasionally reveals a "model" for nonorganic physical deficits. The similarity of the patient's difficulties to his father's was, at the least, a very interesting coincidence that is perhaps of diagnostic significance. (4) Psychogenic speech disturbances occasionally occur in people who are considering or are involved in litigation related to their physical or speech difficulties. In some cases, this can raise concerns about malingering or represent a vehicle for secondary gain in conversion disorder.*

Case 14.7

A 31-year-old woman was admitted through the emergency room with right-sided weakness and mutism. Initial impression was that she had had a stroke. Neurologic exam the following day, however, suggested the presence of give-way weakness of the right extremities, raising suspicions of a functional component to her deficits. Subsequent computed tomography scan was normal. She was referred for speech evaluation.

During the initial part of the evaluation, she was virtually mute, with occasional high-pitched grunting. She appreciated the humor in jokes, and she followed complex commands without error. She communicated normally through writing. When pushed to speak, she ultimately produced some broken syllables with much associated facial grimacing. Symptomatic treatment was undertaken, and within 45 minutes her speech had returned to normal. The clinician concluded that her speech deficit was psychogenic.

Subsequent evaluation in psychiatry, conducted with the help of family members, indicated that she had significant problems with impulse control for some time and long-standing difficulties with low self-esteem and conflict with her mother. She had attempted suicide at age 18. She received a psychiatric diagnosis of conversion disorder and probable borderline personality disorder.

During subsequent inpatient psychiatric treatment, her right-sided weakness resolved and her mood improved. When discharge was discussed, she became hostile and depressed and reported suicidal ideation. She was transferred to a closed psychiatric unit, where she had what were described as temper tantrums with shouting and striking out at others. She was ultimately transferred to outpatient treatment in her hometown.

Commentary. *(1) Conversion disorder can present as muteness, and this may be accompanied by other physical deficits suggestive of focal neurologic impairment. In this case, it initially appeared that the patient had suffered a left hemisphere stroke, with right-sided weakness and muteness due to aphasia or apraxia of speech. (2) Symptomatic speech therapy can produce rapid improvement of speech, helping to rule out organic pathology as the primary explanation for muteness. (3) In some people, conversion disorder seems to occur as a relatively isolated event. In others, it may represent a symptom of more serious and longstanding psychological difficulties.*

SUMMARY

1. Speech can be altered in a variety of ways by psychological disturbances. Such disorders are not unusual within large multidisciplinary medical practices. Of importance, they can be very similar to and difficult to distinguish from organic disease, including neurologic disease and its associated motor speech disorders. Psychogenic and neurogenic speech disorders can also co-occur.

2. Depression, manic depression, and schizophrenia tend to be associated with logically predictable speech characteristics, and such characteristics may actually help to define the psychopathology. It is important to keep in mind that depression occurs frequently in neurologic disease and that the language of schizophrenic patients may be difficult to distinguish from some of the characteristics of aphasia.

3. Speech disorders that reflect responses to life stress, conversion or somatization disorders, or factitious disorders or malingering are most often manifested as changes in voice, fluency, or prosody. Voice disorders probably represent the largest category of psychogenic speech disturbances, and most are characterized by aphonia, hoarseness, or spasmodic dysphonia. Stuttering-like behavior probably represents the next largest category of psychogenic speech disturbance. Articulation and prosodic deficits, infantile speech, and mutism may also be caused by psychological disorders.

4. Many psychogenic speech disorders present in a manner that raises suspicions about neurologic disease. The distinction between the two etiologies can be difficult to make. Details of the history as well as observations made during clinical evaluation are important to diagnosis. The degree to which a speech disturbance can be classified neurologically, consistency of oral mechanism and speech findings, the degree to which the speech deficit is suggestible and distractible, patterns of fatigue of speech, and reversibility of the speech deficit are particularly important for identifying the presence of a psychogenic speech disorder.

5. Symptomatic therapy for suspected psychogenic speech disorders may result in rapid and dramatic speech improvement. Such symptom reversibility helps to rule out neurologic causes and confirm the diagnosis as psychogenic. This establishes the value of symptomatic therapy during diagnostic assessment. The absence of an immediate response to symptomatic therapy, however, does not rule out psychogenic etiology.

6. Because psychogenic speech disturbances can occur in people with neurologic disease, it is important to recognize the lawful manifestations of neurogenic motor speech disorders and features of speech production that are incompatible with neurologic disease. The ability to make such distinctions is probably highly dependent on clinical experience with large numbers and wide varieties of motor speech disorders, as well as familiarity with the varieties of

speech disturbances that may occur secondary to psychological disturbances. The distinction between neurogenic and psychogenic speech disorders not only has implications for the diagnosis and management of the speech disorders themselves but also may contribute importantly to the diagnosis of neurologic and psychiatric disorders.

REFERENCES

American Psychiatric Association: Diagnostic and statistical manual of mental disorders, ed 3 revised, Washington, DC, 1987, American Psychiatric Association,

Aronson AE: Clinical voice disorders. New York, 1990, Thieme.

Aronson AE, Peterson HW, and Litin EM: Psychiatric symptomatology in functional dysphonia and aphonia, J Speech Hear Disord 31:115, 1966.

Attanasio JS: A case of late-onset or acquired stuttering in adult life, J Fluency Disord 12:287, 1987.

Baker JHE and Silver JR: Hysterical paraplegia, J Neurol Neurosurg Psychiatry 50:375, 1987.

Baumgartner J and Duffy JR: Adult onset stuttering: psychogenic and/or neurologic. Miniseminar presented at American Speech-Language-Hearing Association Convention, Detroit, MI, November 1986.

Brookshire RH: A dramatic response to behavior modification by a patient with rapid onset of dysfluent speech. In Helm-Estabrooks N and Aten JL, editors: Difficult diagnoses in communication disorders, Boston, 1989, College-Hill.

Carden NL and Schramel DJ: Observations of conversion reactions seen in troops involved in the Viet Nam conflict, Am J Psychiat 123:21, 1966.

Darby J and Hollien H: Vocal and speech patterns of depressive patients, Folia Phoniatr 29:279, 1977.

Darby JK, Simmons N, and Berger PA: Speech and voice parameters of depression: a pilot study, J Commun Disord 17:75, 1984.

Deal J: Sudden onset of stuttering: a case report, J Speech Hear Disord 47:301, 1982.

Deal J and Cannito MP: Acquired neurogenic dysfluency. In Vogel D and Cannito MP, editors: Treating disordered speech motor control, Austin, TX, 1991, Pro-Ed.

Deal JL and Doro JM: Episodic hysterical stuttering, J Speech Hear Disord 52:299, 1987.

DiSimoni FG, Darley FL, and Aronson, AE: Patterns of dysfunction in schizophrenic patients on an aphasia battery, J Speech Hear Disord 42:498, 1977.

Duffy JR: A puzzling case of adult onset stuttering. In Helm-Estabrooks N and Aten JL, editors: Difficult diagnoses in communication disorders, Boston, 1989, College-Hill Press.

Eames P: Hysteria following brain injury, J Neurol Neurosurg Psychiatry 55:1046, 1992.

Fahn S and Williams DT: Psychogenic dystonia, Adv Neurol, 50:431-455, 1988.

Folks DG, Ford CV, and Regan WM: Conversion symptoms in a general hospital, Psychosomatics 25:285, 1984.

Ford CV and Folks DG: Conversion disorders: an overview, Psychosomatics 26:371, 1985.

Freeman RL and others: The neurology of depression: cognitive and behavioral deficits with focal findings in depression and resolution after electroconvulsive therapy, Arch Neurol 42:289, 1985.

George MK, O'Connel JE, and Batch AJ: Paradoxical vocal cord motion: an unusual cause of stridor, J Laryngol Otol 105:312, 1991.

Gerson SN, Benson DF, and Frazier SH: Diagnosis: schizophrenia versus posterior aphasia, Am J Psychiatry 134:9, 1977.

Hartman DE, Daily WW, and Morin KN: A case of superior laryngeal nerve paresis and psychogenic dysphonia, J Speech Hear Disord, 54:526, 1989.

Head H: An address on the diagnosis of hysteria, BMJ, 1:827, 1922.

Hirschfeld RMA and Goodwin FK: Mood disorders. In Talbott JA, Hales RE, and Yudofsky SC, Textbook of psychiatry, Washington, DC, 1988, American Psychiatric Press.

Kallen D, Marshall RC, and Casey DE: Atypical dysarthria in Munchausen syndrome, Br J Disord Commun 21:377, 1986.

Keane JR: Wrong-way deviation of the tongue with hysterical hemiparesis, Neurology 36:1406, 1986.

Kellman RM and Leopold DA: Paradoxical vocal cord motion: an important cause of stridor, Laryngoscope 92:58, 1982.

Koller W and others: Psychogenic tremors, Neurology 39:1094, 1989.

Lazare A: Current concepts in psychiatry: conversion symptoms, N Engl J Med 305:745, 1981.

Lebrun Y: Mutism, London, 1990, Whurr Publishers.

Lecours AR and Vanier-Clement M: Schizophasia and jargonaphasia, Brain Lang 3:516, 1976.

Mahr G and Leith W: Psychogenic stuttering of adult onset, J Speech Hear Res 35:283, 1992.

Merskey H: Conversion symptoms revised, Semin Neurol 10:221, 1990.

Nicholi AM Jr.: The new Harvard guide to psychiatry, Cambridge, 1988, Belknap Press of Harvard University Press.

Pannbaker M: Dysphonia associated with factitious asthma, Ear Nose Throat J 69:656, 1990.

Patton H and others: Paradoxical vocal cord syndrome with surgical cure, South Med J 80:256, 1987.

Robinson RG and Benson DF: Depression in aphasic patients: frequency, severity, and clinical-pathological correlations, Brain Lang 14:282, 1981.

Robinson RG and others: Mood disorders in stroke patients: importance of location of lesion, Brain 107:81, 1984a.

Robinson RG and others: A two-year longitudinal study of post-stroke mood disorders: dynamic changes in associated variables over the first six months of follow-up, Stroke 15:510, 1984b.

Robinson RG, Lipsey JR, and Price TR: Diagnosis and clinical management of post-stroke depression, Psychosomatics 26:769, 1985.

Rogers D: Psychiatric consequences of basal ganglia disease, Semin Neurol 10:262, 1990.

Roth CR, Aronson AE, and Davis LJ: Clinical studies in psychogenic stuttering of adult onset, J Speech Hear Disord 54:634, 1989.

Sapir S and Aronson AE: Aphonia after closed head injury: aetiologic considerations, Br J Disord Commun 20:289, 1985.

Sapir S and Aronson AE: Coexisting psychogenic and neurogenic dysphonia: a source of diagnostic confusion, Br J Disord Commun 22:73, 1987.

Sapir S and Aronson AE: The relationship between psychopathology and speech and language disorders in neurologic patients, J Speech Hear Disord 55:503, 1990.

Schiffer RB: Depressive syndromes associated with diseases of the central nervous system, Semin Neurol 10:239, 1990.

Starkstein SE and Robinson RG: Aphasia and depression, Aphasiology 2:1, 1988.

Starkstein SE and Robinson RG: Depression following cerebrovascular lesions, Semin Neurol 10:247, 1990.

Stoudemire GA: Somatoform disorders, factitious disorders, and malingering. In Talbott JA, Hales RE, and Yudofsky SC, editors: Textbook of psychiatry, Washington, DC, 1988, American Psychiatric Press.

Teitelbaum ML and McHugh PR: Psychiatric conditions presenting as neurologic disease. In Johnson RT, editor: Current therapy in neurologic disease, ed 3, Philadelphia, 1990, BC Decker.

Thompson TL: Psychosomatic disorders. In Talbott JA, Hales RE, and Yudofsky SC, editors: Textbook of psychiatry, Washington, DC, 1988, American Psychiatric Press.

Tippett DC and Siebens AA: Distinguishing psychogenic from neurogenic dysfluency when neurologic and psychologic factors coexist, J Fluency Disord 16:3, 1991.

Todt EH and Howell RJ: Vocal cues as indices of schizophrenia, J Speech Hear Res 23:517, 1980.

Tomb DA: Psychiatry for the house officer, Baltimore, 1981, Williams and Wilkins.

Uomoto JM: Evaluation of neuropsychological status after traumatic brain injury. In Beukelman DR and Yorkston KM, editors: Communication disorders following traumatic brain injury: management of cognitive, language, and motor impairments, Austin, TX, 1991, Pro-Ed.

Wallen V: Primary stuttering in a 28-year-old adult, J Speech Hear Disord 26:394, 1961.

Williams JBW: Psychiatric classificiation. In Talbott JA, Hales RE, and Yudofsky SC, editors: Textbook of psychiatry, Washington, DC, 1988, American Psychiatric Press.

Ziegler FJ and Imboden JB: Contemporary conversion reactions: II A conceptual model, Arch Gen Psychiatry 6:37, 1962.

15 Differential Diagnosis

Is a speech disorder present? If so, is it neurogenic? If so, what is its type? What are the implications of the type of neurogenic speech disorder for lesion localization? To answer these and related questions, the meaning of speech signs and symptoms must be established. Meaning in this case derives from the application of a knowledge base and clinical skill to the clinical problem.

Sometimes examination findings are unambiguous and have only one possible interpretation. More often, they have two or more possible interpretations, and sometimes diagnosis can be expressed only as an ordering of possibilities. The *process of narrowing possibilities and reaching conclusions about the nature of a deficit is known as differential diagnosis.*

This chapter will summarize the distinctive clinical characteristics of the primary speech disorders that have been discussed in previous chapters. It will also highlight the similarities and differences among the speech disorders that are clinically most difficult to distinguish from one another.

GENERAL GUIDELINES FOR DIFFERENTIAL DIAGNOSIS

A few guidelines should be kept in mind in the context of differential diagnostic efforts. They may help to focus the clinician's thinking and serve as a guide to communicating with the referring professionals who are most interested in the diagnosis.

1. *Speech examination should always lead to an attempt at diagnosis.* Establishing the meaning of clinical observations is essential, especially when diagnosis is the primary purpose of examination. This is often ignored by clinicians who view their only role as that of therapist. However, even when the primary goal of examination is to address management issues, the nature of the problem should be established as clearly as possible because we usually treat what we understand better than what we do not understand.

2. *When the results of examination cannot go beyond description, the reasons should be stated explicitly.* Sometimes a diagnosis cannot be made. This can happen when abnormalities are subtle, atypical, or combine in ways that are incompatible with known patterns of speech deficit in neurologic disease. It can also occur when a patient does not or cannot cooperate with the simplest aspects of examination. When these findings or circumstances occur, they should be stated as reasons for inability to establish a diagnosis.

Even under difficult assessment circumstances or with equivocal or atypical findings, some valuable interpretations sometimes can be made, particularly when the reasons for the evaluation have been made clear by the referral source. For example, if the purpose of examination is to establish if the patient has dysarthria versus a psychogenic speech disorder, enough information may be obtained to establish that a dysarthria is present, even if its type cannot be specified. Conversely, enough speech may be produced to establish that no evidence of dysarthria was detected, even though formal examination may not have been possible. In other cases, it may be possible to state what the problem is not. For example, the clinician may be able to state that the patient has a motor speech disorder whose type is indeterminate but inconsistent with hypokinetic or hyperkinetic dysarthria; such a narrowing of diagnostic possibilities would imply that the source of the speech deficit is probably not in the basal ganglia control circuit.

3. *The clinician should not state a diagnosis when one cannot be determined.* To offer a diagnosis when evidence for it is lacking can be misleading at best and dangerous at worst. There are numerous instances in which the best diagnosis is an undetermined one. In fact, knowing that a speech diagnosis cannot be made can be helpful. For example, a diagnosis of "diagnosis undetermined" may help eliminate diseases in which the presence and nature of a motor speech disorder should be very predictable, or it may help confirm suspicions that neurologic disease may not be present. Relatedly, it may be necessary and very appropriate to provide a degree of confidence in a diagnosis by qualifiers such as "unambiguous," "most likely," "probable," " possible," or "equivocal."

4. *Diagnosis should be related to the suspected or known neurologic diagnosis or lesion localization.* Referring neurologists usually have, at the least, suspicions about lesion localization and etiology. It is appropriate, therefore, to address whether the speech diagnosis is consistent with such suspicions. If it is not, it may raise questions about the neurologic diagnosis or suggest that there is another lesion(s) or disease process at work.

5. *Different speech disturbances can co-occur.* Although a single diagnosis is parsimonious, it is not always correct. Disease does not always respect the divisions we impose on the nervous system. As a result, some neurologic diseases lead to combinations of dysarthria types, apraxia of speech, and other neurogenic speech disturbances. In addition, the presence of one neurologic disease does not preclude the presence of another, so different neurogenic speech disorders can co-occur as a result of co-occurring neurologic diseases. Finally, neurogenic speech disorders can co-occur with non-neurologic but organic speech disorders or with psychogenic speech disturbances. It is important, therefore, to recognize that diagnosis does not end when a single disorder is recognized. The clinician must establish that the recognized disorder can explain all of the deviant speech characteristics that are present. If it cannot, the presence of additional disorders must be considered.

6. *Examination sometimes leads to a conclusion that speech is normal.* A conclusion that speech is normal is not unusual when baseline assessment of speech and language is sought (1) as part of routine screening of speech (for example, screening all patients admitted to a rehabilitation unit), (2) for individuals with neurologic disease frequently associated with speech deficits (for example, amyotrophic lateral sclerosis [ALS]), or (3) when a medical procedure carries risk for speech deficits (for example, baseline assessments of patients who will undergo temporal lobectomy for control of seizure disorders or thalamotomy for control of movement disorders).

A diagnosis of normal speech sometimes requires explanation. Referral for speech evaluation is often based on someone's suspicion or complaint that speech is abnormal in some way, and the concern must be addressed. Possible explanations include, but are not limited to:

a. Speech may have changed but is still in the normal range. This is not uncommon in the early stages of some diseases; the patient hears or feels that speech has changed, but the change is insufficient to be perceived by others or detected on physical examination or by acoustic or physiologic analyses. If the patient can provide a good history and description of the changes they perceive, however, a list of diagnostic possibilities sometimes can be formulated.

b. A change has occurred but not in the motor system in general or speech specifically. For example, some depressed individuals report that speaking is effortful or abnormal. This may reflect the effect of their mood on their energy level for speech, their focus on physical manifestations rather than psychological explanations for the depression, or the effect of other factors not directly related to motor speech.

c. Speech is normal, but psychological factors have triggered a perception of abnormality by the patient. For example, fear of a disease associated with speech difficulty may be triggered by the presence of the disease and speech deficit in a loved one or by exposure to someone with a threatening communicable disease.

d. Speech is normal, but a physically traumatic event has generated a complaint of speech change. This can occur in individuals involved in litigation who may have something to gain from the presence of speech difficulty (malingering or conversion disorder). In most of these instances, however, such individuals have abnormal speech.

e. The referring individual has misperceived a normal speech variant as abnormal.

7. *Fixing a diagnostic label is a convenient shorthand for communicating information.* A diagnostic label can be misleading or of no value if it is applied (a) without thinking of its implications, (b) without explanation to people who may not know its meaning, or (c) to impart an air of knowledge when knowledge is lacking. However, if the meaning of the label is clear to the user, clinical evidence supports its use, and its meaning and implications are made clear in communication of findings, the label can convey information concisely and precisely. To experienced clinicians, a label can convey a gestalt of speech characteristics. To neurologists familiar with the neurologic correlates of motor speech disorders, the label has implications for lesion localization. In some instances, the label may generate predictions about likely management approaches. For example, a diagnosis of hypokinetic dysarthria may suggest that treatment will likely focus on reducing speech rate or increasing vocal loudness. All such implications may be tentative, but in the hands of clinicians who have a common understanding of diagnostic labels they promote effective, efficient communication.

DISTINGUISHING AMONG THE DYSARTHRIAS

There is considerable overlap among the speech characteristics that are present across dysarthria types. For example, imprecise articulation may be present in any of the dysarthrias. This means that although identification of imprecise articulation may help identify the *presence* of dysarthria, it is not very useful in *distinguishing among types* of dysarthria. There are a number of deviant speech characteristics, clusters of deviant speech charac-

teristics, associated physical findings, patient complaints, etiologies, and lesion loci for which there are varying degrees of overlap among the dysarthrias. There also are some speech characteristics and patterns of deficit that are relatively unique and allow clinical distinctions among the dysarthrias. Because the dysarthrias are a predominant focus of this book, it is appropriate to summarize here the commonalties and distinctions among them.

Anatomy and vascular distribution

When the anatomic localization or vascular source of a lesion is known, certain expectations or predictions can be made about the motor speech disorder. This information may aid (or bias) differential diagnosis and help guide judgments about the compatibility of the speech diagnosis with localization.

Table 15–1 summarizes the associations between each of the dysarthrias and the gross anatomic levels of the nervous system and the major vascular supply of each. Although there is considerable anatomic and vascular overlap across dysarthria types, certain distinctions are apparent. They can be summarized as follows:

1. Flaccid and ataxic dysarthria are not associated with supratentorial lesions or with lesions in the distribution of the anterior, middle, or posterior cerebral arteries.

2. Hypokinetic dysarthria is associated only with supratentorial (subcortical) lesions. Posterior fossa lesions and lesions in the distribution of the vertebrobasilar system may cause any type of dysarthria, except hypokinetic.

3. Only flaccid dysarthria is associated with lesions at the spinal and peripheral levels of the nervous system and their associated vascular supplies.

Etiology

When etiology is known, expectations also arise about the type of motor speech disorder that may be present. This can aid (or bias) differential diagnosis and guide judgments about the compatibility of the speech diagnosis with the known or suspected etiology.

Table 15–2 summarizes the types of motor speech disorders that are encountered with a variety of neurologic conditions. Mixed dysarthrias are not included in the table, but any etiology associated with more than a single dysarthria type can be assumed capable of causing a mixed dysarthria containing the individual types listed. The table makes clear that there is much overlap among dysarthria types as a function of etiology,

Table 15–1 Distinctions among motor speech disorders as a function of major anatomic levels of the nervous system and vascular supply*

Anatomic level	Vascular supply	Dysarthria						Apraxia of speech
		Flaccid	Spastic	Ataxic	Hypo-kinetic	Hyper-kinetic	Unilateral UMN	
Supratentorial (cerebral hemispheres, basal ganglia, thalamus)	Carotid system (major cerebral arteries & their branches)	–	+	–	+	+	+	+†
Posterior fossa (pons, medulla, midbrain, cerebellum)	Vertebro-basilar system (vertebral & basilar arteries & their branches)	+	+	+	–	+	+	–
Spinal	Spinal arteries	+	–	–	–	–	–	–
Peripheral	Branches of major extremity vessels	+	–	–	–	–	–	–

+, lesions may produce disorder; –, lesions do not produce disorder; *UMN,* upper motor neuron.
*See Tables 2–1 and 2–2 for a detailed summary of the relationships between motor speech disorders and anatomic levels, the skeleton and meninges, and the ventricular and vascular components of the nervous system.
†Left (dominant) hemisphere only.

but there are also some clear distinctions. These similarities and differences can be summarized as follows:

1. Vascular disease can cause virtually any type of dysarthria. It is a very frequent cause of spastic and unilateral upper motor neuron (UMN) dysarthria, and a common cause of ataxic dysarthria. It may cause flaccid and hyperkinetic dysarthria, but not frequently. Nonhemorrhagic stroke is the most frequent vascular cause of dysarthrias.

2. Degenerative disease can cause any type of dysarthria. It is a very frequent cause of spastic, ataxic, and hypokinetic dysarthria and a common cause of flaccid dysarthria. It may cause hyperkinetic and unilateral UMN dysarthria, but not frequently. Among the degenerative diseases, ALS is a frequent cause of flaccid and spastic dysarthria and not typically associated with any other dysarthria type; thus, the presence of another dysarthria type in someone with a diagnosis of ALS should raise suspicions about an additional disease or questions about the ALS diagnosis. Similarly, Parkinson's disease and parkinsonism are associated only with hypokinetic dysarthria, and certain degenerative cerebellar diseases only with ataxic dysarthria. The presence of other

dysarthria types in those conditions should raise similar doubts about etiology.

3. Traumatic injury can cause any type of dysarthria. In closed head injury, spastic dysarthria may occur more frequently than other types, but any type may be encountered. Penetrating head injuries rarely cause flaccid dysarthria but may cause any central nervous system (CNS) dysarthria. In contrast, skull fracture and neck trauma may cause flaccid dysarthria but not usually any other type of dysarthria.

4. Surgical trauma may cause any type of dysarthria, with the possible exception of hypokinetic dysarthria. Ear, Nose, and Throat (ENT) and cardiac/chest surgery are exclusively associated with flaccid dysarthria. Neurosurgery may cause CNS dysarthrias and is also a possible cause of flaccid dysarthria.

5. Neoplasms rarely cause hyperkinetic dysarthria but can cause other types of dysarthria.

6. Toxic and metabolic disturbances rarely cause flaccid and unilateral UMN dysarthria but are possible causes of other dysarthria types. Toxic and metabolic disturbances, especially those associated with drug abuse and the toxic effects of prescribed medication, cause hyperkinetic and ataxic dysarthria more than any other type.

Table 15–2 Distinctions among motor speech disorders as a function of etiology.

| Etiology | Dysarthria | | | | | | Apraxia of speech |
	Flaccid	Spastic	Ataxic	Hypokinetic	Hyperkinetic	Unilateral UMN	
Vascular	+	+	+	+	+	+	+
Aneurysm rupture	−	+	+	+	−	+	+
Anoxia, cardiac arrest	−	+	+	+	−	−	−
Hypoxic encephalopathy	−	−	+	+	+	−	−
Intracranial arteritis	−	+	+	−	−	+	+
Stroke, hemorrhagic	+	+	+	+	+	+	+
Stroke, nonhemorrhagic	+	+	+	+	+	+	+
Degenerative disease	+	+	+	+	+	+	+
Amyotrophic lateral sclerosis	+	+	−	−	−	−	−
Alzheimer's disease	−	−	−	+	−	−	+
Cerebellar and brainstem degeneration	−	+	+	−	−	−	−
Corticobasal degeneration	−	+	+	+	+	−	+
Dystonia musculorum deformans	−	−	−	−	+	−	−
Freidreich's ataxia	−	+	+	−	−	−	−
Hereditary cerebellar atrophy	−	−	+	−	−	−	−
Hereditary cerebral calcinosis	−	−	+	−	−	−	−
Hereditary degenerative CNS disease	−	+	+	+	+	+	+
Huntington's chorea	−	−	−	−	+	−	−
Leukoencephalopathy	−	+	+	−	−	−	+
Multiple systems atrophy	−	+	+	+	+	−	−
Olivopontocerebellar atrophy	+	+	+	+	−	−	−
Parkinson's disease	−	−	−	+	−	−	−
Parkinsonism	−	−	−	+	−	−	−
Pick's disease	−	−	−	+	−	−	−
Primary lateral sclerosis	−	+	−	−	−	−	−
Primary progressive aphasia	−	−	−	−	−	+	+
Progressive bulbar palsy	+	−	−	−	−	−	−
Progressive supranuclear palsy	−	+	+	+	−	−	−
Shy-Drager syndrome	+	+	+	+	−	−	−
Spinocerebellar degeneration	−	+	+	−	−	−	−
Striatonigral degeneration	−	+	+	+	+	−	−
Traumatic	+	+	+	+	+	+	+
Closed head injury	+	+	+	+	+	+	+
Neck trauma	+	−	−	−	−	−	−
Penetrating head injury	−	+	+	+	+	+	+
Skull fracture	+	−	−	−	−	−	−
Surgical trauma	+	+	+	−	+	+	+
Chest or cardiac	+	−	−	−	−	−	−
Ear, Nose, and Throat	+	−	−	−	−	−	−
Neurosurgical	+	+	+	−	+	+	+
Neoplastic	+	+	+	+	−	+	+
Paraneoplastic syndrome	−	+	+	−	−	−	−
Primary or metastatic	+	+	+	+	−	+	+
Toxic or metabolic	−	+	+	+	+	−	−
Botulism	+	−	−	−	−	−	−
Carbon monoxide	−	+	+	+	−	−	−
Central pontine myelinolysis	−	+	+	−	+	−	−

Table 15–2 Distinctions among motor speech disorders as a function of etiology—cont'd

Etiology	Dysarthria						Apraxia of speech
	Flaccid	Spastic	Ataxic	Hypokinetic	Hyperkinetic	Unilateral UMN	
Dialysis encephalopathy	−	+	+	−	+	−	−
Drug abuse	−	+	+	+	+	−	−
Hepatic encephalopathy	−	+	+	−	+	−	−
Hepatocerebral degeneration	−	+	+	+	+	−	−
Hypoparathyroidism	+	+	−	−	+	−	−
Hypothyroidism	−	−	+	−	−	−	−
Medication effect	−	+	+	+	+	−	−
Wilson's disease	−	+	+	+	−	−	−
Infectious	+	+	+	+	+	+	+
AIDS	+	+	+	−	−	−	−
Creutzfelt-Jakob	+	+	+	+	+	+	+
Herpes zoster	+	−	−	−	−	−	−
Infectious encephalopathy	−	+	+	+	+	−	−
Multifocal leukoencephalopathy	−	+	+	−	−	−	−
Polio	+	−	−	−	−	−	−
Sarcoidosis	+	−	−	−	−	−	−
Sydenham's chorea	−	−	−	−	+	−	−
Inflammatory	−	+	+	−	−	−	+
Encephalitis	−	+	+	+	−	−	+
Meningitis	+	+	+	−	−	−	−
Demyelinating disease	+	+	+	−	+	+	+
Chronic demyelinating polyneuritis	+	−	−	−	−	−	−
Guillain-Barré	+	−	−	−	−	−	−
Multiple sclerosis	+	+	+	−	+	+	+
Anatomic malformation	+	+	+	−	−	−	−
Arnold-chiari	+	+	+	−	−	−	−
Syringobulbia	+	+	+	−	−	−	−
Syringomyelia	+	−	−	−	−	−	−
Neuromuscular junction disease	+	−	−	−	−	−	−
Eaton-Lambert syndrome	+	−	−	−	−	−	−
Myasthenia gravis	+	−	−	−	−	−	−
Muscle disease	+	−	−	−	−	−	−
Muscular dystrophy	+	−	−	−	−	−	−
Myopathy	+	−	−	−	−	−	−
Myotonic dystrophy	+	−	−	−	−	−	−
Neuropathy, undetermined etiology	+	−	−	−	−	−	−
Other	+	+	+	+	+	+	+
Chorea gravidarum	−	−	−	−	+	−	−
Meige's syndrome	−	−	−	−	+	−	−
Myoclonic epilepsy	−	−	−	−	+	−	−
Normal pressure hydrocephalus	−	+	+	−	−	−	−
Radiation necrosis	+	−	+	+	−	−	−
Seizure disorder	−	−	−	−	−	−	+
Tourette's syndrome	−	−	−	−	+	−	−
Undetermined disease	+	+	+	+	+	+	+

+, possible cause; −, rare/never, or uncertain cause; *UMN* upper motor neuron.
This table is based primarily on reviews of Mayo Clinic cases in Chapters 4 through 12, but also on published data when applicable.

7. Infectious and inflammatory conditions are possible but not common causes of dysarthrias. Because their effects are diffuse or have multiple possible foci, they generally do not lead to distinctive expectations regarding dysarthria type. Examples of exceptions include botulism, herpes zoster, and polio (flaccid dysarthria); hypothyroidism (ataxic dysarthria); and Sydenham's chorea (hyperkinetic dysarthria).

8. Demyelinating diseases may cause any type of dysarthria but rarely hypokinetic dysarthria. Guillain-Barré syndrome is associated with flaccid but not other dysarthria types, and multiple sclerosis probably causes ataxic dysarthria more frequently than any other dysarthria type.

9. Anatomic malformations such as Arnold-Chiari, syringobulbia, and syringomyelia are more frequently associated with flaccid dysarthria than any other dysarthria type. Because Arnold-Chiari malformation and syringobulbia can affect posterior fossa structures, however, they may also be associated with spastic or ataxic dysarthria.

10. Neuromuscular junction disorders, muscle disease, and neuropathies are, by definition, disorders of peripheral nerves. As a result, they are exclusively associated with flaccid dysarthria.

11. The "other" conditions listed in Table 15–2 are not common causes of dysarthrias, but some of them are associated with only one dysarthria type.

12. Any type of dysarthria may be present in the absence of an established neurologic diagnosis. The etiology is undetermined very frequently in hyperkinetic dysarthria and often in spastic and ataxic dysarthria.

Oral mechanism findings

Table 15–3 summarizes oral mechanism findings associated with various motor speech disorders. There is considerable overlap across disorders but some findings are much more common in some disorders than others, whereas some are unusual or should not be present in others.

The presence or absence of certain oral mechanism findings is not a requirement for any motor speech disorder diagnosis. They are confirmatory signs only; that is, they help support a diagnosis but are neither diagnostic of nor exclusionary of any type of motor speech disorder. The major distinguishing features of oral mechanism findings can be summarized as follows.

Flaccid dysarthria. Atrophy and fasciculations in speech muscles are frequently but not invariably present in flaccid dysarthria, but they are not expected in any other motor speech disorder. Hypotonia and a hypoactive gag reflex are encountered more commonly in flaccid dysarthria than any other motor speech disorder. Rapid deterioration in the strength of speech muscles during nonspeech tasks is distinctive of myasthenia gravis but should not be encountered in any other flaccid dysarthria or in any other motor speech disorder. Nasal regurgitation is a possible finding in flaccid dysarthria and is unusual in other motor speech disorders.

Spastic dysarthria. Pathologic reflexes (suck, snout, jaw jerk), hyperactive gag reflex, and pseudobulbar affect are common and more frequently found in spastic dysarthria than in any other motor speech disorder. Dysphagia and drooling are probably more common in patients with spastic dysarthria than any other motor speech disorder, but they are not distinctive of spastic dysarthria.

Ataxic dysarthria. A normal oral mechanism examination is not uncommon in speakers with ataxic dysarthria. However, their jaw, face, and lingual nonspeech alternating motion rates (AMRs) frequently may be dysmetric, an observation not commonly made in other motor speech disorders.

Hypokinetic dysarthria. Facial masking, tremulousness of orofacial structures, and reduced range of movement on nonspeech AMR tasks are common in hypokinetic dysarthria. Such abnormalities are uncommon in other motor speech disorders.

Hyperkinetic dysarthria. A number of abnormalities in the oral mechanism may be apparent at rest, during nonspeech sustained postures or movement, and during speech. The presence of quick or slow patterned or unpatterned adventitious movements is a strong confirmatory sign of hyperkinetic dysarthria. It should be kept in mind, however, that some hyperkinesias occur only during speech and that the absence of hyperkinesias at rest or during nonspeech tasks is not necessarily evidence against a diagnosis of hyperkinetic dysarthria. The presence of abnormal, involuntary movements in the orofacial muscles (with the exception of fasciculations, synkinesis, and myokymia in some speakers with flaccid dysarthria) is very uncommon in other motor speech disorders.

Unilateral upper motor neuron dysarthria. Unilateral right or left central facial weakness and lingual weakness without atrophy or fasciculations are common findings. These unilateral findings are unusual in other dysarthria types, although flaccid dysarthria may also be associated with unilateral face and lingual weakness.

Speech characteristics

Differential diagnosis among the dysarthrias is made on the basis of perceived deviant speech characteristics. Experienced clinicians probably arrive at a diagnosis through perception of a gestalt of speech abnormalities, rather than a simple listing of deviant characteristics. However, the gestalt is created by the co-occurrence of individual characteristics whose presence should be documented in support of the diagnosis. Table 15–4 lists the speech characteristics that are most helpful in distinguishing among the dysarthrias and apraxia of speech (AOS). The list is not as exhaustive as those provided in each chapter on the individual dysarthrias because only characteristics that are helpful in distinguishing among the dysarthrias are included. A summary of the distinctive characteristics of each single dysarthria type and its relationship to other dysarthria types follows.

Flaccid dysarthria. Phonatory and resonatory abnormalities are the most common distinguishing features of flaccid dysarthria. Continuous breathiness, diplophonia, audible inspiration, and short phrases—reflecting vocal cord or laryngeal-respiratory weakness—may be prominent when the vagus nerve is involved. They are uncommon or less pronounced in other dysarthria types. Laryngeal stridor may occur in hyperkinetic dysarthria, but it is usually accompanied by other obvious hyperkinesias when it does. Short phrases may be present in spastic and hyperkinetic dysarthria, but they are generally not accompanied by continuous breathiness or other evidence of vocal cord weakness when they are. Breathiness may occur in hypokinetic dysarthria and can be difficult to distinguish from the breathiness of flaccid dysarthria, although diplophonia and hoarseness in flaccid dysarthria may aid the distinction between the two types. Although hypernasality may occur in other dysarthria types—especially spastic and hypokinetic—it is usually most pronounced in flaccid dysarthria. Audible nasal emission and nasal snorting are uncommon in other dysarthria types. Finally, flaccid dysarthria is the only motor speech disorder in which rapid deterioration of speech can occur during continuous speaking (with recovery with rest), as in myasthenia gravis.

Spastic dysarthria. A combination of slow rate, slow and regular speech AMRs, and a strained-strangled voice quality represent the "classic" speech pattern of spastic dysarthria. The co-occurrence of these three characteristics is unexpected in other dysarthria types. Strained-strangled voice quality may occur in hyperkinetic dysarthria (for example, adductor spasmodic dysphonia) but is generally not associated with significant slowing of AMRs in a regular manner or with a dramatic slowing of rate. Slow rate is not uncommon in other dysarthria types but usually is not also accompanied by strained-strangled voice quality. Slow rate and excess and equal stress may make spastic dysarthria difficult to distinguish from ataxic dysarthria, except that ataxic dysarthria is not associated with strained-strangled voice quality.

Ataxic dysarthria. Irregular articulatory breakdowns during connected speech, irregular speech AMRs, and dysprosody are the primary distinctive features of ataxic dysarthria. Hyperkinetic and unilateral UMN dysarthrias may be difficult to distinguish from ataxic dysarthria. However, hyperkinetic dysarthria often is accompanied by adventitious movements of the jaw, face, or tongue, abnormalities not present in ataxic dysarthria. Unilateral UMN dysarthria sometimes has ataxic-like irregular articulatory breakdowns; in such cases, the presence of unilateral lower facial weakness and lingual weakness may aid conclusions about dysarthria type; that is, isolated ataxic dysarthria usually is not associated with asymmetric facial weakness.

Hypokinetic dysarthria. The classic constellation of speech characteristics associated with hypokinetic dysarthria includes monopitch, monoloudness, reduced stress and loudness, a tendency toward rapid or accelerated rate, and rapid and blurred speech AMRs. Hypokinetic dysarthria is the only dysarthria in which rapid rate may occur, and it is rapid rate that is most useful in differential diagnosis. It should be noted, however, that rapid or accelerated rate is not invariably present in hypokinetic dysarthria. Finally, although repeated phonemes and palilalia are not always present in hypokinetic dysarthria, their presence is distinctively associated with hypokinetic dysarthria.

Hyperkinetic dysarthria. Hyperkinetic dysarthria may be manifested in multiple and heterogeneous ways. Of all of the types of dysarthria, it is probably the one in which visual observation during speech helps to define the disorder because involuntary movements of the jaw, face, and tongue during speech so obviously explain many of its deviant auditory perceptual characteristics.

Speech abnormalities such as tremor or myoclonus distinguish hyperkinetic dysarthria from other types by their regularity, whereas unpredictable and variable speech abnormalities associated with chorea, dystonia, and other problems are distinguished by their unpredictability and capacity to interrupt the flow of speech in nonstereotypic

Table 15–3 Distinguishing oral mechanism findings among motor speech disorders

| Physical findings | Dysarthria | | | | | | Apraxia of speech |
	Flaccid	Spastic	Ataxic	Hypokinetic	Hyperkinetic	Unilateral UMN	
Hypoactive gag	+	−	−	−	−	−	−
Hypotonia	+	−	+	−	−	−	−
Atrophy	++	−	−	−	−	−	−
Facial myokymia	++	−	−	−	−	−	−
Fasciculations	++	−	−	−	−	−	−
Rapid deterioration & recovery with rest	++	−	−	−	−	−	−
Synkinesis (eyeblink/lower face)	++	−	−	−	−	−	−
Nasal regurgitation	++	−	−	−	−	−	−
Unilateral palatal weakness	++	−	−	−	−	−	−
Dysphagia	+	+	−	+	+	+	−
Drooling	+	+	−	+	−	+	−
Hyperactive gag	−	++	−	−	−	−	−
Sucking reflex	−	++	−	−	−	−	−
Snout reflex	−	++	−	−	−	−	−
Jaw jerk reflex	−	++	−	−	−	−	−
Pseudobulbar affect	−	++	−	−	−	−	−
Dysmetric jaw, face, tongue AMRs	−	−	++	−	−	−	−
Masked facies	−	−	−	++	−	−	−
Tremulous jaw, lips, tongue	−	−	−	++	−	−	−
Reduced range of motion on AMR tasks	−	+	−	++	−	−	−
Head tremor	−	−	+	+	+	−	−

ways. Hyperkinetic dysarthria is the only dysarthria in which abnormal noises may interrupt speech or be produced when the patient is not speaking.

Hyperkinetic dysarthria is probably most frequently difficult to distinguish from spastic and ataxic dysarthria. The strained-strangled voice quality of spastic dysarthria may occur in hyperkinetic dysarthria, but hyperkinetic dysarthria can affect isolated speech valves, a very unusual occurrence in spastic dysarthria. Variability of breakdowns can make hyperkinetic and ataxic dysarthria sound similar, but the presence of involuntary movements in hyperkinetic dysarthria generally helps to distinguish it from ataxic dysarthria.

Unilateral UMN dysarthria. Unilateral UMN dysarthria may be distinguished from other dysarthria types more by its mildness and somewhat nebulous speech characteristics than by any distinctive characteristics of its own. It is probably most easily confused with flaccid and ataxic dysarthria because of the predominance of imprecise articulation and the occasional occurrence of irregular articulatory breakdowns in it. The fact that it is rarely accompanied by resonance or voice abnormalities may help distinguish it from flaccid dysarthria. There is a tendency for AMRs in unilateral UMN dysarthria to be regular, in spite of the occurrence of irregular articulatory breakdowns during contextual speech; this may help distinguish unilateral UMN dysarthria from ataxic dysarthria because speech AMRs are usually irregular in ataxic dysarthria.

DISTINGUISHING DYSARTHRIAS FROM APRAXIA OF SPEECH

The distinction between dysarthria and AOS, in most cases, is not as difficult as distinguishing among the dysarthrias. Difficulties arise most often in attempting to differentiate AOS from ataxic

Table 15–3 Distinguishing oral mechanism findings among motor speech disorders—cont'd

Physical findings	Dysarthria						Apraxia of speech
	Flaccid	Spastic	Ataxic	Hypokinetic	Hyperkinetic	Unilateral UMN	
Involuntary head, jaw, face, tongue, palate, respiratory movements during sustained postures or during movement	–	–	–	–	++	–	–
Sensory "tricks"	–	–	–	–	++	–	–
Relatively sustained head deviation (torticollis)	–	–	–	–	++	–	–
Myoclonus of palate, pharynx, larynx, lips, nares, tongue, or respiratory muscles	–	–	–	–	++	–	–
Multiple motor tics	–	–	–	–	++	–	–
Jaw, lip, tongue, pharyngeal, or palatal tremor	–	–	–	–	++	–	–
Facial grimacing during speech	–	–	–	–	++	–	–
Unilateral lower face weakness	–	–	–	–	–	++	+
Unilateral lingual weakness without atrophy/ fasciculation	+	–	–	–	–	+	+
Nonverbal oral apraxia	–	–	–	–	–	–	++

+, may be present but not generally distinguishing; ++, distinguishing when present; –, not usually present; *AMR,* alternating motion rate; *UMN,* upper motor neuron.

dysarthria or in attempting to establish if both AOS and a dysarthria are simultaneously present. In the latter case, the separation of apraxic from unilateral UMN dysarthric characteristics often must be made. The following subsections summarize the localization, etiologic, oral mechanism, and speech characteristics of AOS and dysarthria that best distinguish between them.

Anatomy and vascular distribution

Anatomically, AOS is a supratentorial disorder. It is nearly always associated with left hemisphere pathology, except in cases with right hemisphere or mixed language dominance. In contrast, dysarthrias can arise from supratentorial, posterior

fossa, spinal, or peripheral lesions. Similarly, with vascular etiologies AOS is caused by carotid system lesions, usually in the distribution of the left middle cerebral artery, whereas dysarthrias can be associated with lesions in a much wider vascular distribution (see Table 15–1).

In terms of gross localization, therefore, AOS is most like spastic, hypokinetic, hyperkinetic, and unilateral UMN dysarthria. In dysarthria, supratentorial lesions are more often subcortical than cortical, whereas lesions leading to AOS are probably more often cortical than subcortical. Of the supratentorial dysarthrias, unilateral UMN dysarthria is probably most difficult to distinguish from AOS.

Table 15–4 Distinguishing speech characteristics among motor speech disorders

Dimensions	Dysarthria						Apraxia of speech
	Flaccid	Spastic	Ataxic	Hypokinetic	Hyperkinetic	Unilateral UMN	
Hypernasality	++	+	−	+	−	−	−
Breathiness (continuous)	++	−	−	+	−	−	−
Diplophonia	++	−	−	−	−	−	−
Nasal emission (audible)	++	−	−	−	−	−	−
Audible inspiration (stridor)	++	−	−	−	+	−	−
Short phrases	++	+	−	−	+	−	−
Rapid deterioration & recovery with rest	++	−	−	−	−	−	−
Speaking on inhalation	++	−	−	−	−	−	−
Harshness	−	++	−	−	+	−	−
Low pitch	−	++	−	−	+	−	−
Slow rate	−	++	+	−	+	+	+
Strained-strangled quality	−	++	−	−	+	−	−
Pitch breaks	+	++	−	−	−	−	−
Slow & regular AMRs	−	++	−	−	−	−	−
Excess & equal stress	−	+	++	−	−	−	+
Irregular articulatory breakdowns	−	−	++	−	+	+	+
Irregular AMRs	−	−	++	−	++	+	−
Distorted vowels	−	−	++	−	++	−	+
Excess loudness variation	−	−	++	−	++	−	−
Prolonged phonemes	−	−	++	−	+	−	+
Telescoping of syllables	−	−	++	−	−	−	+
Monopitch	+	+	−	++	+	−	+
Reduced stress	−	−	−	++	−	−	−
Monoloudness	+	+	−	++	−	−	+
Reduced loudness	+	−	−	++	−	−	−
Inappropriate silences	−	−	−	++	+	−	−
Short rushes of speech	−	−	−	++	−	−	−
Variable rate	−	−	−	++	+	−	−
Increased rate in segments	−	−	−	++	−	−	−
Increased overall rate	−	−	−	++	−	−	−
Rapid, "blurred" AMRs	−	−	−	++	−	−	−
Repeated phonemes	−	−	−	++	−	−	−
Palilalia	−	−	−	++	−	−	−
Prolonged intervals	−	−	−	−	++	−	+
Sudden forced inspiration/expiration	−	−	−	−	++	−	−

Table 15–4 Distinguishing speech characteristics among motor speech disorders—cont'd

Dimensions	Dysarthria						Apraxia of speech
	Flaccid	Spastic	Ataxic	Hypokinetic	Hyperkinetic	Unilateral UMN	
Voice stoppages/arrests	−	−	−	−	++	−	−
Transient breathiness	−	−	−	−	++	−	−
Voice tremor	−	−	−	−	++	−	−
Myoclonic vowel prolongation	−	−	−	−	++	−	−
Intermittent hypernasality	−	−	−	−	++	−	−
Slow & irregular AMRs	−	−	+	−	−+	−	−
Marked deterioration with increased rate	−	−	−	−	−+	−	−
Inappropriate vocal noises	−	−	−	−	++	−	−
Echolalia	−	−	−	−	++	−	−
Coprolalia	−	−	−	−	++	−	−
Intermittent strained voice/arrests	−	−	−	−	++	−	−
Intermittent breathy/aphonic segments	−	+	−	−	++	−	−
Poorly sequenced SMRs	−	−	−	−	−	−	++
Articulatory groping	−	−	−	−	−	−	++
Articulatory substitutions	−	−	−	−	−	−	++
Attempts at self-correction	−	−	−	−	−	−	++
Regressive articulatory errors	−	−	−	−	−	−	++
Reiterative articulatory errors	−	−	−	−	−	−	++
Metathetic articulatory errors	−	−	−	−	−	−	++
Articulatory additions/ complications	−	−	−	−	−	−	++
Automatic > volitional speech	−	−	−	−	−	−	++
Inconsistent articulatory errors	−	−	+	−	+	−	++
Increased errors with increased length	−	−	−	−	−	−	++

+, may or may not be present, but is not distinguishing by itself; ++, prominent and/or distinguishing (but not necessarily always present); −, rare/uncommonly present, and not distinguishing; *AMR,* alternating motion rate, *SMR,* sequential motion rate; *UMN,* upper motor neuron.

Etiology

Table 15–2 summarizes etiologies associated with AOS and dysarthria in a manner that identifies etiologic similarities and distinctions among them. Apraxia of speech is most often associated with nonhemorrhagic stroke, which can cause virtually any type of dysarthria. Like all dysarthria types, AOS can be caused by degenerative disease, although, as is apparent in Table 15–2, no single degenerative disease is a common cause of AOS, and a large number of degenerative diseases are never or only rarely associated with it. Thus, for example, patients whose only neurologic disorder is ALS, Parkinson's disease, progressive supranuclear palsy, or spinocerebellar degeneration would not be expected to have AOS.

Like nearly all dysarthria types, traumatic injuries, neurosurgery, and neoplasms can produce AOS, although AOS is expected only when the lesion is in the left hemisphere. In contrast to several dysarthria types, AOS is very unusual in toxic and metabolic and infectious disorders, and it generally develops in inflammatory and demyelinating disorders only when they produce dominant hemisphere effects. Like all dysarthria types, except flaccid dysarthria, AOS does not occur in conditions with exclusive effects on the peripheral nervous system (PNS), such as neuromuscular junction disease and muscle disease.

Oral mechanism findings

Table 15–3 summarizes distinct oral mechanism findings among the dysarthrias and AOS. It establishes that AOS can be present in the absence of any abnormal oral mechanism findings, an unusual occurrence for dysarthria (with the possible exceptions of ataxic and hyperkinetic dysarthria). It is often associated with right central facial weakness and, less frequently, with right lingual weakness, both of which occur in unilateral UMN dysarthria, but there is no causal relationship between such weakness and AOS when they co-occur. The one positive oral mechanism finding in AOS that is useful in differential diagnosis is the presence of nonverbal oral apraxia (NVOA) because NVOA is not expected in dysarthria and has no obvious causal relationship with any dysarthria when they do co-occur. Thus, with the exception of NVOA, when any of the other characteristics noted in Table 15–3 are found in a patient with AOS, they probably represent incidental findings or raise the possibility of additional speech disorders.

Speech characteristics

Similar to distinctions among the dysarthrias, the distinction between AOS and dysarthria is dependent on the identification and interpretation of deviant speech characteristics. Table 15–4 makes it clear that AOS and some dysarthria types share several deviant characteristics. Differential diagnosis tends to hinge mostly on the recognition of deviant speech characteristics found in AOS that are not present in dysarthrias.

General Distinctions. Some general distinctions between the dysarthrias and AOS include the following.

1. The speech and oral mechanism examinations usually make it apparent that the deviant characteristics of dysarthria are secondary to neuromuscular alterations, particularly those related to strength, tone, range, and steadiness of movement. Such alterations either are not obvious in AOS or, when they are, do not explain its deviant characteristics (Darley, Aronson, and Brown, 1975; Wertz, 1985).

2. In dysarthria, all components of speech—respiration, phonation, resonance, articulation, and prosody—may be affected. Apraxia of speech is predominantly an articulation and prosodic disorder (Darley, Aronson, and Brown, 1975; Wertz, LaPointe, and Rosenbek, 1984).

3. Dysarthria is infrequently associated with aphasia; AOS is very often associated with aphasia (Wertz, 1985; Wertz, LaPointe, and Rosenbek, 1984).

4. In dysarthria, deviant speech characteristics are generally consistent across utterances and are relatively uninfluenced by the degree of automaticity of the utterance, stimulus modality (spontaneous, reading, imitation), or linguistic variables. In AOS, there may be islands of error-free speech, errors across repetition of identical utterances may vary, automatic speech may be better than propositional speech, and the error rate may be influenced by variables such as word length and frequency of occurrence, meaningfulness, and stimulus modality (Darley, Aronson, and Brown, 1975; Johns and Darley, 1970; Wertz, LaPointe, and Rosenbek, 1984).

5. The predominant errors in dysarthrias are usually related to distortions or simplification of speech gestures. Distortions also are common in AOS, but perceived substitutions as well as additions, repetitions, prolongations, and complications of targeted sounds also occur (Darley, Aronson, and Brown, 1975; Johns and Darley, 1970; Wertz, LaPointe, and Rosenbek, 1984). Variable dysfluencies are probably more common in AOS than in dysarthria.

6. Dysarthric speakers rarely grope for correct articulatory postures or attempt to correct er-

rors. Trial-and-error groping and attempts at self-correction are common in AOS (Darley, Aronson, and Brown, 1975; Johns and Darley, 1970; Wertz, LaPointe, and Rosenbek, 1984).

Some Specific Distinctions. Perusal of Table 15–4 will show that AOS shares a number of deviant speech characteristics with spastic, hyperkinetic, and ataxic dysarthria. Because of this, it may help to address more specifically the distinctions between these dysarthrias and AOS.

1. Although they share a number of common features, AOS is usually not difficult to distinguish from spastic dysarthria. The deviant features of spastic dysarthria are usually highly predictable and consistent, regardless of stimulus or utterance conditions or characteristics. Apraxia of speech is typically much less predictable along several stimulus and response parameters. Spastic dysarthria is classically associated with a strained-harsh dysphonia and frequently with hypernasality, neither of which is usually present in AOS. Oral mechanism findings are also distinguishing. People with spastic dysarthria frequently have dysphagia, drooling, and pseudobulbar affect, as well as pathologic or hyperactive oral motor reflexes. The oral mechanism examination in speakers with AOS may be entirely normal.

2. Although hyperkinetic dysarthria can be predominantly an articulatory or prosodic problem, similar to AOS, the distinction between the two disorders usually is not difficult. The presence of visible involuntary movements in hyperkinetic dysarthria is very common, but such movements are not present in AOS. Hyperkinetic dysarthria is generally not influenced by stimulus or response parameters, but AOS is.

3. Ataxic dysarthria and AOS can be quite difficult to distinguish from each other. This is not unexpected, given the cerebellum's role in motor programming and coordination, the irregular nature of articulatory breakdowns, and the predominance of articulatory and prosodic abnormalities in ataxic dysarthria. Apraxia of speech shares these features. In addition, oral mechanism examination in patients with ataxic dysarthria and AOS may be normal. The most helpful distinguishing speech characteristics between the two disorders are: speech AMRs are usually irregular in ataxic dysarthria but regular in AOS; the sequencing of speech SMRs is usually normal in ataxic dysarthria but abnormal in AOS; irregular articulatory breakdowns and variable prosodic abnormalities are often more pervasive in ataxic dysarthria than in AOS; islands of error-free speech are un-usual in ataxic dysarthria but not unusual in AOS; automatic speech is no better than propositional speech in ataxic dysarthria, but a mismatch between them may exist in AOS; ataxic speakers rarely grope for articulatory postures and do not usually attempt to correct articulatory errors, whereas many speakers with AOS do; and perceived substitutions are not as frequent in ataxic dysarthria as in AOS.

4. Although unilateral UMN dysarthria and AOS do not share a large number of deviant features, they often co-occur with left hemisphere lesions. In such cases, especially when unilateral UMN dysarthria has ataxic-like features, it may be difficult to attribute specific errors or characteristics to one disorder rather than the other. In most instances, such distinctions are not very important to lesion localization (both problems may be localized to the left hemisphere). Relative to management, if the disorders coexist, the AOS is usually the focus of treatment.

DISTINGUISHING MOTOR SPEECH DISORDERS FROM APHASIA
Dysarthria versus aphasia

Distinguishing dysarthria from aphasia should not be difficult. Distinctions between the two categories of disorder on anatomic, vascular, and etiologic grounds are the same as those that distinguish AOS from the dysarthrias. With the exception of right central facial weakness and sometimes right lingual weakness and NVOA, the aphasic patient's oral mechanism exam may be entirely normal. The language difficulties of aphasic patients are nearly always evident in their verbal and reading comprehension and writing, as well as in their verbal expression. In contrast, speakers with dysarthria alone do not have deficits in any input or output modality beyond speech, and their speech is linguistically normal. Their complaints regarding communication center on speech production and not on word retrieval or language formulation or interpretation.

Even when dysarthria and aphasia co-occur, it is generally not difficult to distinguish speech distortions associated with neuromuscular deficits from verbal deficits associated with inefficiencies and errors in language formulation and expression. But, when dysarthria reduces intelligibility, it may be difficult to establish if unintelligible content reflects only the dysarthria or is also a function of aphasic deficits. Delays during speech or attempts to revise utterances, however, may signal the presence of language difficulties. When these traits are not apparent, careful assessment of verbal and reading comprehension and writing can usually establish if aphasia is present. When aphasic difficulties are evident in other modalities, it can be assumed that language deficits are also present in spoken language.

Apraxia of speech versus aphasia

Distinguishing AOS from aphasia can be difficult for several reasons. First, there are no significant differences between the two disorders in their gross anatomic and vascular characteristics and in the disorders that may cause them. Second, although aphasia is fairly frequently present in the absence of AOS, it is uncommon for AOS to be present in the absence of aphasia; the co-occurrence of the two disorders can make distinguishing between them difficult. Third, aphasic patients may make sound errors that are presumably linguistic (phonologic) in nature, whereas apraxic patients make sound errors that presumably reflect motor programming problems. These two types of errors can be difficult to distinguish, and they present the biggest challenge to differential diagnosis. Finally, patients with a prominent AOS and a less severe aphasia may nonetheless make some sound errors that are aphasic in nature, and patients with prominent aphasia and less severe or no apparent AOS may nonetheless make some sound errors that are apraxic in nature.

Table 15–5 summarizes the attributes of AOS and aphasia that may help to distinguish between them. The following points clarify those distinctions.

1. Although AOS is usually accompanied by aphasia, AOS can occur independently of aphasia. When it does, there is no difficulty in verbal comprehension, verbal retention, auditory perception, or reading comprehension, and the linguistic aspects of writing can be normal. In contrast, and by definition, aphasia is a multimodality disorder of language (Darley, Aronson, and Brown, 1975; Halpern, Darley, and Brown, 1973; Wertz, LaPointe, and Rosenbek, 1984).

2. Aphasic verbal deficits may be severe enough to mask the presence of AOS, in that a sufficient and valid speech sample for AOS diagnosis may not be obtainable. Apraxia of speech need not mask identification of aphasia, however. Even if AOS is severe enough to produce muteness, careful assessment of other language modalities can establish if language deficits are present. If AOS is isolated, performance in other language modalities is normal. If aphasia is present, careful examination will detect language deficits.

3. When AOS and aphasia co-occur and the AOS is moderately severe or worse, the patient's profile of difficulty across language modalities

Table 15–5 Distinctions between apraxia of speech and aphasia

	Apraxia of speech	Aphasia
Localization	Left hemisphere, middle cerebral artery Frontal > temporoparietal	Left hemisphere, middle cerebral artery Temporoparietal > frontal
Etiology	Stroke predominant	Stroke predominant
Accompanying deficits	Aphasia very frequent, often Broca's NVOA present > absent Right hemiparesis common	AOS may or may not be present NVOA less often present Right hemiparesis less common
Speech/language	UUMN dysarthria probably common Nonspeech language modalities intact Need not mask detection of aphasia When aphasic, usually nonfluent in character Prosody abnormal	UUMN dysarthria less common Nonspeech language modalities impaired May mask detection of AOS Fluent or nonfluent verbal output Prosody normal
	Distortions frequent Articulatory hesitancy & groping Attempt to correct articulatory errors Errors approximate target Errors influenced by articulatory complexity	Distortions infrequent Articulation effortless Unaware of articulatory errors Errors further from target Errors less affected by complexity

AOS, apraxia of speech; *NVOA,* nonverbal oral apraxia; *UMN,* upper motor neuron; *UUMN,* unilateral upper motor neuron.

is disproportionately severe in the verbal modality. This is often apparent during casual observation and may also be apparent in response profiles across language modalities on standard aphasia examinations. For example, patients with AOS or with AOS plus aphasia often have poorer percentile scores on the verbal subtests of the *Porch Index of Communicative Ability (PICA)* (1981) than in any other modality tested. In addition, the multimodality scoring scale used in the PICA often shows a disproportionate number of "4-7-14" responses on verbal subtests, scores that reflect a predominance of unintelligible, close approximation, or distorted speech responses, a pattern uncommon in aphasic patients who do not have an accompanying AOS.

4. Patients with AOS alone or with AOS plus aphasia often have distinctive profiles on other standard aphasia tests, usually falling into one of the "nonfluent" categories of aphasia. On the *Boston Diagnostic Aphasia Examination* (Goodglass and Kaplan, 1983) and the *Western Aphasia Battery* (Kertesz, 1982), they often are classified as having "Broca's aphasia" and are rarely classified as having one of the so-called transcortical aphasias or fluent aphasias labelled "Wernicke's" or "anomic aphasia." On the *Minnesota Test for the Differential Diagnosis of Aphasia* (Schuell, 1965) aphasic patients with AOS often are classified as having "aphasia with sensorimotor impairment." In contrast, patients with aphasia but no AOS may receive a wider variety of aphasia diagnoses.

5. Nonverbal oral apraxia may occur in AOS and in aphasia without AOS, but NVOA is probably more common when AOS is also present.

6. Apraxia of speech with or without aphasia is probably more commonly associated with unilateral UMN dysarthria than is aphasia without AOS. This probably reflects the tighter alignment of the neuromuscular execution system with motor speech programming mechanisms than with the language mechanism. Similarly, although AOS and aphasia are usually accompanied by right-sided motor findings, the association between right hemiparesis and AOS is probably stronger than that between such deficits and aphasia.

7. In general, AOS tends to be more strongly associated with posterior frontal and insular lesions than lesions in the temporal or parietal lobes, and aphasia without AOS tends to be associated with temporal or temporoparietal lesions.

8. Because "phonologic" errors are most common in Wernicke's and conduction aphasia, it is the distinction between them and AOS that is most difficult. The work of Trost and Canter (1974); Burns and Canter (1977), Canter, Trost, and Burns (1985); and summaries by Darley (1982), Wertz (1985), and Wertz, LaPointe, and Rosenbek (1984) provide some helpful clues to the distinction.

   a. Patients with AOS have articulation and prosodic disturbances, whereas Wernicke's and other fluent aphasic speakers usually do not have pervasive prosodic deficits. Even when substitutions are perceived in AOS, they are often produced in a context of articulatory hesitancy, struggle, and groping. These distortions may lead to a perception that non-English phonemes have been produced. In contrast, aphasic phonologic errors are not usually perceived as distorted; usually occur without articulatory hesitancy, struggle, or groping; and are usually perceived as adequately produced English phonemes.

   b. Apraxic speakers often recognize and attempt to self-correct their articulatory errors. Phonologic errors frequently go unnoticed by aphasic patients without AOS.

   c. Apraxic errors tend to be more predictable and closer to the articulatory target than phonologic errors. For example, the word "banana" may be produced as "bamama" by an apraxic speaker, but as "streeble" by a speaker with Wernicke's aphasia.

   d. Apraxic errors tend to be more frequent in the initial position of syllables or show no particular position bias. Phonologic errors tend to occur more frequently in the final position.

   e. Articulatory complexity of a target response has a greater influence on error frequency in AOS than in aphasic phonologic errors.

9. Treatment that facilitates language production in aphasia is not effective for AOS, and treatment that facilitates speech production in AOS is not effective for aphasia. (Management of AOS will be discussed in Chapter 18).

DISTINGUISHING AMONG FORMS OF NEUROGENIC MUTISM

Distinguishing among the forms of neurogenic mutism can be difficult, but there are a number of nonverbal communicative behaviors and other observations that often permit the nature of neurogenic mutism to be established. Table 15–6 summarizes major distinguishing features among anarthric, AOS, aphasic, and cognitive-affective (abulic) forms of mutism. Etiology is not of particular value to differential diagnosis, except

Table 15–6 Distinctions among major types of mutism

	Motor speech		Language	Cognitive-affective	
	Anarthria	**Apraxia of speech**	**Aphasia**	**Decreased arousal/diffuse cortical dysfunction**	**Akinetic mutism**
Etiology (most common)	Stroke, CHI	Stroke	Stroke	CHI, anoxia, infectious, inflammatory	Stroke, tumor, CHI
Localization	Bilat UMN Bilat LMN Basal ganglia Cerebellum	Left hemisphere	Left hemisphere	Reticular activating system	Frontal lobes– limbic system
Mechanism	Neuromuscular (dysarthria)	Motor program-ming	Language	Arousal Cognitive	Drive, initiative Cognitive
Accompanying deficits	Dysphagia Quadriparesis Weakness Spasticity Rigidity Hyperkinesias Pathologic reflexes	Aphasia NVOA Hemiparesis	Multimodality language deficits Apraxia of speech NVOA Hemiparesis	Coma Unresponsive-ness Altered tone or posture Pathologic reflexes	Abulia Delayed responses Unresponsive-ness Apathy Pathologic reflexes
Retained capacities	Alert Responsive in other modalities	Alert Responsive and accurate in other language modalities Normal chew and swallow	Alert Responsive but inaccurate in other language modalities Normal chew and swallow	Minimal	Alert Normal but slow chew and swallow
Speech and vocal characteristics when present	Severe dysarthria, with severely reduced intelligibility	Limited sound repertoire, few mean-ingful or nonmean-ingful utterances	Automatic social utterances Stereotypic recurrent utterances	Vocalization (cry, groan, shout)	Delayed, unelaborated, concrete responses Aphonic, whispered, reduced in loudness, monotonous

CHI, closed head injury; *UMN*, upper motor neuron; *LMN*, lower motor neuron; *NVOA*, nonverbal oral apraxia.

that conditions that have diffuse or multifocal effects are more likely to be associated with mutism related to cognitive and affective distur-bances than with anarthria, AOS, or aphasia. Con-versely, conditions that produce focal distur-bances, such as stroke, are more likely to produce mutism associated with motor speech or language disturbances.

The following subsections summarize the clues that help distinguish among the forms of mutism.

Anarthria

Anarthric patients usually have significant and obvious neuromuscular deficits in the bulbar muscles that predict the neuromuscular basis for their mutism. Dysphagia, drooling, pseudobulbar affect, and pathologic oromotor reflexes associated with anarthria may not be present at all in apraxic and aphasic mutism and may be absent or less pronounced in mutism that reflects cognitive and affective disturbances. Similarly, quadriplegia or evidence of weakness, spasticity, rigidity, and movement disorders in the limbs (and bulbar muscles) may be prominent in anarthric patients and absent or less evident in other forms of mutism.

It should be noted that anarthria is occasionally present without significant limb motor deficits, which can lead to its misdiagnosis as aphasia, AOS, or even psychogenic mutism. However, the significant dysphagia and other oromotor abnormalities associated with anarthria help clarify diagnosis because anarthric mutism in the absence of nonspeech oromotor abnormalities should not (ever?) be encountered.

Anarthric patients may be normally alert and responsive, even if their alertness and ability to respond are evident only in eye movements (as in locked-in syndrome). Their responses may be initiated fairly rapidly, in contrast to slower response initiation in other forms of mutism, especially cognitive and affective varieties. Finally, when anarthric patients attempt speech, their slowness, restricted range of articulatory movements, low volume, and strained-groaning-effortful phonatory quality help to establish the neuromuscular basis of their disorder.

Apraxia of speech

Apraxic mutism, in contrast to anarthria, may be associated with a normal oral mechanism examination or evidence of only right lingual or central facial weakness. Reflexive facial movements, such as yawning, smiling, and crying, are normal, and there may be no significant drooling or dysphagia. The reflexive cough may be normal and may actually contain traces of normal-sounding phonation, an unusual finding in anarthria.

Mute apraxic patients attempt to perform nonverbal oromotor tasks; if NVOA is present, responses are off-target and reflect groping or efforts at self-correction, but a full range and grossly normal rate of movement during such attempts may be apparent. Right hemiplegia may or may not be present, but a limb apraxia in both upper extremities may be evident. Limb apraxia and NVOA are not commonly encountered in cognitive and affective forms of mutism, although they may be present in mute aphasic patients. In contrast to aphasic and mute patients with cognitive and affective disturbances, the performance of mute apraxic patients in other language modalities may be initiated and completed rapidly and accurately. As a general rule,

however, muteness due to AOS is nearly always accompanied by some degree of aphasia, so difficulty in other language modalities may be evident.

Mute apraxic patients usually attempt to speak and display frustration at their inability to do so, in contrast to the indifference that is common in muteness associated with cognitive and affective disturbances. Finally, the mute apraxic patient may occasionally curse when frustrated or respond reflexively with "hi" or "bye" or a few notes of a song in unison singing, even though they are mute during volitional speech attempts.

Aphasia

The mute aphasic patient may be very much like the mute apraxic patient on oral mechanism examination and reflexive oromotor responses, except that they may not follow verbal directions for such examination as readily because of verbal comprehension deficits. Their aphasia is almost always severe when mutism is present, so they perform poorly on measures of verbal and reading comprehension and writing. Like apraxic patients and in contrast to those with cognitive and affective disturbances, they may respond emotionally to their deficits and other events.

Cognitive-affective disturbances

Mutism associated with cognitive and affective disturbances can be attributed to decreased arousal, alertness, drive, and initiative, as well as to higher level cognitive deficits. When the reticular activating system is impaired, the muteness may be associated with coma or hypoarousal or to complete lack of alertness, eye contact, or responsiveness. These states are dissimilar to those of anarthric, apraxic, or aphasic patients.

When muteness is associated with frontal lobe–limbic system deficits, as in akinetic mutism, the patient may be awake and seemingly alert, and eye contact may be achieved. The patient may eat very slowly and retain food in the mouth, unchewed or simply never swallowed, but swallowing may be adequate once the pharyngeal phase is initiated.

If the akinetically mute patient is responsive, responses are typically delayed, with the delay characterized by apathetic silence or lack of evidence of effort, in contrast to anarthric or mute aphasic or apraxic individuals, who usually attempt to speak. Unresponsiveness or delayed responses are as evident nonverbally and in other language modalities as they are in the failure to speak; such traits are unusual in other forms of neurogenic mutism. When such patients do speak, speech emerges after lengthy delays, is brief and unelaborated, and is whispered, aphonic, or markedly reduced in loudness, as well as prosodically flat. In contrast, articulation may be normal, although sometimes with reduced range of articulatory movement. Such phonatory characteristics, in the presence of good articulation, are less common in individuals emerging from anarthria, AOS, and aphasia.

DISTINGUISHING MOTOR SPEECH DISORDERS FROM OTHER NEUROGENIC SPEECH DISORDERS

Chapter 13 addressed several neurogenic speech disturbances that bear a variety of relationships to dysarthrias and AOS. Aphasia was discussed at that time, and its distinction from motor speech disorders has already been addressed in this chapter. Distinctions between other neurogenic speech disturbances and motor speech disorders will now be addressed. A number of them are summarized in Tables 15–7 and 15–8.

Neurogenic stuttering

The line distinguishing neurogenic stuttering from the dysarthrias and AOS can be drawn in several places because neurogenic dysfluencies are so heterogeneous in their behavioral and neuroanatomic characteristics. When significant dysfluencies are present, the challenge is to decide if they are a component of dysarthria, AOS, or aphasia or if they represent a separate, independent disorder.

This decision has implications for localization and behavioral management. The distinctions among the various neurogenic speech disorders associated with dysfluencies are summarized in Table 15–7.

Dysarthria and neurogenic stuttering. Dysfluencies can occur in dysarthria, probably more frequently in hypokinetic dysarthria than in other types. They should not be associated with flaccid dysarthria, however, and when they are it should be assumed that there is either a CNS-based dysfunction in addition to the lower motor neuron (LMN) lesion(s) causing the flaccid dysarthria or that the dysfluencies are maladaptively compensatory or psychogenic in origin.

Dysfluencies associated with hypokinetic dysarthria tend to occur at the beginning of phrases and are characterized by rapid, sometimes blurred initial sound or syllable repetitions. They are consistent with the rapid or accelerated rate and reduced range of articulatory movement that characterize the gestalt of hypokinetic dysarthria and should be considered one of the defining characteristics of the hypokinetic dysarthria rather than a separate disorder. When dysfluencies are a prominent feature of a hypokinetic dysarthria, it is appropriate to describe the speech disorder as a "hypokinetic dysarthria with prominent dysfluencies." This designation implies that a single speech disorder rather than two is present and that a single lesion or disease process involving the basal ganglia is

Table 15–7 Distinctions among dysfluencies associated with neurogenic stuttering, palilalia, motor speech disorders, and aphasia.

	Neurogenic stuttering	Palilalia	Dysarthria	Apraxia of speech	Aphasia
Localization	CNS motor system (multiple loci) Often bilateral, when persistent	Bilateral basal ganglia	CNS motor system (multiple loci)	Left hemisphere	Left hemisphere
Mechanism	Unknown (? dysequilibrium)	? motor disinhibition	Neuromuscular	Motor programming	Language
Speech characteristics	Sound/syllable/ word dysfluencies only or Dysfluencies disproportionate or not explainable by co-existing motor speech or aphasic disorder	Reiterative word and phrase repetition only Frequently associated with hypokinetic dysarthria	Sound/syllable/ word dysfluencies consistent with characteristics of dysarthria, plus dysarthria	Sound/syllable/ word dysfluencies consistent with characteristics of AOS, plus AOS	Sound/syllable/ word dysfluencies consistent with language deficit, plus language deficits

AOS, apraxia of speech; *CNS,* central nervous system.

responsible for it. Highlighting the dysfluencies in the dysarthria diagnosis may signal a need to address them specifically in management efforts.

Apraxia of speech and neurogenic stuttering. Apraxia of speech may be characterized by hesitations, repetitions, and prolongations of sounds and syllables. These dysfluencies may reflect efforts to establish or revise articulatory targets or movements and may be linked to the searching, groping, off-target speech movements of many apraxic speakers. When they reflect compensatory efforts to correct sound or movement errors, they are best considered as characteristics of AOS and not as a separate disorder. When they are a prominent characteristic of AOS, it is appropriate to describe the disorder as "AOS with prominent dysfluencies," a designation that indicates that a single speech disorder rather than two is present

and that a single lesion or disease process in the left hemisphere is probably responsible for it. Highlighting the dysfluencies in the diagnosis may signal a need to address them specifically during management.

Aphasia and neurogenic stuttering. Dysfluencies may occur in aphasia as a manifestation of word retrieval difficulties or efforts to correct linguistic errors or organize verbal expression. They may be characterized by fillers ("um," "well uh"), hesitations and prolongations, and sound, syllable, word, and even short phrase repetitions. When they are part of the numerous manifestations of aphasic verbal impairments, they should not be singled out as a distinct, separate disorder. When they are prominent, they should be highlighted in the diagnosis, for example, as "aphasia whose verbal output characteristics include prominent dysfluencies," a designation that implies that the aphasia

Table 15–8 Distinctions among abulia, aprosodia, hypokinetic and unilateral UMN dysarthrias, and depression

	Abulia	Aprosodia	Unilateral UMN dysarthria	Hypokinetic dysarthria	Depression
Localization	Frontal-limbic system (bilateral)	Right hemisphere	Upper motor neuron	Basal ganglia control circuit	No structural lesion
Mechanism	Cognitive-affective	Uncertain	Weakness/? incoordination	Rigidity, bradykinesia, hypokinesia	Mood disorder
Speech/language					
Prosody	Reduced (flat, emotionless, apathetic)	Reduced (flat, indifferent, robotlike, stereotypic)	Normal or dysprosodic	Reduced (flat, monopitch, monoloudness)	Reduced (flat, monopitch, monoloudness)
Loudness	Reduced/ hypophonic	Normal	Normal or mildly reduced	Reduced/ hypophonic	Reduced
Articulation	Normal	Normal	Impaired	Impaired	Normal
Rate	Normal or slow	Normal	Normal or mildly slow	Normal, slow, or fast	Slow or normal
Dysfluencies	No	No	No	Sometimes	No
Response latency	Slow	Normal	Normal	Slow or normal	Slow or normal
Content	Brief, unelaborated, concrete	Normal linguistic structure & complexity	Normal linguistic structure & complexity	Normal linguistic structure & complexity	Unelaborated but normal linguistically
Complaints	None	Speech does not convey emotion	Speech imprecise	Speech imprecise, & loudness reduced	No speech complaints

UMN, upper motor neuron.

and dysfluencies share the same etiology and left hemisphere localization. Highlighting the prominence of dysfluencies suggests they may deserve attention during therapy.

Neurogenic stuttering as a distinct diagnosis. When dysfluencies are the only evident speech abnormality or when their characteristics are not compatible with a co-occurring dysarthria, AOS, or aphasia, and when psychogenic explanations for them can be ruled out, they deserve a designation as neurogenic stuttering. The diagnosis of neurogenic stuttering as a distinct entity is more than an academic exercise because it implies the presence of neurologic disease when there may be no other such evidence and may broaden the possible etiologies and anatomic loci of the neuropathology to numerous areas of the nervous system if it is not consistent with dysfluencies associated with AOS, aphasia, or a single type of dysarthria. Relative to management, it identifies a disorder for which intervention may be appropriate.

Palilalia

The differential diagnosis of palilalia is not difficult because the behaviors that define it—compulsive repetition of one's own words and phrases—has little behavioral overlap with motor speech disorders and other neurogenic speech disturbances (see Table 15–7).

The stereotypic prosody, the progressively increased rate, the decreased loudness, the sometimes large number of repetitions, and the definitional limitation of palilalia to word and phrase repetition (as opposed to sound or syllable repetitions) help to distinguish it from dysfluencies associated with AOS, aphasia, and neurogenic stuttering. In addition, when apraxic and aphasic speakers repeat words, they are often accompanied by obvious efforts to articulate or express specific words or meanings, slowed rate, and attempts at self-correction. Palilalic speakers tend to speak rapidly and without effort and show no obvious attempts to inhibit their repetitions.

Palilalia very often occurs with hypokinetic dysarthria, but not invariably. Both disorders usually reflect bilateral basal ganglia pathology. The typical dysfluencies associated with hypokinetic dysarthria involve sound and syllable repetitions, and the repetitions tend to occur at the beginning of utterances or phrases; palilalic repetitions tend to occur at the end of utterances. When word and phrase repetitions occur frequently with hypokinetic dysarthria, it is appropriate to identify the presence of both hypokinetic dysarthria and palilalia.

Echolalia

There is minimal overlap between echolalia and motor speech and other neurogenic speech disorders. Echolalic utterances are motorically normal, so they should not be confused with dysarthria or AOS. In contrast to palilalia, echolalia involves the repetition of others' utterances and not one's own utterances, and it generally does not involve multiple, uninterrupted repetitions. Because echolalia is motorically precise and does not involve sound or syllable dysfluencies, it should not be confused with neurogenic stuttering. Although it may occur with aphasia (and diffuse cognitive deficits), it is not simply a manifestation of aphasia because it is usually associated with diffuse or multifocal lesions that extend beyond the perisylvian language zone.

Cognitive and affective disturbances (abulia)

Cognitive and affective disturbances can lead to mutism (already discussed). At lesser degrees of severity, they may alter speech in ways that can be confused with motor speech disorders, especially hypokinetic dysarthria.

When damage to frontal lobe activating mechanisms leads to abulia, speech initiation may be delayed and then characterized by reduced loudness, hypophonia, and flattened prosody. These characteristics are also encountered in hypokinetic dysarthria. Two general observations can help to distinguish abulic speech from hypokinetic dysarthria. First, the content of the abulic patient's speech is usually brief, unelaborated, and concrete, and the delay in initiating an utterance is unaccompanied by behavioral evidence of effort; speech content in those with hypokinetic dysarthria may be normal in length and linguistic and cognitive complexity, and delays in initiating speech may contain evidence of physical effort to initiate speech. Second, the abulic patient's speech rate is slow or normal and does not accelerate, and articulation is precise and without dysfluency. Hypokinetic dysarthria is often associated with rapid or accelerated rate, speech AMRs may be rapid or blurred, and articulation is imprecise and sometimes dysfluent (see Table 15–8 for summary).

Aprosodia

Aprosodia associated with right hemisphere lesions may be difficult to distinguish from dysarthria and from the speech characteristics of patients with attenuated speech associated with abulia or frontal or limbic pathology. Because aprosodia is not well understood or described, only a few guidelines can be offered for differential diagnosis (see Table 15–8 for summary).

Aprosodia versus dysarthria. Unilateral UMN dysarthria can result from right hemisphere lesions and may explain speech abnormalities without invoking a separate disorder of aprosodia as an explanation for them (see Chapter 13 for a discussion of some of these issues). In addition, the prosodic deficits of patients with hypokinetic dysarthria may resemble those of aprosodic patients with right hemisphere lesions. However, these dysarthrias are often distinguishable from right hemisphere aprosodia on the basis of some of their predominant speech characteristics. Such distinctions may include the following.

1. Aprosodia is characterized by flat, indifferent, robotlike, or stereotypic prosodic patterns, without obvious distortions, irregular articulatory breakdowns, or reductions in loudness or rate. Unilateral UMN dysarthria is primarily an articulatory disorder characterized by imprecise consonants and sometimes by irregular articulatory breakdowns; prosodic deficits, if present, may be more dysprosodic than aprosodic and tied to articulatory imprecision or breakdown. Both prosody and articulation are impaired in hypokinetic dysarthria, loudness may be reduced, and rate is sometimes increased.

2. The aprosodic speaker may be noticeably deficient in the ability to produce correct intonational patterns on imitation or in spontaneous linguistic or affective prosodic tasks. The speaker with unilateral UMN dysarthria may approximate such intonational patterns fairly well.

3. The aprosodic speaker may convey linguistic stress adequately but express affective prosody poorly. The prosodic patterns of people with unilateral UMN or hypokinetic dysarthria generally do not vary as a function of linguistic or affective stimulus or response parameters.

4. Aprosodic patients may complain about their inability to convey felt emotions but rarely complain about articulatory imprecision. Unilateral UMN and hypokinetic dysarthric speakers may have the opposite pattern of complaints.

Aprosodia versus abulia. The flattened prosody of aprosodia may be similar to that of abulic patients with frontal or limbic pathology. The distinction between the two disorders may be made more on the basis of content and general behavior than the speech characteristics themselves, although speech distinctions may also exist. These distinctions may include the following.

1. Aprosodic patients generally have normal response latency and normally long (sometimes excessively long) narrative responses, in contrast to the delayed, unelaborated, and concrete responses of the abulic patient.

2. Aprosodic patients may be quite responsive nonverbally (except when neglect interferes) in contrast to the abulic patient, who may be as slow and impoverished in their nonverbal as in their verbal behavior.

3. Aprosodic patients may state that they feel emotions, and their linguistic content may reflect such emotions. In contrast, the abulic patient's apathy, indifference, and impoverished thought is as evident in the content of their speech as it is in their tone.

4. The aprosodic patient may have normal loudness and is not usually hypophonic. Their prosodic pattern may be stereotypic but not unvarying in loudness, duration, or pitch, and not suggestive of apathy. In contrast, the abulic patient's speech is often markedly reduced in loudness and hypophonic, and prosody may sound truly emotionless or apathetic.

DISTINGUISHING NEUROGENIC FROM PSYCHOGENIC SPEECH DISORDERS

Distinguishing neurogenic from psychogenic speech disorders is very important but sometimes very difficult. The distinction is important because it is an etiologic one that may send medical diagnostic and management efforts down a neurologic versus a psychiatric pathway. The distinction can be difficult because the speech characteristics associated with neurogenic and psychogenic disorders can be quite similar and because neurogenic and psychogenic speech disorders can co-occur.

Psychogenic speech disorders were addressed in Chapter 14. Clues useful to differential diagnosis were reviewed in that chapter, and the reader should refer to it for details that will not be repeated here. In this section, an attempt will be made to summarize the distinctions between the characteristics of some of the more common psychiatric disturbances and the motor speech disorders with which they may be confused. Psychogenic speech disturbances associated with conversion disorders and life stresses will be emphasized because they are the psychogenic etiologies that challenge differential diagnosis most frequently in speech pathology practices.

Depression

Because the speech of depressed people tends to be characterized by monopitch, monoloudness, and reduced stress and loudness, it may raise suspicions about hypokinetic dysarthria. The distinction can be complicated further by the common occurrence of depression in Parkinson's disease.

In addition to nonspeech physical findings on neurologic examination (for example, resting tremor) that help distinguish Parkinson's disease from depression, there are some clues in speech that distinguish the speech of depression from that of hypokinetic dysarthria. Some of them are similar to those that help to distinguish among abulia, aprosodia, and dysarthria (see Table 15–8). The distinctions include the following.

1. Depressed individuals' contextual speech and speech AMRs tend to be slow or normal in rate. Hypokinetic dysarthria may be associated with rapid or accelerated speech and AMR rates.
2. The speech of depression reflects attenuations in loudness and prosody, but articulatory precision is not generally affected. Hypokinetic dysarthria may be characterized by significant articulatory imprecision. In addition, voice quality is generally adequate in depressed people, whereas a harsh, breathy, aphonic quality is often present in hypokinetic dysarthria.
3. The facial expression of depressed people conveys sadness, whereas hypokinetic speakers may appear expressionless or devoid of emotion. Saliva accumulation, drooling, dysphagia, and jaw, lip, and tongue tremulousness are common in hypokinetic dysarthria but not in depression.

Schizophrenia

Schizophrenic speech is not difficult to distinguish from motor speech disorders. It may, however, be difficult to distinguish from that of individuals with Wernicke's aphasia. These distinctions were discussed in Chapter 14.

Conversion disorders and responses to life stress

People with psychogenic speech disorders that reflect conversion reactions or responses to life stress present to medical speech pathologists who work closely with neurologists and otorhinolaryngologists. Many of them have been on a long medical diagnostic journey marked by a search for organic explanations for their speech disorder, and many have been dismissed by physicians with a casual explanation of "there's nothing wrong with you" or "it's all in your head." Some of these patients have undetected neurologic disease, whereas others have undetected, unexplained, or subconsciously avoided psychological disturbances. The diagnosis often becomes evident during a careful history of the speech disorder and psychosocial issues, examination of speech, and efforts to modify the speech disorder. Information derived from these efforts often distinguishes psychogenic from neurogenic speech disturbances.

History. Points about the history that may be of value to distinguishing psychogenic from neurogenic disturbances were addressed in Chapter 14. In general, the following contrasts between the histories of people with psychogenic versus neurogenic speech disorders may be useful in differential diagnosis (see Table 15–9 for summary).

Relative to people with neurogenic speech disorders:

1. The onset of psychogenic speech disorders is more frequently associated with a cold or non-neurological illness or a physically (but non-neurologic) or psychologically traumatic event.
2. Psychogenic speech disorders are more frequently associated with a prior history of unexplained speech disturbance or other physical deficits of unexplained origin.
3. Psychogenic speech disorders are more frequently associated with ongoing psychological stress or conflict, unrelated to those in response to the individual's speech or other physical symptoms. People with neurogenic speech disturbances are more likely to complain of stress generated by their speech and other physical symptoms.
4. Psychogenic speech disorders are more frequently associated with evidence of "gain" from the speech disorder, such as avoidance of confrontation or expression of anger or leave of absence from a job requiring normal speech.
5. People with psychogenic speech disorders are more likely to deny the experience of stress, anxiety, or conflict and the possibility that their speech problems may be related to such psychological states.
6. Unexplained fluctuations in the presence or severity of the speech disorder, especially as a function of stress and anxiety in specific situations, are more likely in psychogenic speech disorders.
7. Indifference to the speech disturbance is more likely in psychogenic speech disorders. It is important to distinguish indifference from stoicism and denial, however, because many people dealing with organic disease respond in a stoic manner. Denial of speech difficulty caused by neurologic disease is not unusual when the problem is mild or before a neurologic diagnosis has been made.

Examination Observations. Chapter 14 summarized important questions that should be addressed during the examination of individuals with suspected psychogenic speech disorders. The thrust of such questions is to determine if the disorder follows the lawful patterns of speech deficits and oral mechanism examination findings that exist for motor speech and other neurogenic speech disorders. Table 15–9 summarizes the answers to these questions as they relate to differential diagnosis. They apply to the differential diagnosis of psychogenic voice disorders (including musculoskeletal tension disorders, conversion aphonias and dysphonias, psychogenic spasmodic dysphonias, and iatrogenic and inertial dysphonias), psychogenic stuttering and mutism, and other psychogenic speech disturbances that may affect

Table 15–9 Distinctions between psychogenic (conversion and stress-related) speech disorders and neurogenic speech disorders

	Relative to neurogenic speech disorders, conversion and stress-related speech disorders tend to be associated with
History	Nonneurologic illness or nonneurologic physical trauma at onset
	Prior history of unexplained speech or other physical deficits
	Ongoing psychological stress or conflict unrelated to speech or other physical symptoms
	Evidence of primary or secondary gain
	Denial of possibility that psychological factors may play a role in the disorder
	Unexplained fluctuations in presence and severity of symptoms or fluctuations as a function of situational emotional content
	Indifference to the speech disturbance
Examination	Speech characteristics that do not fit known patterns of neurogenic speech disorders
	Inconsistencies between speech characteristics and oral mechanism exam findings
	Variability in severity or specific speech characteristics as a function of task or emotional content
	Improvement or worsening of symptoms as a function of clinician suggestion
	Improvement of speech when distracted
	A pattern of speech fatigue inconsistent with common patterns of speech changes with physical fatigue
	Significant, sometimes rapid improvement in speech with symptomatic therapy

articulation, resonance, or prosody. The reader is referred to Chapter 14 for descriptions of the specific characteristics of these psychogenic disturbances and some additional clues that help to distinguish them from neurogenic speech disorders.

It is particularly important to keep in mind that neurogenic and psychogenic speech disturbances can and do co-occur and that distinguishing between them can be very difficult. It is not unusual, for example, to conclude that a patient has both a neurogenic and a psychogenic speech disorder, the psychogenic disorder representing a response to the neurologic disease or specific neurogenic speech disorder. It is also possible for psychogenic and neurogenic speech disorders to coexist as independent, unrelated entities. Missing the coexistence of these disorders can have serious consequences for medical diagnosis as well as for medical and behavioral management.

CASES

A total of 64 cases were discussed at the ends of Chapters 4 through 14. Each illustrated the history, clinical findings, and diagnostic interpretations and conclusions drawn from the examination of people with specific motor speech disorders, related neurogenic speech disorders, or psychogenic speech disorders. The diagnosis in many of the cases was fairly straightforward, in keeping with the intent to illustrate specific disorders discussed in each chapter. However, about half of the cases illustrated problems in differential diagnosis, either during medical workups prior to speech pathology assessment or during the speech

evaluation itself. The reader may wish to reread these cases at this time to develop a sense of the clinical reality of problems in differential diagnosis. They illustrate that differential diagnosis sometimes is fairly straightforward and that at other times the conclusions that are drawn are tentative or uncertain. The following list organizes in a general way some of the more difficult or complex diagnostic cases that were presented in Chapters 4 through 14:

Distinguishing among the dysarthrias: Cases 4.5, 5.1, 5.3, 7.3, 8.3, 8.4, 8.5, and 10.4.

Distinguishing among motor speech disorders and other neurogenic speech disorders: Cases 12.3, 12.4, 12.5, 13.4, 13.5, and 13.7.

Recognizing the presence of more than one neurogenic speech disorder: Cases 7.2, 11.2, 11.3, 13.1, 13.2, and 13.6.

Distinguishing neurogenic from non-neurogenic or psychogenic speech disorders: Cases 4.1, 4.6, 5.2, 6.4, 7.2, 10.3, 10.5, and 14.1 through 14.7.

SUMMARY

1. Differential diagnosis is the process of narrowing diagnostic possibilities and reaching conclusions about the nature of a deficit. It requires the application of knowledge and clinical skill to a specific clinical problem.

2. Speech examination should always lead to an attempt at diagnosis. If a diagnosis is not possible, the reasons should be stated. A diagnosis should never be stated if one cannot be determined.

3. Diagnosis of a neurogenic speech disorder should be related to the suspected or known neurologic diagnosis or lesion localization. This may help to confirm or modify neurologic diagnosis and localization.

4. Different speech disturbances can co-occur, so multiple diagnoses are possible in any given patient. At the same time, referral for speech examination does not guarantee abnormal findings. A diagnosis of normal speech is among the diagnostic possibilities in many cases.

5. Although the fixing of a diagnostic label carries certain risks, it is a convenient shorthand for communicating information concisely and precisely.

6. Distinguishing among the dysarthrias can be difficult because there is considerable overlap among their characteristics and because various combinations can be present within individuals. However, the dysarthrias differ in their anatomic and vascular localization, etiologic distributions, oral mechanism findings, and speech characteristics. Although many deviant speech characteristics are associated with each of the major types of dysarthria, diagnosis is very often derived from the recognition of only a few deviant characteristics that are distinctive of a given dysarthria type.

7. When a distinction between dysarthria and apraxia of speech must be made, distinguishing AOS from ataxic or unilateral UMN dysarthria is usually most difficult. Differential diagnosis most often depends on recognizing deviant speech characteristics commonly associated with AOS that are uncommon in the dysarthrias.

8. The distinction between dysarthrias and aphasia is usually not difficult, but distinguishing AOS from aphasia can be. Although there are some differences between AOS and aphasia in the nature of perceived sound substitutions, the distinction between the two disorders must often rely on confirmatory evidence from oral mechanism and language examinations, the prosodic features of speech, and patients' reactions to their articulatory difficulties.

9. Distinguishing among various forms of neurogenic mutism must generally rely on nonverbal communicative behaviors and other nonspeech observations. The constellation of deficits that accompany mutism and identification of retained capacities are most useful to differential diagnosis.

10. The diagnosis of neurogenic stuttering is dependent upon recognition of dysfluencies and their relationship to any co-occurring dysarthria, AOS, or aphasia, because stuttering-like behavior may occur in all of those conditions. In contrast, the characteristics of palilalia and echolalia are quite distinctive, and it is usually not difficult to distinguish between them and repetitions that may be associated with the dysarthrias, AOS, and aphasia.

11. Distinguishing among the prosodic deficits associated with cognitive and affective disturbances, aprosodia associated with right hemisphere lesions, and certain dysarthria types can be difficult. Certain speech characteristics and the clinical milieu in which they occur are helpful in distinguishing among them, however.

12. Distinguishing neurogenic from psychogenic speech disorders is important because the distinction can have a substantial impact on overall medical diagnosis and on medical and behavioral management. People for whom this distinction is important require a careful psychosocial history and speech examination, each of which can provide important clues to differential diagnosis. The rapid and dramatic improvement of speech during examination of some individuals can confirm a diagnosis of psychogenic speech disorder, even in those with suspected or confirmed neurologic disease.

REFERENCES

Burns MS and Canter GJ: Phonemic behavior of aphasic patients with posterior cerebral lesions, Brain Lang 4:492, 1977.

Canter GJ, Trost JE, and Burns MS: Contrasting speech patterns in apraxia of speech and phonemic paraphasia, Brain Lang 24:204, 1985.

Darley FL: Aphasia, Philadelphia, 1982, WB Saunders.

Darley FL, Aronson AE, and Brown JR: Motor speech disorders, Philadelphia, 1975, WB Saunders.

Goodglass H and Kaplan E: The Boston diagnostic aphasia examination, Philadelphia, 1983, Lea & Febiger.

Halpern H, Darley FL, and Brown JR: Differential language and neurologic characteristics in cerebral involvement, J Speech Hear Disord 38:162, 1973.

Johns DF and Darley FL: Phonemic variability in apraxia of speech, J Speech Hear Res 13:556, 1970.

Kertesz A: Western aphasia battery, New York, 1982, Grune and Stratton.

Porch BE: Porch index of communicative ability, Palo Alto, CA, 1981, Consulting Psychologists Press.

Schuell HM: Minnesota test for differential diagnosis of aphasia, Minneapolis, 1965, University of Minnesota Press.

Trost JE and Canter GJ: Apraxia of speech in patients with Broca's aphasia: a study of phoneme production accuracy and error patterns, Brain Lang 1:63, 1974.

Wertz RT: Neuropathologies of speech and language: an introduction to patient management. In Johns DF, editor: Clinical management of neurogenic communicative disorders, Boston, 1985, Little, Brown.

Wertz RT, LaPointe LL, and Rosenbek JC: Apraxia of speech in adults: the disorder and its management, Orlando, FL, 1984, Grune and Stratton.

PART THREE

Management

16 Managing Motor Speech Disorders: General Principles

Most clinicians and researchers would agree with Rosenbek and LaPointe (1985) that "American speech pathology has spent more of its energy and resources defining and describing the dysarthrias [motor speech disorders] than on developing treatments for them" (p. 101). They also would agree with the observation that in the past many believed that treatment for motor speech disorders was of little value (Netsell and Rosenbek, 1985). In spite of this history, and relatively limited efficacy data, most clinicians today believe that the communication difficulties of many people with motor speech disorders can be managed in beneficial and sometimes very effective ways.

The management of motor speech disorders and related neurogenic and psychogenic speech disturbances will be addressed in the remaining chapters of this book. In this chapter, the broad issues involved in managing motor speech disorders, the primary avenues for their treatment, and principles for their behavioral management will be emphasized.* With this background established, Chapters

17 and 18 will discuss specific approaches to managing the dysarthrias and apraxia of speech, respectively. Chapter 19 addresses the management of related neurogenic speech disturbances. Chapter 20 provides a broad overview of principles and some of the behavioral strategies for managing psychogenic speech disorders.

MANAGEMENT ISSUES AND DECISIONS
The territory

There are several reasons for thinking about *communication* rather than speech when considering the management of motor speech disorders. First, it places the ultimate goal where it belongs—on the ability to transmit thoughts and feelings to others. During most interpersonal communication, this occurs through speech and a variety of extralinguistic, nonverbal cues, but a variety of additional channels exist, including writing and gesturing. Some people with motor speech disorders may need to shift the degree to which they use different channels to convey information. They may need to repeat or answer questions that clarify the meaning of what they say, supplement speech by pointing to the first letter of each spoken word on a letter board, write or type portions of messages, and so on. Second, a focus on

---

*The broad issues, concepts, and techniques of management discussed here and in Chapter 17, although based on the efforts of many individuals, rely heavily of the influential work of Yorkston, Beukelman, and Bell (1988) and Rosenbek and LaPointe (1985).

communication broadens the goals of management. Rather than focusing only on speech, it recognizes that actions other than speech can improve the accuracy and efficiency of communication. Third, it broadens the criteria by which the efficacy of treatment is judged. A focus on communication influences management planning, prognosis, counseling of patients and those in their environment, decisions about whether direct treatment is appropriate, the conduct of management activities, and the point at which formal therapy should be terminated.

Management goals

The primary goal of management is to *maximize the effectiveness, efficiency, and naturalness of communication* (Rosenbek and LaPointe, 1985; Yorkston, Beukelman, and Bell, 1988). Achieving this requires efforts that can take several directions (Wertz, 1985). The key words that represent these directions are *restore, compensate,* and *adjust.* Their meanings are discussed next.

Restore lost function. This effort attempts to reduce impairment. Its likelihood of success is influenced by the etiology and course of the causal disease and by the type and severity of the speech disorder. For example, a person with a mild-moderate unilateral upper motor neuron (UMN) dysarthria due to a single, unilateral stroke two days prior to initial speech assessment has a reasonably good chance of nearly complete return of normal speech on the basis of physiologic recovery alone. A person with an isolated, idiopathic, unilateral vocal cord paralysis might achieve full or nearly complete recovery of voice as a result of nerve regeneration or surgical thyroplasty. People with reduced physiologic support for speech, such as respiratory, laryngeal, or lingual weakness, may benefit from efforts to increase strength to meet the strength demands of speech.

It is crucial that clinicians and patients realize that *full restoration of normal speech is not a realistic treatment goal in most cases.* However, some degree of recovery occurs for many patients and may be enhanced with treatment, especially when etiology is an acute vascular or traumatic event or other etiology in which full or partial physiologic recovery can be expected.

Promote the use of residual function (compensate). Knowing that restoration of normal speech will probably not occur should lead to efforts to compensate for lost abilities. Compensation can take many forms but is exemplified by modifications of rate and prosody; the use of prosthetic devices to amplify voice, reduce nasal airflow, or pace the rate of speech; modifying the physical environment or behavior of people within it in ways that enhance intelligibility; using supplements to speech during verbal efforts (for example, referring to a list of words to indicate a change in topic); and using alternative means of communication, such as an alphabet board or computer-based system.

Reduce the need for lost function (adjust). For those who earn their living by speaking (salesperson, teacher, trial lawyer, broadcaster), a motor speech disorder may mean the end of a career. For others, it may require a reorganization of their work environment or responsibilities or a change in social life-style, such as restricting verbal interactions to individuals or small groups. Depending on the course of the underlying disease, the prognosis for speech recovery, and the severity of the speech disorder, these adjustments may be temporary or permanent. For those with degenerative disease, planning for the progressive loss of speech may be necessary. Management has an important role to play in these adjustments, its primary goal being to maximize speech and communication functions so that the need to reorganize other life functions can be minimized.

Factors influencing management decisions

Unfortunately, many people with motor speech disorders are never referred for management because of ignorance about what can be done to help them. It is also unfortunate that some people receive treatment when they should not or are treated longer than is necessary. There are no firm rules for deciding whether treatment should be pursued, but the decision should be based on a good deal more than receipt of a referral to evaluate or treat someone. One general assumption that can be made is that *not all people with motor speech disorders are candidates for treatment.* The decision to treat or not treat should be based on consideration of the factors discussed next.

Medical diagnosis and prognosis. Did the underlying neurologic disease develop acutely, subacutely, or chronically? Is its predicted course one of complete resolution or improvement with eventual plateauing, or will it be chronic and stable, exacerbating-remitting, or progressive? Is there a medical treatment for the disease that may result in resolution or significant improvement of speech, and will such treatment take place soon and with subsequent rapid benefits? Answers to questions like these help decide whether or not to treat, or when treatment should be reconsidered if it is deferred. The following scenarios illustrate how decisions about treatment can vary as a function of neurologic diagnosis and prognosis.

1. Patients seen for assessment shortly after stroke, who are not yet neurologically stable and whose stamina and alertness are fluctuating, but who have only moderate speech impairment and adequate intelligibility, are probably not treatment candidates. Assuming that their stamina and alertness improve, the prognosis for significant improvement of speech is quite good. If they fail to improve and stabilize neurologically, it is not likely they would be interested or concerned about speech intervention or benefit from it if it were provided. In general—and ignoring a number of other influential factors—the best decision in such cases is to not recommend therapy or to reassess when the patient's physical status and alertness have stabilized.

2. Providing speech treatment before effective medical treatment is rarely justified (Rosenbek and LaPointe, 1985). For example, patients who are about to undergo neurosurgery for the underlying cause of their motor speech disorder (tumor removal, carotid endarterectomy) should have speech management decisions deferred until after surgery. In such cases, if necessary, augmentative or alternative means of communication may be provided prior to surgery, but, if speech is functional for the person's communication needs at the time, full assessment and reconsideration of management are best deferred until after surgery.

3. Patients with degenerative neurologic disease and dysarthria that are expected to worsen may nonetheless benefit from efforts to help maintain intelligibility and anticipate a need for augmentative communication. Patients with significant motor speech impairments who have had strokes and are still in the spontaneous phase of recovery also may be good treatment candidates. Patients whose physiologic recovery from stroke or traumatic brain injury has probably plateaued may similarly benefit from management.

Disability and handicap. The diagnosis of motor speech disorders relies on detecting *impairment, abnormality, or loss of function.* Although the nature of the impairment can influence the specific focus of management, the mere presence of impairment has little to do with a decision to treat or not treat. That decision relies on assessment of disability and handicap. *Disability reflects the degree of inability to speak normally because of the speech impairment.* It can be assessed by measures of speech normalcy, such as intelligibility, rate, and naturalness. *Handicap is the effect of impairment or disability on the ability to accomplish a previously normal role, one that, in the*

absence of handicap, would be played in the future. Handicap is determined by impairment, disability, the patient's communication needs, and societal attitudes. Yorkston, Beukelman, and Bell (1988), who have addressed these definitional issues in detail, point out that impairment, disability, and handicap are not always highly intercorrelated. For example, mild, isolated hypernasality from velopharyngeal weakness (impairment) may have little impact on speech intelligibility (disability), but may represent a major handicap to a television broadcaster. A marked spastic dysarthria (impairment) with subsequent reduced intelligibility (disability) may not be a great handicap to a shy and reclusive retired farmer who never placed great value on social or verbal interaction.

Estimates of disability and handicap also may diverge between patient and family (and clinician). For example, some patients with speech and cognitive impairments may minimize or be oblivious to the degree to which they are not understood by their family, whereas family members are constantly frustrated with how hard they must work to understand the patient. Some patients with uncompromising personal standards or difficulty accepting their impairment and disability may view themselves as unable to perform prior roles (such as leading a meeting), even though their impairment and disability are mild and their potential listeners find little reason for them not to continue to play those roles.

It is important that a clinician's discussions with patients and their families make clear the distinctions among impairment, disability, and handicap when discussing management issues and goals. In general, *intervention will not be recommended if there is negligible disability and no handicap associated with a motor speech impairment.*

Environment and communication partners. Decisions about management must consider the environments in which patients speak and the people to whom they speak. The problems encountered in noisy, poorly lit, bustling places, in which listeners may not know the patient and may have disabilities themselves, are quite different from those faced in quiet, familiar settings in which listeners are cognitively and sensorily intact, are familiar with the patients, care about them, and are sensitive to their disability. Such considerations should play a role in determining not only the need for management but also the needs to be addressed during management. The environment and traits of communication partners may have a significant impact on a patient's prognosis for benefiting from management as well as on specific management goals and approaches.

Motivation and needs. It is essential to address the patient's motivation and need for verbal communication. *The need to communicate may be the most important determinant to a decision to provide treatment* (Netsell and Rosenbek, 1985). Specific needs are determined by many factors, including, but almost certainly not limited to, age; educational level; premorbid personality; intelligence and life-style; personal goals; coexisting motor, sensory, and cognitive deficits; general health issues; and living environment.

It is surprising how frequently a clinician's judgment of disability and handicap does not match that of the patient. Many elderly patients, for example, are very accepting of their impairment and disability, do not feel particularly handicapped, and deny a need for intervention. To say that they are unmotivated is pejorative in many cases. Their judgment is simply based on standards that differ from those of the clinician; this perspective is often borne out by the patient's significant others, who often are in full agreement with the patient. The clinician's responsibility in such cases is to explain what management might accomplish if undertaken and to respect the patients' wishes if they decline the offer.

When a patient is truly unmotivated because of depression, more pressing personal concerns, cognitive impairments, or other problems, then direct intervention should not be recommended. Counseling of significant others may be undertaken instead, with an option to reassess direct management options if the patient's level of motivation changes.

Associated problems. Most people with motor speech disorders have accompanying neurologic deficits. *Motor deficits in the limbs* are very common, but if speech is not so impaired that augmentative or alternative means of communication are required, they may not have a big impact on speech management. Such deficits do influence the priorities of patients, however; some and perhaps many patients with functional verbal abilities are much more concerned about their mobility and ability to manage their basic physical needs than they are about their speech.

Cognitive deficits may significantly influence the conduct of management, and all of the central nervous system (CNS)-based dysarthrias (spastic, ataxic, hypokinetic, hyperkinetic, unilateral UMN, mixed) frequently are accompanied by them. For example, across the cases reviewed for etiology of dysarthria in previous chapters, approximately 30% to 80% had associated cognitive deficits. Such deficits vary widely in severity. They often include difficulties with attention, memory, learning, insight, planning, and motivation. Some patients with motor speech disorders, particularly apraxia of speech and unilateral UMN or spastic dysarthria, may be *aphasic* and have significant difficulties in all language modalities.

The presence of cognitive and language deficits can have a range of influences on communication and efforts to improve it. When they are pronounced, they can magnify the speech disability and handicap, strongly influence communication needs and motivation to speak, and have a major negative influence on the potential to benefit from therapy. They may require that a motor speech disorder take a low priority in rehabilitation efforts or that attention to motor speech be deferred until cognitive deficits improve. They may result in a decision not to address the speech deficit at all. In general, *if accompanying cognitive deficits preclude attention, drive, or motivation to communicate, or result in speech that has no functional communicative value, then the motor speech disorder should not receive direct treatment.*

The health care system. Managing motor speech disorders can be costly, and cost must be weighed in management decisions. It is clear that health care reform in this country, in its financial motivation to do less instead of more, will have an impact on patterns of clinical practice and patient care. Such changes will place great value on the efficacy and efficiency of management. In addition, there may be a shift to an objective standard of decision making in which external templates will override clinicians' and patients' autonomy in management decisions (Siegler, 1993). Clinicians, patients, and their families will be faced with decisions about what can be done to help and how quickly it can be accomplished. Actually, such issues are at the foundation of excellence in clinical practice and should be addressed independent of cost or reimbursement considerations. What is uncertain is the degree to which the decisions of clinicians and their patients will be congruent with the health care system's templates for management. It is likely that some treatment decisions will be influenced by factors beyond the clinician-patient relationship. The challenge to clinicians will be to maintain quality while increasing efficiency and reducing demand on costly resources.

Focus of treatment

In general, the component of speech that should be treated is the one from which the greatest functional benefit will be derived most rapidly, or that will provide the greatest support for improvement in other aspects of speech. For example, improved respiratory support may improve intelligibility rapidly and may also allow subsequent improvements in articulation to have a more obvious additional impact on intelligibility. These issues will be addressed in detail when specific approaches to treatment are discussed.

Duration of treatment and its termination

For how long should treatment be provided? The obvious answer is *for as long as is necessary to accomplish its goals but for as short a time as possible.* This qualifier must be weighed against the notion that intensive protracted treatment sometimes may be necessary to be successful (Abkarian and Dworkin, 1993; Netsell and Rosenbek, 1985).

In general, *no management program should begin without a plan about when it will end.* The clinician and patient should have in mind how long it will take to achieve goals, with an understanding that revision is possible. This temporal plan will help some patients decide if they wish to pursue treatment in the first place. Many, for example, are willing to commit to therapy when told that goals are likely to be reached within a short time. For others, it may assist their need to know how long it will take before they are "on their own" and able to function independently.

Duration of treatment is influenced by many factors. The etiology, the predicted course of recovery, the severity of deficits, the specific goals and techniques of management, patients' motivation and communication needs, the duration of hospitalization, the ability to travel for outpatient services, and health care coverage all have an impact on the duration of treatment.

When management goals are reached or plateauing has occurred, or when patients decide for other reasons that they do not wish further treatment, then treatment should end. After treatment ends, however, it may be important periodically to reassess a patient's speech and communication abilities and needs. For example, patients who plateau in speech progress but might improve further if new potential emerges or if their environment or needs change, should be reassessed periodically to address such changes. Patients with degenerative disease whose speech or communication problems are likely to worsen, but who are functioning optimally at the present time, may be discharged with prescheduled reassessment or the option for reassessment when change takes place.* Whenever reassessment is planned, the clinician and patient should know beforehand what options

for future management exist and what they might be expected to accomplish.

APPROACHES TO MANAGEMENT

There is no single approach to treating motor speech disorders. This statement reflects the significant differences that exist among motor speech disorders in pathophysiology, deviant speech characteristics, and severity, as well as the many other factors that influence management decisions, such as etiology, prognosis, environment, and communication needs.

Approaches to management can be organized in several ways, but they generally can be parsed into three distinguishable but frequently overlapping and sometimes inseparable areas of effort. They include *medical management, prosthetic and instrumental management,* and *behavioral management.* The goal of activities within each of these areas is to improve communication, preferably by improving intelligibility, rate, and naturalness of speech. A broad overview of each of these areas follows. Their specific methods and their effectiveness will be discussed in Chapters 17 and 18.

Medical intervention

Medical management includes pharmacologic and surgical interventions that can directly or indirectly affect speech. In general, medical management should always precede or be provided concurrently with other management approaches because it may maximize physiologic functioning and have a rapid or dramatic effect on speech.

Medical interventions that are specifically designed to improve speech require collaboration between the medical speech pathologist and otolaryngologist, plastic surgeon, or neurologist. The primary responsibility of the medical speech pathologist in such cases is to assess speech carefully and establish the need for medical or surgical intervention; the likelihood that the patient will benefit from such management; the specific benefits to be derived; what the intervention will not accomplish for speech; the need for postprocedure behavioral management and the provision of such management; and clear communication of all this information to the medical subspecialist and patient. It is important to have an understanding of the medical risks and costs of such procedures so that the decision to refer for such management can weigh risks and costs against predicted benefits.

Pharmacologic management. Pharmacologic management is almost always directed at relieving symptoms, but sometimes it effectively "cures" the disorder. Such approaches are directed to the underlying disease process (for example, infection) rather than designed to improve speech per

---

*For example, Yorkston and others (1993) indicate that they follow individuals with amyotrophic lateral sclerosis at two-week to four-month intervals, depending on their needs and rate of disease progression.

se. Thus, neurologic disease that can be managed by drug intervention may improve speech in the process. Because some drugs may improve some symptoms of a disease but not others, improvement in a patient's general condition may not always be matched by improvement in speech. Examples of drugs with indirect effects on speech include antibiotics for the treatment of CNS infection, steroids to treat the inflammatory effects of disease, and anticonvulsants to control seizures.

Some neurologic diseases commonly associated with dysarthrias are effectively managed by drugs, and their benefits can include improved speech. These include, for example, dopaminergic agents for Parkinson's disease, pyridostigmine bromide (Mestinon) for myasthenia gravis, dietary modifications and chelating agents for Wilson's disease, and a variety of drugs that may control movement disorders.* Injection of botulinum toxin (Botox) into certain laryngeal muscles for the treatment of spasmodic dysphonia or into the jaw, face, or neck muscles to treat orofacial dyskinesias or spasmodic torticollis is a prime example of the use of a drug for the sole purpose of altering the functions of specific muscles and sometimes for the sole purpose of improving speech.

Before beginning behavioral management, the clinician should know if the patient is receiving medication for the neurologic problem, if there are plans to initiate such treatment, or if drug therapy has been tried and abandoned. Behavioral management should be delayed until drug therapy that might improve speech is started because such therapy may make behavioral management unnecessary or change its focus. The exceptions are patients whose speech disorders necessitate the use of augmentative or alternative means of communication. Provision of those strategies and devices (usually "low tech") should always be undertaken to permit functional communication until the medication may have its desired effect on speech. It is also important to establish if fluctuations in speech are expected to occur over the course of a medication cycle as, for example, may be the case for patients taking medication for Parkinson's disease; behavioral management may be necessary but directed only to problems that emerge at a particular time during the drug cycle.

Surgical management. Surgery to manage neurologic disease may have direct and indirect ef-

fects on speech. Neurosurgery for aneurysms, hydrocephalus, tumors, seizures, and occluded arteries are examples of procedures directed to the causes of neurologic deficits rather than the deficits themselves. In some cases, surgery may "cure" signs and symptoms. In others, there may be improvement but not resolution, stabilization but not improvement, deterioration, or the development of new deficits. In still others—such as neoplasm resection—gains may be temporary.

Some surgeries are performed for the sole purpose of improving speech. Prime examples are *pharyngeal flap* or *sphincter pharyngoplasty* procedures to improve velopharyngeal function for speech and *thyroplasty* for vocal cord paralysis or weakness.

Prosthetic management

A number of mechanical and electronic prosthetic devices are available to improve speech or assist communication. Some may be temporary, used only until physiologic recovery or the effects of behavioral management allow them to be discarded. Others may be permanent because disability or handicap would be increased without them.

Some prosthetic devices directly modify what happens in the vocal tract during speech and help to promote perceptual normalcy. For example, *a palatal lift prosthesis* may facilitate velopharyngeal closure during speech, with resultant reduced hypernasality and increased intraoral pressure for pressure consonants.

Other prosthetic devices modify speech after it is produced. For example, *voice amplifiers* may increase vocal loudness in speakers whose primary speech difficulty is reduced loudness or inability to increase loudness to overcome noise, distance, or reduced hearing acuity in listeners.

Some prostheses are designed to modify the manner of speech production rather than simply support normal production or modify the speech signal. These devices may actually alter rate or prosody in the direction of abnormality in order to improve intelligibility. Examples include *pacing boards, metronomes,* and *delayed auditory feedback (DAF),* all of which slow speech rate and increase syllabic stress. Certain biofeedback devices may indicate to the patient when speech is failing to meet certain preset standards. For example, a *vocal intensity monitoring device* may provide an audible or visible signal when loudness falls below a preset level that is necessary to maintain intelligibility.

Finally, prostheses are available to augment speech or serve as alternatives to it. They belong under the broad category of *augmentative and alternative communication (AAC)* and are actually tools of behavioral intervention. They include *pic-*

---

*Some medications have side effects that may worsen or alter the character of a dysarthria. For example, a significant proportion of people with Parkinson's disease and hypokinetic dysarthria will develop dyskinesias (including hyperkinetic dysarthria) at some time during their treatment with levodopa (Rosenfield, 1991).

ture, letter, and word boards and more sophisticated *computerized devices* with multiple control and output options, sometimes including *synthesized speech* or the computerized recognition of speech. When limb movements are insufficient to activate AAC devices conventionally, a variety of assistive devices are available to activate them, including *light pointers* that may be worn on the head and *switches* that may be placed on any part of the body that is under volitional control.

Decisions about the need for and benefits to be derived from prosthetic management rest with the speech pathologist. The responsibilities are similar to those for decision making for medical or surgical intervention. Implementation is very often multidisciplinary, frequently requiring the skills of prosthodontists, occupational and physical therapists, rehabilitation engineers, and others. When heavy reliance on AAC is required, it is often essential to involve a speech pathologist who has subspecialty expertise in that area, at least on a consultative basis.

Behavioral management

Behavioral management includes all intervention efforts that are neither medical nor prosthetic. As already stated, medical, prosthetic, and behavioral interventions are not mutually exclusive, and some patients require all approaches. Behavioral management is probably provided to a larger proportion of people with motor speech disorders than is medical or prosthetic management.

Behavioral management has a wide variety of goals and may take many forms. Its primary goal, however, is to *maximize communication* by whatever means will produce the most rapid, effective, and natural results. For many patients, this requires a direct attack on speech. For others, it requires a combination of speech and AAC strategies or the sole use of avenues other than speech for communication.

The goals of behavioral management can be accomplished in a number of ways, including *improving physiologic support for speech, modifying speech through compensatory speaking strategies, developing alternative and augmentative means of communication, and controlling the environment and communicative interactions* (Rosenbek and LaPointe, 1985; Yorkston, Beukelman, and Bell, 1988). Approaches to behavioral intervention can be parsed in a number of ways. The most basic divisions include *speaker-oriented approaches* and *communication-oriented approaches*.

Speaker-oriented approaches work to restore or compensate for impaired speech functions. Their goal is to improve communication by *improving the speaker.* In contrast, communication-oriented approaches work to improve communication by altering speaking strategies, the behavior of listeners, or the environment in which communication occurs; their goal is to improve communication by *modifying aspects of the communicative interaction.* Treatment of mild impairments tends to be speaker-oriented; treatment of severe impairments tends to be communication-oriented. Both approaches may be employed at all severity levels, however.

Speaker-oriented approaches. Speaker-oriented treatment focuses primarily on *improving speech intelligibility* and secondarily on *improving the efficiency, naturalness, and quality* of communication. These goals are shared with communication-oriented approaches, but motor speech is the focus of speaker-oriented approaches. These goals are accomplished by *reducing impairment* by increasing physiologic support for speech or through *compensation* by making maximum use of residual physiologic support (Rosenbek and LaPointe, 1985; Yorkston, Beukelman, and Bell, 1988). Both methods are used with many patients.

Efforts to reduce impairment by increasing physiologic support attempt to remediate the deficits in posture, strength, and tone that underlie the speech disorder. Brookshire (1992) calls such approaches *indirect* because they may be conducted independent of speech. Activities may include sensory stimulation, strengthening exercises, the modification of muscle tone, altering posture and positioning, and improving respiratory capacity and efficiency. Rosenbek and LaPointe (1985) believe these efforts should be among the first goals of treatment, and they point out that medical and prosthetic management may be important components of them.

Making maximum use of residual physiologic support is characterized as a *behavioral compensation method* by Yorkston, Beukelman, and Bell (1988) and as a *direct approach* by Brookshire (1992) because it focuses directly on modifying respiration, phonation, resonance, articulation, or prosody in order to compensate for residual impairment (these compensations can include medical and prosthetic management). This approach assumes that some patients are more disabled or handicapped by their speech impairment than need be because they are not making maximum use of their residual physiologic capacity. Rosenbek and LaPointe (1985) point out that patients may fail to use such compensation spontaneously because they lack the knowledge to do so, wish to persist in speaking as they did in the past, have difficulty doing consciously what was once a subconscious process, have cognitive deficits that limit their capacity to learn and employ new strategies, or are anxious, depressed, or unmotivated. Some of these traits may actually preclude treatment, others may limit progress, and others can be overcome during treatment.

Compensatory approaches also focus on improving *efficiency* and *naturalness. Efficiency means increasing rate of communication without sacrificing intelligibility.* This may be done by manipulating speech directly, by adopting certain augmentative strategies, by altering language content or style, by manipulating the environment, or by developing strategies for efficiently handling breakdowns in intelligibility when they occur.

Focusing on *naturalness* involves attention to prosody. As Yorkston, Beukelman, and Bell (1988) note, working on prosody may be important at all severity levels because it contributes to the identification of speech segments and provides clues to meaning. Rate, rhythm, intonation, and stress carry important syntactic information and increase substantially the amount of redundancy in the speech signal. Thus, efforts to increase naturalness can be part of efforts to increase intelligibility.

In their efforts to speak more adequately or in response to physiologic limitations or abnormalities, some patients develop *maladaptive behaviors* or persist in using an adaptive strategy long after it is necessary or helpful. For example, some patients with vocal cord paralysis or respiratory weakness may speak on inhalation to normalize phrase length. Some use phrase lengths that are shorter than necessary or longer than can be physiologically supported. Such behaviors can substantially affect intelligibility, efficiency, or naturalness of speech. Their elimination may result in dramatic improvements in speech.

Communication-oriented approaches. Communication-oriented treatment may improve communication even when speech itself does not improve. It includes a variety of modifications ranging from altering the number of listeners, the amount of noise, speaker-listener distance, and eye contact to informing new listeners about the speech problem, its cause, and the speaker's preferred method of communicating. It also includes identification of the most effective strategies for repairing breakdowns in communication; for example, repeating utterances, rephrasing, spelling, writing, and answering clarifying questions.

Communication strategies may change from one speaking environment to another or from one listener to another. They often require negotiation, practice, and demonstration (proof) that one strategy works better than another. Some of these environmental manipulations and speaking strategies must be managed by the patient, but others are the primary responsibility of listeners.

Augmentative and alternative communication

A motor speech disorder can severely limit the degree to which speech and the gestures that normally accompany it transmit messages intelligibly and efficiently. The affected person may need to augment or substitute other means of communication for speech, either temporarily or permanently. The area of clinical practice that focuses on meeting these needs has come to be known as *augmentative and alternative communication (AAC).* Activities associated with AAC are part of behavioral management strategies but also include prosthetic management because they often rely on the use of aids—physical objects or devices—for the transmission or receipt of messages. These activities lead to the development of an AAC *system,* which is "an integrated group of components, including the symbols, aids, strategies and techniques used by individuals to enhance communication" (ASHA, 1991, p. 10).

The development and refinement of AAC in the last 10 to 15 years have been dramatic, and there has been a significant impact on many people with motor speech disorders. Augmentative and alternative communication can be considered a subspecialty area of practice within the profession of speech-language pathology. It holds Special Interest Division status within the American Speech-Language-Hearing Association.

The tools of AAC are heterogeneous. They include gestural communication that may not require the use of any additional physical aid, such as eye gaze, body postures, and facial, head, and hand gestures. They include a variety of symbols beyond the spoken word, such as pictures, photos, icons, printed words and letters, objects, signs or pantomime, Braille, and Morse code, and a variety of aids to facilitate message transmission, such as communication books or boards, a wide array of mechanical and electronic devices, and computers.

The use of AAC in the management of motor speech disorders can be highly variable across and even within individuals. For those whose expected disease course is one of improvement, AAC may be relied on heavily before recovery begins and then faded as recovery takes place.* For people with degenerative disease, there may be no need for AAC early, but total reliance on it may be

---

*Abkarian and Dworkin (1993) have stressed the importance of periodically readdressing patients' potential for developing functional speech after an effective alternative means of communication has been established. This is particularly important when onset is acute and recovery with plateauing is expected, as in stroke or traumatic brain injury.

necessary in the later stages.* For those with chronic and stable disorders, AAC strategies may remain constant, although changes in technology may permit refinements over time. For example, voice recognition devices may play an increasingly important role for some speakers who are poorly intelligible but capable of some variety in speech production that retains consistency over time (Fried-Oken, 1985).

The decision to use AAC strategies is based on careful assessment of speech and communication abilities and needs, prognosis, and the individual's potential to benefit from them. Use of AAC may be minimal for many patients; for example, a person may learn to identify the first letter of each word they say because it improves intelligibility, and they may drop that strategy as soon as intelligibility is adequate without it. In contrast, patients with locked-in syndrome may rely entirely on alternatives to speech, using eye gaze or forehead movements to identify symbols or trigger switches that will transmit messages.

It is beyond the scope of this book to provide a comprehensive review of AAC systems and techniques. Chapter 17 will discuss a few augmentative techniques that are useful in managing people with motor speech disorders. Several excellent, clinically relevant overviews and in-depth discussions of AAC are available (for example, Beukelman, and Mirenda, 1992; Yorkston, 1992; Yorkston, Beukelman, and Bell, 1988). They are valuable resources for clinicians who work with patients in need of a range of AAC systems.

Counseling and support

Behavioral management includes important counseling and supportive roles. There may be a need to provide information about why certain aspects of speech are not normal and may not ever be normal, what can be done to remediate the underlying impairment or compensate for it, what kind of efforts it will take, and the likely outcome of those efforts. For people with degenerative disease, it may include discussion about what may happen to speech over the course of the disease and what can be done to maintain speech intelligibility and communicative effectiveness as deterioration takes place. Obviously, the prognosis determines the degree to which such information generates feelings of optimism or hope for improvement, a need to accept permanent limitations, or a need to prepare for a loss of the ability to communicate easily and naturally.

These responsibilities require knowledge, confidence, sensitivity, and empathy. Sensitivity and empathy are particularly important traits, but are difficult to quantify. They tend to be born to many good clinicians but, paradoxically, sometimes are difficult to maintain as knowledge and experience are accumulated, especially in a health care environment that increasingly bases its rewards on efficiency and quantifiable results. Clinicians who provide this very human form of care—improving or maintaining communication—often have to struggle against a "body shop" mentality of care, and keep in mind that their patients may not ever have known anyone else with their particular problem, that they are *living with and not just working with* their problems, and that they are interested in success and not just the probability of success in treatment. There is no formula for developing or maintaining these traits,* except perhaps to remember that the manner in which care is provided may be as important from the patient's perspective as the actual outcome of efforts to improve speech or communication.

PRINCIPLES AND GUIDELINES FOR BEHAVIORAL MANAGEMENT

Some general principles and guidelines can be applied to the organization and conduct of behavioral management. They relate to decisions about when to start treatment, influences on treatment planning, baseline data, the focus of treatment, principles of motor learning, and the organization and format of treatment sessions. Many of them derive from consideration of factors that have already been discussed. Some of them are more relevant to the management of dysarthrias than to apraxia of speech; the differences will be apparent in Chapters 17 and 18.

Management should start early

Behavioral management should not begin until the patient is medically stable, that is, not in medical danger, physical distress or pain, or otherwise limited in attention or responsiveness. It should also not begin until medical management is complete or underway, unless medical management will be delayed for a prolonged time.

With the preceding qualifications in mind, it is generally agreed that early treatment is desirable. For example, it appears that the success of stroke rehabilitation (in the broad sense) is more strongly

---

*Yorkston and others (1993) indicate that they begin to explore AAC options for people with ALS when speech rate slows and intelligibility becomes inconsistent in adverse speaking situations.

The Healer's Art (1985), by Eric Cassell, sensitively examines many of the "human elements" that play a role in the relationship between patient and physician. The issues it addresses apply to all healthcare professionals whose responsibilities include personal interactions with patients.

related to early intervention than it is to the duration of intervention (Ottenbacher and Jannell, 1993). Although there are no data to support the notion of early versus deferred behavioral treatment of motor speech disorders, there is face validity to the notions that early intervention may slow deterioration of speech in degenerative diseases and that it may prevent the development of maladaptive speaking strategies in disorders that will improve or become chronic (Darley, Aronson, and Brown, 1975; Rosenbek and LaPointe, 1985). When factors such as efficiency of management and the desirability of bringing individuals to a maximum level of function as soon as possible are also considered, early treatment is almost always preferable to deferred treatment.

Medical and speech diagnoses are relevant to management

It is generally true that the better we understand a problem, the better we are able to manage it. Thus, medical and speech diagnoses should contribute to decisions about how to focus management.

Medical diagnosis. Many medical diseases have a known course and therefore have prognostic implications for speech. Some diseases are associated with an identifiable pathophysiology that explains many or most features of the speech disorder; when this is the case, it can help set broad management goals. If a disease is confined to a single part of the motor system or a single pathophysiologic process (for example, weakness, incoordination, hyperkinesia), it tells us in a general way what goals and tasks are or are not likely to be relevant to efforts to improve speech. For example, knowing a patient has a degenerative disease makes it unlikely that efforts to restore physiologic function should be part of the management program; this knowledge makes maintenance rather than improvement of speech a legitimate goal. Similarly, efforts to increase strength would be counterproductive for those with flaccid dysarthria due to myasthenia gravis; that is, strengthening exercises would induce weakness rather than increase strength.

Speech diagnosis. Optimal treatment derives from fitting our understanding of the determinants of abnormal speech patterns to available treatments (Netsell, 1984). The diagnosis of a specific dysarthria type or apraxia of speech implies a specific underlying neuromuscular deficit or problem of movement programming. Diagnosis in this sense has meaning for treatment. For example, because flaccid dysarthria is the result of weakness and reduced muscle tone, treatment efforts might attempt to increase strength. Because ataxic dysarthria reflects incoordination, treatment might focus on facilitating coordination or compensating for

incoordination; efforts to improve strength would be misdirected. In Chapter 17, treatment approaches that may be particularly relevant to specific dysarthria types will be discussed. Similarly, distinguishing dysarthrias from apraxia of speech is crucial because apraxia of speech requires a different approach to management; this will become apparent in Chapter 18.

In spite of its value, a diagnostic label cannot establish the focus of management completely. Identifying specific deviant speech characteristics, their relationship to each component of speech production, and their relationship to each other is also necessary. Relating speech characteristics to dysfunction in various muscle groups helps determine the component of the speech system that should receive attention. For example, reduced loudness is usually linked to deficits at the respiratory or laryngeal level and hypernasality to deficits at the velopharyngeal level.

Speech impairments should also be related to each other because a hierarchical organization of symptoms may enhance treatment efficiency. In this context, a hierarchy refers to hypotheses about causal relationships among speech characteristics or the degree to which a deviant speech characteristic at one level of the mechanism may lead to the emergence of deviant speech characteristics at other levels. For example, imprecise articulation may result from rapid rate, and short phrases may result from breathiness stemming from laryngeal weakness.

Rosenbek and LaPointe (1985) point out that the ability to establish hierarchies of symptoms can help determine where to begin treatment. In general, *treatment should begin as close to the bottom of the hierarchy—as close to the source or cause—as possible, because change at that level is most likely to have the biggest effect on intelligibility.* For example, establishing that imprecise articulation is secondary to nasal emission caused by palatal weakness may lead to management of velopharyngeal function, with resultant reduction in hypernasality, nasal emission, *and* articulatory imprecision. Establishing that short phrases and reduced loudness are linked to reduced respiratory support and not to laryngeal weakness may lead to efforts to improve respiration, with resultant increases in loudness and phrase length.

The preceding examples suggest that the bottom of the hierarchy tends to be related to the vertical level of the speech mechanism; that is, focus on a vertically lower level of the speech system tends to have an impact on upstream events to a greater degree than focus on upstream events influences events downstream. Thus, initial focus on respiration, when it can be related to speech symptoms, may yield more immediate and dramatic change than an initial focus at higher levels of the system. Of course, if physiologic support cannot be improved at a lower level, then treatment should move to compensation at that level or to a higher level. This tendency does not always hold, however. A more appropriate general rule for focusing treatment is that *treatment should begin with the component whose improvement will have the most effect on other components.* In general, "effect" refers to the impact of treatment on intelligibility (Wertz, 1985).

Identifying features that are readily modified with minimal instruction is also useful in establishing the initial focus of treatment. For example, what happens if patients slow their rate, attempt to speak more forcefully, inhale more deeply before speaking, or speak with their nares occluded? For some patients, immediate improvement is apparent in response to such simple instructions. Such improvement may not guarantee long-term gains, but what changes with minimal effort tends to be easiest to change habitually.

Baseline data are necessary for establishing goals and measuring change

Before behavioral management begins, the clinician should have baseline data that are relevant to the ultimate goals of treatment and to the specific tasks that will be the initial focus of therapy. Diagnosis and an inventory of deviant speech characteristics are generally insufficient as baseline data for measuring change during treatment. Diagnosis is independent of severity of impairment, disability, or handicap, and ratings of deviant speech characteristics on a severity scale have an uncertain relationship to more direct measures of disability and handicap.

Baseline data should include quantitative ratings or more specific measures of word and sentence intelligibility and efficiency of communication (see Chapter 3). These measures can serve as the standard for measuring change, for judging the effectiveness of treatment, and for decision making about altering or terminating treatment.

Although other factors are not necessarily quantifiable, it is important to inventory patients' communicative needs and goals,* their motivation to improve, their daily speaking environment, communication strategies they and their listeners find useful, and characteristics of their listeners. The potential influence of cognitive and sensory or

*Yorkston, Bombardier, and Hammen (1994) have presented and discussed a 100-item questionnaire that is useful for gathering information about patients' perspectives on their disabilities and handicaps.

motor deficits on prognosis and treatment activities must also be considered.

Finally, it is important to obtain baseline data on specific treatment tasks. For example, if the goal is to increase respiratory control by learning to generate 5 cm of water pressure for 5 seconds by blowing through a straw into a glass, it makes sense to establish the degree to which the patient cannot do this before treatment. Then measured progress is task-specific, and progress on the task can be related to the overall goals of improving intelligibility and efficiency. It should be recognized, however, that *progress on a specific task may not and need not always lead to a temporally concurrent change in intelligibility or efficiency.* It is possible that small amounts of progress on a number of different tasks aimed at different levels of the speech system must add together before a change in intelligibility or efficiency becomes apparent (see Simpson, Till, and Goff, 1988; and McHenry, Wilson, and Minton, 1994) for case study reports that seem to illustrate this possibility).

Increasing physiologic support often should be the initial focus of treatment

Treatment should usually begin by improving functions that support speech (Rosenbek and LaPointe, 1985). Thus, modifying posture and increasing strength, speed, range, and muscle tone, if relevant to speech deficits, should be attended to first to ensure maximum physiologic capacity for speech. When this is achieved, then efforts at compensation can be made through prosthetic and other forms of behavioral management.

Compensation requires that speech production become conscious

Darley, Aronson, and Brown (1975) included the notion of *purposeful activity* among their basic principles of treatment. They stressed the need to make speech highly conscious, recognizing that doing so requires a major shift in the speaker's orientation to the speech act, one in which being heard and understood takes precedence over quick and emotive expression. Conscious control requires constant monitoring and self-criticism, at least during early stages of therapy, as well as recognition by the clinician and patient that maximum effort rarely can be maintained constantly.

Principles of motor learning should influence management

The patient's understanding of the management process is important, but simply knowing that something is necessary seldom leads automatically to improved speech. Physical and psychological "work" are also essential.

Motor learning includes *cognitive, associative,* and *autonomous or automatic stages* (Fitts, 1964, as reviewed by Rosenbaum, 1991). The cognitive stage includes understanding the nature of the problem, knowing why it is necessary to do certain things to achieve a goal, and learning the procedures that are to be followed. In the context of behavioral management, this stage may include understanding what is required for speech to improve (for example, understanding that rate must be slowed to improve intelligibility) and understanding the procedures that will be followed to achieve that improvement.

The associative stage includes the transition from conscious to more automatic control through trial and error, with feedback especially important for learning what does and does not work. It is unclear if people with motor speech disorders can ever get beyond the associative stage of learning, but the goal of behavioral management should be to bring the patient at least to the associative stage.

During the autonomous or automatic stage, a skill can be performed quickly, with little conscious effort. Feedback is less crucial, and, if truly automatic, performance is possible even when the person is involved in another task.

The structure and organization of therapy can benefit from what is known about the acquisition of motor skills in normal individuals. The following points represent some "principles" that seem most relevant in this regard. The reader is cautioned that the validity of some of these principles for treating motor speech disorders is uncertain.* However, they can serve as valuable guidelines for management until their validity as principles is formally assessed.

---

*In fact, the validity of some principles of motor learning in nonimpaired people is not firmly established. Schmidt and Bjork (1992), in a comprehensive and compelling discussion of commonly accepted principles of training, argue that "certain conceptualizations about how and when to practice are at best incomplete, and at worst incorrect" (p. 207). Of particular relevance, they point out that manipulations that facilitate performance during training sometimes can be detrimental in the long run and that manipulations that degrade speed of acquisition during training can actually facilitate long-term carryover. At the least, these issues indicate that the short-term effects on speech of applying some of the principles discussed here (particularly those related to instruction and to consistent and variable practice) may not accurately predict long-term effects and that the effectiveness of a technique must be assessed by measures of long-term retention and generalization as well as its more immediate effects on the rate and degree of skill acquisition during therapy tasks. Put another way, clinicians should not assume that techniques that maximize performance during therapy necessarily facilitate the ultimate goal of treatment: long-term retention of improved performance within a variety of natural communicative contexts.

Improving speech requires speaking. People with motor speech disorders must speak to improve their speech. This is self-evident but must be kept in mind, considering people's tendency to talk less when their impairment makes speaking difficult, triggers a change in self-concept, or generates negative reactions from listeners. In nonimpaired individuals, disuse leads to muscle atrophy, and gains derived from exercise are lost when exercise ceases. The importance of speech "exercise" may be greatest during the recovery or improvement phase of management, as it is generally agreed that less activity is necessary to maintain a skill once it has been achieved (Saxon, 1993).

It is possible that mental practice—imagining the performance of the task—can contribute to motor learning. Rosenbaum (1991) indicates that, in general, *mental practice is more effective than no practice, but is less effective than physical practice.* He suggests that a judicious mixture of mental and physical practice may reduce the amount of physical practice needed to achieve a given level of performance. The contribution of mental practice to improvement of motor speech disorders is largely unexplored; it may have greater potential relevance to the management of apraxia of speech than dysarthria.

Drill is essential. Drill is the systematic practice of specially selected and ordered exercises (Rosenbek and LaPointe, 1985). Drill implies repetitiveness and tedium, but most patients do not mind it if tasks are selected in ways that ensure success.

Multiple opportunities for practice are probably important. Rosenbek and LaPointe (1985) indicate that treatment should be frequent in its early stages, preferably twice per day. Yorkston, Beukelman, and Bell (1988) recommend 10 minutes of practice once or twice per day, presumably beyond the formal treatment session(s).

The immediate effects of *brief periods of practice distributed over time* may be better than lengthy periods of massed practice (Singer, 1980: Wertz, LaPointe, and Rosenbek, 1984). This may be particularly true for motor speech disorders, in which fatigue with extended periods of speaking is often a problem. This suggests that drill be conducted for short periods of time, but frequently. Alternating drill with short periods of rest or nondrill activities may help to combat the effects of fatigue.

Instruction improves performance. Most patients do not improve simply by talking. They often need some instruction and demonstration about what to do. Hammen and Yorkston (1994), for example, demonstrated that instructing dysarthric speakers to be "more forceful" resulted in increased intraoral pressure during speech. The ability to alter speech with instruction is taken by many clinicians to be a positive prognostic sign, although this assumption has not been tested formally.

Self-learning is valuable. Although instruction may set the stage for learning, there is evidence that *discovery learning, in which the individual determines how best to achieve goals, may lead to better retention and generalization than learning that is highly prompted* (Singer, 1980; Wertz, LaPointe, and Rosenbek, 1984). Thus, a balance must be struck between clinician-provided instruction and allowing patients to instruct themselves. The best strategy may be to set a general goal (for example, slow rate), allow the patient to discover how best to accomplish it, and provide instruction when the patient is unsuccessful. Instruction generally should be faded as soon as possible, perhaps even if it slows the rate of improvement on a therapy task; that is, it is possible that slower progress without instruction may lead to better long-term carryover (Schmidt and Bjork, 1992).

Feedback is essential to motor learning. Knowledge of results is crucial to motor learning, especially in its early stages (Rosenbaum, 1991; Singer, 1980). It is most effective when it is provided immediately and is precise relative to immediate treatment goals (Yorkston, Beukelman, and Bell, 1988). Feedback may be provided by the clinician (or other people) or be instrumental.

Clinician-provided feedback is most appropriate when the immediate goal is intelligibility or some aspect of performance for which other feedback is not available. It appears that the more specific the listener feedback is, the more likely it is to influence subsequent responses. For example, dysarthric speakers are more likely to modify voice onset time in response to feedback in which the type and locus of errors are specified than when feedback simply indicates that a message is not understood (Till and Toye, 1988). The long-term effects of such feedback during therapy, however, are unknown.

Feedback provided during group therapy by other individuals with dysarthrias has been reported as more potent and "appreciated" than clinician-provided feedback by some patients (Thomas and Keith, 1989). Reviewing audiotapes or videotapes can also demonstrate to patients the effects of adopting certain strategies for speaking and repairing communication breakdowns. It is also useful to show the patient evidence of progress over time (for example, improvement of intelligibility scores). Such feedback is motivational and psychologically reinforcing, and it may be very useful when discussing the continuation, modification, or termination of treatment.

Instrumental feedback or biofeedback can be useful when a specific motor behavior or acoustic result is the focus of treatment. A mirror may provide information about range of jaw movement, a hand on the abdomen may provide feedback about range of inspiratory or expiratory effort, a volume unit (VU) meter may indicate loudness, an acoustic display may pace or reflect rate or stress or loudness, an electromyogram (EMG) may signal excessive or insufficient muscle contraction, and so on. The precision and immediacy of instrumental feedback can facilitate online adjustments in speech. Such feedback is more directly linked to motor behavior than is the more "cognitive" nature of feedback about completed performance.

It is generally accepted that immediate, accurate, and frequent feedback (including biofeedback) facilitates performance when a skill is being acquired. However, Schmidt and Bjork (1992) review data on motor and verbal learning that suggest that highly frequent feedback during acquisition may actually degrade performance on long-term retention and generalization. The reasons are unclear, but Schmidt and Bjork speculate that frequent feedback may become part of the task, so that performance is degraded later when feedback is removed or altered, or that external feedback may block processing of kinesthetic feedback, leading to less effective error detection when external feedback is removed. Thus, less frequent feedback or feedback provided in summary form may have better long-term effects than frequent, immediate feedback.

"Specificity of training." A general principle of strength training is that it should be as specific as possible to the direction, velocity, and range of motion of the ultimate goals to which training is directed (Gonyea and Sale, 1982). This principle makes good sense when applied to motor speech disorders and may apply to more than strength training. Treatment tasks should have some logical relevance to speech, and movements practiced should be representative of those needed for speech, even when they are nonspeech in nature.

In general, *treatment should not begin with any skill below the most advanced skill that can be demonstrated during assessment* (Netsell, 1984). This means that, for many patients, speech and not nonspeech tasks should be the focus of treatment activities. Relatedly, treatment should focus on changing motor abilities only as far as is necessary to achieve the goals of treatment (Yorkston, Beukelman, and Bell, 1988). For example, working on respiratory support beyond what is necessary for normal phrase length and loudness is generally inappropriate.

Consistent practice and variable practice have value. *Consistent practice* refers to repeated practice on a single task. A single task can be defined in a number of ways. It might involve production or repetitive production of a single sound, sounds with the same manner of production (stops), single-syllable words, three-word sentences with stress on the first syllable, and so on. *Variable practice* involves practice on a range of related tasks, such as slow rate on a mixture of single-syllable and multisyllabic words and sentences, sentences of varying length with stress placed at a variety of locations within the sentence, and so on. Both types of practice can be beneficial.

Rosenbaum (1991) indicates that responses frequently are not allowed to vary early in motor learning. This reduction in "degrees of freedom" promotes consistency of response by limiting what must be attended to and controlled. It also appears that when a series of responses is produced over and over again as quickly as possible that speed is higher when responses are identical over repetitions than when they vary. This suggests that consistent practice may facilitate speed and, perhaps, automaticity of responses. It should be kept in mind, however, that this kind of drill is a poor representation of natural speaking conditions.

Increasing task variability during practice tends to depress performance during training—relative to consistent practice—but it tends to lead to better retention and generalization to different contexts (Schmidt, 1991; Schmidt and Bjork, 1992). The reason may be that an *average* representation of experience is more readily developed with variable practice because changing contexts force trial-to-trial changes and encourage "additional information processing activities about the lawful relationships among the task variants" (Schmidt and Bjork, 1992, p. 214). In addition, efficiency and naturalness tend to increase with practice, perhaps moreso when degrees of freedom are allowed to vary and more than a single stereotyped response is allowed to achieve the same or variable motor goals (Rosenbaum, 1991).

These notions suggest that consistent practice may be most effective early in motor learning or when impairment is severe and the capacity to vary responses is limited. Variable practice may be more valuable in promoting generalization and naturalness and when recovery is sufficient to require that new responses be distinguished from preceding responses. This is especially relevant to the unique character of speech, language, and communication—the production of novel utterances that have not been practiced previously.

Increasing strength. Little is known about optimal strategies for increasing strength in the oral muscles. Even less is known about the necessity and effectiveness of attempts to do so within the context of managing motor speech disorders. In general, efforts to develop strength as part of motor speech disorders management are somewhat controversial.

It is generally felt that strengthening exercises should not be excessively emphasized. However, efforts to increase strength may have positive effects in some patients, especially severely impaired patients whose physiologic support for speech is significantly compromised (Brookshire, 1992). A few observations about strength training in normal individuals may help to guide clinical decisions about strength training for dysarthric speakers (strength training is not appropriate for apraxia of speech).

1. *Strength can be increased only by overloading muscle in some way.* Strength increases when muscle mass (the size and number of muscle fibers) is increased or when neural control (the recruitment and firing rates of motor units) increases. These increases can be achieved by low-resistance, high-repetition exercise or by high-resistance, low-repetition exercise. Because growth of muscle may be dependent on the tension developed within muscle with exercise, low-repetition, high-resistance exercise may be better for muscle growth (Gonyea and Sale, 1982).

2. *Exercise may be isometric or isotonic.* Isometric exercise involves exertion against stationary resistance; isotonic exercise requires movement of the structure to be strengthened. Isotonic exercise may be preferable for speech therapy because it comes closer to meeting "specificity of training" principles and because it requires agility and range of movement, both of which may be more important to speech than is strength. Brookshire (1992) points out that isotonic exercise requiring increased range and accuracy of movement can also strengthen muscles. He suggests that patients move to isotonic exercise as soon as muscles are strong enough to carry out exercise at low levels of speed and efficiency.

3. *Strengthening exercise requires repetition.* Rosenbek and LaPointe (1985) recommend sets of 5 to 10 repetitions with rest between sets, with approximately 1 to 2 minutes devoted to each muscle group. Although exercise at maximal levels (true weight training) should not exceed two or three times per week, more frequent training at less than maximal levels is justifiable (Gonyea and Sale, 1982). To be effective, muscle activity should be greater than that required by normal, nontreatment activi-

ties, but probably not so great that exhaustion occurs (Rosenbek and LaPointe, 1985). Striking this balance means that training at submaximal levels probably can take place daily.

4. *Once strengthening has been achieved, less activity is needed to maintain strength.* When strength is sufficient to support demands for speech, strengthening exercises can probably be discontinued in favor of activities that are speech-specific; that is, speaking may be sufficient at that point to maintain strength for speaking.

5. It is important to recognize that if maximum strength is required on some treatment tasks, it is not for the purpose of having the patient use maximum strength or effort all of the time. *Ultimately, speaking should demand less than maximum effort because maximum effort can rarely be maintained for extended periods* (Rosenbek and LaPointe, 1985; Wertz, 1985).

Speed-accuracy trade-off. Emphasizing speed tends to reduce accuracy, while emphasizing accuracy reduces speed (Singer, 1980; Wertz, LaPointe, and Rosenbek, 1984). This suggests that the early stages of treatment for most patients may emphasize speed *or* accuracy, but not both.

Accuracy should be emphasized initially for most patients because of its impact on intelligibility. In fact, accuracy is achieved initially by many patients through a reduction of speech rate. Increasing speed tends to be addressed only when acceptable intelligibility is achieved, and rate increases constantly must be weighed against the possible trade-off with intelligibility.

Organization of sessions

Frequency. Treatment sessions should be frequent, especially early in the course of treatment. Many clinicians suggest two sessions per day, which is quite possible in most inpatient settings. When only one formal session is possible, practice at home should be required, preferably frequently but for only short periods.

Task ordering. How should treatment tasks be sequenced within sessions? Little is known about this topic for motor speech disorders management, but clues are available from the aphasia treatment literature.

Studies of aphasic patients suggest that easy tasks should precede difficult ones and that treatment sessions should start with easy or familiar tasks, proceed to novel or more difficult tasks, and end with tasks that ensure success (Brookshire, 1971, 1972, 1976, 1992; Gardner and Brookshire, 1972; Rosenbek and LaPointe, 1985). In addition, within treatment sessions some time should be spent on activities that focus on maximizing the

ability to communicate (Yorkston, Beukelman, and Bell, 1988); that is, even if most tasks are non-speech in nature, some time should always be devoted to the ultimate goal, the improvement of communication.

Error rates. Brookshire (1992) recommends that error rates be kept low in aphasia therapy. High error rates tend to promote failure, may induce fatigue, and do not promote learning. Starting treatment at a level where performance is slightly deficient but never completely inadequate is probably most appropriate. Working on a given task in which performance is 60% to 80% correct and immediate is usually a good starting point; it means success is achieved frequently but that some degree of effort must be exerted to succeed.

When 90% or more of responses are completely adequate (for example, accurate, immediate, and without self-corrected errors), task difficulty should be increased (Brookshire, 1992; LaPointe, 1977). It is also reasonable in some cases to train beyond a criterion of 90% (require maintenance of criterion over several sessions) because overlearning may lead to better retention (Singer, 1980; Wertz, LaPointe, and Rosenbek, 1984)

Fatigue. Physical exercise prior to language therapy negatively affects the performance of aphasic patients, especially on speaking and writing tasks (Marshall and King, 1973). It is reasonable to assume that such effects exist for people with motor speech disorders, especially because the focus of their treatment is motoric. This suggests that therapy may be most productive early in the day, or before or at least not immediately after physical or occupational therapy. Relatedly, therapy may be most successful when benefits from drugs designed to manage the underlying disease are at a point of peak benefit.

Individual versus group therapy. There are no data to establish the advantages of individual versus group treatment for motor speech disorders. Clinicians generally prefer individual therapy, especially early in the course of treatment. The advantages of individual work include the ease of focusing on specific aspects of performance, the opportunity to obtain a maximum number of responses, and the opportunity to alter treatment activities quickly as a function of response adequacy. Most of what is known about treatment efficacy comes from the study of individual treatment.

Group therapy may be desirable for patients with milder degrees of disability and for those who are ready to work on carryover of skills and strategies learned during individual work (Thomas and Keith, 1989). This is especially true if family members or other caregivers are group members because the group can engage in communication-oriented activities in which all members of the interaction have an opportunity to practice their own responsibilities. Group sessions that include several patients provide an opportunity for carryover, a chance for patients to observe the strategies used by others that they must also use, and an opportunity to receive feedback from peers. It is also an opportunity to share common experiences, frustrations, and successes.

TREATMENT EFFICACY

We do not know nearly as much about the effectiveness of treatment as we should. This fact is disappointing and should drive efforts to increase efficacy research.

Our lack of knowledge is not unusual. For example, it has been estimated that data from controlled trials to support the efficacy of *medical* intervention, in general, is available for only about 15% of interventions (Eddy, 1992; Little, 1993). In contrast, Little (1993) points out that disinformation from advertising, vested interests, and poor science is available to support anything. One hopes that the management of motor speech disorders someday will be conducted with universally firm evidence of efficacy, that ineffective and inefficient treatments will be discarded, and that new treatments will be embraced because of factual rather than fictitious information.

There is a general sense among clinicians that treatments for dysarthria and apraxia of speech help patients to speak more intelligibly or communicate more efficiently and that treatment benefits can extend even to people with chronic or degenerative conditions (Netsell, 1984; Netsell and Rosenbek, 1985). These beliefs come from unpublished clinical experience, anecdotal reports, a fairly substantial number of well-controlled (and uncontrolled) case studies, and studies of aggregated cases that document gains in response to a variety of treatment approaches for a variety of dysarthria types and apraxia of speech.

In general, it seems that more is known about the effectiveness of surgical, pharmacologic, and prosthetic treatments for motor speech disorders than about their behavioral management. There are probably several reasons for this. Effective medical and prosthetic approaches tend to have immediate and more rapidly dramatic effects on speech; their results are, therefore, more readily apparent and easier to measure. When they do not work, the outcome is known more rapidly, the reason for their failure may be apparent, and subsequent modifications or new treatments can be pursued. Behavioral management takes time, experimental control often is difficult to achieve, the precise reasons for success or failure often are not readily apparent, effects are not always dramatic or stable, and replication of results can be difficult. Nonetheless, a substantial number of case studies of behavioral management at least suggest treatment efficacy.

Yorkston, Beukelman, and Bell (1988) point out that group treatment studies are conspicuously lacking in the literature on behavioral management. Perhaps more significant than a lack of group studies of single treatments is a lack of data on the comparative merits of various treatment approaches (Netsell, 1984). Kent (1994) has suggested that, for the present, it may be sufficient to know that a procedure works. He implies, however, that we should be making greater efforts to determine the efficiency of various procedures, the degree of benefit derived from them, whether one treatment approach is better than another, and whether some approaches are better for some patients than for others.

It is important to recognize, when reviewing the literature on treatment efficacy, that clinicians, researchers, and editors are disinclined to publish negative results. This tendency is unfortunate because the scientific purpose of treatment studies is to establish *if* a treatment is effective, not to prove that a treatment *is* effective. *It is as important to establish what does not work and who does not benefit from treatment as it is to establish what does and who does.* At this point in time, Wertz's (1978) statement about aphasia treatment—"we have yet to demonstrate what works when and with whom" (p. 91)—seems applicable to our understanding of motor speech disorders treatment.

Chapters 17 and 18 will discuss specific treatment approaches for the dysarthrias and apraxia of speech, respectively. Reference will be made within those chapters to work that has provided evidence of treatment efficacy, whenever such evidence is available.

SUMMARY

1. The goal of management of motor speech disorders is to improve communication. This may be an exclusive emphasis on improving speech intelligibility, efficiency, and naturalness, but it may also include the development of augmentative or alternative means of communication.
2. Management may focus on restoring, compensating, or adjusting to impaired speech functions. The degree to which management emphasizes restoration, compensation, and adjustment depends on many factors. Many

patients engage in efforts to achieve all of these goals.

3. Not all people with motor speech disorders are candidates for treatment. A decision to treat is based on a number of factors, including medical diagnosis and handicap, the environment in which communication will take place and the characteristics of the patient's communication partners, the patient's motivation and needs for communication, and the presence and nature of additional problems that may affect communication, such as memory and learning impairments and sensory and motor deficits. The changing status of the health care system will also affect management decisions.

4. Treatment should be provided for as long as is necessary to achieve treatment goals, but it should be accomplished in as short a time and in as cost-effective a manner as possible. Management should not begin without a plan for when it will end. It should be terminated when goals are reached, when plateauing has occurred, or when the patient decides he or she does not wish further management. Follow-up reassessment is appropriate in many cases.

5. Approaches to management may be medical, prosthetic, and behavioral. Medical management includes pharmacologic and surgical interventions, some of which may be conducted for the sole purpose of improving speech and others that are intended to treat the general effects of the causal condition. Prosthetic management includes a number of mechanical and electronic devices, some of which improve speech and intelligibility and others that augment or substitute for verbal communication.

6. Behavioral intervention may be speaker-oriented or communication-oriented. Speaker-oriented approaches focus on improving intelligibility, efficiency, and naturalness of communication by reducing or compensating for underlying impairment. Communication-oriented approaches emphasize environmental modifications and strategies for interacting and repairing breakdowns in communication when they occur. Alternative and augmentative communication systems represent a wide variety of nonspeech symbols, aids, strategies, and techniques that enhance communication and are an important temporary or permanent part of management for many patients with motor speech disorders.

7. Management includes important counseling and supportive roles for the clinician. These roles are as important as efforts to improve speech and communication in many cases.

8. Universal prescriptions for managing motor speech disorders are not possible, but some general principles can be applied to many patients. They include the importance of starting management early, recognition of the relevance of medical and speech diagnoses to management, the need to acquire baseline data to set goals and measure change, and the value of increasing physiologic support early in treatment. Actual treatment activities must recognize the patient's need to make speech a conscious activity; the value of principles of motor learning in the organization of treatment tasks; the importance of drill; the value of instruction, self-learning, and feedback; and the value of consistent and variable practice. When strength training is appropriate, which often it is not, principles of strength training should be employed.

9. Treatment should generally occur frequently. Sessions should be organized to move from easy to more difficult tasks and to end with success. Error rates during treatment should be low but not so low that the patient does not have to work to succeed. Treatment sessions are most effective when the patient is not fatigued. Individual and group therapy may be appropriate, although empiric data that establish the relative advantages of each approach are unavailable.

10. Efficacy data for motor speech disorders come mostly from individual and aggregated case reports. In general, they support a conclusion that management of motor speech disorders can be efficacious. Very little is known about the relative merits of different approaches to treatment or the specific disorders and other patient characteristics for which specific approaches are most effective. This state of knowledge may not be substantially different from what we understand about the effectiveness of medical interventions in general, especially interventions that focus on the modification of voluntary behaviors. Increased efforts to improve our understanding of the effectiveness of management for motor speech disorders are essential if the quality and efficiency of management are to improve.

REFERENCES

Abkarian GG and Dworkin JP: Treating severe motor speech disorders: give speech a chance, J Med Speech-Lang Pathol 1:285, 1993.

American Speech-Language-Hearing Association: Report: augmentative and alternative communication, *ASHA,* 33(suppl. 5), 9-12, 1991.

Beukelman D and Mirenda P: Augmentative and alternative communication: management of severe communication disorders in children and adults, Baltimore, 1992, Paul H Brooks Publishing.

Brookshire RH: Effects of trial time and inter-trial interval on naming by aphasic subjects, J Commun Disord 3:289, 1971.

Brookshire RH: Effects of task difficulty on the naming performance of aphasic subjects, J Speech Hear Res 15:551, 1972.

Brookshire RH: Effects of task difficulty on sentence comprehension performance of aphasic subjects, J Commun Disord 9:167, 1976.

Brookshire RH: An introduction to neurogenic communication disorders, ed 4, St Louis, 1992, Mosby–Year Book.

Cassell EJ: The healer's art, Cambridge, MA, 1985, MIT Press.

Darley FL, Aronson AE, and Brown JR: Motor speech disorders, Philadelphia, 1975, WB Saunders.

Eddy DM: Medicine, money and mathematics, Bull Am Coll Surg 77:36, 1992.

Fitts PM: Perceptual motor skill learning. In AW Melton, editor: Categories of human learning, New York, 1964, Academic Press.

Fried-Oken M: Voice recognition device as a computer interface for motor and speech impaired people, Arch Phys Med Rehabil 66:678, 1985.

Gardner B and Brookshire RH: Effects of unisensory and multisensory presentation of stimuli upon naming by aphasic patients, Lang Speech 15:342, 1972.

Gonyea WJ and Sale D: Physiology of weight-lifting exercise, Arch Phys Med Rehabil 63:235, 1982.

Hammen VL and Yorkston KM: Effect of instruction on selected aerodynamic parameters in subjects with dysarthria and control subjects. In Till JA, Yorkston KM, and Beukelman DR, editors: Motor speech disorders: advances in assessment and treatment, Baltimore, 1994, Paul H Brookes Publishing.

Kent RD: The clinical science of motor speech disorders: a personal assessment. In Till JA, Yorkston KM, and Beukelman DR, editors: Motor speech disorders: advances in assessment and treatment, Baltimore, 1994, Paul H Brookes Publishing.

LaPointe LL: Base-10 programmed stimulation: task specification, scoring, and plotting performance in aphasia therapy, J Speech Hear Disord 42:90, 1977.

Little JM: Communication and the humanities: the nature of the nexus, Mayo Clin Proc 68:921, 1993.

Marshall RC and King PS: Effects of fatigue produced in isokinetic exercise on the communication ability of aphasic adults, J Speech Hear Res 16:222, 1973.

McHenry MA, Wilson RL, and Minton JT: Management of multiple physiologic system deficits following traumatic brain injury, J Med Speech-Language Pathol 2:59, 1994.

Netsell R: A neurobiologic view of the dysarthrias. In McNeil MR, Rosenbek JC, and Aronson AE, editors: The dysarthrias: physiology, acoustics, perception, management, San Diego, 1984, College-Hill.

Netsell R and Rosenbek J: Treating the dysarthrias. Speech and language evaluation in neurology: adult disorders, New York, 1985, Grune and Stratton.

Ottenbacher KJ and Jannell S: The results of clinical trials in stroke rehabilitation research, Arch Neurol 50:37, 1993.

Rosenbaum DA: Human motor control, San Diego, 1991, Academic Press.

Rosenbek JC and LaPointe LL: The dysarthrias: description, diagnosis, and treatment. In Johns DF, editor: Clinical management of neurogenic communication disorders, Boston, 1985, Little, Brown.

Rosenfield DB: Pharmacologic approaches to speech motor disorders. In Vogel D and Cannito MP, editors: Treating disordered speech motor control, Austin, TX, 1991, Pro-Ed.

Saxon K: Exercise physiology and vocal rehabilitation. Miniseminar presented at the annual convention of the American Speech-Language-Hearing Association, Anaheim, CA, November 1993.

Schmidt RA: Frequent augmented feedback can degrade learning: evidence and interpretations. In Stelmach GE and Requin J, editors: Tutorials in motor neuroscience, Dordrecht, The Netherlands, 1991, Kluwer.

Schmidt RA and Bjork RA: New conceptualizations in practice: common principles in three paradigms suggest new concepts for training, Psychol Sci 3:207, 1992.

Siegler M: Falling off the pedestal: what is happening to the traditional doctor-patient relationship? Mayo Clinic Proc 68:461, 1993.

Simpson MB, Till JA, and Goff AM: Long-term treatment of severe dysarthria: a case study, J Speech Hear Disord, 43:433, 1988.

Singer RN: Motor learning and human performance: an application to motor skills and movement behaviors, New York, 1980, Macmillan.

Thomas JE and Keith RL: Group therapy for dysarthric speakers. Paper presented at the American Speech-Language-Hearing Association Convention, 1989.

Till JA and Toye AR: Acoustic and phonetic effects of two types of verbal feedback in dysarthric subjects, J Speech Hear Disord 53:449, 1988.

Wertz RT: Neuropathologies of speech and language: an introduction to patient management. In Johns DF, editor: Clinical management of neurogenic communicative disorders, ed 2, Boston, 1985, Little, Brown.

Wertz RT, LaPointe LL, and Rosenbek JC: Apraxia of speech in adults: the disorders and its management, New York, 1984, Grune and Stratton.

Yorkston KM: Augmentative communication in the medical setting, Tucson, 1992, Communication Skills Builders.

Yorkston KM, Beukelman D, and Bell K: Clinical management of dysarthric speakers, San Diego, 1988, College-Hill.

Yorkston KM, Bombardier C, and Hammen VL: Dysarthria from the viewpoint of individuals with dysarthria. In Till JA, Yorkston KM, and Beukelman DR, editors: Motor speech disorders: advances in assessment and treatment, Baltimore, 1994, Paul H Brookes Publishing.

Yorkston KM and others: Speech deterioration in amyotrophic lateral sclerosis: implications for the timing of intervention, J Med Speech-Lang Pathol 1:35, 1993.

17 Managing the Dysarthrias

It has been said, "There is no special treatment for the dysarthric disturbance of speech" (Mohr, 1991, p. 209). It is unclear if this statement is meant to imply that treatment for dysarthria is homogeneous and provided without regard for severity and the specific nature of the speech disturbance, or that nothing can be done to help dysarthric speakers. Neither implication, however, is true. There are a substantial number of ways in which clinicians manage dysarthria, and much of the diversity is a function of type and severity of the disorder. And, although efficacy data are limited, there are data that document the effectiveness of several approaches to management.

This chapter addresses the management of people with dysarthria. It assumes that the reader has read Chapter 16 and is aware of the basic issues and general approaches to managing motor speech disorders. It is also assumed that the reader has an appreciation of the general principles and guidelines for behavioral management because most of them are directly applicable to dysarthria management.

This chapter will first address speaker-oriented approaches to intervention. Medical, prosthetic, and behavioral interventions directed at modifying respiration, phonation, resonance, articulation, and the rate, prosody, and naturalness of dysarthric speech are the focus of this first section. Next, the degree to which specific speaker-oriented management strategies apply to each of the dysarthria types will be addressed. It makes it clear that treatment does not vary only as a function of

severity, that not all available management approaches are appropriate for all dysarthria types, and that some approaches may be contraindicated for some dysarthria types. It will also illustrate the value of differential diagnosis to management; that is, because differential diagnosis implies an understanding of underlying pathophysiology, it helps determine to some extent the most relevant approaches to treatment.

The last section of the chapter will focus on communication-oriented approaches. Such approaches are relatively independent of dysarthria type and are more strongly tied to individuals' communication needs and desires and to the severity of their disabilities.

The efficacy of the approaches discussed here will be addressed during discussion of each approach, when efficacy data are available. The availability or lack of efficacy data should serve as a gauge for the enthusiasm or caution with which these approaches should be embraced.

SPEAKER-ORIENTED TREATMENT
Respiration

Darley, Aronson, and Brown (1975) felt that respiration usually does not require attention in treatment because respiratory demands for speech are not great and because improving function at the phonatory, resonatory, and articulatory valves generally promotes efficient use of the airstream. Similarly, Yorkston, Beukelman, and Bell (1988) indicate that the presence of abnormal respiratory function does not necessarily mean that respiration is not adequate for speech. They suggest that *if a patient has adequate loudness and the capacity for flexible breath patterning during speech, then respiration does not require attention.*

Many dysarthric speakers do not need to attend specifically to respiration. However, poor respiration may impact on other speech functions, especially phonation, and work on it may be necessary to maximize consistent subglottal air pressure for speech without inducing significant fatigue and to ensure appropriate breath group lengths for speech (Yorkston, Beukelman, and Bell, 1988). At the least, *treatment planning should explicitly address the possible need to attend to respiration.* When the need exists, management efforts are primarily behavioral and prosthetic.*

Increasing respiratory support. Netsell and Rosenbek (1985) indicate that they do not focus directly on respiration if a patient can generate steady subglottal air pressure of 5 to 10 cm of water for 5 seconds. Yorkston, Beukelman, and Bell (1988) suggest that work to increase respiratory support may be appropriate for patients who cannot generate 3 cm of water pressure on speech or speechlike tasks, cannot sustain consistent air pressure for two seconds, or are unable to produce more than one word per breath group during speech.

Nonspeech respiratory exercises are probably unnecessary and inappropriate when speech exercise can accomplish the treatment goal. Some patients, however, may need to work on respiration in isolation before they can engage in speech tasks. Examples of tasks that may improve respiratory support for such patients include the following.

1. *Producing consistent subglottal air pressure.* Nonspeech tasks include blowing into a water glass manometer (see Figure 3–5) with a goal of sustaining 5 cm of pressure for 5 seconds ("5 for 5") (Hixon, Hawley, and Wilson, 1982; Linebaugh, 1983; Netsell and Daniel, 1979; Netsell and Hixon, 1978). An air pressure transducer with a target cursor and responses displayed on an oscilloscope or computer screen can be used for the same purpose; they may provide more easily seen and monitored feedback about performance.

   A related speech task might include *maximum vowel prolongation,* with duration and loudness goals. Feedback can be provided by the clinician, a tape recorder's volume unit

(VU) meter, or a Visipitch or similar acoustic feedback device (Yorkston, Beukelman, and Bell, 1988). Murry (1983) suggests that practice exhaling at a steady rate for several seconds, sometimes with glottal frication and eventually with voicing, may help promote respiratory control. Steady vocal output for 5 seconds would be the goal of such activities, followed by producing several syllables on one exhalation.

Linebaugh's (1983) concept of the *"optimal breath group"* has special relevance for speech respiratory control. An optimal breath group is *the number of syllables that a patient can produce comfortably on one breath.* Establishing this can help teach patients to keep utterances within the optimal breath group and may establish a baseline against which attempts can be made to increase breath group length. Contextual speech tasks may include gradually *increasing the length of phrases and sentences* that can be uttered in a single breath group without significant decreases in loudness or acceleration of rate.

Pushing, pulling, and bearing down during speech or nonspeech tasks may help to increase respiratory drive for speech. *Controlled exhalation tasks,* in which a uniform stream of air is exhaled slowly over time, may help increase respiratory capacity and enhance control of exhalation for speech (Brookshire, 1992).

2. *Postural adjustments.* Posture may be important for maintaining adequate physiologic support for respiration. Patients who need to make postural adjustments for speech may benefit from adjustable beds, wheelchairs, and chairs with adjustable backs (Yorkston, Beukelman, and Bell, 1988).

   Some patients with greater expiratory than inspiratory difficulty for speech may do considerably better in the supine than sitting position because of its stabilizing effects and because gravity and abdominal contents may help push the diaphragm into the thoracic cavity and assist expiration (Netsell and Rosenbek, 1985). This positioning may generate sufficient additional subglottal pressure to enhance loudness and reduce vocal effort in some cases.

   Putnam and Hixon (1984) point out that patients with amyotrophic lateral sclerosis (ALS) and lung disease tend to do worse in the supine position because of their significant inspiratory problems. Such patients may do better in the upright position because gravity may help lower the diaphragm into the abdomen on inspiration.

---

*Detailed discussion and specific treatment techniques and procedures for managing respiratory function in dysarthria can be found in Dworkin (1991), Rosenbek and LaPointe (1985), and Yorkston, Beukelman, and Bell (1988).

Prosthetic assistance. Prostheses that provide postural support during respiration or that help control expiration can be useful during speech. *Abdominal binders or corsets* can enhance posture, support weak stomach muscles, and improve respiratory support and air flow with reduced effort, especially for people with spinal cord injuries who may have intact diaphragmatic function but weak expiratory muscles (Aten, 1983; Rosenbek and LaPointe, 1985; Yorkston, Beukelman, and Bell, 1988). The risk of abdominal binding is that it may restrict inspiration and cause pneumonia (Rosenbek and LaPointe, 1985). Medical approval and supervision are important when binding is used. The duration of each period of use generally should be limited.

Leaning into a flat surface during expiration or using an *expiratory board or paddle* mounted on a wheelchair and swung into position at the abdominal level may help increase respiratory force for speech (Rosenbek and LaPointe, 1985). Yorkston, Beukelman, and Bell (1988) observed, however, that people who may need such assistance often lack sufficient trunk strength or balance to use it well. Some patients with adequate arm strength can push in on the abdomen with one hand during expiration and obtain similar assistance.

Behavioral compensation. Some patients simply need to practice *inhaling more deeply* or *using more force when exhaling* during speech (Hammen and Yorkston, 1994; McHenry, Wilson, and Minton, 1994). Working to inhale more deeply may take advantage of elastic recoil forces of the lungs during expiration in weak patients. Working to increase inspiratory range may be tied to attempts to sustain isolated sounds for 5 seconds while keeping intensity and quality constant (Rosenbek and LaPointe, 1985).

The higher expiratory pressures permitted by inhaling more deeply, if unchecked during exhalation, may lead to excessive loudness bursts, rapid air wastage, and no functional improvement in speech. Netsell (1992) has stressed the importance of *inspiratory checking* in this regard, which is the use of inspiratory muscles to "check" or control exhalatory forces to maintain steady subglottal pressure. The key instruction for this is to "take a deep breath and *let it out slowly when speaking.*" Netsell reported a dramatic increase in syllables per breath group and intelligibility in a patient who was able to follow this instruction.

Some patients initiate speech at variable points in the respiratory cycle and need to learn to be more consistent in inspiratory control. Similarly, some patients need to terminate speech earlier in the expiratory cycle if they speak at low lung volume levels that are insufficient to sustain adequate loudness (Yorkston, Beukelman, and Bell, 1988). For example, patients with Parkinson's disease and chest wall rigidity may find it easier to use short phrases per breath group rather than long phrases over which loudness may decrease or excessive energy is expended (Solomon and Hixon, 1993).

Sometimes, patients adopt maladaptive compensatory breathing strategies. For example, they may produce only one word per breath group when, in fact, they have respiratory support adequate for lengthier breath groups. A clue to this maladaptive strategy is the ability to sustain a vowel for significantly longer than syllable-level breath groups. This faulty strategy often is easily overcome by pointing it out to the patient and providing an opportunity to practice more appropriate respiratory patterns.

Hixon, Putnam, and Sharp (1983) have discussed two compensatory modes of breathing for speech that may be useful for people with flaccid paralysis of the rib cage, diaphragm, and abdomen. The first of these techniques is known as *neck breathing,* in which the sternocleidomastoid, scalene, and trapezius muscles of the neck are used to bring about to-and-fro displacement of the rib cage for inspiration. The second, known as *glossopharyngeal breathing* (or "frog breathing") is a self-generated positive-pressure strategy in which the larynx and upper airway structures are used to pump small volumes of air into the lungs in a stepwise fashion. A patient described by Hixon, Putnam, and Sharp used these strategies well enough to be judged normal in intelligibility, in spite of respiratory weakness sufficient to put him at ventilatory risk and require breathing assistance much of the time. His voice quality was mildly strained, fricative duration was shortened, and stops were sometimes substituted for fricatives; all of these characteristics probably reflected compensatory efforts to decrease rate of airflow and improve expiratory efficiency. The authors pointed out that such compensatory breathing patterns may be adopted automatically; their subject spontaneously adopted neck breathing and was taught glossopharyngeal breathing.

People who have impaired bulbar muscle function as well as respiratory weakness may not have the strength or coordination for respiratory compensations; therefore, the benefits of these breathing modes may be limited to patients with isolated respiratory impairment. Also, because of the prolonged inspiratory phase of breathing required for neck and glossopharyngeal breathing, the clinician should consult a physician knowledgeable about pulmonary function to get medical clearance for their use.

Phonation—medical treatments

Several medical interventions are available for improving laryngeal function in dysarthric speakers. Many are appropriate for only certain types of dysarthria.

Laryngoplasty. Medialization laryngoplasty or *type I thyroplasty* is a type of *phonosurgery* or *laryngeal framework surgery* that attempts to improve phonation in people with vocal cord paralysis or weakness. It involves placing cartilaginous or alloplastic implant material between the thyroid cartilage and inner thyroid perichondrium at the level of the vocal cord on the involved side, in effect displacing the paralyzed cord medially and facilitating vocal cord approximation—particularly anterior approximation—during phonation (Isshiki, Okamura, and Ishikawa, 1975; Koufman, 1986, 1988). The procedure is reversible, so medialization can be undone if vocal cord function returns. People with unilateral paralysis who undergo the procedure may have good improvement in pitch, loudness, and intonation, and they are generally satisfied with the results. Breathiness, harshness, and vocal fatigue may persist, however (Gray and others, 1991). Bilateral medialization has been used for dysphonia due to vocal cord bowing, and it may have potential for managing abductor spasmodic dysphonia (Koufman, 1988).

Teflon/collagen injection. Injection of Teflon into the submucosal tissue of a paralyzed vocal cord has been a popular procedure for managing vocal cord paralysis. Injected into the middle third of the cord, it increases bulk and narrows the glottis. It is generally not used until about one year postonset because removal of Teflon is not possible without compromising normal vocal cord anatomy. Its value is questionable for vocal cord bowing or when neurologic involvement goes beyond the recurrent laryngeal nerve (Koufman, 1988). McFarlane and others (1991) found that the results of behavioral voice treatment were superior to Teflon injection on preinjection and postinjection comparisons across several perceptual voice parameters. They suggested that voice therapy may be justified while waiting for spontaneous recovery from vocal cord paralysis when the patient has a competent cough and no problems with aspiration.

Collagen may be used for the same purpose as Teflon and may be preferable to it; it is structurally similar to natural collagen in the vocal folds and is subject to only limited absorption. It has been documented to reduce aspiration and airflow, im-

prove glottal efficiency and intensity, and generally improve the dysphonia associated with vocal cord paralysis (Ford and Bless, 1986; Remacle and others, 1989).

Recurrent laryngeal nerve resection. Unilateral resection of the recurrent laryngeal nerve has been used to treat adductor spasmodic dysphonia. By paralyzing one of the vocal cords, the procedure, in effect, prevents their hyperadduction and reduces laryngospasm. Preoperative lidocaine injection of the recurrent laryngeal nerve to induce temporary paralysis of the vocal cord is a useful method for estimating the effects of resection. Until recently, it was the preferred method for managing adductor spasmodic dysphonia of neurogenic origin. However, 15% to 65% of procedures "fail" by three years postsurgery, apparently because of increased hyperadduction of the nonparalyzed cord, ventricular folds, or supraglottic pharyngeal constrictors (Aronson, 1990). The procedure, in most settings, has given way to botulinum toxin injection in recent years.

Botulinum toxin injection. Unilateral or bilateral injection of botulinum toxin (Botox) into the thyroarytenoid muscle has become the preferred method for treating neurogenic adductor spasmodic dysphonia and idiopathic adductor spasmodic dysphonia that resist behavioral management. There are a large number of reports of its efficacy. The toxin blocks the release of acetylcholine from presynaptic nerve endings, in effect denervating some of the thyroarytenoid muscle fibers. Because the vocal folds are not completely paralyzed, they can be approximated, but with less than the degree of hyperadduction prior to injection. The effect takes place in 24 to 72 hours after injection and lasts for about three months, with return of symptoms occurring because new nerve sprouts develop and reinnervate the muscle (Aronson, 1990). Unilateral or bilateral injections can be successful, but bilateral injection is generally preferred. The injection can be given to individuals with failed recurrent laryngeal nerve resection.

Side effects of injection include transient breathiness and mild dysphagia for fluids, which may last for days to weeks. The course of improvement and eventual regression is variable, with maximum gains generally occurring 5 to 10 weeks after injection and average onset of decline about 3 to 4 months postinjection (Aronson, 1990; Aronson and others, 1993; Whurr and others, 1993). Aronson and others (1993) point out that, as a group, patients are very pleased with the results, often rating the reduction of physical effort for speech as more beneficial than the actual improvement in voice. Injection of the thyroarytenoid or posterior cricoarytenoid muscles, or both muscle groups, has been used for patients with abductor spasmodic dysphonia with success, but the experience with such injections has been relatively limited (Blitzer and others, 1992; Ludlow and others, 1991; Rontal and others, 1991).

Pharmacologic management. Some medications are occasionally effective in managing the phonatory impairments associated with dysarthrias. They are generally directed at specific dysarthria types. They will be discussed when management of specific dysarthria types is addressed.

Phonation—prosthetic management

A *vocal intensity controller* may be used to warn patients of excessive or inadequate intensity. Rubow and Swift (1985) described a loudness monitoring device that samples vocal intensity from a throat microphone and provides feedback if intensity is below a predetermined threshold. They documented the successful use of the device as an aid in speaking situations outside the clinical setting in a patient who had mild-moderate Parkinson's disease. An example of a simple feedback device for increasing loudness is the VU meter on a tape recorder, adjusted by the clinician to set new goals for loudness.

Patients with adequate articulation but significantly decreased vocal loudness may benefit from a *portable amplification system* (Figure 17–1) in which the speaker is located on the body, chair, or bed, or in which the voice is transmitted by FM signal to a speaker at a distance. Patients who are aphonic, severely breathy, or lacking sufficient respiratory support for speech, but who have good articulation skills, may benefit from the use of any one of a number of *artificial larynges.* Patients with movement disorders or significant neck weakness may benefit from *neck braces* or *cervical collars* that stabilize the head and neck during speech (Rosenbek and LaPointe, 1985).

Phonation—behavioral management

The primary goal of working on phonation is usually to increase utterance length per breath group and to obtain loudness levels that are sufficient for the social context. Patients with unilateral or bilateral vocal cord weakness or paralysis may benefit from *effort closure techniques.* These include grunting and controlled coughing, pushing, lifting, and pulling (Aronson, 1990; Rosenbek and LaPointe, 1985; Yorkston, Beukelman, and Bell, 1988). These effortful movements presumably maximize vocal cord adduction and may ultimately improve vocal cord strength. Patients with vocal cord weakness may also benefit from learning to *initiate phonation at the beginning of exhalation,* a strategy that can reduce air wastage and

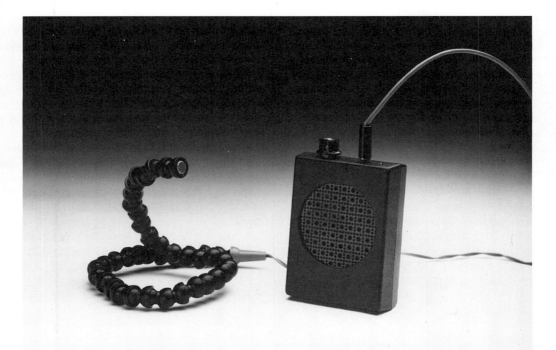

Figure 17–1 Portable amplification system with speaker and adjustable neck collar microphone. (Courtesy of The Radio Engineers Co.)

fatigue and possibly increase loudness and phrase length.

Some patients improve quality and loudness by *turning the head* to the left or right when speaking or by *lateral digital manipulation* of the thyroid cartilage; such postures may increase tension within the weak vocal cord and facilitate glottal closure (Aronson, 1990; McFarlane and others, 1991). However, Rosenbek and LaPointe (1985) note that such mechanical manipulation is cosmetically undesirable and may not lead to any true improvement in vocal cord adduction. In general, head turning and digital displacement should be considered compensatory, perhaps reserved for occasions when there is a clear situational demand for increased loudness.

Behavioral treatment of voice quality often is not undertaken because it is so difficult to modify and may not contribute greatly to improving intelligibility. However, some suggest that strained voice quality can be decreased if pitch is increased, the head is rotated back, and speech is initiated at high lung volume (that is, after a deep breath). Smitheran and Hixon (1981) discussed a patient who benefited from such strategies. They suggested that the lower diaphragm position associated with increased lung volume induced passive vocal cord abduction by tugging on the trachea. Others suggest that traditional relaxation exercise and laryngeal massage used for nonneurologic hyperfunctional voice disorders may also be of help in some dysarthric speakers with strained voices (Brookshire, 1992; Rosenbek and LaPointe, 1985). Patients with vocal cord hyperadduction may also benefit from learning to initiate phonation with a breathy onset or sigh in order to avoid stenosis (Darley, Aronson, and Brown, 1975).

Some additional phonatory treatment tasks will be addressed within the discussion on improving intonation and prosody.

Resonance

Managing velopharyngeal inadequacy is important for some dysarthric speakers. Excessive nasal airflow can result in air wastage during speech and can place extra demands on marginally adequate respiratory and laryngeal functions. Damping effects of the nasal cavity may reduce overall loudness, and nasal emission may reduce the perceptual distinctiveness of consonants requiring intraoral pressure.

A crude but often effective way of determining the impact of velopharyngeal inadequacy on speech intelligibility, loudness, phrase length, and articulatory precision is to compare speech with the nares occluded (by fingers or a nose clip) versus unoccluded, or with the patient upright versus supine (patients with marked palatal weakness may be aided by the effect of gravity on palatal position in the supine position). Marked improvement under facilitated conditions may signal the need to focus on velopharyngeal function early in management.

Surgical management. Pharyngeal flap surgery (usually a superiorly based flap) is the preferred method for managing velopharyngeal incompetence in people with repaired palatal clefts. It has also been used to manage velopharyngeal incompetence in dysarthric speakers, although with mixed results that generally seem less favorable than prosthetic management (for example, Gonzalez and Aronson, 1970; Hardy and others, 1961; Heller and others, 1974; Minami and others, 1975). Johns (1985), however, summarizing his experience with a substantial number of dysarthric speakers with velopharyngeal incompetence who had superiorly based pharyngeal flaps—many after behavior and prosthetic management failed—concluded that surgical management may help some dysarthric patients. In general, however, available data and clinical opinion indicate that palatal lift prosthesis management is preferable to surgical management for dysarthric individuals.

Teflon injection into the posterior pharyngeal wall has been used to manage velopharyngeal inadequacy in some dysarthric speakers (for example, Lewy, Cole, and Wepman, 1965). However, the procedure has not been well investigated and is not frequently used.

Prosthetic management. Yorkston, Beukelman, and Bell (1988) indicate that there are more case reports of successful management of velopharyngeal function than of any other aspect of dysarthria management. Most focus on successful prosthetic management in the form of *palatal lift prostheses*.

A palatal lift prosthesis (Figure 17–2) consists of a palatal portion that is attached to the teeth and a lift portion that extends posteriorly to lift the palate in the direction of velopharyngeal closure. Fitting of a lift requires adequate dentition to retain the device. Some patients must first adapt to wearing only the palatal portion, with the lift built in stages until adaptation and maximum benefit occur.

The best candidates for palatal lifts are those with significant velopharyngeal weakness whose deficits at other levels of the speech system are minimal or would be minimized by more adequate velopharyngeal closure; whose deficits are stable or not degenerating rapidly; who have sufficient supporting dentition; who do not have significant spasticity or a hyperactive gag reflex; who are motivated to improve speech and willing to tolerate the time to fit and adapt to the device; and who

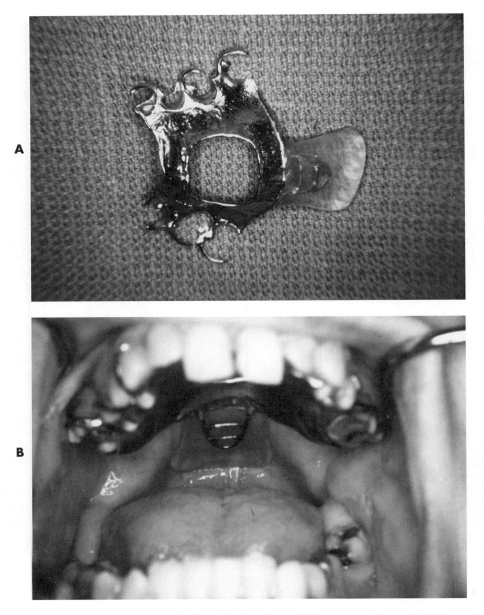

Figure 17–2 Palatal lift prosthesis: **A,** palatal portion with fasteners and extended lift portion; **B,** in place.

are able to insert and remove the lift without assistance. The fundamental question the clinician must address is whether a patient's intelligibility or efficiency will improve significantly if velopharyngeal closure can be provided by a palatal lift. Patients whose respiratory, phonatory, and articulatory abilities are significantly impaired may not derive functional benefit. In contrast, some patients who wear a palatal lift eventually develop improved palatal function for speech without the prosthesis, perhaps through stimulation of neuromuscular responses by the lift and the successful

exercise it provides (Dworkin and Johns, 1980; Johns, 1985).

The success of palatal lift prostheses—as indicated by increased intelligibility, decreased hypernasality, and improved articulation—has been reported for patients with flaccid, spastic, and mixed flaccid-spastic dysarthrias (for example, Aten and others, 1984; Gonzalez and Aronson, 1970; Hardy and others, 1969; Kerman, Singer, and Davidoff, 1973; Lawshe and others, 1971; McHenry, Wilson, and Minton, 1994; Yorkston and others, 1989). Etiologies in these successful cases have been quite variable, including stroke, traumatic brain injury (TBI), ALS, cerebral palsy, and polio.

Problems encountered in palatal lift fitting and use include inadequate retention of the lift because of poor dental support; hyperactive gag responses that are unresponsive to desensitization or appliance modification; a spastic or stiff palate that does not tolerate the lift; and lack of cooperation (Dworkin and Johns, 1980; Rosenbek and LaPointe, 1985). There are reports of edentulous patients for whom a lift was successfully fitted to an upper denture. For example, Aten and others (1984) reported successfully fitting lifts in several edentulous patients; the lift portion was attached to a maxillary retainer or existing dentures with wire connectors instead of the traditional solid acrylic material. Brand, Matsko, and Avart (1988) discussed a patient whose considerable difficulty in retaining a palatal lift was dramatically reduced by applying a topical anesthetic (lidocaine gel) to the surface of the lift to reduce sensation. The patient was then able to retain the lift, with benefits to speech, for several hours at a time, and the gel was reapplied as part of cleaning and reinsertion procedures.

Behavioral management. Behavioral management of velopharyngeal function and resonance seems to generate mixed opinions and results. Rosenbek and LaPointe (1985) indicate that they usually work to increase overall speaking effort, articulation, and prosody and pay little attention to the palate because it has less of an impact on intelligibility than other functions. This is probably the case when velopharyngeal problems do not significantly outweigh problems at other levels of the speech system.

Johns (1985) notes that some clinicians advocate facilitation techniques such as pressure, icing, brushing, stroking, and electrical stimulation or vibration of velar muscles to stimulate velopharyngeal function in people with flaccid dysarthria. Similarly, inhibition techniques such as prolonged icing, pressure to muscle insertion points, slow and irregular stroking and brushing, and desensitization of the velopharyngeal muscles have been advocated to bring about more normal muscle function in people with spastic dysarthria. Others emphasize strengthening exercises, such as blowing and sucking, to improve velopharyngeal movement. Such nonspeech approaches have a certain appeal because of their direct physical attack on muscles and the hope that such physical manipulations can alter function. However, Dworkin and Johns (1980), Netsell and Rosenbek (1985), and Brookshire (1992) feel that neither stimulation nor strengthening exercises are likely to help velopharyngeal function in dysarthric speakers. Dworkin

and Johns (1980) indicate that such techniques are especially suspect when the speaker has problems with more than velopharyngeal function for speech and that even when they seem to produce some improvement it is usually insufficient to eliminate the eventual need for prosthetic or surgical management. Johns (1985) concluded that "the general consensus seems to be that these exercises are disappointing and generally ineffective" (p. 158).

Although controlled study of the effectiveness of palatal stimulation and strengthening techniques may be warranted, their use at this time does not seem justified, given the conclusions that have been drawn by experienced clinicians. The possible stimulating effects of a palatal lift prosthesis may represent an exception, however; at the same time, the purpose of a palatal lift is as a prosthesis, not as a stimulant to permanent changes in palatal function for speech.*

Some speakers may benefit from feedback from a mirror, nasal flow transducer, or nasendoscope during efforts to decrease nasal air flow and hypernasality (Rosenbek and LaPointe, 1985). Modifications in speaking strategies that may improve resonance and reduce nasal air flow include: exaggerated jaw movement to increase oral opening during speech; increasing loudness; and reducing the duration of stops, fricatives, and affricates to reduce demands for intraoral pressure.

Speaking in the supine position may facilitate velopharyngeal closure, although there should be no expectation that adopting this posture will eventually lead to better velopharyngeal function in the upright position. Some patients may improve intelligibility by manually occluding the nares or wearing a nose clip; although this is not usually done on a constant basis, it may represent an effective strategy for improving intelligibility when a statement has not been understood. Relatedly, Stewart and Rieger (1994) recently described the fabrication and use of a relatively visually unobtrusive nasal obturator that can be inserted into the nares for the purpose of occluding nasal airflow during speech. They described its use in

---

*Recently, Kuehn and Wachtel (1994) reported the use of continuous positive airway pressure (CPAP) in the treatment of palatal weakness. Sometimes used for people with obstructive sleep apnea, CPAP delivers positive airflow into the nasal cavities through a hose and nasal mask assembly. It was used to develop a resistance exercise program in which velopharyngeal muscles were challenged to overcome the positive airway pressure to achieve velopharyngeal closure during speech. The authors reported two successfully treated cases, one of which resulted in a significant and lasting reduction in hypernasality and allowed a palatal lift to be discarded. It is possible that the success of this program is related to careful subject selection and to the specificity of its strength training to speech.

facilitating speech improvement in a person with flaccid dysarthria resulting from TBI.

Articulation

Focus on articulation has traditionally been viewed as a major part of dysarthria treatment. This is probably not the case for many patients today, especially if efforts to improve articulation by slowing rate and modifying prosody are placed outside the realm of articulation activities. Thus, although the goal of many treatment efforts is to improve accuracy and precision of sound production, it is often accomplished by focusing on functions other than those directly related to place and manner of articulation.

Surgical management. Neural anastomosis is occasionally pursued to restore function to a nerve. In dysarthric patients, this procedure most often involves attempts to restore function to the facial nerve, for both cosmetic and functional purposes. This usually involves connecting a branch of the XIIth nerve to the damaged VIIth nerve. Anastomosis of the facial and accessory nerve, or with the facial nerve on the unaffected side, has also been conducted, but the VII to XII anastomosis is generally preferred (Mingrino and Zuccarello, 1981). Mingrino and Zuccarello point out that the hypoglossal-facial anastomosis sometimes leads to facial synkinesis during speech, a result that might be socially embarrassing and interfere with articulation.

The procedure is usually pursued in people with normal hypoglossal function and no clear evidence of dysarthria because lingual weakness usually develops after surgery (Daniel and Guitar, 1978; Hammerschlag and others, 1987; Yorkston, 1989). Thus, the procedure's goal of improving facial appearance and movement is not typically done to improve speech, but it does not appear to carry great risks to speech if tongue function is normal before surgery.

Yorkston (1989) reported the case of a woman who had a VII to XII anastomosis subsequent to a brainstem stroke that had also left her with lingual involvement, reduced speech rate, and about 90% intelligibility. Immediately after surgery, intelligibility dropped, rate decreased slightly, and lingual consonant precision deteriorated; she also had difficulty managing saliva and the oral phase of swallowing. Over a seven-month period, intelligibility and rate returned to baseline levels, and swallowing and saliva difficulties resolved. It thus appears that the procedure is not without risk to speech for individuals with lingual involvement prior to surgery, although losses may be overcome if the preexisting dysarthria is mild. Yorkston recommended that such surgery be pursued with extreme caution for patients more involved than the case she reported and that presurgical counseling clearly review the risks to speech and swallowing.

Botox injection, in addition to its usefulness in treating spasmodic dysphonia, also can be an effective treatment for hemifacial spasm, spasmodic torticollis, and oral mandibular dystonia (Brin and others, 1987; Jankovic, 1989; Tolosa, Marti, and Kulisevsky, 1988). To the extent that the injection decreases abnormal movement in these disorders, it should decrease its associated hyperkinetic dysarthria. Schulz and Ludlow (1991) examined the effect on speech in three patients with focal dystonias affecting orofacial and mandibular muscles who had Botox injections of the genioglossus, styloglossus, medial pterygoid, masseter, anterior belly of the digastricus, or risorius muscles. Their acoustic analyses following injection revealed improvements in word and sentence duration and reduction of inappropriate silences.

Pharmacologic management. There are a number of pharmacologic possibilities that may have an impact on articulation, but they have received little formal investigation. Antispasticity medications such as chlordiazepoxide (Librium), diazepam (Valium), dantrolene (Dantrium), and baclofen (Lioresal) are sometimes effective in decreasing limb spasticity (Merritt, 1981), but their effects on articulation are uncertain. Choreiform movements are sometimes decreased with reserpine, haloperidol (Haldol), or Lioresal. Haldol may be helpful in managing symptoms of Tourette's syndrome. Propranolol (Inderal) may be effective in decreasing tremor, as may primidone (Mysoline). Inderal may also help spasmodic dysphonia due to tremor, as may Mysoline and carbamazepine (Tegretol); some patients respond to Lioresal or a combination of trihexyphenidyl (Artane) and lithium (Rosenfield, 1991).

Prosthetic management. Prostheses to aid articulation are limited. A *bite block* is a small piece of material (acrylic, putty) that is custom fitted to be held between the lateral upper and lower teeth (Dworkin, 1991; Netsell, 1985). Speaking with a bite block in place may help patients whose jaw control is disproportionately impaired relative to other articulators. Netsell (1985) noted that "some clients become immediately and strikingly intelligible" (p. 105) with a bite block in place and reported this effect in a patient with Parkinson's disease; he also noted that it may help patients with spastic or hyperkinetic (dystonia) dysarthria.

A bite block may be of particular use to patients with jaw opening dystonia who are often able—temporarily, at least—to inhibit jaw opening by clenching the teeth or biting on an object during speech. Its usefulness is probably contraindicated for flaccid dysarthria because jaw movement may be necessary to compensate for weakness in other articulators. However, Linebaugh (1983) and Netsell and Rosenbek (1985) suggest that a bite block may represent a method for "forcing" increased lip and tongue movement in some patients by taking jaw movement out of the speech loop and removing its capacity to compensate for weak or otherwise reduced lip and tongue movements.

Behavioral management. Behavioral management of articulation includes strength training, relaxation, stretching, biofeedback, and traditional articulation methods. Patients requiring focus on articulation almost always receive traditional treatments; other techniques are probably less universally appropriate.

1. *Strengthening*—The use of *strength training* to improve articulation is controversial. It is certainly possible to engage in activities that might increase strength in articulators. The jaw can be opened, closed, lateralized, and pushed forward against resistance; the lips can be rounded, spread, puffed, and closed isometrically with or without clinician-provided resistance; the tongue can be protruded and lateralized against resistance or pushed against the alveolus, cheeks, or a tongue blade, and so on. Patients with marked weakness or limited movement may simply be asked to perform movements without resistance. Such exercise can be done with instrumentation designed to measure force and strength, especially when it is capable of providing feedback about results.

   An important issue is whether strengthening exercise during nonspeech activities is necessary at all for most patients. Yorkston, Beukelman, and Bell (1988) noted the absence of data on the effect of strengthening exercises on articulatory adequacy and concluded that there are probably only a small number of patients for whom strengthening exercises are appropriate. That strengthening exercise may be unnecessary is supported by the facts that the tongue and lips use only 10% to 30% of their maximum forces for speech, and the jaw only 2%, and that up to one third of motor nerve fibers can be lost before functional impairments are encountered (Barlow and Abbs, 1983; DePaul and Brooks, 1993). DePaul and Brooks (1993) concluded from their study of patients with ALS that weakness is not directly related to intelligibility, possibly because many orofacial muscles can trade off or compensate for weakness, and because only low levels of force are required for speech.

In general, nonspeech strengthening exercises should be used only after establishing that weakness is clearly related to speech impairment and disability. If a clinician makes a commitment to improving strength during nonspeech activities, the effort should be a concerted one. For example, Linebaugh (1983) suggests that strengthening exercises be done in 5 sets of 10 repetitions each, 3 to 5 times per session, with 5 to 10 exercise periods per day.

2. *Relaxation*—Some clinicians suggest that *relaxation exercises* may help to improve muscle tone in patients with spasticity or rigidity. For example, shaking the head and the open jaw to create lateral movements of the jaw may help loosen jaw movements for speech; chewing movements to promote relaxation may help decrease mild muscle hypertonus in the jaw and tongue (Rosenbek and LaPointe, 1985). The problem with such exercises is that the movements necessary to accomplish them (jaw shaking) are often as impaired as those they are designed to improve (jaw movement for speech). Rosenbek and LaPointe (1985) suggest that most clinicians should work on speech movements rather than relaxation.

3. *Stretching*—The notion of stretching is one of the foundations for managing spasticity in the limbs. It is generally recommended that stretching in the limbs be steady, continuous, prolonged, and directional, with avoidance of sudden changes in force or direction because oscillating forces can stimulate muscle spindle activity and promote spasticity.

   Stretching exercise has been noted to prevent joint and muscle contractions and also modulate spasticity (Merritt, 1981). For example, there is evidence that passive range of movement with terminal stretch applied to finger flexion muscles temporarily improves control of finger extension movement in patients with spastic hemiparesis, perhaps by improving joint mobility (Carey, 1990); stretching exercises can improve range of motion of voluntary hip adduction (Odéen, 1981). Range-of-motion limb exercises that are not vigorous or fatiguing are also recommended for patients with ALS, to stretch their unaffected muscles and prevent joint stiffness and muscle contraction (Sinaki, 1987).

   These findings for the limbs raise the possibility that stretching exercises, such as sustained maximum jaw opening; sustained maximum tongue protrusion, retraction, or lateralization; or sustained maximum lip retraction, pursing, and puffing may have some effect on increasing range of motion and decreasing the effects of spasticity on speech. Because stretch of articulators is necessarily voluntary and not passive, it may also contribute to increasing strength. Stretching may be most applicable for those with spasticity and rigidity; the possible strengthening effect of stretch might help some patients with weakness.

4. *Biofeedback*—Some evidence suggests that hypertonicity (for example, dystonia) in speech muscles can be modified by *biofeedback*. Netsell and Cleeland (1973) used biofeedback from the upper lip to modify a constant stiff and retracted upper lip that interfered with bilabial stop production in a parkinsonian individual with upper lip hypertonicity. The patient learned to reduce lip retraction to the point that it occurred only during speech, and some normal bilabials during structured and conversational speech were possible. Hand, Burns, and Ireland (1979) also discussed a biofeedback program to reduce lip hypertonia and retraction in a parkinsonian patient with severe dysarthria. The biofeedback training was successful in reducing excessive muscle activity for postural and some simple speech tasks but was less effective for more complex utterances. Rubow and others (1984) documented impressive results of electromyogram (EMG) feedback to reduce hemifacial spasm that distorted the face and generated overflow to the tongue and larynx during speech. Their patient learned to decrease frontalis and hemifacial spasm with and eventually without EMG feedback. Speech markedly improved even though biofeedback training was not provided during speech activity, and gains were maintained at 1-month and 15-month follow-up.

Nemec and Cohen (1984) used biofeedback to reduce tension and facilitate restoration of voluntary mandibular control in a patient with spastic dysarthria. Biofeedback helped develop maintenance of jaw elevation, with subsequent reduction of drooling and improved speech intelligibility.

Daniel and Guitar (1978) also used surface EMG biofeedback from the lip to increase muscle activity during speech and nonspeech activities five years after a VII to XII anastomosis in one speaker. Facial gestures during speech and nonspeech activities improved and were maintained. Speech was not perceptually abnormal before treatment, however, except for some slight distortion on a few consonant clusters.

5. *Traditional approaches*—Rosenbek and LaPointe (1985) emphasized the importance of traditional methods of articulation therapy for dysarthric speakers; including (1) *integral stimulation* (watch and listen imitation tasks), (2) *phonetic placement* (hands-on assistance in attaining targets and movements, pictured illustrations of articulatory targets, and the like), and (3) *phonetic derivation* (using an intact nonspeech gesture to establish a target, such as blowing to facilitate production of /u/).

Articulation work often emphasizes the *exaggeration of consonants* to prevent their slighting and improve precision, especially in the medial and final position of syllables (Darley, Aronson, and Brown, 1975; Netsell and Rosenbek, 1985). Instruction to increase effort and slow rate may facilitate efforts at exaggeration. Although some patients need to work on sounds in isolation before they can integrate them into syllables and words, it is generally agreed that articulatory drills should emphasize movements and syllables and not simply fixed positions (Brookshire, 1992; Rosenbek and LaPointe, 1985).

Some patients need to learn compensatory articulatory movements. They may include, for example, use of the tongue blade instead of tongue tip when the tongue is markedly weak, or lingual-dental contact instead of bilabial closure when lip weakness or hypertonicity is significant. Patients with poor laryngeal control who are unable to adjust voice onset time to distinguish voiced from voiceless consonants may learn to release final consonants or to shorten vowels preceding final consonants to signal voiceless sounds.

A careful inventory of articulatory errors that contribute to decreased intelligibility is important to the ordering of stimuli in treatment. In general, stops and nasals are easier than fricatives and affricates, especially when respiratory support is decreased. When the palate is weak, nasals, vowels, and glides are generally easier than consonants requiring intraoral pressure. Phonetic environment also must be considered in stimulus preparation. For example, producing lingual alveolar consonants is generally facilitated in high vowel environments as opposed to environments in which the jaw is relatively open or the tongue retracted.

Working on *minimal contrasts* may be particularly helpful in achieving control over consonants, especially when moving from single-syllable to longer productions (for example, contrasting productions of "pay-may," "pie-bye," "chew-shoe," "stop-top"). It is important during such *contrastive drill tasks* that the patient know that the purpose is to make the distinction between the minimal contrasts as clear as possible. Such tasks can involve contrasts between consonants or vowels and can be used with word, phrase, or sentence stimuli in order to increase or decrease difficulty.* In general, meaningful stimuli are preferred over nonsense syllables, although this rule may be compromised for work on minimal contrasts at the syllable level.

Yorkston, Beukelman, and Bell (1988) discussed the usefulness of *intelligibility drills* that may be most applicable during work on articulation, rate, and prosody. These drills involve *referential tasks* in which the clinician-listener is naive to the target produced by the patient. The materials can be, for example, randomized word lists, sentences, or pictures to be described. The listeners' task is to tell the speaker what they heard. These drills are useful because they promote discovery learning—patients do not receive instruction, they discover how to make their speech intelligible; focus on the primary goal of treatment, improved intelligibility; can be adjusted to ensure success— that is, even markedly impaired speakers can be given materials that can result in a high, but not perfect, degree of intelligibility; facilitate the development of strategies to repair breakdowns in intelligibility by both speaker and listener.

Rate

Rate may be the most powerful single, behaviorally modifiable variable for improving intelligibility (Yorkston, Dowden, and Beukelman, 1992).

Rate modification is used with many dysarthric speakers because it frequently facilitates articulatory precision and intelligibility by allowing time for full range of movement, increased time for coordination, and improved linguistic phrasing. Reducing rate may also be easier to achieve than other motor goals, given the physiologic limitations imposed by many dysarthrias. There are many ways to achieve reduced rate. Some employ prosthetic devices, whereas others use more natural methods. Some impose rigid rate reductions while sacrificing prosody and naturalness, whereas others do not.

Yorkston, Beukelman, and Bell (1988) stress that rate reduction that does not improve intelligibility should not be used because it reduces naturalness. The perceptual integrity of consonants and vowels may also deteriorate at extremely slow rates (Turner and Weismer, 1993). This suggests that rate reduction must utilize *pause time* as much as reduced articulatory rate to achieve its desired effects. *Pauses* are very important to variations in speech rate and are probably particularly important to modifying rate in dysarthria (Rosenbek and

LaPointe, 1985; Yorkston, Beukelman, and Bell, 1988). Pauses may represent up to 50% of total utterance time (Goldman-Eisler, 1961; Henderson, Goldman-Eisler, and Skarbek, 1966), they carry considerable information about syntactic boundaries, and they are more modifiable than the duration of actual speech production.

Prosthetic management. Several prosthetic devices may aid rate reduction. Among the most useful for well-selected patients is *delayed auditory feedback (DAF)*. It is an instrumental procedure in which the rate at which an individual's speech is fed back (through earphones) to them is delayed by varying intervals that can be set by the clinician or patient (Figure 17–3). The effect of the delay is to slow speech rate and, presumably, increase articulation time and accuracy. Delayed auditory feedback requires little training; the speaker must attend to the feedback but other learning is unnecessary, and its effect is usually rapidly apparent. It may be effective when other rate-control techniques fail and may have temporary value in demonstrating to patients that slowing speech rate has positive effects on intelligibility (Rosenbek and LaPointe, 1985). Effective delays generally range from 50 to 150 milliseconds.

Yorkston, Beukelman, and Bell (1988) suggest that a "rigid rate control" technique like DAF should be used when techniques that more adequately preserve prosody and naturalness are ineffective. The DAF technique does tend to disrupt naturalness, it may be cosmetically unacceptable to some speakers, and adaptation to its effects may occur. It may not be very effective in conversations in which utterances are short, so it may not be appropriate for patients who are capable of or choose only to make statements that are brief and unelaborated.

Several reports have documented the success of DAF for patients with hypokinetic dysarthria (Adams, 1994; Downie, Low, and Lindsay, 1981; Hanson and Metter, 1980, 1983; Yorkston, Beukelman, and Bell, 1988). Improvement was usually achieved rapidly and dramatically, and it lasted for months to years. Weaning from DAF while maintaining benefits generally was not possible, but adaptation to beneficial effects generally was not reported. Benefits included marked reductions in speech rate, increased loudness, reduced phonetic errors, increased acoustic distinctiveness, increased amplitude of lip and jaw movements, and improved intelligibility. The benefits for several of the reported cases were maintained outside the clinical setting, with very obvious functional and social benefits in several cases.

Pacing devices such as a *pacing board* (Figure 17–4), initially described by Helm (1979), re-

---

*Keith and Thomas' (1989) *Speech Practice Manual* contains a variety of stimulus materials that are designed for contrastive drill and related articulation tasks.

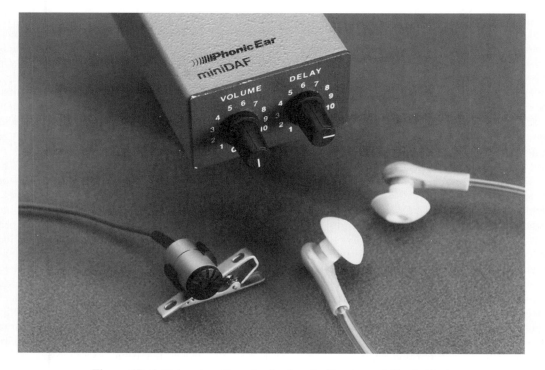

Figure 17–3 Delayed auditory feedback unit. (Courtesy of Phonic Ear.)

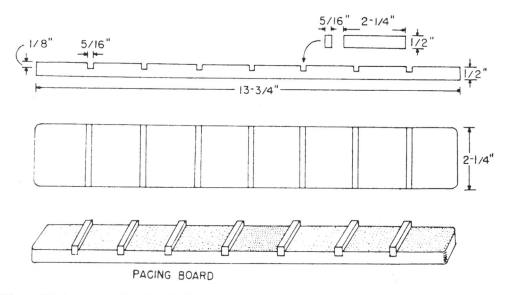

PACING BOARD

Figure 17–4 A pacing board, with dimensions, for rate control. (From Helm N: Management of palilalia with a pacing board, J Speech Hear Disord 44:350, 1979.)

quires the patient to point sequentially to each slot on a board as each word or syllable is produced. This promotes rate reduction and a syllable-by-syllable approach to speaking. It seems particularly appropriate for some people with hypokinetic dysarthria whose rate is rapid or accelerated. Helm described a patient with Parkinson's disease and palilalia who was unresponsive to verbal instruc-

tion to slow his rate or to tap his hand to pace his rate, but who was, with reminders, able to speak in a syllable-by-syllable manner with reduced palilalia when using the pacing board. Other pacing devices, such as metronomes and flashing lights, may produce similar results.

Beukelman and Yorkston (1977) described a rate-control technique that may be an ideal transition from augmented to unaugmented communication (or vice versa) for some patients. It requires the speaker to *point to the first letter of each spoken word* on an alphabet board (*"alphabet board supplementation"*) (Figure 17–5). Their results with two dysarthric speakers were impressive. The rate of unaided and aided (first-letter approach) speech was about four times faster than rate of communication when the entire word was spelled on a letter board. The aided speech was only one third to one half as rapid as unaided speech, but intelligibility was noticeably better, with the speakers able to converse at 100% intelligibility. The effect seemed attributable to a combination of rate reduction and the information provided by the first letter of each word. Crow and Enderby (1989) also demonstrated the technique's effectiveness for six patients with a variety of dysarthria types. In comparison to unaided conditions (speech only), when the first-letter approach was used, intelligibility improved significantly for words and sentences. Articulatory accuracy, as judged by sound intelligibility, was also markedly better. The rate of communication using the first-letter approach was only about one third that of unaided speech. Because listeners did not see the letter the speaker was pointing to, the improvements in intelligibility could be attributed to rate reduction and not information provided by letter cues.

Nonprosthetic rate reduction strategies. Nonprosthetic strategies for decreasing rate include the following.
1. *Hand or finger tapping* in pace with syllable production. It should be noted, however, that many parkinsonian patients accelerate their hand tapping as well as their speech rate and that ataxic patients may be uncoordinated in tapping. Some patients are able to speak in a syllable-by-syllable fashion simply by being told to do so, although they may need considerable practice to make the strategy habitual.
2. Using *visual feedback* from a computer screen or storage oscilloscope to pace rate. Berry and Goshorn (1983) used oscilloscopic feedback with one ataxic speaker to set the duration of utterances; he was asked to speak at a rate that would "fill the screen" during reading tasks. The approach led to decreased rate and increased intelligibility. Increased pause time during speech probably contributed to improvement. Of interest, increased pause time was adopted spontaneously by the speaker to slow rate.
3. *Rhythmic cuing* (Yorkston and Beukelman, 1981) is a technique in which the clinician points to words in a written passage in a rhythmic fashion, giving more time to prominent words and pauses at syntactic boundaries. The approach has been computerized (Beukelman, Yorkston, and Tice, 1988), with a cursor setting the target rate, which permits selection of a precise rate and allows independent practice. Yorkston, Beukelman, and Bell (1988) documented the effectiveness of the technique for a person with Friedreich's ataxia.

It may be that external pacing of rate is more effective when it is "metered" and each word is given equal time, as opposed to "rhythmic," in which timing patterns more closely simulate

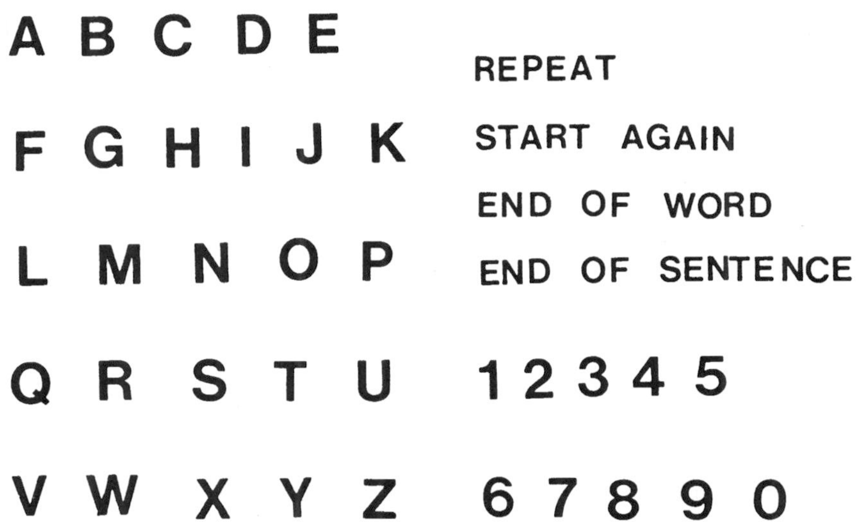

A B C D E   REPEAT

F G H I J K   START AGAIN

                  END OF WORD

L M N O P   END OF SENTENCE

Q R S T U   1 2 3 4 5

V W X Y Z   6 7 8 9 0

Figure 17–5 Alphabet board for alternative or augmentative communication. (From Yorkston KM, Beukelman D, and Bell K: Clinical management of dysarthric speakers, San Diego, 1988, College-Hill.)

natural speech. Yorkston and others (1990) found that ataxic and hypokinetic speakers' intelligibility improved during reading to a greater extent when pacing was metered than when it was rhythmic. Of interest, ratings of naturalness were not worse at paced rates than at unpaced speech rates, although metered rates were associated with poorer ratings of naturalness than rhythmic rates. This highlights the sacrifices and trade-offs that must be made between intelligibility and naturalness when rate is modified.

Prosody and naturalness

Work on prosody can be appropriate at all severity levels. Rosenbek and LaPointe (1985) believe that working on stress should be an early part of treatment and that it can begin once respiration and articulation are sufficient to support connected utterances. The goal of this effort is to maximize the accuracy of prosodic patterns and their naturalness (Yorkston, Beukelman, and Bell, 1988).

Naturalness can be defined as "a perceptually derived, overall description of prosodic adequacy" (Yorkston, Beukelman, and Bell, 1988, p. 356). When naturalness is compromised by prosodic abnormalities, it is often perceived as monotonous or unpredictably variable. Prosodic features may be out of sync with syntactic structures, such as inhalation that does not occur at natural syntactic boundaries. Pitch, loudness, and durational characteristics that signal stress may send contradictory messages when variations in each of them do not co-occur in ways that naturally signal stress.

Yorkston, Beukelman, and Bell (1988) suggest that acoustic analyses may be helpful in managing prosodic deficits. Displaying fundamental frequency, intensity, and durational contours of words and phrases may provide information about how a speaker is signaling stress and also the source of perceived unnaturalness. It may also serve as a feedback device during management. Caligiuri and Murry (1983) obtained some empiric support for the value of acoustic and physiologic feedback in treatment. They provided oscilloscopic feedback to three dysarthric speakers about intensity, duration, and intraoral pressure and noted gains in rate and prosody that were generally superior to those derived from auditory perceptual feedback alone.

Following are some strategies that may be useful in modifying prosody and increasing naturalness.

1. Working at the level of the *breath group*—the prosodic pattern during a single exhalation—is important because the breath group is a basic unit of prosody. In normal speakers, a breath group is more dependent on syntax than on the physiologic requirements of respiration. The duration of the breath group in speech is highly variable as a function of syntax; it may be less than two seconds and as long as eight seconds (Fonagy and Magdics, 1960). In addition, when asked to increase speech rate, normal speakers usually reduce pauses and only minimally increase articulation rate. In contrast, dysarthric speakers may pause more frequently because of physiologic limitations; subsequently, their breath groups may be very short and not associated with syntactic boundaries (Bellaire, Yorkston, and Beukelman, 1986). Therefore, some patients may need to work to increase breath control (respiratory and phonatory control) to extend breath groups, a goal that requires increasing physiologic capacity or more adequately using available capacity.

Physiologic limitations may reduce breath group length. Some speakers may need to learn to *chunk utterances into natural syntactic units,* within the limits of their physiologic capacity; that is, speakers capable of only four or five words per breath group may learn to use pauses at logical syntactic boundaries within the limited breath group, removing one potential source of confusion to listeners.

2. Rosenbek and LaPointe (1985) emphasize the value of *contrastive stress tasks.* These can use scripted responses in which segmental information does not vary, but stress patterns do. For example, the core response "John loves Mary" may be produced in response to questions like "Does Jim love Mary?" "Does John hate Mary?" and "Does John love Jane?" Similar tasks can be used to practice intonation for questions versus statement forms ("John loves Mary" versus "John loves Mary?") or expressions of mood ("John loves Mary" with happy versus sad versus surprised affect). Obviously, vocabulary, syntax, and length need not be as stereotyped as these examples.

Referential tasks, in which the patient reads randomized phrases or sentences containing prespecified stress targets that are unknown to the clinician, may help promote discovery learning of ways to signal stress, as well as a way to evaluate the effectiveness of actively taught stress strategies; that is, if the clinician can identify the targeted stressed word, the patient has succeeded.

3. Some patients can signal stress by modifying pitch or loudness or duration, but cannot use all parameters at the same time. Some use one parameter better than any other. Yorkston and others (1984) and Linebaugh and Wolfe (1984)

point out that the manner in which naturalness is impaired may vary both within and across dysarthria types and that a single strategy for modifying stress probably does not exist. Tasks in which the patient is required to stress specified words and phrases may help identify the feature spontaneously used to signal stress; that feature may then become the focus of stress drills. Yorkston, Beukelman, and Bell (1988) and Yorkston and others (1984) indicate, for example, that ataxic speakers are often encouraged to prolong syllables and insert pauses at appropriate times to signal stress. The strategy seems easier than pitch and loudness variations, and exaggerating duration seems to be perceived as less bizarre than exaggerating pitch or loudness. Pitch and loudness variation sometimes also become more natural when durational adjustments are used effectively.

4. Some patients benefit from work *across breath groups.* Bellaire, Yorkston, and Beukelman (1986) discussed a patient with a monotonous stress pattern and slow rate who signaled stress within breath groups adequately but who inhaled on 93% of his pauses during reading (compared to about 65% for normal speakers). He was physiologically more capable, however; for example, his mean number of words per breath group was about five, but he was able to produce 25 words on a single breath when counting. Treatment focused on increasing the frequency of pauses without inhalation and increasing the number of words per breath group. Materials consisted of reading sentences and paragraphs marked for pauses and inhalation, with gradual fading of cues. The speaker accomplished the treatment goals and developed greater variability in words per breath group. This led to reduced perception of monopitch, suggesting that breath groups of equal length may contribute to perceptions of monopitch. The case illustrates the value of obtaining information on both habitual and maximum performance as a way of identifying problems and potential for benefiting from treatment.

5. Working on prosody may have beneficial effects on rate control. For example, Simmons (1983) noted that work on loudness and pitch variation and word and stress patterns in an ataxic speaker resulted in a reduction of speaking rate, even though rate was not a focus of treatment.

6. Yorkston, Beukelman, and Bell (1988) stress the need to work on highly structured tasks and then make the transition to spontaneous speech, perhaps through the use of short dialogues or scripts of conversation. They note that patients

should learn to critique their own production and that audiotape and videotape review may be very useful in this regard.

SPEAKER-ORIENTED TREATMENT FOR SPECIFIC DYSARTHRIA TYPES

A number of treatment approaches are applicable to almost any dysarthria type. The value of others varies according to dysarthria type as a function of either the underlying pathophysiology or the predominance of particular speech characteristics. As a result, some speaker-oriented techniques are appropriate for only certain dysarthria types or are likely to be used much more frequently for some dysarthria types than for others. Some treatment approaches are inappropriate for some dysarthria types.

The purpose of this section is to highlight those speaker-oriented approaches that are used exclusively or predominantly—or that may be contraindicated—with certain dysarthria types. Table 17–1 summarizes behavioral, prosthetic, medical-surgical, and pharmacologic techniques that are particularly useful, frequently used, or logically relevant to the management of specific dysarthria types, as well as those techniques that are contraindicated or of uncertain usefulness for particular dysarthria types.

Flaccid dysarthria

Because flaccid dysarthria is associated with weakness, its unique treatments tend to be designed to increase strength or compensate for weakness. These include treatments aimed at the respiratory, laryngeal, resonatory, and articulatory components of speech.

Patients with respiratory weakness may benefit from efforts to increase physiologic support for speech breathing. Therefore, activities designed to increase subglottal air pressure on nonspeech tasks; increase loudness, breath group duration, and words per breath group; and establish maximum breath groups for speech are often appropriate. Pushing/pulling exercises to increase respiratory support and drive, postural adjustments, and compensatory efforts such as deep inhalation, controlled exhalation, and increased force are often emphasized. Patients with relatively isolated, severe respiratory weakness are probably the only dysarthric speakers who might be taught to use neck breathing or glossopharyngeal breathing for speech.

Patients with adductor vocal cord weakness or paralysis may be candidates for medialization laryngoplasty or Teflon/collagen injection of the vocal cords, procedures more appropriate for flaccid dysarthria than any other dysarthria type. More frequently than any other dysarthria type, flaccid dysarthric speakers have management attention focused on resonance and velopharyngeal function. They are the best candidates for palatal lift prostheses and pharyngeal flap surgery. They also are the group most likely to benefit from postural adjustments or nares occlusion to prevent excessive nasal flow during speech. Strengthening exercises to improve velopharyngeal function for speech are more likely to be effective for flaccid than other dysarthria types.

Patients with facial nerve paralysis are the only dysarthric patients likely to have facial nerve anastomosis surgery. As a result, they may be the only group to receive EMG feedback training to improve facial movement following such surgery, and they are the only group to be at risk for the possible negative effects on tongue function of

Table 17–1 Treatment approaches and their relationship to various dysarthria types

Approach	Dysarthria Type					
	Flaccid	Spastic	Ataxic	Hypokinetic	Hyperkinetic	Unilateral UMN
Behavioral	+	+	+	+	+	+
Respiration	+	+	+	+	−	−
"5 for 5" respiratory tasks	+	+	+	+	−	−
Pushing-pulling exercise	++	−	−	−	−	−
Supine-reclining postures	+	+	−	−	−	−
Manual push on abdomen	+	−	−	+	−	−
Inhale more deeply	+	+	−	+	−	−
Speak at onset of exhalation	+	+	+	+	−	−
Inspiratory checking	+	−	+	+	−	−
Neck breathing	++	−	−	−	−	−
Glossopharyngeal breathing	++	−	−	−	−	−
Maximum vowel prolongation	+	+	+	+	−	−
Controlled exhalation tasks	+	+	+	+	−	−
Terminate speech earlier during exhalatory cycle	+	+	+	+	−	−
Optimal breath group	+	+	+	+	−	−
Increase sentence length	+	+	+	+	−	−
Increase vocal strain	+	−	−	+	−	−
Shorten fricative duration	+	−	−	−	−	−
Shorten phrases	+	+	+	+	−	−
Phonation	+	+	−	+	+	−
Relaxation, massage	−	+	−	−	+	−
Turn head during speech	++	−	−	−	−	−
Lateralize thyroid cartilage	++	−	−	−	−	−
Head back, increased pitch, deep breath	−	+	−	−	−	−
Effort closure techniques	++	−	−	++	−	−
Abrupt glottal attack	++	−	−	++	−	−
Intense, high-level phonatory effort	++	−	−	++	−	−
Breathy onset	−	++	−	−	++	−
Speak at onset of exhalation	+	+	+	+	−	−
Continuous voicing of consonants	−	−	−	−	++	−
Optimal breath group	+	+	+	+	−	−
Resonance	+	+	−	+	−	−
Blowing-sucking exercise	+	+	−	−	−	−
CPAP	++	−	−	−	−	−
Supine positioning	+	+	−	−	−	−
Occlude nares	+	+	−	−	−	−
Exaggerate jaw movement	+	−	−	+	−	−
Increase loudness	+	+	−	+	−	−
Reduce pressure consonant duration	++	−	−	−	−	−

Continued.

Table 17–1 Treatment approaches and their relationship to various dysarthria types—cont'd

Approach	Dysarthria Type					
	Flaccid	Spastic	Ataxic	Hypokinetic	Hyperkinetic	Unilateral UMN
Articulation	+	+	+	+	+	+
Strengthening exercises	++	–	–	–	–	+
Relaxation exercise	–	+	–	–	+	–
Stretching	+	+	–	+	–	–
Biofeedback	+	+	+	+	+	+
Sensory tricks	–	–	–	–	++	–
Conservation of strength	+	+	–	+	–	–
Exaggerate consonants	+	+	+	+	–	+
Integral stimulation	+	+	+	+	–	+
Phonetic placement	+	+	+	+	–	+
Phonetic derivation	+	+	+	+	–	+
Minimal contrasts	+	+	+	+	–	+
Alternative place, manner, voicing strategies	+	+	–	–	–	–
Intelligibility drills	+	+	+	+	+	+
Referential tasks	+	+	+	+	+	+
Rate	+	+	+	+	+	+
Rate reduction	+	+	+	+	+	+
Hand or finger tapping	+	+	+	+	–	+
Rhythmic or metered cuing	–	+	+	+	–	+
Visual feedback	+	+	+	+	+	+
Modify pauses	+	+	+	+	–	+
Identify first letter on board	+	+	+	+	+	+
Prosody & naturalness	+	+	+	+	+	+
Breath group duration	+	+	+	+	+	+
Modify syllable duration and pause time	+	+	+	+	+	–
Across breath group tasks	+	+	+	+	–	–
Chunk by syntactic units	+	+	+	+	–	–
Contrastive stress tasks	+	+	+	+	+	+
Referential stress tasks	+	+	+	+	+	+
Prosthetic	+	+	+	+	+	–
Abdominal binders and corsets	++	–	–	–	–	–
Expiratory board or paddle	++	–	–	+	–	–
Vocal intensity controller	+	+	–	+	–	–
Vocal amplifier	+	+	–	+	–	–

such a procedure. Flaccid dysarthria associated with lingual and lip weakness may benefit from the use of a bite block during treatment designed to increase tongue or lip movement for speech, but a bite block would never be a permanent prosthesis for improving speech in flaccid dysarthria.

Behavioral speech treatment is contraindicated for people with flaccid dysarthria resulting from myasthenia gravis. Such patients are managed most effectively surgically (thymectomy) or pharmacologically (pyridostigmine bromide [Mestinon], adrenal corticosteroids). The best that can be done for speech beyond medical treatments is to teach conservation of strength by limiting speak-

ing to durations that do not produce significant fatigue. Most patients with myasthenia gravis do this on their own.

Spastic dysarthria

Some techniques that are appropriate for flaccid dysarthria are contraindicated for spastic dysarthria because they would increase rather than decrease impairment. Behaviorally, for example, pushing, pulling, and other effort closure techniques to enhance vocal cord adduction are contraindicated because hyperadduction is generally already a problem for the spastic speaker. Surgical procedures to medialize the vocal cords (medialization laryngo-

Table 17–1 Treatment approaches and their relationship to various dysarthria types—cont'd

Approach	Dysarthria Type					
	Flaccid	Spastic	Ataxic	Hypokinetic	Hyperkinetic	Unilateral UMN
Artificial larynges	++	–	–	–	–	–
Palatal lift	++	+	–	–	–	–
DAF	–	–	–	++	–	–
Pacing board	–	–	–	++	–	–
Metronome	–	–	–	++	–	–
Bite block	+	–	–	–	++	–
Nose clip or nasal obturator	+	+	–	–	–	–
Jaw sling	++	–	–	–	–	–
Neck brace or cervical collar	+	–	+	–	+	–
Medical-surgical	+	+	–	+	+	–
Medialization laryngoplasty	++	–	–	+	–	–
Teflon or collagen injection	++	–	–	+	–	–
Recurrent laryngeal nerve resection	–	–	–	–	++	–
Botox injection	–	–	–	–	++	–
Pharyngeal flap	++	+	–	–	–	–
Neural anastomosis (VII-XII)	+	–	–	–	–	–
Pharmacologic	+	+	–	+	+	–
Artane (trihexyphenidyl)	–	–	–	–	+	–
Dantrium (dantrolene sodium)	–	+	–	–	–	–
Elavil (amitriptyline)	–	+	–	–	–	–
Haldol (haloperidol)	–	–	–	–	+	–
Inderal (propranolol)	–	–	–	–	+	–
Klonopin (clonazepam)	–	–	–	+	+	–
L-Dopa (levodopa)	–	–	–	++	–	–
Librium (chlordiazepoxide)	–	+	–	–	–	–
Lioresal (baclofen)	–	+	–	–	+	–
Lithane, Eskalith (lithium carbonate)	–	–	–	–	+	–
Mestinon (pyridostigmine bromide)	++	–	–	–	–	–
Mysoline (primidone)	–	–	–	–	+	–
Neptazine (methazolamide)	–	–	–	–	+	–
Reserpine	–	–	–	–	+	–
Sinemet (carbidopa-levodopa)	–	–	–	++	+	–
Tegretol (carbamazepine)	–	–	–	–	+	–
Valium (diazepam)	–	+	–	–	–	–
Xanax (alprazolam)	–	–	–	–	+	–

+, may be appropriate; ++, uniquely appropriate but not necessarily for all patients; –, contraindicated, rarely necessary, or uncertain; *CPAP,* continuous positive airway pressure; *DAF,* delayed auditory feedback; *UMN,* upper motor neuron.

plasty and Teflon/collagen injection) would be contraindicated for the same reasons.

Medication to reduce the effects of spasticity seem to be more effective for the limbs than the bulbar muscles; actually, the effect of antispasticity medications on speech has received little attention. An anecdotal report by Dworkin (1991) suggests that Dantrium may reduce the strained voice quality in some patients.

Speakers with spastic dysarthria may benefit from relaxation exercises more than those with other dysarthria types, but whether such relaxation actually facilitates speech is a matter of conjecture. Similarly, stretching exercise of the articulators has some face validity for speakers with spastic

dysarthria but has not been investigated.

The management of pseudobulbar affect, or pathologic crying and laughter, deserves mention because it occurs more commonly in spastic dysarthria than any other dysarthria type and because it can interfere significantly with verbal communication. In patients for whom pseudobulbar affect is a significant problem, low doses of amitriptyline may be effective in relieving the behavior. For example, dramatic improvement of pathological laughter and crying in response to the drug has been reported in a double-blind cross-over study comparing amitriptyline with placebo in eight patients with multiple sclerosis (Schiffer, Herndon, and Rudick, 1985). It is also possible that the problem may respond to behavior modification techniques in some patients. Brookshire (1970) described a patient whose crying was so frequent that it precluded therapy for his dysarthria; he would cry whenever asked to repeat or speak more clearly. A program was developed in which head turning that usually preceded crying was modified and eliminated by verbal reinforcement of incompatible behavior. Crying was greatly reduced and intelligible speech was achieved with subsequent therapy. Aten (1983) referred to a patient who was able to dramatically modify the frequency and duration of labile periods. These reports suggest that some aspects of this apparently involuntary behavior may be under voluntary control, at least in some patients. Working to modify such behavior when medication is ineffective or inappropriate seems justified when it is pervasive enough to interfere consistently with speech or therapy activities. For some patients with spastic dysarthria, treating the laughter and crying may be the first goal of treatment.

Ataxic dysarthria

Efforts to increase physiologic support by increasing muscle strength or reducing muscle tone are generally unnecessary and inappropriate for ataxic speakers. Similarly, surgical or prosthetic efforts to improve phonation or resonance are unnecessary because they are not related to the motor problems of ataxic speakers. In general, the focus of treatment activities is behavioral, with activities centered on improving motor *control* and *coordination.*

Although some patients benefit from isolated work on respiratory control, particularly controlled exhalation over time (Murry, 1983; Rosenbek and LaPointe, 1985), most of the focus is generally on *modifying rate and prosody* to improve intelligibility and, when possible, further modifying rate and prosody to improve naturalness. For example, several clinicians explicitly note that ataxic speakers may benefit from using durational adjustments as their primary method of signaling stress (Yorkston, Beukelman, and Bell, 1988; Yorkston and others, 1984). Several studies of ataxic speakers have reported improved intelligibility or naturalness with behavioral techniques that emphasized rate, loudness, or pitch control (Berry and Goshorn, 1983; Caligiuri and Murry, 1983; Simmons, 1983; Yorkston, Dowden, and Beukelman, 1992; Yorkston and others, 1990).

Hypokinetic dysarthria

The treatment of hypokinetic dysarthria resembles that for flaccid dysarthria, but the overlap is far from complete. There are also some behavioral treatment approaches that have been developed specifically for hypokinetic dysarthria.

Some hypokinetic speakers have a prominent dysphonia that may be related to bowing or weakness of the vocal cords. When it is severe and the prominent manifestation of the dysarthria, medialization laryngoplasty or Teflon or collagen injection may result in improved voice.

Many hypokinetic speakers with rapid or accelerated rate are prime candidates for rate-control efforts, at least partially because articulatory hypokinesia may be reduced at slower speaking rates (Caligiuri, 1989). Rigid rate-control approaches may be necessary for many patients, and several reports document the success of devices such as DAF and pacing boards (Adams, 1994; Hanson and Metter, 1980, 1983; Helm, 1979). Similarly, the reduced loudness associated with hypokinetic dysarthria may respond favorably to vocal intensity monitors and feedback devices (Rubow and Swift, 1985) or to voice amplifiers when loudness cannot be improved behaviorally and other aspects of speech production are relatively preserved.

In the past, behavioral therapy for patients with Parkinson's disease has been viewed with pessimism (Sarno, 1968), the common opinion being that the dysarthria might respond favorably within treatment sessions but that little carryover is ever achieved (Ramig, in press). It is very likely that this is indeed the case for some patients, but recent evidence suggests that intensive, focused treatment can be beneficial and lasting for others. Some of these treatments appear to improve physiologic functions for speech. They are usually intensive (for example, 6 to 9 hours over 6 weeks; 10 hours over 2 weeks; 35 to 40 hours over 2 weeks) and tend to include work on prosody and loudness, as well as on rate control and articulation (Johnson and Pring, 1990; Moore and Scudder, 1989; Robertson and Thomson, 1984; Scott and Caird, 1981, 1983). Carryover for three to six months posttreatment has been noted in some studies, although gains are not always completely maintained. Investigators usually note the importance of follow-up activities after the initial intensive treatment program.

Evidence suggests that physical therapy or a general program of physical exercise has a beneficial effect on a variety of measures of motor performance in patients with Parkinson's disease (Formisano and others, 1992; Palmer and others, 1986). Exercise also seems to have some value for speech, as attested to by the studies of speech therapy referred to in the preceding paragraph.

Ramig and colleagues recently have developed a promising program for patients with Parkinson's disease (Ramig, in press). The approach emphasizes *voice therapy* that attempts to modify laryngeal pathophysiology through exercise designed to increase loudness and decrease breathiness. The distinctive characteristics of this treatment program seem to be its *intensity* (four times per week for one month); requirement for *energetic, high levels of physical effort* to increase vocal loudness and vocal cord adduction; and *exclusive focus on phonatory effort*. Activities may include pushing exercises and directed efforts to "speak loud" or "shout." Homework exercise is an important part of the program. Exercise is intense (for example, maximum loud, steady vowel duration tasks, 10 to 15 minutes per session) and includes vowel, word, phrase, sentence, and conversation production tasks. The goal is to achieve adequate loudness during 85% of utterances. Careful study has documented that vocal loudness and intelligibility increase, monotony decreases, and articulation improves. When compared to an untreated control group, significant increases in maximum vowel duration, maximum phonation range, and fundamental frequency in reading have been documented in treated patients following treatment, and three- to-six-month follow-up data indicate maintenance of gains. Videoendoscopic and electroglottographic evaluations have documented increased vocal fold adduction following treatment in some subjects (Ramig, 1992; Ramig, Horii, and Bonitati, 1991). It appears that depression and lack of motivation may be important variables that limit the success of the treatment in some patients (Ramig, Horii, and Bonitati, 1991). The data to date support the efficacy of this intensive voice therapy for at least some patients with Parkinson's disease.

The major drugs to treat Parkinson's disease—L-dopa and carbidopa-levodopa (Sinemet) generally appear to have positive effects on hypokinetic dysarthria (Mlcoch, 1992; Rigrodsky and Morrison, 1970; Wolfe and others, 1975), with improvement ranging from equivocal to dramatic, but usually not as great as in other areas of physical functioning. It is important to keep in mind that the effects of these drugs can fluctuate as a function of the drug cycle. For example, Caligiuri (1989) documented variability across patients and fluctuation in improvements in the velocity and amplitude of lip movements over a 2 to 3 hour period in five people taking Sinemet. Therefore, the positive effects of Sinemet on speech seem to be variable within the drug cycle and somewhat heterogeneous across patients. In addition, a high percentage of patients develop hyperkinesia at some time during treatment with levodopa, with fluctuations over the course of the drug cycle. It is possible, therefore, to see a patient whose hypoki-netic dysarthria improves, then evolves to a hyperkinetic or mixed hypokinetic-hyperkinetic dysarthria, and then returns to baseline within a single dosage period.

Clonazepam (Klonopin) also seems to be an effective drug for treating hypokinetic dysarthria in some patients. For example, 9 of 11 parkinsonian patients in a double-blind study with the drug had sufficient functional improvement of speech (mostly in rate and pause characteristics and consonant precision) that they decided to continue the drug after completion of the study (Biary, Pimental, and Langenberg, 1988). A number of other drugs can be effective in treating Parkinson's disease, but their effects on speech have received little attention.

Hyperkinetic dysarthria

The most effective management approaches for hyperkinetic dysarthria are surgical and pharmacologic (Beukelman, 1983). The underlying pathophysiology of hyperkinetic dysarthria logically predicts this because the abnormal movements that cause the speech disturbance are not under voluntary control. Fortunately, an increasing number of nonbehavioral treatments provide relief for the speech deficits associated with some of the hyperkinetic dysarthrias, including Botox injection for the treatment of spasmodic dysphonias, oromandibular dystonias, and spasmodic torticollis, as well as some medications that reduce symptoms for some of these same problems.

Medication is occasionally helpful in the management of movement disorders that affect phonation but usually not dramatically so. Inderal, an effective drug for treating essential tremor in the limbs (Findley and Koller, 1987), only infrequently leads to a significant reduction of head or voice tremor or the spasmodic dysphonia of essential voice tremor (Koller, Graner, and Mlcoch, 1985). Recently, methazolamide (Neptazine) has been reported as effective in relieving essential tremor, particularly head or voice tremor (Muenter and others, 1991). Mysoline and Tegretol may also reduce voice tremor in some patients, according to Rosenfield (1991). Small amounts of alcohol frequently decrease the amplitude of essential voice tremor (Koller, Graner, and Mlcoch, 1985), although its use obviously must be judicious and limited to appropriate social situations.

Artane has been used with significant benefit to speech in a patient with laryngeal and respiratory dystonia (Ludlow, Sedora, and Fujita, 1989). Lioresal, combinations of Artane and lithium, and alprazolam (Xanax) are said to occasionally reduce symptoms of oromandibular dystonia and spasmodic dysphonia (Rosenfield, 1991). Similarly, Lioresal, reserpine, and Haldol "may reduce chorea-induced dysarthria, but their effect is often minimal" (Rosenfield, 1991, p. 130). Haldol is also often used in the treatment of Tourette's syndrome. Clonazepam (Klonopin) is reportedly effective in diminishing the dysarthria associated with action myoclonus (Aronson, O'Neill, and Kelly, 1984).

A few behavioral and prosthetic approaches may help some patients with certain types of hyperkinetic dysarthria, although most of them provide only temporary and less than optimal relief.

1. Some patients with mandibular dystonias or other hyperkinesias affecting jaw movement benefit from the use of a bite block (or pipe or other socially acceptable device held in the mouth) that may inhibit or limit adventitious jaw movements during speech, with resultant improvement in articulation and rate.

2. Some patients with focal dystonias of the jaw, tongue, or face spontaneously discover sensory tricks (postural adjustments) that inhibit adventitious movements and facilitate speech. It is usually worth searching for such sensory tricks in patients who have not discovered them on their own. If the discovered tricks are socially acceptable, they may provide relief and improvement of speech, at least under some circumstances; unfortunately, they are rarely maximal or lasting solutions.

3. Patients with the hyperkinetic dysarthria of action myoclonus usually discover on their own that speech improves if rate is slowed. When they do not, actively taught rate-reduction strategies can be beneficial.

4. Some patients with adductor spasmodic dysphonia benefit from increasing vocal pitch or adopting a breathy onset of phonation. Similarly, some patients with abductor spasmodic dysphonia may reduce the abductor spasm by adopting a hard glottal onset of phonation and voicing voiceless consonants, which reduces requirements for the cord abduction that may trigger abductor spasms (Aronson, 1990). These strategies are most often beneficial when the disorder is mild and when demands for excellent speech are not great. Unfortunately, for most patients it is very difficult to maintain such compensatory strategies, the benefits are less than optimally acceptable, and they are often lost if the disorder progresses.

5. Case reports of the effectiveness of EMG feedback in modifying lip dystonia and hemifacial spasm have already been noted. The limited number of such reports warrant caution in assuming that the technique can provide sig-

nificant benefit to most patients in a cost-effective and efficient manner that significantly alters intelligibility and efficiency of speech. For example, Beukelman (1983) has commented anecdotally on his limited success with such treatment. Biofeedback for treating movement disorders deserves continued study, but its use should not be considered an accepted, common treatment for orofacial movement disorders at this time.

Unilateral upper motor neuron dysarthria

There have been no formal reports of treatment for unilateral UMN dysarthria, although Duffy and Folger's (1986) retrospective study noted that therapy was recommended for a substantial number of patients who had the disorder and that many improved over the course of treatment. Because the disorder is usually relatively mild, patients with it are not generally candidates for medical or prosthetic management. Behavioral approaches usually focus on rate, prosody, and articulation, and compensation may receive more emphasis than efforts to restore physiologic support. Some patients seem to benefit from mirror work to monitor drooling or squirreling of food in the cheek on the weak side.* Efforts to strengthen the unilateral face and tongue weakness that often accompany the disorder might be justified, although most clinicians probably focus more directly on speech than on nonspeech oromotor exercise.

COMMUNICATION-ORIENTED TREATMENT

What can be done to enhance communication between dysarthric speakers and their listeners when direct medical, prosthetic, and behavioral approaches to restoring or compensating for speech deficits have failed, have had their desired effect, are in progress, or must be deferred, and yet reduced intelligibility or efficiency of communication is present? Solutions are to be found in the adoption of strategies that focus on interactions between listeners and speakers and the environments in which they occur. These strategies are *independent of dysarthria type*. They are strongly dependent on degree of disability and handicap, accompanying deficits, the environment in which communication occurs, and the dysarthric person's communication partners. They are based on the fact that a good deal more than the acoustic attributes of speech determine whether a message is understood. Many of them can be

---

*I am indebted to Jack Thomas for this observation.

implemented by patients alone, by their listeners alone, or by cooperation between speakers and listeners.

Speaker strategies

Speakers can do a number of things to enhance the redundancy and predictability of their speech, especially when they do not have language or other cognitive problems. They include the following.

Convey how communication should take place. This is especially important for speakers who must use augmentative means of communication. This ground rule may be conveyed to novel listeners at the outset of an interaction. It may state that the speaker has a neurologic impairment that makes speaking difficult and that communication will be easiest if, for example, the speaker points to the first letter of each word as the word is spoken. The speaker may instruct the listener to repeat each word or utterance as soon as it is completed in order to confirm comprehension; for example, to wait until a sentence is completed before asking for clarification, to ask for clarification as soon as something is misunderstood, or to be sure to watch the patient. These directions can be mounted on a lap board or presented on a card.

Set the context. For example, the availability of semantic or contextual information (for example, animal names, things you buy in a grocery store) can significantly enhance word and sentence intelligibility in severely dysarthric speakers. The effect is particularly pronounced for single word utterances, with nearly 30% to fivefold increases in intelligibility with contextual cues reported by some investigators (Dongilli, 1994; Yorkston, Dowden, and Beukelman, 1992).

Setting the context may involve indicating the topic of conversation explicitly—with speech or by identifying a topic from a list on a word board. Knowing the topic allows predictions to be made about context before the specific message is initiated. This technique may be particularly valuable when the speaker shifts topics during an interaction.

Modify content and length. Some dysarthric speakers improve intelligibility by increasing redundancy or elaboration in their utterances. Others may need to be more concise, simplifying or limiting content and length to the essentials of the message (Vogel and Miller, 1991). This may be especially relevant when answering questions. For example, learning to say "coffee" when asked if one would like coffee or tea is far more efficient than saying "I've had too much coffee already today but I suppose one more cup won't hurt." Normal speakers can afford to elaborate and ex-plain simple things—many dysarthric speakers cannot. Vogel and Miller (1991) point out that some speakers also need to modify their use of idiomatic expressions and metaphors and focus on more literal meanings. Some speakers adopt these changes automatically. Others may have difficulty, especially when such changes represent a major alteration in style and projection of personality or when cognitive deficits are present. A compromise for such individuals may be to reserve style shifts to situations in which communication has broken down.

Adjusting length may also improve intelligibility. It appears that speakers with severely reduced intelligibility are more intelligible on words than sentences, but that less severely impaired speakers are more intelligible in sentences than words (Dongilli, 1994; Yorkston and Beukelman, 1978). It is likely that listeners benefit from redundancy within sentences when word intelligibility reaches a critical threshold.

Monitor listener comprehension. This can be done by maintaining eye contact with listeners and asking if the message has been understood. In general, the more rapidly a failure to comprehend is perceived, the more efficiently repairs can be made.

Alphabet board supplementation. This practice has already been discussed. Its use should be introduced to novel listeners so they know to watch the speaker as well as the letter board. Yorkston, Beukelman, and Bell (1988) note that the speaker must control these interactions and that using control phrases on the letter board may be helpful in this regard (for example, "end of word," "end of sentence," "start again") (see Figure 17–5).

Listener strategies

Listeners can do a number of things to enhance speaker intelligibility and efficiency. Some of these only they can accomplish, whereas others may be undertaken by the speaker as well. Because many dysarthric speakers are disabled in ways other than speech, listeners/caregivers may need to take responsibility for many environmental modifications that may facilitate communication. These strategies include the following.

Modify the physical environment. Many of these modifications were discussed by Berry and Sanders (1983) as "environmental education." These modifications may include *reducing sources of noise* or *increasing signal-noise ratio* (turning off or muting the television and radio, closing windows, using rugs and drapes to dampen noise, speaking away from fans and air conditioners); *avoiding noisy dark settings* when communication is essential or desirable (crowded, darkly lit restaurants); *maintaining eye contact, direct face-to-face contact;* and *limiting distance from the speaker.*

Maximize listener hearing and visual acuity. Listeners who wear hearing aids and glasses should wear them; their possible need for such sensory aids should be investigated.

Learn active listening. Listeners must learn to confirm their understanding or lack thereof in an ongoing, active way with many dysarthric speakers. Normal expectations that redundancy during discourse eventually will clarify meaning may not hold. Repeating or clarifying far downstream may be inefficient and time-consuming at best, or abort the communicative attempt at worst. Listeners must often learn to increase their attention and vigilance to the speaker, constantly establish for themselves that they are comprehending the message, or initiate a response that will repair a breakdown in intelligibility rapidly. For some listeners, this skill needs to be trained and practiced, and its value relative to efficiency of communication demonstrated to them.

Interaction strategies

There are a number of things that speakers and listeners can do together to facilitate intelligibility and improve communication efficiency. Sometimes these strategies need to be negotiated to accommodate the needs, desires, and assets and liabilities of the speakers and their listeners. They often need to be trained and practiced. Some relate to maximizing intelligibility and efficiency on the first attempt. Many relate to "breakdown resolution strategies" or establishing intelligibility when a message is not understood. These strategies may include the following.

Maintain eye contact by listener and speaker. The exception is when certain augmentative strategies are used. For example, when the speaker supplements speech with a letter or word board or other augmentative device, the listener should look at the letter board and listen to speech.

Establish methods of feedback. Some speakers prefer to complete an utterance without interruption, while others desire feedback as soon as a listener does not understand something. Vogel and Miller (1991) suggest that if a listener gesturally signals a lack of understanding at the time it occurs, the speaker can decide whether to revise immediately or hope that the remainder of their utterance will improve comprehension.

Till and Toye (1988) found that dysarthric speakers changed aspects of production more effectively when feedback identified the locus and type of error than when it was general (for example, "Pardon me?"), as long as the speaker had

the capacity to correct the error. Therefore, the more precise feedback is about when and where errors occur, the more likely repetition or revision is to be effective. This precision may be specific to the location of a word, but it may take other forms. For example, a listener who has grasped little or nothing may ask the speaker to identify the topic (who or what is being talked about), or they may summarize what they have understood and establish what is missing for them ("I know you're going somewhere tomorrow, but I don't know where").

When speakers are interrupted with a general indication that intelligibility has broken down, their adjustments often include total repetition, partial repetition of a phrase, partial repetition with elaboration, or total repetition with elaboration (Ansel and others, 1983). Ansel and others noted that their dysarthric speakers did not always seem aware that listeners were having problems and speculated that the speakers may have become desensitized to breakdowns. This possibility argues for explicit feedback from listeners, especially when breakdowns are frequent. Yorkston, Beukelman, and Bell (1988) recommend that feedback should be immediate and that it establish what has been understood so that speakers can be specific in their attempts at repair.

Many speakers spontaneously improve speech when informed that intelligibility has broken down, but some do not. Listeners who know what speakers are capable of doing with help may be able to provide explicit cues about what is likely to work (slow down, use one word at a time, tap it out, speak louder, take a deep breath, or give the first letter, for example). That such explicit feedback will be given can be established as a general rule of interaction that is negotiated between listener and speaker. This is particularly useful for speakers who are unable to use their maximum capacity all of the time because of physiologic or cognitive limitations, but who can use it when cued. When communication partners are very familiar with each other, a simple gesture may be sufficient to trigger the need to increase effort or adopt a specific compensatory strategy. Finally, Yorkston, Beukelman, and Bell (1988) point out that when a repair attempt fails, a strategy with guaranteed success should then be used (for example, spelling).

During treatment sessions, many patients respond favorably when the clinician consistently uses the manner of speaking the patient is being asked to adopt during conversational interaction. This provides a natural model and paces the interaction in a way that promotes more consistent responses from the patient. Thus, for example, the clinician may slow their own rate, increase pause duration, tap their hand with each syllable spoken, or take a deep breath at phrase boundaries.*

Referential communication tasks during treatment are very valuable for establishing feedback strategies because they allow patients and their listeners to discover what works best and provide an opportunity to practice feedback and repair strategies. Review of videotapes of communicative interaction also may be a valuable source of feedback about the effectiveness of communicative strategies.

Establish what works best when. Combinations of communication strategies are often appropriate. For example, speech may be quite adequate when exchanging social greetings and represent the most rapid and efficient means of doing so. The same speaker, however, may need to spell out more elaborate or novel messages or use a letter or word board to introduce new topics.

Communicative strategies may also vary considerably across listeners. Speech without augmentation is most often possible with familiar listeners, whereas augmentative strategies are often necessary with novel listeners or under adverse environmental circumstances.

SUMMARY

1. There are a variety of speaker-oriented and communication-oriented approaches to managing the dysarthrias. Although evidence of their efficacy is relatively limited, a substantial number of reports document the effectiveness of a number of management approaches and techniques.

2. Speaker-oriented approaches to managing dysarthria may focus on restoration or compensation for impairments in respiration, phonation, resonance, articulation, rate, and prosody. A number of medical-surgical, prosthetic, and behavioral approaches are available for improving respiratory, phonatory, resonatory, and articulatory functions for speech. Prosthetic and behavioral management approaches are generally used to improve rate and prosody.

3. Many of the techniques used in speaker-oriented treatments can be applied to patients with a variety of dysarthria types. However, some approaches and techniques are much more useful for some dysarthria types than others, some are useful for only a single dysarthria type, and some are contraindicated for use with some types. Differences in management across dysarthria types exist for medical-surgical, prosthetic, and behavioral approaches.

4. Communication-oriented approaches to treatment include a number of strategies that can be adopted by speakers and listeners. Although such approaches do not result in modification of speech production per se, they can contribute substantially to improving the intelligibility of messages and the efficiency with which they are transmitted. Communication-oriented approaches to treatment are independent of dysarthria type, but they are strongly dependent on degree of disability and handicap, the presence and severity of deficits that may accompany motor speech disorders, the environment in which communication takes place, and the characteristics of dysarthric individuals' communication partners.

REFERENCES

Adams SG: Accelerating speech in a case of hypokinetic dysarthria: descriptions and treatment. In Till JA, Yorkston KM, and Beukelman DR, editors: Motor speech disorders: advances in assessment and treatment, Baltimore, 1994, Paul H Brookes Publishing.

Ansel BM, McNeil MR, Hunker CJ, and Bless DM: The frequency of verbal and acoustic adjustments used by cerebral palsied dysarthric adults when faced with communicative failure. In Berry W, editor: Clinical dysarthria, 1983, Boston, College-Hill.

Aronson AE: Clinical voice disorders, New York, 1990, Thieme.

Aronson AE, O'Neill BP, and Kelly JJ: The dysarthria of action myoclonus: a new clinical entity. Paper presented at the Clinical Dysarthria Conference, February, 1984.

Aronson AE and others: Botulinum toxin injection for adductor spastic dysphonia: patient self-ratings of voice and phonatory effort after three successive injections, Laryngoscope 103:683, 1993.

Aten JL: Treatment of spastic dysarthria. In Perkins WH, editor: Current therapy of communication disorders: dysarthria and apraxia, New York, 1983, Thieme-Stratton.

Aten JL and others: Efficacy of modified palatal lifts for improved resonance. In McNeil M, Rosenbek J, and Aronson A, editors: The dysarthrias: physiology, acoustics, perception, management, Austin, TX, 1984, Pro-Ed.

Barlow SM and Abbs JH: Force transducers for the evaluation of labial, lingual, and mandibular function in dysarthria, J Speech Hear Res 26:616, 1983.

Bellaire K, Yorkston KM, and Beukelman DR: Modification of breath patterning to increase naturalness of a mildly dysarthric speaker, J Commun Disord 19:271, 1986.

Berry W and Goshorn E: Immediate visual feedback in the treatment of apraxia of ataxic dysarthria: a case study. In Berry W, editor: Clinical dysarthria, Boston, 1983, College-Hill.

Berry WR and Sanders SB: Environmental education: the universal management approach for adults with dysarthria. In Berry WR, editor: Clinical dysarthria, Boston, 1983, College-Hill.

Beukelman DR: Treatment of hyperkinetic dysarthria. In Perkins WH, editor: Current therapy of communication disorders: dysarthria and apraxia, New York, 1983, Thieme-Stratton.

Beukelman DR and Yorkston K: A communication system for the severely dysarthric speaker with an intact language system, J Speech Hear Disord 42:265, 1977.

---

*Again, I am indebted to Jack Thomas for this observation.

Beukelman DR, Yorkston KM, and Tice RL: Pacer/tally for pacing speech and tallying responses, Tucson, AZ, 1988, Communication Skill Builders.

Biary N, Pimental PA, and Langenberg PW: A double-blind trial of clonazepam in the treatment of parkinsonian dysarthria, Neurology 38:255, 1988.

Blitzer A and others: Abductor laryngeal dystonia: a series treated with botulinum toxin, Laryngoscope 102:163, 1992.

Brand HA, Matsko TA, and Avart HN: Speech prosthesis retention problems in dysarthria: case report, Arch Phys Med Rehabil 69:213, 1988.

Brin MF and others: Localized injections of botulinum toxin for the treatment of focal dystonia and hemifacial spasm, Mov Disord 2:237, 1987.

Brookshire RH: Control of "involuntary" crying behavior emitted by a multiple sclerosis patient, J Commun Disord 3:171, 1970.

Brookshire RH: An introduction to neurogenic communication disorders, ed 4, St Louis, 1992, Mosby–Year Book.

Caligiuri MP: Short-term fluctuations in orofacial motor control in Parkinson's disease. In Yorkston KM and Beukelman DR, editors: Recent advances in clinical dysarthria, Boston, 1989, College-Hill.

Caligiuri MP and Murry T: The use of visual feedback to enhance prosodic control in dysarthria. In Berry W, editor: Clinical dysarthria, Boston, 1983, College-Hill.

Carey J: Manual stretch: effect on finger movement control and force control in stroke subjects with spastic extrinsic finger flexion muscles, Arch Phys Med Rehabil 71:888, 1990.

Crow E and Enderby P: The effects of an alphabet chart on the speaking rate and intelligibility of speakers with dysarthria. In Yorkston KM and Beukelman DR, editors: Recent advances in clinical dysarthria, Austin, TX, 1989, Pro-Ed.

Daniel R and Guitar B: EMG feedback and recovery of facial and speech gestures following neural anastomosis, J Speech Hear Disord 43:9, 1978.

Darley FL, Aronson AE, and Brown JR: Motor speech disorders, Philadelphia, 1975, WB Saunders.

DePaul R and Brooks B: Multiple orofacial indices in amyotrophic lateral sclerosis, J Speech Hear Res 36:1158, 1993.

Dongilli PA: Semantic context and speech intelligibility. In Till JA, Yorkston KM, and Beukelman DR, editors: Motor speech disorders: advances in assessment and treatment, Baltimore, 1994, Paul H Brookes Publishing.

Downie AW, Low JM, and Lindsay DD: Speech disorders in parkinsonism: usefulness of delayed auditory feedback in selected cases, Br J Disord Commun 16:135, 1981.

Duffy JR and Folger WN: Dysarthria in unilateral central nervous system lesions. Paper presented at the annual convention of the American Speech-Language-Hearing Association, Detroit, November 1986.

Dworkin JP: Motor speech disorders: a treatment guide, St Louis, 1991, Mosby–Year Book.

Dworkin JP and Johns DF: Management of velopharyngeal incompetence in dysarthria: a historical review, Clin Otolaryngol 5:61, 1980.

Findley LJ and Koller WC: Essential tremor: a review, Neurology 37:1194, 1987.

Fonagy I and Magdics K: Speech of utterance in phrases of different lengths, Lang Speech 3:179, 1960.

Ford CN and Bless DM: A preliminary study of injectable collagen in human vocal fold augmentation, Otolaryngol Head Neck Surg 94:104, 1986.

Formisano R and others: Rehabilitation and Parkinson's disease, Scand J Rehabil Med 24:157, 1992.

Goldman-Eisler F: The significance of changes in the rate of articulation, Lang Speech 4:171, 1961.

Gonzalez JB and Aronson AE: Palatal lift prosthesis for treatment of anatomic and neurologic palatopharyngeal insufficiency, Cleft Palate J 7:91, 1970.

Gray S and others: Vocal evaluation of thyroplasty surgery in the treatment of unilateral vocal cord paralysis, NCVS Status Progress Report 1:87, 1991.

Hammen VL and Yorkston KM: Effect of instruction on selected aerodynamic parameters in subjects with dysarthria and control subjects. In Till JA, Yorkston KM, and Beukelman DR, editors: Motor speech disorders: advances in assessment and treatment, Baltimore, 1994, Paul H Brookes Publishing.

Hammerschlag PE and others: Hypoglossal-facial nerve anastomosis and electromyographic feedback rehabilitation, Laryngoscope 97:705, 1987.

Hand CR, Burns M, and Ireland E: Treatment of hypertonicity in muscles of lip retraction, Biofeedback Self Regul 4:171, 1979.

Hanson WR and Metter E: DAF as instrumental treatment for dysarthria in progressive supranuclear palsy: a case report, J Speech Hear Disord 45:268, 1980.

Hanson WR and Metter E: DAF speech rate modification in Parkinson's disease: a report of two cases. In Berry W, editor: Clinical dysarthria, Boston, 1983, College-Hill.

Hardy JC and others: Surgical management of palatal paresis and speech problems in cerebral palsy: a preliminary report, J Speech Hear Disord 26:320, 1961.

Hardy JC and others: Management of velopharyngeal dysfunction in cerebral palsy, J Speech Hear Disord 34:123, 1969.

Heller JC and others: Velopharyngeal insufficiency in patients with neurologic, emotional and mental disorders, J Speech Hear Disord 39:350, 1974.

Helm N: Management of palilalia with a pacing board, J Speech Hear Disord 44:350, 1979.

Henderson A, Goldman-Eisler F, and Skarbek A: Sequential temporal patterns in spontaneous speech, Lang Speech 9:207, 1966.

Hixon TJ, Hawley JL, and Wilson KJ: An around-the-house device for the clinical determination of respiratory driving pressure: a note on making the simple even simpler, J Speech Hear Disord 47:413, 1982.

Hixon TJ, Putnam A, and Sharp J: Speech production with flaccid paralysis of the rib cage, diaphragm, and abdomen, J Speech Hear Disord 48:315, 1983.

Isshiki N, Okamura H, and Ishikawa T: Thyroplasty type 1 (lateral compression) for dysphonia due to vocal cord paralysis or atrophy, Acta Otolaryngol (Stockh) 80:465, 1975.

Jankovic J: Blepharospasm and oromandibular-laryngeal-cervical dystonia: a controlled trial of botulinum A toxin therapy. In Fahn S, editor: Advances in neurology, vol 50, dystonia 2, New York, 1989, Raven Press.

Johns DF: Surgical and prosthetic management of neurogenic velopharyngeal incompetency in dysarthria. In Johns DF, editor: Clinical management of neurogenic communication disorders, New York, 1985, Little, Brown.

Johnson JA and Pring TR: Speech therapy and Parkinson's disease: a review and further data, Br J Disord Commun 25:183, 1990.

Keith RL and Thomas JE: Speech practice material for dysarthria, apraxia, and disorders of articulation, Toronto, 1989, BC Decker.

Kerman PC, Singer LS, and Davidoff A: Palatal lift and speech therapy for velopharyngeal incompetence, Arch Phys Med Rehabil 54:271, 1973.

Koller W, Graner D, and Mlcoch A: Essential voice tremor: treatment with propranolol, Neurology 35:106, 1985.

Koufman JA: Laryngoplasty for vocal cord medialization: an alternative to teflon, Laryngoscope 96:726, 1986.

Koufman JA: Laryngoplastic phonosurgery. In Johnson JT, editor: Instructional courses, American Academy of Otolaryngology—head and neck surgery, St Louis, 1988, Mosby–Year Book.

Kuehn DP and Wachtel JM: CPAP therapy for treating hypernasality following closed head injury. In Till JA, Yorkston KM, and Beukelman DR, editors: Motor speech disorders: advances in assessment and treatment, Baltimore, 1994, Paul H Brookes Publishing.

Lawshe BS and others: Management of a patient with velopharyngeal incompetency of undetermined origin: a clinical report, J Speech Hear Disord 36:547, 1971.

Lewy RB, Cole R, and Wepman J: Teflon injection in the correction of velopharyngeal insufficiency, Ann Otol Rhinol Laryngol 74:874, 1965.

Linebaugh CW: Treatment of flaccid dysarthria. In Perkins WH, editor: Current therapy of communication disorders: dysarthria and apraxia, New York, 1983, Thieme-Stratton.

Linebaugh CW and Wolfe VE: Relationships between articulation rate, intelligibility, and naturalness in spastic and ataxic speakers. In McNeil MR, Rosenbek JC, and Aronson AE, editors: The dysarthrias: physiology, acoustics, perception, and management, San Diego, 1984, College-Hill.

Ludlow CL and others: Successful treatment of selected cases of abductor spasmodic dysphonia using botulinum toxin injection, Otolaryngol Head Neck Surg 104:849, 1991.

Ludlow CL, Sedora SE, and Fujita M: Inspiratory speech with respiratory dystonia. In Helm-Estabrooks N and Aten JL, editors: Difficult diagnoses in communication disorders, Boston, 1989, College-Hill.

McFarlane SC and others: Unilateral vocal fold paralysis: perceived vocal quality following three methods of treatment, Am J Speech Lang Pathol 1:45, 1991.

McHenry MA, Wilson RL, and Minton JT: Management of multiple physiologic system deficits following traumatic brain injury, J Med Speech Lang Pathol 2:59, 1994.

Merritt JL: Management of spasticity in spinal cord injury, Mayo Clin Proc 56:614, 1981.

Minami RT and others: Velopharyngeal incompetency without overt cleft palate, Plast Reconstr Surg 55:573, 1975.

Mingrino S and Zuccarello M: Anastomosis of the facial nerve with accessory or hypoglossal nerves. In Samii M and Jannetta PJ, editors: The cranial nerves, New York, 1981, Springer-Verlag.

Mlcoch AG: Diagnosis and treatment of parkinsonian dysarthria. In Koller WC, editor: Handbook of Parkinson's disease, New York, 1992, Marcel Decker.

Mohr JP: Disorders of speech and language. In Wilson JD and others, editors: Hanson's principles of internal medicine, ed 12, New York, 1991, McGraw-Hill.

Moore CA and Scudder RR: Coordination of jaw muscle activity in parkinsonian movement: description and response to traditional treatment. In Yorkston KM and Beukelman DR, editors: Recent advances in clinical dysarthria, Boston, 1989, College-Hill.

Muenter MD and others: Treatment of essential tremor with methazolamide, Mayo Clin Proc 66:991, 1991.

Murry T: The production of stress in three types of dysarthric speech. In Berry WR, editor: Clinical dysarthria, San Diego, 1983, College-Hill.

Nemec RE and Cohen K: EMG biofeedback in the modification of hypertonia in spastic dysarthria: a case report, Arch Phys Med Rehabil 65:103, 1984.

Netsell R: Construction and use of a bite-block for use in evaluation and treatment of speech disorders, J Speech Hear Disord 50:103, 1985.

Netsell R: Inspiratory checking in therapy for individuals with speech breathing dysfunction, Presentation at American Speech-Language-Hearing Association Annual Convention, 1992.

Netsell R and Cleeland CS: Modification of lip hypertonia in dysarthria using EMG feedback, J Speech Hear Disord 38:131, 1973.

Netsell R and Daniel B: Dysarthria in adults. Physiologic approach to rehabilitation, Arch Phys Med Rehabil 60:502, 1979.

Netsell R and Hixon JT: A noninvasive method of clinically estimating subglottal air pressure, J Speech Hear Disord 43:326, 1978.

Netsell R and Rosenbek J: Treating the dysarthrias. Speech and language evaluation in neurology: adult disorders, New York, 1985, Grune and Stratton.

Odéen IN: Reduction of muscular hypertonus by long-term muscle strength, Scand J Rehabil Med 13:93, 1981.

Palmer S and others: Exercise therapy for Parkinson's disease, Arch Phys Med Rehabil 67:741, 1986.

Putnam AHB and Hixon TJ: Respiratory kinematics in speakers with motor neuron disease. In McNeil M, Rosenbek J, and Aronson AE, editors: The dysarthrias, San Diego, 1984, College-Hill.

Ramig LO: The role of phonation in speech intelligibility: a review and preliminary data from patients with Parkinson's disease. In Kent RD, editor: Intelligibility in speech disorders, Amsterdam, 1992, John Benjamin.

Ramig LO: Speech therapy for patients with Parkinson's disease. In Koller W and Paulson G, editors: Therapy of Parkinson's disease, New York, in press, Marcel Dekker.

Ramig LO, Horii Y, and Bonitati C: The efficacy of voice therapy for patients with Parkinson's disease, NCVS Status Progress Report, 1:61, 1991.

Remacle M and others: Initial long-term results of collagen injection for vocal and laryngeal rehabilitation, Arch Otorhinol 246:403, 1989.

Rigrodsky S and Morrison EB: Speech changes in parkinsonism during L-dopa therapy: preliminary findings, J Geriat Soc 18:142, 1970.

Robertson SJ and Thomson F: Speech therapy in Parkinson's disease: a study of the efficacy and long-term effects of intensive treatment, Br J Disord Commun 19:213, 1984.

Rontal M and others: A method for the treatment of abductor spasmodic dysphonia with botulinum toxin injections: a preliminary report, Laryngoscope 101:911, 1991.

Rosenbek JC and LaPointe LL: The dysarthrias: description, diagnosis, and treatment. In Johns DF, editor: Clinical management of neurogenic communication disorders, Boston, 1985, Little, Brown.

Rosenfield DB: Pharmacologic approaches to speech motor disorders. In Vogel D and Cannito MP, editors: Treating disordered speech motor control, Austin, TX, 1991, Pro-Ed.

Rubow R and Swift E: A microcomputer-based wearable biofeedback device to improve transfer of treatment in parkinsonian dysarthria, J Speech Hear Disord 50:178, 1985.

Rubow RT and others: Reduction of hemifacial spasm and dysarthria following EMG biofeedback, J Speech Hear Disord 49:26, 1984.

Sarno MT: Speech impairment in Parkinson's disease, Arch Phys Med Rehabil 49:269, 1968.

Schiffer RB, Herndon RM, and Rudick RA: Treatment of pathologic laughing and weeping with amitriptyline, N Engl J Med 312:1480, 1985.

Schulz GM and Ludlow CL: Botulinum treatment for orolingual-mandibular dystonia: speech effects. In Moore CA, Yorkston KM, and Beukelman DR, editors: Dysarthria and apraxia of speech: perspectives on management, Baltimore, MD, 1991, Paul H Brookes Publishing.

Scott S and Caird FI: Speech therapy for Parkinson's disease, J Neurol Neurosurg Psychiatry 46:140-144, 1983.

Scott S and Caird FI: Speech therapy for patients with Parkinson's disease, BMJ 283:1088, 1981.

Simmons N: Acoustic analysis of ataxic dysarthria: an approach to monitoring treatment. In Berry W, editor: Clinical dysarthria, San Diego, 1983, College-Hill.

Sinaki M: Physical therapy and rehabilitation techniques for patients with amyotrophic lateral sclerosis. In Cosi V and others, editors: Amyotrophic lateral sclerosis, New York, 1987, Plenum.

Smitheran J and Hixon T: A clinical method for estimating laryngeal airway resistance during vowel production, J Speech Hear Disord 46:138, 1981.

Solomon NP and Hixon TJ: Speech breathing in Parkinson's disease, J Speech Hear Res 36:294, 1993.

Stewart DS and Rieger WJ: A device for the management of velopharyngeal incompetence, J Med Speech Lang Pathol 2:149, 1994.

Till JA and Toye AR: Acoustic phonetic effects of two types of verbal feedback in dysarthric speakers, J Speech Hear Disord 53:449, 1988.

Tolosa E, Marti MJ, and Kulisevsky J: Botulinum toxin injection therapy for hemifacial spasm. In Jankovic J and Tolosa E, editors: Advances in neurology, vol 49, facial dyskinesias, New York, 1988, Raven Press.

Turner GS and Weismer G: Characteristics of speaking rate in the dysarthria associated with amyotrophic lateral sclerosis, J Speech Hear Res 36:1134, 1993.

Vogel D and Miller L: A top-down approach to treatment of dysarthric speech. In Vogel D and Cannito MP, editors: Treating disordered speech motor control: for clinicians, by clinicians, Austin, TX, 1991, Pro-Ed.

Whurr R and others: The use of botulinum toxin in the treatment of adductor spasmodic dysphonia, J Neurol Neurosurg Psychiatry 56:526, 1993.

Wolfe VI and others: Speech changes in Parkinson's disease during treatment with l-dopa, J Commun Disord 8:271, 1975.

Yorkston KM: Facial anastomosis in a dysarthric speaker. In Helm-Estrabrooks N and Aten JL, editors: Difficult diagnoses in adult communication disorders, Boston, 1989, College-Hill.

Yorkston KM and Beukelman DR: A comparison of techniques for measuring intelligibility of dysarthric speech, J Commun Disord 11:499, 1978.

Yorkston KM and Beukelman DR: Ataxic dysarthria: treatment sequences based on intelligibility and prosodic considerations, J Speech Hear Disord 46:398, 1981.

Yorkston KM, Beukelman D, and Bell K: Clinical management of dysarthric speakers, San Diego, 1988, College-Hill.

Yorkston KM, Dowden PA, and Beukelman DR: Intelligibility measurement as a tool in the clinical management of dysarthric speakers. In Kent RD, editor: Intelligibility in speech disorders, Philadelphia, 1992, John Benjamins.

Yorkston KM and others: Assessment of stress patterning. In McNeil MR, Rosenbek JC, and Aronson AE, editors: The dysarthrias: physiology, acoustics, perception, management, San Diego, 1984, College-Hill.

Yorkston KM and others: The effect of rate control on the intelligibility and naturalness of dysarthric speech, J Speech Hear Disord 55:550, 1990.

Yorkston KM and others: The effects of palatal lift fitting on the perceived articulatory adequacy of dysarthric speakers. In Yorkston KM and Beukelman DR, editors: Recent advances in clinical dysarthria, Austin, TX, 1989, Pro-Ed.

18 Managing Apraxia of Speech

Like management of the dysarthrias, the management of apraxia of speech (AOS) has received less attention than efforts to describe and understand its nature. This is understandable, especially given the history of debate over the very existence of AOS as a unique speech disorder and the ongoing debate about its underlying nature. In spite of this, the last 25 years have seen a number of methods developed for treating AOS. These approaches—although bearing some resemblance to those used for the dysarthrias—have been based on careful observation and study of the unique clinical characteristics of the disorder, the conditions under which it worsens or improves, and an assumption that AOS reflects a disturbance of motor speech programming.

This chapter provides an overview of methods used to improve speech and communication in people with AOS. The general management issues and decisions, approaches to management, and principles and guidelines for behavior management that are applicable to motor speech disorders in general will be reviewed briefly, with emphasis on factors that are especially relevant to AOS. Specific management approaches will then be discussed.

GENERAL PERSPECTIVES

It first may be helpful to return briefly to the discussion in Chapter 16 of general issues and decisions involved in managing motor speech disorders. This will help to establish the manner and degree to which managing AOS corresponds to or departs from the management of dysarthrias. It is clear that the two groups of motor speech disorders share many things relative to management. Most of the important differences lie in specific techniques of treatment.

Management territory and goals

The general orientation and primary goal of managing AOS is to maximize the effectiveness, efficiency, and naturalness of communication. The reasons for this are identical to those discussed in Chapter 16 for motor speech disorders in general. Similarly, management also focuses on restoring or compensating for impaired functions and on adjusting to or modifying the need for normal speech. The only difference between managing dysarthrias and AOS along these lines is the nature of the activities aimed at restoring lost functions; for dysarthria, an attempt is made to improve physiologic support for adequately planned and programmed speech, whereas for AOS, management focuses on reestablishing the programs or ability to program speech movements that can then be carried out by an intact neuromuscular apparatus. Both disorders affect speech movements, but the different underlying nature of each dictates differences in specific treatment activities or their criteria for success.

Factors influencing management decisions

The general factors that influence management decisions for dysarthria and AOS are identical. The rule that not all people with motor speech disorders are candidates for treatment applies equally to AOS and the dysarthrias, and the factors that influence decisions to treat or not are highly similar.

The influence of aphasia on treatment for AOS decisions deserves special mention. Aphasia is present in a high proportion of those with AOS by virtue of the overlap of lesion sites that are associated with the two disorders. Aphasia influences AOS treatment in at least three important ways. First, because aphasia affects language functions in all modalities, it can affect the patient's ability to comprehend spoken and written stimuli during treatment. Second, because aphasia affects verbal expression, it may be very difficult to distinguish aphasic from apraxic errors during AOS treatment activities. Third, and most important to decisions about whether to treat the AOS, the aphasia may be so severe that verbal communication would not be functional even if motor speech programming ability were intact. When deciding whether to focus some proportion of treatment efforts on AOS in a patient with aphasia, therefore, a clinician must ask, "How well would this person be able to communicate if they did not have AOS?" If the answer is that communication would not be functional because of the aphasia (or nonaphasic cognitive communication deficits or dysarthria), then treatment of the AOS should not be undertaken or should be deferred until language abilities are sufficient to generate linguistically adequate verbal messages. This judgment can be very difficult and often must rely on careful assessment of verbal and reading comprehension, writing or typing, or other nonverbal means of communication (for example, pantomime, signing).

The reader is cautioned that the specific approaches to treating AOS discussed later in this chapter do not address the influence of aphasia on AOS treatment. To do so would detract from the goal of understanding AOS treatment. The reader thus will be faced with the pervasive problem of textbook descriptions not precisely matching clinical reality. This problem exists, however, because all of the variations in people's behaviors and problems cannot be captured in print, or at least this writer does not know how to do so. If the "theme" and principles of treatment can be under-stood, however, they can be adapted to the realities of clinical practice by the experienced, thoughtful, and creative clinician.

Focus, duration, and termination of treatment

Treatment for AOS should focus on those tasks that provide the greatest functional benefit most rapidly or that will provide the best foundation for improvement over the course of treatment. The general issues surrounding the duration of treatment and its termination that were discussed in Chapter 16 also apply to the management of AOS.

APPROACHES TO MANAGEMENT

The parsing of management approaches into medical, prosthetic, and behavioral categories begins to shape some of the distinctions that exist between dysarthria and AOS management. In contrast to managing dysarthria—for which there are numerous medical, prosthetic, and behavioral treatments—managing AOS is primarily a behavioral enterprise.

Medical intervention

There are no medical interventions specifically designed to improve AOS for which there is evidence of efficacy. Pharmacologic intervention may be used for people with AOS to treat the underlying etiology or prevent further impairment (for example, antibiotics for infection, anticoagulants to prevent stroke, anticonvulsants to prevent seizures) and may—indirectly—result in speech improvement or prevent deterioration.

A few recent studies have examined the use of the dopamine agonist bromocriptine (presumably to aid the initiation of speech by altering limbic system activity) in the treatment of transcortical motor aphasia, Broca's aphasia, or nonfluent aphasia (Albert and others, 1988; Bachman and Morgan, 1988; MacLennan and others, 1991; Sabe, Leiguarda, and Starkstein, 1992). The results have been mixed, encouraging enough to warrant continued study but sufficiently weak or inconclusive to make use of the drug in aphasia treatment premature. The degree to which such studies have implications for treating AOS is unknown, but examining the effects of a variety of drugs that may influence speech initiation appears warranted. Just as Bachman and Albert (1990) suggest that "certain features of aphasia may be amenable to pharmacologic manipulation" (p. 411), the same *may* be true for AOS. As yet, however, there are no data to establish that this is the case.

Like dysarthria, AOS may benefit from surgery to manage underlying neurologic disease (aneurysm repair, endarterectomy, tumor removal), but the surgical procedure is not designed to manage

AOS per se. There are no surgical procedures specifically designed to improve AOS, and surgeries available for managing the dysarthrias (for example, pharyngeal flap, Teflon or collagen injection, thyroplasty) are not appropriate for managing AOS.

Prosthetic management and augmentative and alternative communication

The use of mechanical and prosthetic devices is appropriate for some people with AOS, but generally far less frequently than for dysarthric individuals. Their use is nearly always temporary, primarily intended to stimulate improved speech without the prosthesis.

Prostheses that modify vocal tract events during speech (for example, a palatal lift) or modify the acoustic signal after it is produced (for example, a voice amplifier) are rarely appropriate, because AOS usually is not characterized by deviations in resonance or loudness that are consistent or pervasive enough to be aided by available prosthetic devices. There are occasional exceptions, however. For example, Marshall, Gandour, and Windsor (1988) discussed a patient who was unable to phonate or articulate normally because of an apraxia of phonation but who was able to articulate normally when using an electrolarynx. This suggests that an electrolarynx may be worth a trial for persistently mute apraxic patients (Simpson and Clark, 1989) who are not responsive to traditional treatment approaches or for the occasional patient whose apraxia affects phonation to a much greater degree than articulation.

Some apraxic patients benefit from prostheses that assist rate reduction or the pacing of word production, although some devices have negligible or negative effects. For example, Shane and Darley (1978) failed to find a beneficial effect of a metronome on articulatory accuracy in apraxic speakers. They speculated that external cues for pacing and setting the rate of speech may be less effective than self-generated ones, such as finger tapping or a pacing board; however, their investigation examined the immediate effects of the metronome, not its effects over the course of a treatment program. This distinction may be important because Dworkin, Abkarian, and Johns (1988) used a metronome to pace all speech and oromotor control task activities in a successful single-subject treatment study; although alternative explanations for the success of their program are possible, the authors concluded that their results support the effectiveness of metronome pacing.

Delayed auditory feedback (DAF), in spite of its established benefits for some dysarthric patients, does not seem to be a viable form of instrumental feedback for AOS. Rosenbek (1985) suggests that DAF would be helpful only to patients capable of phrase and sentence-level utterances, and Chapin and others (1981) found that DAF actually disrupted speech in patients with Broca's aphasia. It may be that, although apraxic speakers may benefit from enhanced feedback or instrumental pacing, they cannot tolerate any *distortion* of feedback, such as that associated with DAF. At this time, there are no data to suggest that DAF is beneficial for those with AOS.

Some forms of biofeedback have facilitated improvement in some apraxic speakers. McNeil, Prescott, and Lemme (1976) noted improvment in four apraxic patients under conditions of muscle relaxation induced by electromyogram (EMG) biofeedback from the frontalis muscle. Rubow and others (1982) reported improved single-word imitative production in a patient provided vibrotactile stimulation to the right index finger during a clinician's verbal model. Improvement with vibrotactile and auditory cue stimulation was greater than in response to auditory cues alone. The investigators suggested that the stimuli provided an organizational framework for the sequencing of speech movements and represented an example of gestural or intersystemic reorganization (to be discussed under Behavioral Management).

A pacing board may help apraxic speakers slow rate and produce words and phrases in a syllable-by-syllable fashion to facilitate articulatory accuracy. Wertz, LaPointe, and Rosenbek (1984) note that stress and rhythm may require attention when a pacing board is used because board use tends to promote stereotypic prosody.

The variety of prostheses used as part of augmentative and alternative communication (AAC) systems are as appropriate for those with AOS as for those with dysarthria. These tools of behavioral intervention—including pictures, letter and word boards, electronic and computerized devices—can be very useful for some patients with AOS, although the degree of accompanying aphasia may preclude or place limits on the sophistication of linguistic messages that can be communicated through them. Several studies have documented the success of AAC strategies (Amerind sign language, Blissymbols, HandiVoice) for people with AOS, occasionally with some carryover of treatment effects to improved verbal communication (Dowden, Marshall, and Tompkins, 1981; Rabidoux, Florence, and McCauslin, 1980; Lane and Samples, 1981; Skelly and others, 1974).

Behavioral management

Behavioral intervention is at the heart of managing AOS. Like the management of dysarthria, behavioral approaches can be speaker-oriented or communication-oriented.

Communication-oriented approaches—those efforts at improving communication in the absence of changes in speech—are as applicable to AOS as they are to dysarthria. The strategies, although individually determined and clearly influenced by accompanying aphasia, are identical to those that may be used for dysarthric patients. They will not be discussed further in this chapter. The reader should consult Chapter 17 for an overview of communication-oriented approaches.

Speaker-oriented approaches—those that seek to improve speech itself—emphasize improved intelligibility, efficiency, and naturalness of communication. Their goals are achieved through efforts to improve the ability to program speech or compensate for residual inadequacies in the programming of speech. In most instances, treatment activities focus on speech itself, although they sometimes are directed to nonspeech oromotor tasks, not to improve physiologic support (as in dysarthria treatment), but to improve the ability to program nonspeech oromotor movements as a necessary precurser to similar gains for speech.

Because AOS is predominantly a disorder of articulation and prosody, behavioral treatment focuses on articulation and prosody. Focus on resonance is rarely appropriate or necessary, and work on respiration and phonation is rarely undertaken for any but the most severely impaired patients.

Most of the remainder of this chapter will focus on speaker-oriented approaches to AOS management. It begins with a review of the principles and guidelines for behavioral management that are especially important to managing AOS. Specific treatment approaches will then be addressed.

PRINCIPLES AND GUIDELINES FOR BEHAVIORAL MANAGEMENT

Many of the principles and guidelines for managing motor speech disorders that were discussed in Chapter 16 apply without qualification to the management of AOS. They do not require repeating here. A few points deserve minor qualification or emphasis, and others deserve special recognition.

Management should start early, as it should for dysarthria. It should be noted, however, that recommending treatment is not precluded by extended time postonset, especially for patients who have not received any treatment or whose treatment has not focused on their AOS. Several single-case or small group studies have established treatment benefits for patients who are in the chronic stage poststroke (for example, Deal and Florence, 1978; Dworkin, Abkarian, and Johns, 1988; Southwood, 1987; Stevens and Glaser,

1983). For patients with degenerative disease, treatment will most likely focus on compensatory strategies for maintaining intelligibility and current or future needs for AAC.

Baseline data

General measures of intelligibility and efficiency of communication (see Chapter 3), establishing the presence and degree of associated deficits, and obtaining an inventory of the patient's communication needs and goals, motivation, speaking environment and communication partners, difficult and easy communication situations, and their perception of others' reaction to their problem are as important to planning AOS treatment as they are for dysarthria. Beyond these things, *it is essential that a careful inventory of the nature of articulatory errors and accurate articulatory responses be acquired,* as well as information on *factors that influence the accuracy and adequacy of speech.* This is because successful responses during AOS treatment tasks often are highly dependent on the selection and ordering of treatment stimuli (Rosenbek, 1985). Tasks for assessing motor speech programming capacity (Table 3–6), published tests for the diagnosis of AOS, tasks for assessing nonverbal oral movement control and sequencing (Table 3–2), and, possibly, the Word Intelligibility Test (Kent and others, 1989, reviewed in Chapter 3) can provide a useful data base in this regard, although the problems of some patients may require an individually tailored inventory. In general, it is important to establish the degree to which a patient's errors correspond to the "typical" articulatory and prosodic characteristics of AOS (see boxes pp. 270, 271) and the variables that influence error frequency. For example, based on averages, the following "typical" patterns may be helpful to ordering stimuli in treatment:

1. Automatic or reactive speech is easier than volitional, purposive speech.
2. Oral-nasal distinctions are easier than voicing distinctions, which are easier than manner distinctions, which are easier than place distinctions.
3. Bilabial and lingual-alveolar places of articulation are easier than other places of articulation.
4. Consonant singletons are easier than clusters.
5. High-frequency words are easier than low-frequency words, and meaningful words are easier than nonsense words.
6. Single-syllable words are easier than multisyllabic words, and single words are easier than phrases or sentences.
7. Combined visual and auditory stimulation (watch and listen) lead to more accurate responses than auditory or visual stimulation alone.

8. Production of stressed words is easier than production of unstressed words.

These are but a few of the variables that should be addressed when acquiring baseline information. They are invaluable to the initial selection and ordering of treatment stimuli.

Physiologic support

Treatment for AOS does not require efforts to improve posture or increase strength, speed, range, and tone; that is, it does not require efforts to increase physiologic support for speech (Square and Martin, 1994; Wertz, LaPointe, and Rosenbek, 1984). For some severely impaired patients who are mute or unable to produce differentiated sounds under any circumstances, however, treatment may necessitate efforts to improve volitional control of nonspeech movements of speech structures; for example, establishing voluntary control of mouth opening and closing, lip pursing and rounding, tongue protrusion and elevation, deep inhalation or prolonged exhalation. These tasks would be used under the assumption (untested) that development of such control will pave the way for improved programming of speech movements.

Principles of motor learning

Principles of motor learning are crucial to AOS treatment, and they are embedded in the treatment principles for virtually all of the specific approaches to AOS treatment. The following paragraphs summarize those principles of motor learning that seem most relevant to AOS.

Drill. Virtually every specific behavioral treatment approach for AOS emphasizes drill. The need for intensive and systematic drill is highlighted by clinicians' sense that the poor speech of apraxic talkers may reflect more than inefficiency in speech programming. Many apraxic patients actually seem to have "lost" some of the "preprogrammed subroutines" for movement sequences that make normal speech so automatic and effortless. Thus, Darley, Aronson, and Brown (1975) observed that apraxic speakers seem to have "forgotten" how to perform speech movements, and Wertz, LaPointe, and Rosenbek (1984) indicated that AOS treatment is "the structured *relearning* of skilled speech movements" (p. 162). As articulated by Rosenbek and others (1973), an essential principle of treatment for AOS is that *systematic intensive and extensive drill is necessary to regain or learn lost speech skills.* Drill becomes systematic when responses are based on careful selection and ordering of stimuli that ensure a high level of success at each step of the treatment program. Drill is intensive and extensive when many responses occur during each of frequent treatment sessions.

Self-learning and instruction. Self-learning is accomplished by many apraxic speakers, especially if their impairment is not severe; what they learn on their own often cannot be improved upon by clinician instruction. As early as possible in treatment, patients should be urged to monitor their speech, grope for correct targets, and self-correct errors (Rosenbek and others, 1973; Wertz, LaPointe, and Rosenbek, 1984). Rau and Golper (1989) have emphasized the importance of identifying the productive self-cueing strategies used by patients and then helping them to use them consciously in a variety of situations.

Apraxic speakers, particularly those whose treatment must begin at the sound, syllable, or word level may need help in knowing how to produce speech movements. Sometimes this takes the form of simple "watch and listen" imitation tasks in which the clinician shows what is to be done. Sometimes more explicit instruction or explanation is required. Techniques of phonetic placement and phonetic derivation are often useful for teaching sound production, and instruction and cues for modifying rate and stress are often essential. In addition, instruction is a necessary component of some of the highly structured treatment programs that will be discussed shortly. In all instances, instruction should be faded as soon as learning has occurred.

Feedback. Wertz, LaPointe, and Rosenbek (1984) consider knowledge of results a general principle of AOS treatment. Many apraxic patients can judge the accuracy of their responses reliably and accurately, and they should be encouraged at the outset to do so, with efforts at self-correction when they judge responses as inadequate. Clinician-provided feedback is also reinforcing and encouraging. It may be especially important when working on nonspeech tasks, on speech tasks in which targets are noncategorical (such as tasks emphasizing stress or rate), or when intelligibility is the immediate goal.

Instrumental feedback and biofeedback may also be useful. A mirror may help some patients develop a strong visual image of correct movement or targets (Rosenbek, 1985; Rosenbek and others, 1973), although some patients do not benefit or are confused by such feedback. The use of EMG biofeedback and vibrotactile stimulation for some patients (McNeil, Prescott, and Lemme, 1976; Rubow and others, 1982) has already been discussed.*

Specificity of training. In general, when a patient has fairly frequent success at the word or

---

*The caveats about the value of feedback (and the validity of motor learning principles in general) discussed in Chapter 16 should be considered in the conduct of treatment for AOS.

phrase level, it is neither necessary nor appropriate to focus on nonspeech, sound-level, or nonsense syllable production tasks; words and phrases are motivating and much more meaningful and specific to the ultimate goal of treatment than are their motor precursors. However, some patients cannot say words or syllables, and some cannot even produce a few sounds. When AOS is marked or severe and initial attempts to improve speech have failed, focusing on syllable, sound, or even nonspeech tasks may be necessary, and some patients may respond more adequately on syllable-level tasks when syllables are meaningless. Thus, learning to plan, execute, evaluate, and self-correct nonverbal oral movements, sounds in isolation, and meaningless syllables may be a necessary precursor to meaningful speech for severely impaired patients (this statement receives some indirect support from Rosenbek's, [1985] impression that oral nonverbal ability is a useful prognostic sign for AOS).

Dabul and Bollier (1976) placed emphasis on sound and nonsense syllable mastery, including their rapid repetition, before moving to meaningful speech, and Dworkin (1991) recommends the inclusion of nonspeech oromotor planning activities as part of his recommended sequence of activities for AOS. It should be noted, however, that Dworkin, Abkarian, and Johns (1988) found that nonspeech oromotor and speech alternating motion rate (AMR) tasks did not generalize to speech tasks in a patient who ultimately benefited from a comprehensive AOS treatment program.

For mute apraxic patients, vegetative actions such as grunting, coughing, laughing, and singing may need to be reflexively elicited and then shaped toward volitional control as a precursor to voluntary or automatic speech production (Simpson and Clark, 1989). It is important to keep in mind that the purpose of nonspeech tasks is not to increase strength or other parameters of physiologic support for speech—their goal is to improve the programming of volitional oral movements.

Consistent and variable practice. The use of consistent practice can be found in many approaches to AOS treatment. For example, Dabul and Bollier (1976) and Dworkin, Abkarian, and Johns (1988) have used multiple trials of multiple repetitions of individual nonsense syllables or nonspeech oromotor movements in treatment. A number of treatment programs include successive productions of verbal responses without intervening stimuli (Rosenbek and others, 1973; Stevens, 1989). These consistent practice efforts tend to give way to variable practice in which the patient is required to program more elements into responses,

with syllable-to-syllable or response-to-response variability. Therefore, for example, repetition of a syllable ("see") may merge into phonetic contrast tasks in which variability of responses must be programmed and produced, either with minimal ("sue/zoo"), intermediate ("sue/moo"), or greater contrasts ("tomato/tornado").

Consistent and variable practice may include contrastive stress tasks as well, in which stereotypic stress patterns in sentences of identical length and structure ("*John* likes Mary," "*Mary* likes John") give way to stress tasks with variable stress placement in phrases of varying length and structure ("John *likes* Mary," "Mary likes to *sing* in church").

Speed-accuracy trade-off. The speed-accuracy trade-off applies to AOS treatment, with reduced rate nearly always emphasized early in treatment, giving way to attempts to increase speed as accuracy increases.* Rate reduction can take several forms. Wertz, LaPointe, and Rosenbek (1984) suggest that patients need to learn to be silent in order to have their response "in mind" before responding. They also indicate that for all but the most automatic of utterances, slow, deliberate, closed-loop control of speech must be used. This may take the form of a syllable-by-syllable approach to production or a conscious prolongation of vocalic nuclei (Southwood, 1987).

The value of rate reduction may derive from a different source for apraxic than dysarthric speakers. For example, Adams, Weismer, and Kent's (1993) examination of normal speakers' rate and movement velocity profiles suggests that alterations in rate are associated with changes in motor control strategies; that is, rapid rate seems to involve "unitary" movements that may be predominantly preprogrammed, whereas slow rates appear comprised of multiple submovements that may be influenced by feedback mechanisms. For many apraxic speakers who seem to have lost—or lost access to—preprogrammed subroutines, rate reduction may facilitate feedback and the "relearning" of the submovements necessary for accurate speech.

Once accurate articulation is achieved during treatment, increased rate should be pursued. This can be done within AMR-like tasks at the syllable, word, or phrase level, within contrastive stress tasks at the phrase level, during sentence and paragraph reading tasks, and so on.

Although never formally assessed for efficacy, divided attention tasks may be useful for mildly

---

*Some apraxic speakers may actually do better when they speak rapidly, without making conscious efforts to "think" about how they are producing speech.

impaired patients in order to assess and challenge the degree to which speech programming is approaching an automatic stage of learning. For example, how well can a patient maintain normal phrase rate when asked to recall a picture, letter, or color presented before or during their production? Such tasks might also serve as a final criterion step before moving to another level of response difficulty in treatment. For example, a patient who is able to produce multisyllabic words accurately could then be required to produce them in the context of a divided attention task and would be allowed to move to the phrase level of production only upon being able to maintain acceptable accuracy of multisyllabic words during the divided attention task.

BEHAVIORAL MANAGEMENT APPROACHES

A number of specific speaker-oriented approaches for managing AOS have been developed, for which there are single-subject design data, case study, or anecdotal reports of effectiveness. These approaches are more like than different from one another and are distinguished primarily by the nature of stimuli used to elicit speech. *They all share an emphasis on careful stimulus selection, an orderly progression of treatment tasks, and the use of intensive and systematic drill.*

Imitation is an integral part of most treatment programs (Wertz, LaPointe, and Rosenbek, 1984), especially during treatment's early stages. There are several reasons for this. First, imitation requires volitional responses to clearly established targets whose parameters can be carefully selected to ensure an appropriate level of success. Second, stimuli to be imitated provide a "map" for programming the response (for example, auditory and visual cues) that is facilitory for most patients. Third, it is efficient and parsimonious because it simplifies drill, facilitates obtaining a maximum number of responses, reduces demand for "creative" cognitive and linguistic efforts by the patient, and bypasses some of the language deficits that affect comprehension and formulation in patients who are aphasic as well as apraxic. Most programs also include steps that move beyond imitation to spontaneous speech; they recognize that imitation is less specific to the training goal than normal interactive communication and that achieving neuromotor control for imitation may not carry over to spontaneous speech (Rosenbek, 1984).

Most speaker-oriented behavioral treatment approaches employ the concepts of *intersystemic* or *intrasystemic reorganization.* Both of these concepts recognize that behavioral treatment for AOS requires some kind of reorganization of the way in which programming for speech is accomplished.

Intrasystemic reorganization (discussed in detail by Rosenbek, 1985; and Wertz, LaPointe, and Rosenbek, 1984) refers to attempts to improve a performance by emphasizing a more primitive or automatic level of function *or* a higher level of control. Making speech more volitional or conscious (for example, through imitation) is an example of higher level control. Eliciting automatic responses such as counting, singing, yawning, or overlearned social phrases are examples of more primitive intrasystemic activities. *Phonetic placement* and *phonetic derivation* techniques (used easily in imitation tasks) probably combine both higher-level and lower-level functions. For example, using tongue protrusion to help shape production of "th" uses a simple, lower-level movement in a highly volitional way to derive correct phonetic placement for a sound. Phonetic placement and derivation techniques are very useful for many patients but may be ineffective for those with a significant accompanying nonverbal oral apraxia.

Intersystemic reorganization refers to the use of nonspeech activity to facilitate speech. Its use receives some support from studies of limb movement. For example, the *"magnet effect"* refers to the tendency for the tempo of one movement to influence the tempo of another, with the sustaining of a mutual phase relationship. Simultaneous movements (such as arm or limb movement with speech) generally can be performed accurately as long as there is a harmonic relationship between them, and interference occurs when simultaneous movements are not compatible (Swinnen, Walter, and Shapiro, 1988). Swinnen, Walter, and Shapiro also point out that the programming of a particular activity in the brain may "spread out" in cerebral space and affect other movements that are being programmed. *Gestural reorganization* (Luria, 1970; Rosenbek, 1983, 1985; Wertz, LaPointe, and Rosenbek, 1984) is a prime example of an attempt to use nonspeech movements to facilitate speech. It may include strategies such as hand or finger tapping, foot tapping, head movements, and the use of a pacing board to facilitate rate reduction and rhythm and stress patterns during speech. In patients whose gestural control of such activities is better than speech, the dominance of the gesture is intended to help organize the control of speech.

In the following subsections, specific treatment approaches will be reviewed. We will begin with the "eight-step continuum" of Rosenbek and colleagues because it has been for some time a prototypic model for treating AOS, one that can be applied across many severity levels. It possesses—by design—considerable flexibility. If its "theme" is understood, the clinician will know how to think about the organization of AOS treatment for many patients. Following that discussion, several other approaches or programs will be reviewed. The acronyms associated with them should not be construed as providing them with greater status or evidence of efficacy than other approaches and techniques that have not been formally titled. They deserve attention because they focus on a particular method of stimulation or nature of responding. Finally, a general potpourri of techniques for facilitating speech production will be reviewed.

The eight-step continuum for treating apraxia of speech

Rosenbek and colleagues, in their "A Treatment for Apraxia of Speech in Adults" (1973), described an eight-step task continuum that they had found effective for teaching words, phrases, or sentences to three severely impaired patients. The themes and general principles of treatment articulated in their article are reflected in most other treatment approaches in use today. They noted the importance of *task continua* to ensure high levels of success, the importance of *intensive and extensive drill,* the need to work on *meaningful and useful communication* as soon as possible, and the importance of *self-correction.* They also recognized the importance of selecting and ordering stimuli on the basis of the pattern of phonetic breakdowns observed in patients. Fundamental to their program, moreover, they stressed the importance of *integral stimulation** (watch and listen) in the early steps of treatment, with gradual fading of auditory and visual cues. The overall theme of their program is one in which stimulus prompts are initially maximal and gradually faded, and response requirements are gradually increased. A brief summary of the eight steps follows. Note that they may use stimuli at the syllable, word, phrase, or sentence level.

Step 1—Integral stimulation in which the clinician presents a target stimulus, which the patient then imitates while watching and listening to the clinician's simultaneous production.

*Step 2—*Same as step 1, but the patient's response is delayed and the clinician mimes the response (without sound) during the patient's response; that is, the simultaneous auditory cue is faded.

*Step 3—*Integral stimulation followed by imitation without any simultaneous cues from the clinician.

*Step 4—*Integral stimulation with several successive productions without any intervening stimuli and without simultaneous cues.

*Step 5—*Written stimuli are presented without auditory or visual cues, followed by patient's production while looking at the written stimuli.

*Step 6—*Written stimuli, with delayed production following removal of the written stimuli.

*Step 7—*A response is elicited with an appropriate question. For example, instead of imitating "I'd like a cup of coffee," the patient is asked to respond with the target phrase to the query, "Would you like anything?"

*Step 8—*The response is elicited in an appropriate role-playing situation.

The authors point out that not all patients need to go through all steps and that some steps may be bypassed because they may be particularly difficult. They also noted that phonetic derivation and placement techniques should be employed when integral stimulation fails.

Deal and Florence (1978) presented a modification of the task continuum by deleting some steps, by setting more rigid criteria for progressing from one step to another, and by incorporating some steps into a program in the home environment. They reported four cases for whom their modifications were successful.

Prompts for restructuring oral muscular phonetic targets

The prompts for restructuring oral muscular phonetic targets (PROMPT) approach to treatment was initially developed by Chumpelik (1984) for children with developmental apraxia of speech, but it has subsequently been applied to adults (Square, Chumpelik, and Adams, 1985; Square and others, 1986). Its distinctive feature is its use of tactile cues to provide touch pressure, kinesthetic, and proprioceptive cues to facilitate speech production. In this sense, the clinician who provides the cues acts as an "external programmer" for speech, providing intersystemic cues for spatial and temporal aspects of speech production (Square-Storer and Hayden, 1989).

The PROMPT approach uses highly structured finger placements on the patient's face and neck to signal articulatory target positions, as well as cues about other movement characteristics, such as manner of articulation, degree of jaw movement, and syllable and segment duration. For example, the thumb placed on the side of the nose may signal a requirement for nasality while, at the same

---

*Watch and listen strategies are not always best. LaPointe and Horner (1976) found that some patients responded more adequately when they only listened or only read stimuli than when they watched and listened to the clinician's model or listened and read a target word.

time, another finger signals place of production, such as bilabial contact; the duration of the cues signals sound duration. By chaining together a series of PROMPTs, movements between phonemes may be facilitated. Square-Storer and Hayden (1989) indicate that "extensive training and practice are required in order to competently and efficiently administer this form of treatment" (p. 192).

It is likely that patients with chronic, severe AOS whose spontaneous verbal output is very limited and for whom traditional methods of treatment have failed are the most appropriate patients for this approach (Square-Storer and Hayden, 1989). Improvements in speech in response to PROMPT have been reported for a small number of patients (Square-Storer and Hayden, 1989; Square, Chumpelik, and Adams, 1985; Square and others, 1986).

Melodic intonation therapy

Melodic information therapy (MIT) is a formal treatment program originally intended for patients with severe nonfluent aphasia (Sparks, Helm, and Albert, 1974; Sparks and Holland, 1976). It has been used by some clinicians to treat AOS, with proponents of MIT recognizing that such use is appropriate (Sparks and Deck, 1994). The program's distinctive feature is its reliance on singing and a variant of it in which intoned utterances are based on the melody, rhythm, and patterns of stress in a spoken model provided to the patient. Its systematic, structured approach and many of its principles are similar to the integral stimulation approach described by Rosenbek and colleagues (1973).

Repetition forms the core of MIT, although its use is faded during progression through the program. Other principles include the use of a variety of high probability utterances with semantic value to the patient, working at levels that ensure a high degree of success, the use of verbal and gestural cues (but avoidance of picture or written cues, which are considered distracting), and twice daily treatment sessions. Because MIT is a departure from the normal speaking mode, it has been recommended that concurrent treatment of speech not be used during MIT (Sparks and Deck, 1994).

Good candidates for MIT have been fairly carefully described. They include those with *good verbal comprehension, preserved self-criticism, a paucity of spontaneous verbal output,* and *nonfluent speech characteristics,* including distorted, pause-filled utterances with attempts at self-correction of articulation errors (some patients may have stereotyped, perseverative utterances). Good candidates have a "typical" Broca's aphasia language profile and often a significant nonverbal oral apraxia. Sparks and Deck (1994) point out that—given the criteria for MIT—it is appropriate for only a portion of the aphasic population. The stated criteria suggest that such patients usually (? always) have an AOS—as AOS has been described in this book—that is clearly worse than any aphasia that may be present. Some clinicians suggest that MIT may be appropriate for those who fail to respond to more traditional "integral stimulation" or "eight-step" approaches (Square-Storer, 1989).

An MIT program begins with the gradual teaching of preselected (but flexible) hand-tapping rhythms, eventually with simultaneous humming, in unison with the clinician, with gradual fading of the clinician's model. When these basics are acquired, meaningful linguistic material is added. Eventually, clinician cues and patient hand tapping are faded, and imitation gives way to the answering of questions by the patient. The singing employed avoids the use of familiar tunes but emphasizes exaggerated pitch, tempo, and rhythm, with tempo lengthened and pitch varied to create a lyrical, melodic pattern, and rhythm and stress are exaggerated for the purpose of emphasis. When this singing style can be used for the accurate repetition of verbal materials, it is modified to "*sprechgesang,*" or "spoken song," a prosodic pattern lying between singing and speech. Detailed descriptions of the MIT program have been provided by Sparks and Deck (1986; 1994). Some clinicians have successfully modified MIT to meet the special needs of their patients (Dunham and Newhoff, 1979; Marshall and Holtzapple, 1976).

Sparks and Deck (1986) suggest that about 75% of carefully selected patients can benefit from MIT. Such patients probably have marked to severe AOS and relatively mild aphasia, so it is probable that only a small segment of the aphasic and AOS population can benefit from MIT. It probably should be chosen as a treatment approach only when more traditional approaches have been unsuccessful; for example, Wertz, LaPointe, and Rosenbek (1984) suggest that methods that focus only on rhythm may be less efficient than other approaches. It is possible that MIT may provide some patients with imitation skills that allow them also then to benefit from other treatment techniques (Tonkovich and Peach, 1989). Although case studies have recorded the effectiveness of MIT for some patients, Brookshire (1992) notes that there are no controlled experimental data that document MIT effectiveness relative to other AOS treatments. Unfortunately, this point is true for all AOS treatments.

Multiple input phoneme therapy

Multiple input phoneme therapy (MIPT) is a treatment approach designed for severely aphasic and apraxic patients whose repetition abilities are severely impaired and whose verbalizations are characterized by repetitive verbal stereotypies (Stevens, 1989; Stevens and Glaser, 1983). Its purpose is to shape from the perseverative verbal stereotypies, or involuntary utterances, a variety of utterances that may eventually be used volitionally.

Initially MIPT requires the reduction of the patient's struggle to speak voluntarily with resultant involuntary stereotypic responses (for example, the patient may say only "two-two-two" with varying inflections). The first step is to identify the most frequently occurring stereotypic utterance, which becomes the initial target of treatment. The patient then watches the clinician slowly produce the target 8 to 10 times, emphasizing the initial phoneme and, with the patient, tapping simultaneously with the patient's ipsilesional arm. The patient then joins the clinician in several repetitions of the utterance. Following this, the clinician fades voice but continues to mouth the utterance and tap as the patient repeats the target. These steps are then repeated for other stereotypic utterances. When this process is complete, new single-syllable words are created, using the same initial phoneme of the stereotypy (for example, "two" may become "tie," "toe," "tune," "tulip," and so on). Targets are then broadened to all phonemes, and then to clusters, multisyllabic words, phrases, and short sentences. Eventually, repetition is faded and responses are elicited by reading cues, picture naming, and assisted phrase production.

Stevens (1989) provides a description of MIPT that conveys the theme of the approach quite adequately. Stevens and Glaser (1983) reported five cases whose verbal stereotypies were decreased and whose verbal expressive abilities increased during MIPT. Stevens (1989) summarized the result of a Veterans Administration pilot project in which a group of five patients receiving 50 sessions of MIPT improved from pretreatment to posttreatment in comparison to five patients who received "traditional procedures" for aphasia and apraxia who failed to improve from pretreatment to posttreatment. Improvement occurred on standard aphasia tests, including spoken communication tasks.

Voluntary control of involuntary utterances

Voluntary control of involuntary utterances (VCIU) was originally described by Helm and Baresi (1980) as a method for modifying the speech of aphasic patients with moderately intact comprehension and nonfluent speech who were not responsive to integral stimulation approaches or MIT. Its target population and general theme are similar to that of MIPT, although its specific methods are different. For example, VCIU relies on visual (written) and verbal input in its initial steps, whereas MIPT relies on auditory and verbal input.

The approach begins by identifying any real word(s) that the patient has uttered in any context (socially, imitatively, or any other), even if the word was inaccurate or inappropriate for that context. The word(s) is then written on a card for oral reading. If the word is then read correctly, it is retained; if it is replaced by another word when read (for example, the written word "dog" is read as "cat"), the original stimulus is discarded and the "voluntary" response is retained. The clinician also may present patients who have very limited repertoires of utterances written words that the patient may be able to read; Helm-Estabrooks (1983) suggests that emotion-laden words (such as "love," "die," "damn") are particularly successful. Other likely candidates, especially for apraxic patients, tend to be short consonant-vowel or consonant-vowel-consonant (CVC), high-frequency words with simple initial consonants (for example, "no," "bye," "good"). These strategies are used to build a list of written words the patient can read voluntarily. The next step is to have the patient produce the words in a confrontation or responsive naming mode. Thus, a picture of a "dog" may be presented with a request that it be named. For a nonpicturable word such as "bad," the patient may be asked, "What is the opposite of good?" Success at this level is followed by conversational activities that elicit target words. New words uttered during any of these steps are added to the list of utterances that receive attention.

One attractive aspect of VCIU is its reliance on the patient's spontaneous utterances to establish the stimuli for treatment, thus facilitating a high level of success, even for severely impaired patients. For this reason, the technique may be quite useful to "getting speech going" for apraxic patients with severely limited verbal output.

Efficacy data are limited. Helm and Baresi (1980) presented anecdotal data for three patients who developed more than 250 voluntary utterances and improved performance on a standard aphasia test, and they reported carryover gains to daily activities. Helm-Estabrooks (1983) anecdotally noted improved spontaneous speech and improved functional communication in two patients with subcortical aphasia with whom VCIU was used.

Additional approaches and techniques

The general concepts of intersystemic and intrasystemic reorganization and gestural reorganization, the usefulness of imitation and phonetic placement and derivation techniques, and the themes conveyed by integral stimulation, PROMPT, MIT, MIPT, and VCIU approaches to treatment capture the scope and essence of behavioral management for AOS. The following subsections briefly discuss some additional approaches and specific techniques that have been found useful in management. They are not exhaustive but do help to round out the management theme for AOS.

Techniques for the speechless apraxic patient. When AOS is characterized by muteness or extremely limited or unreliable ability to vocalize—whether or not aphasia is present—there are some techniques that often get speech going. In general, it is best to begin with those that elicit meaningful speech, rather than focusing on nonverbal activities. The following techniques will often elicit vocalization and sometimes intelligible words and phrases, even in patients who have been mute.

1. *Automatic speech tasks* such as counting or saying the days of the week may elicit speech when all other volitional attempts to speak result in failure. When this is effective, patients are sometimes also able to recite portions of overlearned poems, pledges, nursery rhymes, or prayers.

2. Apraxic patients without severe aphasia may be able to complete predictable *carrier phrases* ("I'd like a cup of _____ ," "The American flag is red, white, and _____ ").

3. *Singing.* Some patients may be able to sing familiar songs ("Happy Birthday," "Jingle Bells"), sometimes only the tune without intelligible words, but sometimes with good or excellent approximation of the lyrics, even when they cannot vocalize under other conditions. Sometimes this ability to sing familiar tunes can be used as a primary mode of treatment to facilitate production of communicative words and phrases (Keith and Aronson, 1975).

4. When phonation cannot be elicited with automatic speech tasks, but the mouth is opened in an attempt, a quick *push on the abdomen* may trigger vocal cord closure and phonation and provide a foundation for voluntary phonation. Similarly, if a reflexive yawn or cough can be induced, phonation may emerge with it or be shaped from it. Some patients can produce a vowel when the clinician's hand is placed on the larynx and they are asked to say "ah"; pressure or lowering of the thyroid cartilage may facilitate phonation.

5. As already noted, an *artificial larynx* may facilitate articulation (or phonation) in some mute apraxic patients (Marshall, Gandour, and Windsor, 1988).

6. *Pairing a highly used symbolic gesture with its associated sound or word* may elicit vocalization in a speechless apraxic patient. For example, waving "hi" or "bye" (especially in an appropriate context) or encouraging patients to use the gesture themselves may elicit the appropriate verbal response. Other automatic social questions and answers are also useful in triggering automatic responses ("How are you?" "Okay," "Fine"). Placing the index finger to the lip to say "sh" may elicit the sound, blowing out a match may be shaped to a phonated vowel, and so on.

Patients who remain mute or unable to produce intelligible syllables may need to work on nonspeech oromotor movements with the same degree of drill and systematic progression that characterize speech tasks. For example, Dworkin, Abkarian, and Johns (1988) employed activities such as raising and lowering the tongue repetitively—with a bite block in place—to the beat of a metronome to develop oromotor control in an apraxic patient. A number of nonspeech oromotor planning exercises for the tongue, lips, jaw, and respiratory control have been described by Dworkin (1991).

Techniques at the volitional sound, syllable, and word level. For patients whose AOS has them working at the volitional sound, syllable, or single word level, phonetic placement and derivation techniques and gestural reorganization may be very helpful. The PROMPT, MIPT, and VCIU approaches are often used at this level. A number of useful general techniques that may be employed at this stage can supplement integral stimulation and other treatment programs.

Some clinicians stress the importance, for some patients, of working at the sound or meaningless syllable level of production. Wertz, LaPointe, and Rosenbek (1984) note that some patients do better if meaning is removed from treatment tasks, and Darley, Aronson, and Brown (1975) recognized the need for some patients to work on isolated sounds that could then be shaped to syllables and words. For example, humming "m" could give way to the addition of a vowel to form "ma," which then would be repeated multiple times. This might be followed by the addition of a variety of vowels, then CVC syllables ("mom"), then two-word phrases ("my mom"), and so on. Dabul and Bollier (1976) emphasized the importance of sound mastery and then the rapid (AMR) repetition of nonmeaningful syllables as building blocks for meaningful speech. They presented data for two chronic patients with AOS who benefited from such a program. Dworkin (1991) describes a number of vowel and syllable exercises that are useful for drillwork at this level.

The *key word technique* (Wertz, LaPointe, and Rosenbek, 1984) is used by many clinicians, and it probably represents the basis for formal approaches such as MIPT and VCIU. The technique takes words that are uttered accurately and automatically and requires the patient to repeat them frequently in order to establish voluntary control. The patient may also be asked to answer questions with the word, read the word, and so on. Then the initial sound of the word, for example, is used to build new utterances. For example, patients who can say "fine" in response to "how are you" may be asked to repeat "fine" multiple times after the clinician and then attempt words such as "fire," "five," "fight."

Cueing strategies are particularly relevant for sound, syllable, and word level activities, with phonetic derivation and placement being especially useful cues. At the word level, there seems to be a hierarchy of effective cues, although they usually need to be individually determined (Rau and Golper, 1989). In addition to biofeedback, cues that facilitate accurate responses at the word level may include word imitation (watch and listen); sentence completion; first sound of the target word; the printed target word; description of function; presentation of associated words (Darley, Aronson, and Brown, 1975; Linebaugh and Lehner, 1977; Love and Webb, 1977; Rau and Golper, 1989; Wertz, LaPointe, and Rosenbek, 1984). Rau and Golper (1989) emphasize the importance of developing cueing hierarchies on an individual basis, use of the most minimal cue that elicits an adequate response, and the value of teaching patients to self-cue rather than rely on clinician-provided cues.

Some response parameters that may be used at the syllable and word level (and beyond) that may facilitate or challenge response adequacy include prolongation of initial consonants; prolongation of vowels and syllables; clinician-imposed or patient-imposed delays before responding; rehearsal before responding; and immediate responding (Bugbee and Nichols, 1980; Warren, 1977). Similar to cueing strategies, the value of these response parameter modifications should be individually determined.

Techniques at the multiple syllable utterance level. Phonetic contrast, rate control, stress, and prosody become important when patients begin to move beyond the single-syllable response level and, as has been discussed, may be very important components of integral stimulation programs and MIT.

Practice in the use of *phonetic contrasts* when moving beyond the single-syllable level may be important for some patients in order to establish articulatory control across syllables. Such contrasts may reflect minimal differences in voicing ("bye-pie"), place ("key-tea"), and manner ("to-chew"); vowels ("toe-to"); singletons versus clusters ("sing-sting"), and so on (Darley, Aronson, and Brown, 1975; Rosenbek, 1983; Square and Martin, 1994).

Rate modification plays a significant role at the multisyllabic word, phrase, or sentence level. A pacing board, metronome, hand or finger tapping, and other intersystemic gestural rate control strategies may be helpful, as well as slowing rate without cues from other modalities. For example, Simmons (1978) reported that the simple use of "finger counting," in which a finger was held up for each word uttered, improved the adequacy of speech in an aphasic and severely apraxic patient who had plateaued after receiving a number of different treatment approaches. Southwood (1987) reported improved articulation in two patients who were instructed to prolong the vowel in each syllable and stretch out words in each phrase.

Many clinicians note the *powerful facilitory effects of stress and rhythm on articulation* in AOS treatment (Horner, 1983; Rosenbek, 1983; Square and Martin, 1994; Wertz, LaPointe, Rosenbek, 1984). *Contrastive stress tasks,* with or without accompanying gestural cues for stress, such as those described in Chapter 17, are very applicable to patients with AOS, both because they slow rate and because they take advantage of the facilitory effects of rhythm on speech. In some instances, these rate and rhythm efforts are so powerful that patients are able to succeed at the multisyllabic word or phrase level even when they have done poorly at the sound, syllable, and word level. Wertz, LaPointe, and Rosenbek (1984) provide a detailed description of the construction of contrastive stress tasks that include imitation, question-and-answer dialogue with stress on a target word, and more complex utterances with different locations for target words or multiple stressed target words. Written stimuli may be useful at the sentence level when the patient is moved beyond imitation, with targeted stressed words highlighted in the text. Horner (1983) notes that frequently used phrases ("Time to go," "How are you?") may be useful in stabilizing stress, pause, and intonation skills.

For mildly impaired patients, treatment generally abandons imitation tasks and emphasizes spontaneous conversational interaction, with the patient bearing responsibility for self-cueing and monitoring. Tasks may include putting target words into sentences, answering open-ended questions, and generating narratives about picture stimuli, articles, or movies.

Efficacy

The preceding discussion of AOS treatment referred to a number of case reports and single-subject design studies that suggest that a variety of programs and techniques can be effective in managing AOS. There seems to be a consensus that treatment of AOS, especially when aphasia is not present or prominent, is effective. Rosenbek (1983) stated that "about 90% of those patients with an apraxia more severe than their aphasia regained some functional communication" (p. 56) and that the prognosis for recovery of functional communication in such patients is excellent with treatment. In contrast, Brookshire (1992) suggests that only a small proportion of patients with AOS whose problems remain severe at three months postonset of stroke will regain functional communication; most such patients have a significant aphasic language impairment.

Wertz (1984) indicates that "what we know about what works for the apraxic patient comes from single subject and small sample designs" (p. 258). He discussed the efficacy of treatment for aphasic patients who had AOS in the Veterans Administration cooperative study on aphasia therapy and noted that 14 of 19 patients with AOS in the study improved and that 4 of 5 of those who did not improve had received group treatment with no direct manipulation of their AOS. These data represent circumstantial evidence that treatment of aphasic patients with AOS is beneficial and that AOS responds better to treatment that directly attacks it, rather than to general language stimulation provided within group settings.

A good deal more needs to be learned about the efficacy of treatment for AOS. It seems particularly important to establish the relative value of the various approaches that have been developed so that treatment may be provided in the most efficient and beneficial ways. For example, if EMG feedback and vibrotactile stimulation are proven effective for a larger number of patients than thus far demonstrated, are they more useful than treatments that do not require expensive equipment and perhaps more time for them to be effective? Is MIT more effective than integral stimulation approaches for some patients with AOS, and, if so, which patients? Are nonspeech oromotor exercises necessary precursors to the development of adequate speech in severely impaired patients with AOS, or should treatment be deferred for such patients until potential emerges for benefiting from direct work on speech? The answers to questions like these will not be obtained without difficulty.

SUMMARY

1. Treatment of AOS and treatment of the dysarthrias are similar in a number of ways, but they are not identical. Differences in treatment between these two categories of motor speech disorders derive mostly from differences in their underlying nature.

2. The co-occurrence of aphasia with AOS often has an important bearing on AOS treatment. Aphasia can affect a patient's comprehension during treatment activities, can complicate interpretation of speech errors, and can limit gains in functional speaking abilities. For some patients, the severity of an accompanying aphasia may preclude treatment of AOS.

3. There are no surgical or pharmacologic interventions with demonstrated efficacy for managing AOS. Prostheses for modifying the vocal tract or the acoustic signal, such as palatal lifts and vocal amplifiers, are generally not appropriate for people with AOS. Rate control devices, biofeedback, and AAC prostheses are applicable to AOS treatment.

4. Communication-oriented approaches to treatment are appropriate for people with AOS and are generally identical to those used in the management of dysarthria.

5. Speaker-oriented behavioral approaches to AOS focus primarily on articulation and prosody. A careful inventory of articulatory characteristics and factors that influence the accuracy and adequacy of speech is essential to systematic treatment planning. For some patients, the initial focus of treatment may be activities that promote nonspeech oromotor control.

6. Systematic, intensive, and extensive drill is an essential component of all speaker-oriented behavioral approaches to AOS. Self-learning, feedback, specificity of training, consistent and variable practice, and speed-accuracy trade-offs are important motor learning concepts in AOS treatment.

7. Several specific speaker-oriented approaches have been developed for AOS. They share an emphasis on careful stimulus selection, orderly progression of treatment tasks, and the use of intensive and systematic drill. Most also employ intersystemic and intrasystemic reorganization concepts in their techniques. Rosenbek and colleagues' "eight-step continuum" for treating AOS is the prototypic treatment for AOS; it or modifications of it are probably used more frequently than any other approach to the disorder. Additional specific treatment approaches such as PROMPT (prompts for restructuring oral muscular phonetic targets), MIT (melodic intonation therapy), MIPT (multiple input phoneme therapy), and VCIU (voluntary control of involuntary utterances) represent additional formalized approaches that may

be useful for some patients with AOS. A large number of techniques that are not tied to any specific treatment program are recognized as effective for facilitating speech at various points along the AOS severity continuum.

8. Efficacy data and clinical impressions suggest that a variety of programs and techniques can be effective in managing AOS, especially when aphasia is not present or prominent. Very little is known about the comparative effectiveness and efficiency of the various approaches and techniques, however.

REFERENCES

Adams SG, Weismer G, and Kent RD: Speaking rate and speech movement velocity profiles, J Speech Hear Res 36:41, 1993.

Albert ML and others: Pharmacotherapy of aphasia, Neurology 38:877, 1988.

Bachman DL and Albert ML: The pharmacotherapy of aphasia: historical perspective and directions for future research, Aphasiology 4:407, 1990.

Bachman DL and Morgan A: The role of pharmacotherapy in the treatment of aphasia: preliminary results, Aphasiology 2:225, 1988.

Brookshire RH: An introduction to neurogenic communication disorders, ed 4, St Louis, 1992, Mosby–Year Book.

Bugbee JK and Nichols AC: Rehearsal as a self-correction strategy for patients with apraxia of speech. In Brookshire RH, editor: Clinical aphasiology conference proceedings, Minneapolis, 1980, BRK Publishers.

Chapin C and others: Speech production mechanisms in aphasia: a delayed auditory feedback study, Brain Lang 14:106, 1981.

Chumpelik (Hayden) D: The PROMPT system of therapy. In Aram D, editor: Seminars Speech Lang 5:139, 1984.

Dabul B and Bollier B: Therapeutic approaches to apraxia, J Speech Hear Disord 41:268, 1976.

Darley FL, Aronson AE, and Brown JR: Motor speech disorders, Philadelphia, 1975, WB Saunders.

Deal J and Florance CL: Modification of the eight-step continuum for treatment of apraxia of speech in adults, J Speech Hear Disord 43:89, 1978.

Dowden PA, Marshall RC, and Tompkins CA: Amerind sign as a communicative facilitator for aphasic and apractic patients. In Brookshire RH, editor: Clinical aphasiology conference proceedings, Minneapolis, 1981, BRK Publishers.

Dunham MJ and Newhoff M: Melodic intonation therapy: rewriting the song. In Brookshire RH, editor: Clinical aphasiology conference proceedings, Minneapolis, 1979, BRK Publishers.

Dworkin JP: Motor speech disorders: a treatment guide, St Louis, 1991, Mosby–Year Book.

Dworkin JP, Abkarian CG, and Johns DF: Apraxia of speech: the effectiveness of a treatment regimen, J Speech Hear Disord 53:280, 1988.

Helm NA and Barresi B: Voluntary control of involuntary utterances: a treatment approach for severe aphasia. In Brookshire R, editor: Clinical aphasiology conference proceedings, Minneapolis, 1980, BRK Publishers.

Helm-Estabrooks N: Treatment of subcortical aphasia. In Perkins W, editor: Language handicaps in adults, New York, 1983, Thieme-Stratton.

Horner J: Treatment of Broca's aphasia. In Perkins WH, editor: Language handicaps in adults, New York, 1983, Thieme-Stratton.

Keith RL and Aronson AE: Singing as therapy for apraxia of speech and aphasia: report of a case, Brain Lang 2:483, 1975.

Kent RD and others: Toward phonetic intelligibility testing in dysarthria, J Speech Hear Disord 54:482, 1989.

Lane VW and Samples JM: Facilitating communication skills in adult apraxics: application of Blissymbols in a group setting, J Commun Disord 14:157, 1981.

LaPointe LL and Horner L: Repeated trials of words by patients with neurogenic phonological selection-sequencing impairment (apraxia of speech). In Brookshire RH, editor: Clinical aphasiology conference proceedings, Portland, OR, 1976, BRK Publishers.

Linebaugh C and Lehner L: Cueing hierarchies and word retrieval: a therapy program. In Brookshire RH, editor: Clinical aphasiology conference proceedings, Minneapolis, 1977, BRK Publishers.

Love R and Webb WG: The efficacy of cueing techniques in Broca's aphasia, J Speech Hear Disord 42:170, 1977.

Luria AR: Traumatic aphasia, The Hague, 1970, Mouton.

MacLennan DL and others: The effects of bromocriptine on speech and language function in a man with transcortical motor aphasia. In Prescott TE, editor: Clinical aphasiology, vol 20, Austin, TX, 1991, Pro-Ed.

Marshall N and Holtzapple P: Melodic intonation therapy: variations on a theme. In Brookshire RH, editor: Clinical aphasiology conference proceedings, Minneapolis, 1976, BRK Publishers.

Marshall RC, Gandour J, and Windsor J: Selective impairment of phonation: a case study, Brain Lang 35:313, 1988.

McNeil MR, Prescott, TE, and Lemme ML: An application of electromyographic feedback to aphasia/apraxia treatment. In Brookshire RH, editor: Clinical aphasiology conference proceedings, Minneapolis, 1976, BRK Publishers.

Rabidoux PC, Florance CL, and McCauslin LS: The use of the handivoice in the treatment of a severely apractic patient. In Brookshire R, editor: Clinical aphasiology conference proceedings, Minneapolis, 1980, BRK Publishers.

Rau MT and Golper LAC: Cueing strategies. In Square-Storer P, editor: Acquired apraxia of speech in aphasic adults, Philadelphia, 1989, Taylor and Francis.

Rosenbek JC: Treatment for apraxia of speech in adults. In Perkins WH, editor: Dysarthria and apraxia, New York, 1983, Thieme-Stratton.

Rosenbek JC: Advances in the evaluation and treatment of speech apraxia. In Rose FC, editor: Advances in neurology, vol 42, Progress in aphasiology, New York, 1984, Raven Press.

Rosenbek JC: Treating apraxia of speech. In Johns DF, editor: Clinical management of neurogenic communicative disorders, Boston, 1985, Little, Brown and Co.

Rosenbek JC and others: A treatment for apraxia of speech in adults, J Speech Hear Disord 38:462, 1973.

Rubow RT and others: Vibrotactile stimulation for intersystemic reorganization in the treatment of apraxia of speech, Arch Phys Med Rehabil 63:150, 1982.

Sabe L, Leiguarda R, and Starkstein S: An open-label trial of bromocriptine in nonfluent aphasia, Neurology 42:1637, 1992.

Shane H and Darley FL: The effect of auditory rhythmic stimulation on articulatory accuracy in apraxia of speech, Cortex 14:444, 1978.

Simmons NN: Finger counting as an intersystemic reorganizer in apraxia of speech. In Brookshire RH, editor: Clinical aphasiology conference proceedings, Minneapolis, 1978, BRK Publishers.

Simpson MB and Clark AR: Clinical management of apractic mutism. In Square-Storer P: Acquired apraxia of speech in aphasic adults, London, 1989, Taylor and Francis.

Skelly M and others: American Indian sign (Amerind) as a facilitation of verbalization for the oral verbal apraxia. J Speech Hear Disord 39:445, 1974.

Southwood H: The use of prolonged speech in the treatment of apraxia of speech. In Brookshire R, editor: Clinical aphasiology, Minneapolis, 1987, BRK Publishers.

Sparks RW and Deck JW: Melodic intonation therapy. In Chapey R, editor: Language intervention strategies in adult aphasia, ed 2, Baltimore, 1986, Williams and Wilkins.

Sparks RW and Deck JW: Melodic intonation therapy. In Chapey R, editor: Language intervention strategies in adult aphasia, ed 3, Baltimore 1994, Williams and Wilkins.

Sparks RW, Helm N, and Albert M: Aphasia rehabilitation resulting from melodic intonation therapy, Cortex 10:303, 1974.

Sparks RW and Holland A: Method: melodic intonation therapy, J Speech Hear Disord 41:287, 1976.

Square P, Chumpelik (Hayden) D, and Adams S: Efficacy of the PROMPT system of therapy for the treatment of acquired apraxia of speech. In Brookshire R, editor: Clinical aphasiology conference proceedings, Minneapolis, 1985, BRK Publishers.

Square P and others: Efficacy of the PROMPT system of therapy for the treatment for the apraxia of speech: a follow-up investigation. In Brookshire R, editor: Clinical aphasiology conference proceedings, Minneapolis, 1986, BRK Publishers.

Square PA and Martin RE: The nature and treatment of neuromotor speech disorders in aphasia. In Chapey R, editor: Language intervention strategies in adult aphasia, Baltimore, 1994, Williams and Wilkins.

Square-Storer PA: Traditional therapies for apraxia of speech—reviewed and rationalized. In Square-Storer P, editor: Acquired apraxia of speech in aphasic adults, London, 1989, Lawrence Erlbaum.

Square-Storer PA and Hayden (Chumpelik) D: PROMPT treatment. In Square-Storer P, editor: Acquired apraxia of speech in aphasic adults, London 1989, Lawrence Erlbaum.

Stevens ER: Multiple input phoneme therapy. In Square-Storer P, editor: Acquired apraxia of speech in aphasic adults, Philadelphia, 1989, Taylor and Francis.

Stevens E and Glaser L: Multiple input phoneme therapy in the treatment of severe expressive aphasia. In Brookshire RH, editor: Clinical aphasiology conference proceedings, Minneapolis, 1983, BRK Publishers.

Swinnen S, Walter CB, and Shapiro DC: The coordination of limb movements with different kinematic patterns, Brain Cogn 8:326, 1988.

Tonkovich JC and Peach RK: What to treat: apraxia of speech, aphasia, or both. In Square-Storer P, editor: Acquired apraxia of speech in aphasic adults: theoretical and clinical issues, London, 1989, Lawrence Erlbaum.

Warren RL: Rehearsal for naming in apraxia of speech. In Brookshire RH, editor: Clinical aphasiology conference proceedings, Minneapolis, 1977, BRK Publishers.

Wertz RT: Response to treatment in patients with apraxia of speech. In Rosenbek J, McNeil M, and Aronson A, editors: Apraxia of speech: physiology, acoustics, linguistics, management, San Diego, 1984, College-Hill Press.

Wertz RT, LaPointe LL, and Rosenbek JC: Apraxia of speech in adults: the disorder and its management, New York, 1984, Grune and Stratton.

19 Managing Other Neurogenic Speech Disturbances

Neurogenic speech disturbances that are not traditionally categorized under the headings of dysarthria or apraxia of speech (AOS) may or may not be legitimate targets of rehabilitation efforts. When they are a reflection of, or are embedded within, a larger constellation of affective, cognitive, or linguistic deficits, their direct treatment may be inappropriate or unnecessary. When they are the only or primary impairment, or when they represent a major source of disability, their direct treatment may be appropriate and necessary.

Management of the "other neurogenic speech disturbances" that were discussed in Chapter 13 is the subject of this chapter. The emphasis will be on *speech production deficits* and not the affective, cognitive, or linguistic disturbances that may underlie the speech characteristics of these problems. To do otherwise would go considerably beyond the scope of this book. Thus, for example, the management of word retrieval and phonologic errors in people with aphasia will not be discussed because such behaviors reflect problems with language and not speech production per se.

It is important to recognize that very little is known about the behavioral management of these speech disturbances. Our lack of knowledge extends beyond a paucity of efficacy data and includes a relative lack of anecdotal suggestions about management for many of these problems. This probably partly reflects the low incidence of some of these problems (for example, isolated neurogenic stuttering or pseudoforeign accent). For others, it reflects the fact that remediation efforts are usually directed at deficits underlying the speech problem rather than the speech symptom itself (for example, for the language problems of aphasia, the cognitive or affective

deficits that may underlie attenuated speech or hypophonia, and echolalia).

NEUROGENIC STUTTERING

As noted in Chapter 13, neurogenic stuttering (NS) is a heterogeneous disorder that may exist as a separate entity or be embedded within the constellation of symptoms that represent dysarthria, AOS, or aphasia. When the dysfluencies are manifestations of a dysarthria or AOS, and when their prominence is not disproportionate to other manifestations of those motor speech disorders, the management of the speech disorder will probably be consistent with the principles and techniques generally used to treat dysarthrias and AOS; they have already been discussed in Chapters 16 through 18 and will not be repeated here. When dysfluencies are prominent, predominant, and disabling, they may require attention and may benefit from some of the strategies that seem to be effective in managing NS.

Neurogenic stuttering may be mild and transient, and resolve spontaneously following stroke in many patients (Helm-Estabrooks, 1986; Peach, 1984; Rosenbek, 1984; Rosenbek and others, 1978). This course implies that supportive reassurance that fluency will improve spontaneously may be the most appropriate management strategy early postonset and that such reassurance may reduce anxiety that could inhibit improvement. The problem, of course, is uncertainty about the prognosis in specific cases. It seems reasonable to introduce direct treatment if the problem persists for more than a few days to a week postonset, especially if the NS is the only or the most disabling communication problem.

The strategies for managing NS center around medical intervention and behavioral treatment. Behavioral treatment includes rate reduction-strategies, self-monitoring, and other techniques, many of which are used in the treatment of developmental stuttering.

Medical management

As noted in Chapter 13, the onset of NS has been associated with the use of prescribed and illicit drugs. Remission of NS has also occurred with drug withdrawal or a change in drug regimens. For example, Baratz and Mesulam (1981) reported a reduction in stuttering in a woman with a seizure disorder from posttraumatic bilateral brain injury when phenytoin (Dilantin) and phenobarbital were instituted; the seizures and stuttering returned but diminished again when the regimen was changed to Dilantin and carbamazepine (Tegretol). Mc-Clean and McLean (1985) reported a case in which stuttering began after Dilantin was introduced to control posttraumatic seizures. Dysfluencies decreased after discontinuing Dilantin and substituting Tegretol. The authors were careful to note that they did not have experimental control over the drugs, so conclusions about their true treatment effect must be considered tentative. Finally, Rentschler, Driver, and Callaway (1984) discussed a patient whose stuttering began following an overdose of clorazepate (Tranxene) and, possibly, chlordiazepoxide (Librium) but who had periods of greatly improved fluency that were usually related to alcohol and marijuana use. There was probably a very strong psychiatric contribution to the stuttering and its fluctuations in this case, however, making the effects of the drugs and the psychological factors impossible to sort out.

These limited observations suggest that drugs may play a role in causing or reducing NS symptoms. It seems reasonable to address their possible causal role in people who develop NS and to address the possibility of modifying drug regimens to control or reduce dysfluencies in some patients. In most cases such issues should be addressed and any changes in drug regimen stabilized before introducing behavioral treatment.

Donnan (1979) reported a case whose stuttering and right-sided motor and sensory problems developed in association with vascular problems and then remitted following a left carotid endarterectomy; fluency was maintained at two months postonset. Rosenbek (1984) concluded that such neurosurgery may have palliative effects on NS by improving cerebral blood flow (perhaps restoring equilibrium to the motor system). This suggests that behavioral management for NS should be deferred when neurosurgery is pending.

Behavioral management

Canter (1971) suggested that treatment of NS tends to be successful. Rosenbek (1984) was not similarly confident. Market and others (1990), in their survey study of clinicians who had encountered acquired stuttering that was not considered part of aphasia or a motor speech disorder, reported that treatment outcome was rated favorably for 82% of treated cases. (Note, however, that these anecdotal reports are uncontrolled for the effects of spontaneous recovery and other influences on outcome.)

In general, behavioral treatment strategies focus on rate reduction, self-monitoring, and other techniques that are frequently associated with the management of developmental stuttering.

Rate reduction strategies. Techniques designed to decrease rate seem common to nearly all reports of successful management of NS. Market and others (1990) reported that 78% of surveyed clinicians used slow rate as a treatment technique. The techniques seem no different than those already described for management of motor speech disorders.

Rosenbek and others (1978) reported that one of their seven cases with NS was treated.* He had otherwise normal speech and language, and treatment began one day after a right hemisphere stroke. The program was one of syllable-timed speech that slowed rate to 50 words per minute. Four days and six treatment sessions later, he was fluent; he remained so at one month post onset. Obviously, this patient's gains cannot be attributed to the treatment, as spontaneous recovery may have led to the same outcome.

Helm-Estabrooks (1986) notes that many people with NS have difficulty maintaining slow rate without a pacing device, and she suggests that tactile pacing, such as a pacing board (or finger counting, tapping, or the like), may be most effective.† Delayed auditory feedback (DAF) also may be helpful, especially when dysfluencies are associated with the accelerated or rapid rate of hypokinetic dysarthria (Downie, Low, and Lind-

---

*They also noted that one patient's dysfluencies improved after two weeks of treatment for dysarthria and that two patients who received treatment for speech and language problems other than their NS did not improve their NS.
†Helm and Butler (1977) reported a case whose severe NS as a result of multiple strokes did not respond to a pacing board approach but did improve with transcutaneous nerve stimulation applied to the left hand during speech.

say, 1981), but it may be counterproductive or disruptive for patients with AOS or aphasia. It is likely that many of the other rate-reduction strategies discussed in Chapter 17 are applicable to the behavioral management of NS.

Self-monitoring. Whitney and Goldstein (1989) reported a dramatic decrease in dysfluencies in three patients with mild aphasia who were trained to self-monitor their dysfluencies. Dysfluencies included audible pauses ("uh," "well"), word or phrase break-offs or revisions ("Water is bein' thrown/comin' off"), and part-word ("Di-dishes"), word, or phrase repetitions. Their approach may be applicable to patients whose NS or dysfluencies are strongly tied to aphasic verbal language deficits, and it is possible that they can be applied to other types of NS as well.

The training used by Whitney and Goldstein can be summarized as follows: (1) the clinician read a baseline transcription of the patient's dysfluencies to the patient, identifying each dysfluency (target behavior); (2) the patient listened and identified each target behavior, with feedback from the clinician about accuracy; (3) the patient self-monitored dysfluencies (by pressing a counter) during picture description tasks, with similar feedback from the clinician; (4) the patient self-monitored independently without clinician feedback. Using a well-controlled, multiple-baseline, single-subject experimental design, the authors documented dramatic decreases in dysfluencies, with generalization to nontreatment tasks. Of interest, the actual accuracy of self-monitoring was low during treatment, so accurate monitoring did not seem crucial to the program's success. Although rate was slowed by the technique, communication was more efficient and was rated positively by patients and unfamiliar listeners because utterances were not interrupted by dysfluencies. The authors concluded that self-monitoring seemed to provide a "delay strategy," presumably for word retrieval efforts, even though delay was not actively taught. They also noted that one patient had AOS that may have explained some of his dysfluencies and that the delay strategy may have aided speech programming. The simplicity, efficiency, and effectiveness of this approach make it a viable way to manage the dysfluencies of mildly aphasic people and perhaps apraxic patients, and it probably justifies examining its effectiveness for other types of NS as well.

Other approaches. "Traditional" approaches for managing developmental stuttering have been applied to NS, with anecdotal reports of success (Market and others, 1990). Meyers, Hall, and Aram (1990), in treating a 7-year-old whose dysfluencies emerged during recovery from aphasia secondary to a left hemisphere stroke, focused on easy-onset phonation and desensitization to decrease anxiety associated with dysfluencies. Improvement occurred during four months of treatment, and residual dysfluencies were related to mild word-finding problems.

Observations that miming, singing, and reading may be associated with improved fluency (Fleet and Heilman, 1985) suggest that such tasks may be used to facilitate fluency in some patients. Rousey, Arjunan, and Rousey (1986) reported the success of an intensive one-week (eight hours per day) treatment program that included several traditional techniques for a patient whose stuttering was associated with a traumatic brain injury (TBI). (The description of this case raises the possibility that the stuttering was psychogenic, however.)

Finally, Helm-Estabrooks (1986) anecdotally reported the success of biofeedback and relaxation treatment for a patient with moderately severe NS associated with multiple strokes. Electrodes were placed over the masseter muscle, with subsequent visual and auditory feedback to reduce masseter muscle tension. A four-month, twice-weekly program of biofeedback, speech therapy, and home practice reduced the dysfluencies to a "mild" degree by the time of discharge.

PALILALIA

The word and phrase repetitions that characterize palilalia may not be a very prominent component of the constellation of problems that affect communication in some people with the disorder. For example, occasional word and phrase repetitions may be produced by patients with hypokinetic dysarthria, but their reduced loudness, accelerated rate, and imprecise articulation may be much more pervasive, obvious, disabling, and disruptive to intelligibility. In such patients, the dysarthria should be treated first, with a good possibility that palilalia will be decreased by the approaches used to manage the dysarthria. Similarly, when palilalia occurs in patients with significant cognitive impairments, deficits in attention, motivation, and memory may make it unlikely that efforts to reduce the palilalia will be successful.

When the palilalia is prominent, pervasive, and disabling and when the patient's cognitive abilities are sufficiently intact to allow cooperation and learning from treatment efforts, attempts to reduce the reiterative utterances are necessary and justified. Unfortunately, very little has been written about how to treat palilalia, and very little is known about the effectiveness of such treatment. In general, it is probably most appropriate to rely on principles and techniques that are appropriate for managing hypokinetic dysarthria and neurogenic stuttering, as well as careful analysis of conditions that increase or decrease the palilalia. With this in mind, the following principles and techniques may help in the management of palilalia:

1. If the patient has Parkinson's disease (PD) that is being managed with medication, determining if palilalia fluctuates over the medication's cycle is important. Institution of drug treatment may decrease palilalia and eliminate the need for behavioral management. If, as has been reported by Ackerman, Ziegler, and Oertel (1989), palilalia occurs during peak dose levels of antiparkinsonism medication and associated hyperkinesias, modification in medication may reduce the palilalia. Boller, Albert, and Denes (1975) noted that palilalia was "brought under some control" (p. 97) by chlorpromazine (Thorazine) in one patient with chorea and evidence of bilateral basal ganglia, cortical, and cerebellar lesions; the palilalia worsened when the medication was withheld.

2. Because palilalia and hypokinetic dysarthria frequently co-occur, approaches to managing hypokinetic dysarthria may reduce palilalia without attention to the palilalia per se or may be effective in directed efforts to decrease palilalia. Rate-reduction techniques seem particularly applicable (LaPointe, 1989). Helm's (1979) initial description of a pacing board for a patient with parkinsonism was designed primarily to modify palilalia; her description represents the only reported behavioral treatment for palilalia. Helm's patient had not been responsive to verbal instruction, hand tapping, or a metronome to reduce rate, but his use of the board resulted in a syllable-by-syllable pattern "with no palilalia" (p. 352) that he was able to use—with reminders—for conversations on the hospital ward. Hand or finger tapping, DAF, rhythmic cueing, and alphabet board supplementation, which slow rate and have some reported success for people with hypokinetic dysarthria, are other possible treatment techniques. Self-monitoring treatment, similar to that described by Whitney and Goldstein (1989) for dysfluencies associated with aphasia (previous section), may also be worthy of investigation.

3. Careful analysis of the speaking modes in which palilalia is most and least frequent may assist the ordering of treatment tasks. For example, reading and repetition tend to be associated with fewer reiterations than conversation, narratives, and elicited speech, suggesting that treatment efforts for patients with such profiles might profitably begin with repetition or reading and then progress to elicited or narrative speech tasks.

ECHOLALIA

The unsolicited repetition or partial repetition of others' utterances that characterize echolalia is typically normal motorically and usually associated with severe aphasia or generalized impairments of cognition and diffuse or multifocal cortical pathology. The associated language and other cognitive deficits represent the true barriers to the formulation and expression of speech. In a sense, echolalia in such patients represents a residual relatively *intact* ability, even though its expression in most circumstances is inappropriate. When behavioral management is appropriate for such patients and echolalia is pervasive, it may be necessary to inhibit or reduce the echolalia before the underlying language and other cognitive deficits can be addressed. However, methods for doing so have not been described, and the outcome of behavioral treatment for the communication impairments of patients with pervasive echolalia has not been reported.

COGNITIVE AND AFFECTIVE DISTURBANCES

The management of attenuations of speech that derive from cognitive and affective disturbances will not be addressed in detail here because the fundamental problem in such disturbances is not one of speech per se. Behavioral management of the underlying cognitive and affective deficits usually does not focus on the motor aspects of speech production. Improvement in the underlying cognitive and affective impairments is usually reflected in increased speed of verbal responding, increased loudness, and more normal voice quality and prosody.

In Chapter 13 the similarity between the hypophonia and reduced loudness associated with frontal lobe–limbic system pathology and the hypokinetic dysarthria due to basal ganglia pathology was discussed. This association raises the possibility that some of the vocal "exercise" programs described in Chapter 17 for managing hypokinetic dysarthria might benefit patients with hypophonia associated with abulia, perhaps as part of treatment efforts to increase their general levels of effort and drive. Although speculative, attempts to modify vocal production may also be justified on the basis of Sapir and Aronson's (1985) report of two patients with posttraumatic aphonia (with no vocal cord pathology or motor speech disorder) who regained normal phonation (but not normal prosody) after a session of symptomatic therapy using techniques applied to people with conversion aphonia. Sapir and Aronson suggested that the persisting aphonia may have been due to an emotional response to trauma or to "inertial aphonia" that persisted beyond the effects of the initial organic cause of the aphonia (vocal cord weakness or paralysis, effects of intubation, apraxia of phonation). At the least, their observations suggest that a trial of behavioral efforts to improve loudness and phonation may be justified in patients with frontal lobe pathology and hypophonia or aphonia, particularly when onset is acute and the degree of speech attenuation is disproportionate to other cognitive or affective deficits.

APHASIA

Aphasia can have prominent effects on spoken language, which are often manifested as deficits in grammar and syntax, delays, hesitancy, dysfluencies and errors associated with word retrieval problems, and phonologic errors. These difficulties affect the form, content, rate, prosody, and fluency of speech, but they result from the underlying language formulation deficits and not from abnormalities in motor speech programming or execution. Their management is directed at the inefficiencies in language and not the physical production of speech. When significant AOS accompanies aphasia—which it often does—management of the AOS may complicate the management of aphasia (and vice versa), take precedence over it, be conducted concurrently with it, or be deferred because of it. It is essential to recognize that the management of aphasia and AOS (and dysarthria) are quite different from each other and that treatment of one disorder cannot be expected to remediate deficits in the other.

The literature on the management of aphasia is extensive, considerably larger than that for motor speech disorders. Discussion of aphasia management is beyond the scope of this book, although management of dysfluencies associated with it was discussed under the heading of neurogenic stuttering. It is important to keep in mind that the management of aphasia and the disorder's effects on communication abilities can have substantial influence on the management of patients with motor speech disorders.*

PSEUDOFOREIGN ACCENT

The rare and unusual disorder of pseudoforeign accent associated with neurologic disease has been described in a limited number of case reports. No

published report has discussed its behavioral management. The disorder may resolve fairly rapidly in some patients (for example, two of the four cases reported by Berthier and others, 1991) and, therefore, may not require behavioral management. However, too little is known about the problem to predict who will and will not recover from it. It is also apparent that some people find the problem to be socially handicapping even when it does not affect speech intelligibility.

The frequent association of pseudoforeign accent with aphasia and AOS, the possibility that the perception of accent is conveyed by grammatic and syntactic deficits attributable to aphasia, and the articulatory and prosodic errors associated with a variant of AOS suggest that the "accent" may be managed at least partially during traditional treatment activities for aphasia and AOS. It may be quite appropriate to adapt principles and techniques for managing AOS (Chapter 18) to efforts to modify the voice, place and manner distortions, substitutions, and alophonic variations in consonant production that contribute to the perception of accent. Similarly, and perhaps more important, focus on vowel "errors" that convey accent may be necessary, extending in some cases to vowel articulation drill activities.

The crucial role of prosody in conveying accent suggests that treatment of pseudoforeign accent may require special attention to the techniques for improving prosody, stress, rhythm, and naturalness that were discussed for the management of dysarthria and AOS in Chapters 17 and 18, respectively. When such techniques are exhausted—or in conjunction with them—materials that are used for reducing foreign accent in neurologically normal nonnative English speakers may be useful.

APROSODIA

As discussed in Chapter 13, the aprosodia associated with right hemisphere damage (RHD) is not well understood, and its relationship to other perceptual and cognitive disturbances that may affect communication in people with right hemisphere lesions has not been clearly established. This lack of understanding, as well as uncertainty about the frequency of significant, lasting, and unique prosodic deficits in people with RHD, suggests that information about management of aprosodia is limited. Indeed, this is the case.

Robin, Klouda, and Hug (1991) state, "There are no reports of treatments for primary prosodic disturbances for focal cerebral lesions in general" (p. 253). Brookshire (1992) points out that the literature on treatment of any communication impairment associated with RHD is "primarily anecdote and opinion, without much empirical sup-

---

*Some valuable recent texts that address the manifestations and management of aphasia include Brookshire (1992); Chapey (1994); Davis (1993); and Rosenbek, LaPointe, and Wertz (1989).

port" (p. 196). Myers (1994), recognizing the existence of problems producing emotional prosody and linguistic stress in RHD patients, nonetheless states, "Treatment for prosodic deficits is not considered . . . to be a priority in patient management, since these deficits are probably the least of the patient's communication problems" (p. 529). She further suggests that uncertainty about the source of prosodic production deficits may make treatment of them nonproductive.

When an individual with RHD has significant deficits in prosodic production that are isolated or disproportionately severe in comparison to other communication deficits, when these deficits persist beyond the acute phase of the causative illness, and when the individual or significant others are aware of and concerned about the disorder, direct treatment of aprosodia should be considered. At the least, patients and their significant others may benefit from counseling about the nature of the problem (to the extent that the clinician understands it). For example, knowing that the lack of emotion conveyed by prosody does not reflect an absence of true emotional feeling, and that "tone of voice" cannot be relied upon to convey emotions, may help avoid many misinterpretations that may be made about a patient's affective state and may encourage the patient and others to rely more heavily on linguistic content rather than on intonation as an index of feelings. It may be useful to focus on strategies for verbal expression that explicitly identify emotional states; for example, "My arm is not getting any better" may sound like a simple statement of fact when in fact the patient's intent is to convey the feeling that "I'm upset and depressed that my arm is not getting any better." Similarly, family members may learn to ask, "How do you feel about that?" or "Does that make you happy or sad?" when a statement or topic is likely to be associated with strong emotions.

When direct modification of prosody seems appropriate, many of the techniques emphasizing prosody that are used for treating dysarthrias and apraxia of speech—discussed in Chapters 17 and 18—may be useful. Robin, Klouda, and Hug (1991), for example, emphasize the use of contrastive stress tasks using emotional (for example, happy versus sad) or linguistic stress as the basis for contrasts. They suggest that linguistic stress may be emphasized initially because it may be less impaired than emotional prosody. They also suggest that imitation of a clinician's model, in combination with instrumental feedback about pitch, duration, and loudness, may be useful in the early steps of a treatment program. Instrumental analysis may also help to determine if problems with pitch, loudness, or duration lie at the heart of the

disturbance and establish which of those parameters is most easily modified by the patient in a direction that facilitates prosodic accuracy.

SUMMARY

1. When neurogenic speech disturbances other than dysarthrias and apraxia of speech represent the only or primary impairment of communication, or when they represent a major source of disability, their treatment may be appropriate and necessary. However, very little is known about the treatment of such speech production deficits.

2. Because neurogenic stuttering may be associated with drug effects, particularly anticonvulsants and psychotropic drugs, modifications of drug regimens may be helpful in reducing dysfluencies. Behavioral treatment of neurogenic stuttering usually should be deferred until after any pending neurosurgery. The literature suggests that neurogenic dysfluencies may be modified by rate reduction strategies that are effective for modifying rate in people with dysarthria or apraxia of speech. Training in the self-monitoring of dysfluencies has been shown to reduce dysfluencies in some aphasic patients. Traditional approaches for managing developmental stuttering, as well as biofeedback and relaxation treatment, represent other possible treatment strategies for neurogenic stuttering.

3. Very little is known about the treatment of palilalia, but approaches that are appropriate for hypokinetic dysarthria and neurogenic stuttering may be applicable to its management in some cases. Palilalic patients with Parkinson's disease may improve with the institution of drug management.

4. Echolalia and other speech abnormalities associated with primary cognitive and affective disturbances are generally not approached by attempts to modify the motor aspects of speech production. Hypophonia associated wtih frontal lobe–limbic system pathology may, in some cases, benefit from vocal exercise to increase loudness, similar to that used for some patients with hypokinetic dysarthria. Behavioral efforts to improve loudness and phonation may be most appropriate when the degree of speech attenuation is disproportionate to other cognitive or affective deficits.

5. Deficits in verbal expression associated with aphasia reflect the underlying language disturbance and therefore are not appropriately managed by focusing on speech production per se. Dysfluencies associated with aphasia may require intervention.

6. Management of pseudoforeign accent is unexplored. Because of its association with aphasia and apraxia of speech, however, management of those disorders may improve the accent. Techniques for improving prosody, stress, rhythm, and naturalness that are appropriate for managing dysarthria and apraxia of speech may be of value, as may be some techniques used for reducing foreign accent in nonneurologically impaired speakers.

7. Very little is known about the management of aprosodia in patients with right hemisphere lesions. Counseling about the nature of the deficit may help patients and their significant others, as may some actively taught strategies for expressing or clarifying emotional feelings when they are inadequately conveyed by prosody. Techniques used in managing prosodic impairments in dysarthric and apraxic patients also may be of value. Managing aprosodia may be important for only a small percentage of patients with right hemisphere lesions because the problem may be transient or of less functional importance than other perceptual and cognitive deficits that affect communication.

REFERENCES

Ackerman H, Ziegler W, and Oertel W: Palilalia as a symptom of L-dopa induced hyperkinesia, J Neurol Neurosurg Psychiatry 52:805, 1989.

Baratz R and Mesulam M: Adult onset stuttering treated with anticonvulsants, Arch Neurol 38:132, 1981.

Berthier ML and others: Foreign accent syndrome: behavioral and anatomic findings in recovered and non-recovered patients, Aphasiology 5:129, 1991.

Boller F, Albert M, and Denes F: Palilalia, Br J Disord Commun 10:92, 1975.

Brookshire RH: An introduction to neurogenic communication disorders, ed 4, St Louis, 1992, Mosby–Year Book.

Canter G: Observations on neurogenic stuttering: a contribution to differential diagnosis, Br J Disord Commun 6:139, 1971.

Chapey R, editor: Language intervention strategies in adult aphasia, edition 3, Baltimore, 1994 Williams and Wilkins.

Davis GA: A survey of adult aphasia and related language disorders, edition 2, Englewood Cliffs, NJ, 1993, Prentice-Hall.

Donnan GA: Stuttering as a manifestation of stroke, Med J Aust 1:44, 1979.

Downie AW, Low JM, and Lindsay DD: Speech disorders in parkinsonism: use of delayed auditory feedback in selected cases, J Neurol Neurosurg Psychiatry 44:852, 1981.

Fleet WS and Heilman KM: Acquired stuttering from a right hemisphere lesion in a right-hander, Neurology 35:1343, 1985.

Helm NA: Management of palilalia with a pacing board, J Speech Hearing Disord 44:350, 1979.

Helm NA and Butler RB: Transcutaneous nerve stimualtion in acquired speech disorder, Lancet 3:1177, 1977.

Helm-Estabrooks N: Diagnosis and management of neurogenic stuttering in adults. In The atypical stutterer: principles and practices of rehabilitation, St Louis, 1986, Academic Press.

LaPointe LL: Progressive echolalia and echopraxic: what could it be? What could it be? In Helm-Estabrooks N and Aten JL, editors: Difficult diagnoses in adult communication disorders, Boston, 1989 College-Hill.

Market KE and others: Acquired stuttering: descriptive data and treatment outcome, J Fluency Disord 15:21, 1990.

McClean MD and McLean A: Case report of stuttering acquired in association with phenytoin use for post-head-injury seizures, J Fluency Disord 10:241, 1985.

Meyers SC, Hall NE, and Aram DM: Fluency and language recovery in a child with a left hemisphere lesion, J Fluency Disord 15:159, 1990.

Myers PS: Communication disorders associated with right hemisphere brain damage. In Chapey R, editor: Language intervention strategies in adult aphasia, ed 3, Baltimore, 1994, Williams and Wilkins.

Peach RK: Acquired neurogenic stuttering, Grand Rounds Communic Disord 9:177, 1984.

Rentschler GJ, Driver LE, and Callaway EA: The onset of stuttering following drug overdose, J Fluency Disord 9:265, 1984.

Robin DA, Klouda GV, and Hug LN: Neurogenic disorders of prosody. In Vogel D and Cannito MP, editors: Treating disordered speech motor control, Austin, TX, 1991, Pro-Ed.

Rosenbek JC: Stuttering secondary to nervous system damage. In Curlee RF and Perkins WH, editors: Nature and treatment of stuttering: new directions, San Diego, 1984, College-Hill.

Rosenbek JC, LaPointe LL, and Wertz RT: Aphasia: a clinical approach, Boston, 1989, College-Hill.

Rosenbek JC and others: Stuttering following brain damage, Brain Lang 6:82, 1978.

Rousey CG, Arjunan KN, and Rousey CL: Successful treatment of stuttering following closed head injury, J Fluency Disord 11:257, 1986.

Sapir S and Aronson AE: Aphonia after closed head injury: aetiologic considerations, Br J Disord Commun 20:289, 1985.

Whitney JL and Goldstein H: Using self-monitoring to reduce dysfluencies in speakers with mild aphasia, J Speech Hear Disord 54:576, 1989.

20 Managing Acquired Psychogenic Speech Disorders

Psychogenic speech disturbances can be disabling and handicapping because of the barriers they introduce to communicative interaction and because of the psychological difficulties they represent. Their diagnosis as psychogenic—discussed in Chapters 14 and 15—is essential to setting the direction of treatment and is usually derived from the medical and psychosocial history and from careful assessment of the speech disturbance itself.

People with changes in speech due to major depression, schizophrenia, and other serious psychiatric disturbances generally are not referred for speech evaluation or treatment. In such cases, speech abnormality is not usually a presenting complaint and is rarely a direct focus of treatment. In contrast, changes in speech that reflect a conversion disorder or response to life stresses may be a presenting complaint and the focus of concerted medical efforts at diagnosis and management. Gratifyingly, a significant proportion of people with these latter types of speech disturbances seem responsive to treatment provided by the speech pathologist. Such positive outcomes obviously benefit the affected person, and they can be very satisfying to the clinician who provides the treatment.

This chapter will emphasize general principles, guidelines, and techniques for managing psychogenic speech disorders. Many of them are derived from the literature on voice disorders because treatment of psychogenic voice disorders is more fully developed and refined than is treatment of other psychogenic speech disorders and because psychogenic voice disorders probably represent the largest subcategory of psychogenic speech disturbances seen in speech pathology practices.* Because there do not appear to be clear differences in the histories and psychosocial dynamics among people with different types of psychogenic speech disorders and because their various speech symptoms seem to respond equally well to very similar techniques, the general principles and techniques discussed in the next section will form the foun-

---

*For example, psychogenic voice disorders represented 80% of the psychogenic speech disorders in the Mayo Clinic cases reviewed in Chapter 14.

dation for treating all psychogenic speech disorders. Following discussion of them, management of several specific types of psychogenic speech disturbances will be addressed.

GENERAL PRINCIPLES AND GUIDELINES

The personality traits of individuals afflicted by psychogenic speech disorders, the life events that help to trigger and maintain the disorders, the specific characteristics of the abnormal speech, and the degree to which additional influential organic and psychological variables are at work are too heterogeneous to permit simple prescriptive treatment for these disorders. In this section, general principles and guidelines that seem important for management will be addressed. They help to set the clinician's attitude about management, and they highlight the major issues that must be addressed in decision-making and management activities.

Many people with psychogenic speech disorders can be managed effectively by the speech pathologist

There is an odd and persistent belief among some clinicians that psychogenic speech disorders are not within their scope of practice or, if they are, that the clinician's role is to treat the symptoms while avoiding the psychosocial history and its relationship to the speech disorder. The psychosocial issues and perhaps even symptom management are seen as the responsibility of the psychiatrist or psychologist because they are, after all, experts in problems of "the mind." This belief is analogous to arguing that motor speech disorders should not be managed by the speech pathologist because the neurologist is the expert in problems of "the brain." These arguments ignore the expertise of speech clinicians in the diagnosis and management of neurogenic and psychogenic speech disorders and their ability to determine when consultation from other medical subspecialties should be pursued—along with, or instead of, speech therapy—for optimal patient care.

One source of concern about managing the symptoms of a psychogenic speech disorder—especially conversion disorder—without psychiatric treatment is that the underlying psychological disorder will simply generate a different symptom if the speech symptom is removed. Few psychiatrists today subscribe to this view, and there are many reported cases in which speech symptom resolution is not associated with adverse effects or the subsequent appearance of different conversion symptoms (Aronson, 1990a; Roth, Aronson, and Davis, 1989). Aronson also suggests that premature referral to psychiatry may guarantee failure to improve speech because the speech symptom is often dissociated from awareness on the part of the patient of any emotional problem; thus referral may be rejected by the patient. In addition, symptom removal often requires explicit attention to modifying symptoms, something most psychiatrists are not trained to do. Patients are more likely to be receptive to psychiatric referral after speech has improved because the etiology has then been established as nonorganic and hopefully the possible links between the speech problem and psychological issues have been discussed.

Psychiatric referral is neither invariably necessary nor appropriate following successful speech treatment. Psychogenic speech disorders can occur as a way of handling acute emotional distress or stress in people who are otherwise psychologically healthy. In some cases, the experienced speech clinician and the patient may conclude that further intervention is unnecessary.* This receives some support from psychiatrists who note that psychoanalysis is not appropriate for the majority of patients with conversion disorders (Nemiah, 1988; Tomb, 1981) and that treatment and remission of conversion symptoms can occur in a variety of ways, including through behavioral management and "brief supportive therapy" (Ford and Folks, 1985; Stoudemire, 1988).† Therefore, the speech pathologist has an important diagnostic and management role to play, and in many cases the role is a central one.

Prognosis for recovery usually is good

The prospects for recovery from psychogenic speech disorders, especially with treatment, appear to be good, even when neurologic disease is present. In general, for example, patients with conversion disorders tend to improve over the course of weeks or months, and spontaneous remission may be the rule rather than the exception (Stoudemire, 1988; Tomb, 1981). The prognosis for recovery from a conversion disorder is felt to be especially good when it is of recent onset, when there is an identifiable precipitating stressful event, when premorbid health is good, and when there is an absence of serious psychopathology. Prognosis becomes complicated when these conditions are

---

*For example, Aronson, Peterson, and Litin (1966) reported than none of 27 patients they studied with conversion aphonia or dysphonia had serious psychopathology warranting immediate psychiatric help.

†Baker and Silver (1987) found that patients with "hysterical paraplegia," originally thought to have paraplegia from physical trauma, responded rapidly to treatment. The most successful management was "a firm diagnosis, a confident prediction of improvement and sympathy, interest and common sense" (p. 381).

not met, especially when severe psychopathology is present (Ford and Folks, 1985; Lazare, 1981; Stoudemire, 1988; Teitelbaum and McHugh, 1990).

Conversion aphonias and dysphonias may normalize in minutes or over several therapy sessions in many patients (Aronson, 1990a; Boone, 1977; Stemple, 1993). Recovery may be more of a problem for patients in whom increased musculoskeletal tension represents their lifelong pattern of responding to stress; although normal voice may be readily achieved in symptomatic therapy, the gain may be short-lived unless the habitual pattern of responding to stress can be changed. The same may be true for patients with conversion disorder, if the underlying cause is still active and the patient remains unwilling or unable to acknowledge or deal with it more directly; in such cases, psychotherapy or time may be necessary instead of, or prior to, symptomatic speech therapy. Case (1991) also suggests that people with psychogenic voice problems that are situation-specific (for example, only at work) are unlikely to respond to symptomatic treatment and may be in need of psychotherapy. Sapir and Aronson (1990) summarize prognostic expectations by stating that "in our experience, prognosis for improvement with speech therapy is excellent for conversion disorders, good for anxiety-induced speech disorders, and guarded for depression-related speech disorders" (p. 506).

A good prognosis is not precluded by the presence of neurologic disease. For example, rapid improvement of acquired psychogenic stuttering and aphonias and dysphonias has been reported in people with a variety of neurologic diseases, some with co-occurring neurogenic speech or language disorders (Brookshire, 1989; Baumgartner and Duffy, 1986; Sapir and Aronson, 1985 & 1987; Tippett and Siebens, 1991).*

To summarize, based on general impressions about recovery from conversion disorders and frequent reports of effective treatment of psychogenic speech disorders, the prognosis for recovery from them generally can be considered

good. Clinicians are thus justified in bringing a positive, optimistic attitude to their management of people with psychogenic speech disorders.

Symptoms and explanations must be addressed

Effective management requires that the clinician be prepared to address the patient's symptoms as well as the psychological explanations for them, although neither is always necessary or possible. For example, speech may normalize in some patients as they reveal their psychosocial history and "discover" the psychological trigger for their symptoms; others respond to symptomatic treatment without ever identifying plausible explanatory factors. However, these two components of management must be kept in mind by the clinician during diagnosis and any subsequent treatment sessions.

Underlying explanations for the speech disorder may be addressed at various levels. The most basic is during the psychosocial history, in which potential causal mechanisms may be brought to light. This can be accomplished by reviewing the events surrounding the onset of the speech disorder from both physical and psychological perspectives. Patients' answers will help set the sequence of subsequent events, for example, whether to move quickly to symptomatic management or to delve immediately and more deeply into psychosocial issues.

After symptomatic treatment—especially if it is successful—the relationship between the speech symptoms and their emotional causes should be addressed. Techniques for doing this will be discussed in the next section. What is essential to remember, however, is that the psychosocial history and its relationship to the speech problem are crucial for both diagnosis and treatment (Aronson, 1990b).

The patient's belief that the problem is organic must be addressed

People with psychogenic speech disorders usually believe their problem has an organic basis. This belief may stem from the inaccessibility of the psychological dynamics that have produced the speech problem, and it is often reinforced by multiple medical tests—and sometimes treatments—that are undertaken to investigate possible neurologic and other organic causes. Rather than dispelling fears of organic disease, negative medical evaluations sometimes generate uncertainty and increase anxiety about the possible seriousness of the condition; this may be particularly true for patients who are afraid of having a disease that has affected a family member or others close to them.

---

*It should be noted that the literature may lead to an overestimate of the "true" proportion of cases that recover from psychogenic speech disorders in response to speech therapy; that is, it is much more likely that positive rather than negative treatment results will be reported, especially for conditions in which the best external criterion for establishing the accuracy of diagnosis is a rapid positive response to symptomatic treatment. Put another way, patients who do not respond to symptomatic treatment may not be reported as treatment failures because the lack of positive response may produce doubt about whether the disorder is psychogenic in the first place, especially when neurologic disease is present.

Unfortunately, acceptance of the nonorganic basis for their symptoms is rarely dispelled by professionals who dismiss them by saying "the problem is all in your head" without having explored the psychosocial history and without further explanation. This kind of confrontation rarely works and often promotes an adversarial relationship or patient withdrawal (Lazare, 1981; Stoudemire, 1988; Tomb, 1981).

Even when a specific cause cannot be found, the nonorganic basis for the speech problem should be addressed. The degree to which this is done directly or indirectly will vary as a function of the evidence for a specific causal mechanism, the patient's willingness to discuss psychological issues, and the clinician's degree of certainty about the psychogenic etiology. In some cases, discussion of this issue takes place before any attempt at symptomatic therapy. In others, discussion is deferred until after speech has improved. Often, the idea of nonorganic causes is introduced briefly before symptoms are managed and then in more detail after improvement has occurred. The gradual unfolding of these issues is nearly always more effective than telling the patient abruptly that their problem has no organic basis.

The process of developing acceptance of the problem as nonorganic is not synonymous with identifying it as psychogenic and discovering its exact psychodynamics. This may happen in some cases, but a primary goal of this principle is to have the patient accept that there are no organic barriers that preclude the possibility of speech improvement and maintenance of improvement once it has occurred. For many patients, the triggering events are no longer active and may have been forgotten or be inaccessible to them; these patients are particularly "ready" to improve. Many readily accept an explanation that the cause is not clear but that there are no "active" organic explanations for the problem. This may be particularly effective for patients whose speech problems developed at the time of a physical injury or organic illness that subsequently resolved. By accepting that organic barriers to normal speech are not currently present, the way is paved for symptomatic therapy, improvement, and maintenance of normal speech.

Treatment should be attempted within the diagnostic session

When the clinician is reasonably certain that the etiology is psychogenic and that the speech disorder should be treated symptomatically, treatment should be attempted immediately. This is important because the majority of people can be helped

considerably or completely within the diagnostic session or within one or two subsequent therapy sessions (Aronson, 1990a; Boone, 1977; Stemple, 1993). This aggressive approach can accomplish several things: if treatment results in significant improvement, the diagnosis of the disorder as psychogenic will be confirmed; the confirmed diagnosis may alter or modify previously planned medical and psychiatric evaluations; the patient is likely to accept that the problem is not organic and may be receptive to addressing the psychological causes for the disorder; many patients will be very pleased (although often perplexed) at the rapid return of their speech and be in a position to resume their life in a more normal way, especially if the underlying psychological causes are no longer active; and patient and medical resources, costs, and energy will be saved.

Clinician attitude and manner of relating to the patient are crucial

In 1922 Henry Head said, "No one is a greater failure than the medical officer who wishes all hysterics could be shot at dawn. On the other hand, the firm diplomatist with subtle and demonstrable reasons why the patient can stand, walk, or feel, often produces miraculous cures" (p. 829). This reference to the attitude of physicians toward people with conversion disorders, if not literally true, captures what people with physical manifestations of psychological problems feel from people who dismiss them as having "nothing wrong" or a problem that is "all in your head." Such pronouncements, especially when made in the absence of any exploration of the psychosocial history or when unaccompanied by any supportive recommendations, are rarely accepted by the patient and usually do not put an end to their search for organic explanations. At best, such attitudes reflect ignorance, discomfort, or impatience in dealing with psychological issues or a belief that problems that are psychological in origin are not "legitimate" medical problems. They may also reflect insensitivity or a lack of respect for the effects that stress, anxiety, and conflict can exert on people's lives. The basic attitude with which to approach people with physical deficits caused by psychogenic disturbances should be that their problem is "real and no less genuine an illness than any other, despite the absence of organic pathology" (Teitelbaum and McHugh, 1990, p. 418).

Clinician attitude is crucial to evaluation and management, and the attitude should be clear to the patient. There can be no prescription for the style in which these attitudes are expressed, for style is a highly personal trait, but it is important that the following attitudes and beliefs be conveyed.

1. *Respect* for patients' concern about the possible organic cause for their problem and recognition of the legitimacy of their symptoms and the frustrations and limitations imposed by them. For example, much can be done to develop a therapeutic alliance with a patient by responding to "all the doctors say there's nothing wrong with me" with "that seems a foolish thing to say. You can't talk normally—of course, there's something wrong!"

2. *Reassurance and optimism* about the negative findings of medical workups. Reviewing with seriousness and confidence the results of general and subspecialty medical workups and concluding that an absence of an organic explanation is encouraging rather than worrisome can set the stage for effective symptomatic treatment and discussion of possible psychological explanations.

3. *Support and approval* for the patient's desire and ability to improve. Some patients are indifferent to an invitation to work to improve their speech or make excuses about why they are unable to do so; they usually do not respond to symptomatic treatment or discussion of psychological issues. Many others state that they want to improve and are willing to work to do it when asked directly if that is their desire. An explicit invitation to work hard to improve speech places responsibility with the patient to play an active role in therapy, puts them in a position to take credit for their improvement, and begins to establish their capacity to do well in the future, independent of reliance on formal symptomatic therapy.

4. *Empathy and compassion* for the ordinary or extraordinary psychological burdens the patient is willing to reveal and discuss. Assuming the patient is "ready" to improve, the manner in which psychological issues are discussed is crucial. It has much to do with kindness, an attitude that respects the reality and seriousness of the problem in spite of the lack of organic explanation, and one that involves as much as possible the patient's participation in the process of exploration of underlying psychological issues.

5. *Assertiveness and confidence* that symptomatic therapy can be effective. The literature indicates that "suggestion" is a common denominator in successful treatment of conversion disorders (Baker and Silver, 1987; Stoudemire, 1988; Teitelbaum and McHugh, 1990), mean-

ing that it is important to convey a belief that the symptoms will remit; it is also reasonable to suggest that speech problems often improve *rapidly* with some hard work. Because symptomatic therapy involves trial-and-error techniques, it must be conducted with an air of confidence that each technique has the capacity to be effective. As treatment progresses, it is also important that the clinician immediately acknowledges changes in speech and enlists the patient's recognition of the same.

6. *Honesty.* The patient should be told directly when the clinician does not understand completely the reasons for the speech problem or why it has or has not improved, but the uncertainty should be conveyed with confidence. This can be done with prefaces like "We don't always understand how these things develop" or "I don't know for certain why or how this problem developed, but it does seem that there's no physical barrier present that is in the way of your speech improving." Often, after symptomatic therapy has resulted in a return to normal speech, a patient asks what caused the problem or why it improved so rapidly; this then allows the clinician to say, "I'm not sure; let's explore that." This represents an ideal opportunity to discuss psychosocial issues.

7. *Pleasure and respect* for the patient's efforts and progress during symptomatic therapy and, when appropriate, their courage in confronting the psychological issues that are tied to their symptoms. This opens the door to discussing the future.

The future must be discussed

When symptomatic therapy results in a return of normal speech, discussing the future is still important. If the emotional issues that triggered the speech disturbance are no longer active or are resolving, discussion of the relationship between them and the speech disorder may establish that psychiatric referral or further symptomatic treatment is unnecessary. As Aronson (1990a) points out, the experienced clinician usually develops a sense about whether psychiatric referral is necessary. It is essential to involve the patient in this decision and also to review other ways available to them for dealing with similar psychological burdens in the future. Reassurance that the speech problem may never recur can usually be given, but the patient should be urged to contact the clinician if the problem returns.

Whether or not speech has improved, if major ongoing psychological issues are present, discussion about the need for psychiatric or psychological referral should be pursued. Patients who have revealed the presence of such issues and have confronted their impact and importance are usually willing to accept such referral. Those who deny the presence of these factors or their relevance to their current physical symptoms often resist such recommendations.

When symptomatic therapy succeeds, the patient must usually leave with an explanation for it

Tied to discussion of the future is the need of most patients for an explanation for their recovery, if not an explanation for the cause of the problem. Explanations vary greatly. They depend on the degree to which causal mechanisms have been discovered, the patient has insight into them, their social and cultural beliefs and customs, and so on. It is nearly always important to explore with patients what their significant others, colleagues at work, and other people have thought about the problem and what they are likely to think about its resolution. Patients frequently ask how they can explain their improvement to others, partly as a way of admitting they do not understand it well themselves, but also as a way of saying they need a strategy for "saving face."

Unfortunately, there is a fairly pervasive attitude in our society that psychological difficulties, particularly those that produce unusual physical symptoms (for example, aphonia or stuttering-like behavior), are a sign of weakness or intrinsic instability. These attitudes may be exacerbated when symptoms resolve rapidly. As a result, saving face is important to patients' future ability to cope in their social environment and, perhaps, to their ability to maintain their gains. Without an adequate explanation, the patient may be unable or unwilling to maintain normal speech because of the possible psychosocial penalties for doing so. It is therefore important to work with patients to develop plausible explanations that they understand and that will be acceptable to those they know who will desire or demand an explanation. There is no formula for such explanations, but they should be structured to support the legitimacy of the symptoms, the inability of the patient to improve in the past, and the patient's active participation in resolving the speech problem.

Not everyone wishes to be helped, is ready to be helped, or can be helped

Contraindications to pursuing symptomatic therapy are relatively uncommon among patients referred for speech evaluation in rehabilitation and multidisciplinary medical practices. There are,

however, some circumstances in which symptomatic therapy should not be pursued or is unlikely to be successful.

Some patients who are referred for evaluation do not come with a desire to be helped. Some assertively or angrily state that they think such assessment is nonsensical because the problem is certainly due to some threatening organic disease. They may reject any attempt to address their psychosocial history and any effort to modify their speech symptoms, even when approached empathetically and with confidence that symptomatic therapy may help them. These patients generally are not candidates for symptomatic therapy. If the experienced clinician is certain of this, symptomatic efforts should be aborted early. The best that can be done is to document the reasons for concluding that the speech disorder is nonorganic.

Some patients initially do not resist examination but may become threatened by inquiries about psychological issues or the prospect that symptomatic therapy might resolve the speech symptom. They may give numerous excuses for not participating in treatment, such as lack of time or other pending medical tests, or they may display severe pain in response to touch or manipulation of speech structures by the clinician. They may become hostile or angry at attempts to discuss emotional issues or work on speech symptoms. Many of these patients are not ready to be helped by symptomatic therapy.

Some patients have psychogenic speech disturbances that are present transiently and unpredictably or are situation-specific (for example, present only during or after an encounter with an estranged spouse). Symptomatic therapy is unlikely to be successful with such patients and may be impossible if speech is normal during speech evaluation. Assessment during an episode of speech difficulty may be of value to establish the nonorganic nature of the problem and to see if speech improvement can be achieved with symptomatic therapy, but the gains are unlikely to be lasting if psychological issues are not dealt with. Case (1991) suggests that these patients should be referred for psychiatric assessment.

Sometimes a patient is oblivious to or denies the presence of speech abnormality, in spite of floridly abnormal speech. Others may reveal ongoing events or residual effects of prior psychologically traumatic events that are so profoundly disturbing that symptomatic therapy would be inconsequential or even risky if it provided a mechanism for further repressing or denying the trauma. Symptomatic therapy in these cases should be deferred until psychiatric evaluation has established that it is appropriate or necessary.

GENERAL TREATMENT TECHNIQUES

A number of treatment techniques were implied in the preceding discussion. They, as well as some additional techniques, will be discussed here to provide a sense of how to approach management. Treatment within the diagnostic session will be emphasized, but the techniques discussed here can be applied over a number of sessions.

The emphasis on single-session treatment is not intended to imply that psychogenic speech disorders are always effectively treated in one or a few sessions, or that people with such disorders might not require a more extended period of time to achieve a return to normal speech. It is not entirely clear why some patients respond very rapidly to symptomatic therapy and others require treatment and recovery over time, although it seems that gradual improvement is more often the course for people with more serious psychiatric difficulties, some requiring inpatient psychiatric care. For others, the need to save face may require that they recover in a manner that more closely resembles recovery from organic disease.

The sequence of assessment and management

Speech evaluation and subsequent management are *best conducted following all medical evaluations that are directly relevant to establishing the nature of the speech disorder.* For most patients, this means that *speech assessment should follow Ear, Nose, and Throat or neurologic examinations, or both.* Preceding medical examinations allow the clinician to review those findings, reassure the patient that there is no apparent organic explanation for the speech problem, and introduce the notion that there are no physical barriers to improving speech.

It is often effective to ask patients to review what they have been told by examining physicians because the clinician can then reinterpret or reinforce the patient's understanding of the meaning of such findings. For example, in response to the patient's "They said that everything looks normal," the clinician may respond, "That's good news, isn't it!" In response to "Just like everyone else, they can't find the reason for this; one doctor told me there's absolutely nothing wrong with me," the clinician might respond, "Well, there's obviously something wrong because you're not talking very well, but the fact that there's nothing physically threatening going on is encouraging, isn't it?"

Patients for whom medical examinations have not yet been conducted are more likely to maintain a belief that their problem is organic and thus be less willing to accept the clinician's conclusion that it probably is not. In fact, the clinician may require such information to be confident that the problem is nonorganic. The clinician may decide that it is better to defer symptomatic treatment until after medical assessments are complete, although some patients do respond well to symptomatic treatment prior to such assessments. When they do, it may nonetheless be important to complete medical assessments even after resolution of the speech problem, especially if it is apparent that the patient may still fear organic disease.

When there is evidence of neurologic or other organic disease, but the speech disorder is wholly or partly psychogenic, the clinician must then use medical assessment results as a basis for addressing the relationship between the organic findings and the speech disorder. It is necessary to establish that, in spite of organic factors, there are no major barriers to improving those aspects of the speech problem that cannot be explained by organic disease. This is obviously more difficult to convey but it can be accomplished. ("Although you have multiple sclerosis, it's very unlikely that MS would affect speech in this way. Even though the MS might have played some role in triggering your speech problem, I think it's very possible that right now it won't prevent you from making significant improvements in your speech.")

The psychosocial history

The psychosocial history can be obtained during a review of the history of the current illness. The facts of the history determine the direction and sequence of inquiry. The interview may begin with a review of the circumstances surrounding the onset of the speech problem. Was onset associated with an obvious illness, physically traumatic event, surgery, or a suspected or confirmed neurologic event? Was the speech problem immediately apparent, or was there a delay between the physical event and onset of speech difficulty? If so, what was going on at or shortly before the time the speech problem began? What was the speech problem like at onset? How has it changed and what conditions make it better or worse? Has it ever remitted, even for short periods of time? Answers to these questions help determine the degree to which the speech problem is associated with actual or perceived organic illness and the degree to which the patient is convinced the problem is organic.

When the physical facts of the problem have been reviewed and especially when there is no evidence of a possible organic cause, patients can be asked about their jobs, family situation, and social life. The clinician can then ask how things have been going and were going in each of those areas when the speech problem began. The patient may not have been asked such questions before, in spite of numerous medical consultations. For some, this inquiry will be welcome; to others, it will be perceived as inappropriate or threatening. It is generally the case, however, that patients rarely reveal information about their personal lives without being asked, especially when they fail to see a connection between nonorganic factors and their physical symptoms.

Some patients reveal potentially significant psychosocial problems, but many deny any difficulties and insist that life is happy and stable. If they nonetheless seem receptive to inquiries about these issues, it is often appropriate to ask directly what stresses, conflicts, or pressures they are under or were under when the speech problem began. Sometimes etiologically significant psychosocial problems are immediately revealed in response to questions like "What was going on that might have been upsetting or concerning to you at the time your speech problem began?" or "Were you or are you having any difficulties at home or at work?" Sometimes this leads to immediate discussion of the possible connection between the speech problem and psychological factors, occasionally producing catharsis and resolution of the speech problem; more often the clinician simply tucks the information away for later discussion.

Patients sometimes respond aggressively, angrily, or sarcastically to inquiries about their psychosocial history. Statements like "You think I'm crazy [just like everybody else], don't you?" can be responded to with something like "Not at all. It's just important to understand all of the things that can influence problems like this, and we know that stress and conflict are sometimes important," "No, but what is it that other people have said about that?" or "What do you think about that?" The patient's belief about the possibility of psychological explanations will determine the extent to which discussion of such issues should be pursued at the time. If there is resistance or denial, it is often best to proceed to speech assessment and symptomatic treatment.

When patients do reveal evidence of psychologically significant events, they may ask if the clinician sees a connection between them and the speech disorder. It is helpful to ask the patient's opinion in this regard. If their answer demonstrates recognition of a possible causal relationship, the clinician should support and perhaps elaborate upon the explanation, acknowledging that psychological issues can affect physical symptoms, even in people without serious psychiatric difficulty who are under great stress or conflict. At the same time, it is often important to acknowledge that such problems are often complicated and difficult to understand.

There is no need for the clinician to explore in an explicit way the connection between the psychosocial history and the speech disorder during history taking. Sometimes this happens in a very natural way, but often it does not. What is important is to gather some initial facts that contribute to hypotheses about causal mechanisms and the patient's beliefs about the disturbance, willingness to discuss psychological issues, and capacity for insight. The actual drawing together of the psychosocial data and speech symptoms are often deferred until after or during symptomatic treatment. It is most important that this information be gathered with an attitude that conveys concern, an interest in all aspects of the patient's history, and a desire to understand the problem and help manage it.

Addressing beliefs about organicity

The medical and psychosocial history should establish the degree to which the patient believes the problem has an organic basis. It is often valuable to ask directly, "What do you believe is the cause of this problem?" when it is not readily apparent or when the clinician is ready to address the issue. When no possible physical explanations are readily apparent, it is valid to say so or to state that "right now it's difficult to know just what has caused this problem" and, after the basic speech mechanism examination is complete, to indicate that "at this point I don't see or hear anything that should prevent your speech from improving. It may be that something [the cold, the surgery, the physical trauma, the stroke] happened when this problem began that prevented you from speaking normally, but right now there's no evidence that that's still active or that it should prevent improvement in your speech." At this point, the notion of symptomatic treatment can be introduced. Further discussion of the organicity of the problem can be deferred until after an assertive attempt at symptomatic treatment is complete.

Symptomatic therapy

Symptomatic treatment should be introduced with the notion that a concerted effort to improve speech can result in significant and often rapid improvement. This can be followed by an explicit invitation to the patient ("Should we give it a try?") and a confident, pleased response when the patient accepts.

The direction of symptomatic efforts is determined by the specific abnormal speech characteristics. Several general techniques are very frequently applicable.

1. Identify for the patient the behaviors that represent the disorder (for example, tight and effortful voice; whispering; facial grimacing; neck extension; eye blinking; speaking only one syllable per breath group; general muscle tension; sound repetitions, slow speech rate, and consistent articulatory substitutions). Very often, these characteristics reflect excessive or misdirected muscular efforts.

2. After the behaviors are identified, it is appropriate to indicate to the patient that they reflect a well-intentioned effort to speak but are actually physically exhausting and acting as a barrier to more normal speech ("You're working so hard to talk, that you're unable to speak naturally"). The patient can then be told that together you will attempt to redirect or reduce the amount of effort in speaking.

3. Have the patient do something with speech that approximates a normal or at least a different response. This effort may range from a grunt to a sigh to a prolonged sound to a single syllable. It should be reinforced if adequate and modified if accompanied by struggle or abnormal quality. It often helps to have patients do something different, even if it is not normal, from what they have been doing habitually. For example, if they are grimacing, point out the behavior and have them do something else instead (open their eyes widely). Any change should be reinforced. Patients are told to listen to and feel the difference from their habitual response and then prompted to repeat the new response. When consistent, responses should be shaped toward normal or toward a lengthier normal response (for example, moving from a vowel to a syllable or word).

   Patients often express or display signs of fatigue, exhaustion, or discomfort during these efforts. They should be reinforced for working hard, praised for each small gain, and told that speaking may become easier than it has been within a short time. It may help to tell them that the first steps are the hardest and that success often builds momentum, with progress becoming rapid after the initial period of hard work. Failed techniques should be accompanied by explanations that it is often necessary to try several things, each of which might work, but some more adequately than others. The clinician should not let the patient's physical discomfort inhibit assertive efforts to work for change. The patient should have a sense that the clinician is willing to commit considerable physical effort to work for change.

4. Talk to the patient about what has and is going on during symptomatic efforts. Statements such as "You've been trying hard to speak well but your efforts have not been quite in the right direction. It's as if a train has been knocked off track [perhaps by your cold, accident, etc.]. You've been trying by yourself to get it back on track but haven't quite known how. What we're doing here is putting you back on the track in a way that will make it easier to do what you're trying so hard to do," can motivate continued effort and begin to address possible causal mechanisms at the same time.

5. *Physical contact may be very important to symptomatic therapy.* Laryngeal manipulation and massage can be a very effective way of reducing musculoskeletal tension and modifying voice in psychogenic voice disorders. The physical benefits of relieving musculoskeletal tension are clearly significant for many patients, but the physical contact between clinician and patient may also have considerable psychological value by "bonding" them together in the therapeutic effort and providing evidence that something physical is being done to induce change. Physical contact may be important in the management of other psychogenic speech disorders as well, both for its value in identifying points of excessive musculoskeletal tension (the face, jaw, eyes, hands) and for its psychological value. Touch may thus be an invaluable tool both physically and psychologically. It is important that it is done naturally and confidently.

6. As speech begins to improve and the clinician senses that symptomatic treatment will be successful, it is appropriate to accelerate enthusiasm about the patient's progress. Gradual withdrawal of physical manipulation or touch can take place, with increased expectations that the patient can modify speech without physical assistance.

7. When speech has normalized or improved noticeably, the patients can be asked to read a paragraph and get a "feel" for their improved speech. The clinician can interrupt to ask some general questions; the patient's improved speech during such responses should be pointed out. These transition points are passed very rapidly by some patients. Others may need to proceed much more gradually. It is crucial that the clinician repeatedly let the patient know that each step of improvement reflects a capacity for normal speech and that the patient's effort is the major factor determining the outcome.

As normalization takes place, many patients begin to ask, "What can I do to keep my speech like this?" or "How can I get my speech back if I lose it again?" The clinician can indicate that the patient is very likely to maintain gains without any special help, now that a feel for normal speech has been regained.

Addressing the nature of the problem and its improvement

How the nature of the problem is addressed is highly dependent on the degree to which the clinician understands the problem. If the patient has good insight into causal stresses, and there is a logical link between them and the speech problem, a frank discussion of the role of stress, anxiety, and conflict in the production of physical symptoms may be accepted and understood. For patients with a clear history of an organic trigger for the problem, an explanation may be more difficult. It may include the notion that a physical event was initially responsible for triggering the speech abnormality, but that the speech problem persisted when the organic event was no longer active, either because the patient developed faulty habits that could not be overcome or because psychological issues expressed themselves in speech abnormalities.

It is important at this point to address the role of ongoing stress and anxiety because it bears on patients' sense of security about whether their speech gains will last and whether they need to deal in a more active way with psychosocial issues. It often is also valuable, in the presence of the clinician, to have patients speak with their spouses or significant others who may have accompanied them. This establishes for patient and clinician that the improved speech can be maintained with people they know. In some cases, it may be appropriate to review with the patient and significant other the dynamics of the problem and its resolution. This is particularly valuable for patients who may have difficulty explaining these things to others on their own.

Addressing the future

When speech assessment and subsequent symptomatic therapy are complete, the future should be addressed. In general, discussion should address: the likelihood that speech will remain normal or return to normal; the need to address directly the psychological issues that were or are related to the speech problem; and how to explain the problem and its resolution to others. Multiple permutations of these issues may need to be addressed. The following scenarios provide some examples.

1. When symptomatic therapy results in a return of normal speech that is maintained with ease, it is important to establish how the patient feels he or she will do in the future relative to speech. Many patients believe speech will remain normal without future symptomatic help. In most instances, this belief is correct. If triggering psychogenic factors have been identified by the patient, if patients understand their role in the speech problem, and if the factors seem no longer to be active, then the clinician can review the sequence of events from onset to symptom resolution and discuss how the patient can deal with similar issues in the future. Directly addressing the patient's need for professional counseling regarding dealing with stress, conflict, or the specific events that triggered a speech problem, is important, not necessarily because this will lead to an immediate decision to pursue psychiatric help, but at least to establish that such counseling may be of benefit in the future.

   It is often valuable to discuss the patient's concerns about how to explain the problem and its resolution to others, as well as others' likely responses to such explanations. Ideally, the patient will leave the session with a plan for explaining and achieving closure with others about the speech problem and its resolution, and for dealing with similar psychosocial stresses and conflicts in the future.

2. When symptomatic therapy results in a return of normal speech that the patient is maintaining with ease, but the patient has failed to identify any psychosocial factors that could be related to the problem, the future is less certain. The clinician may be left to speculate about the significance of what is known from the history or to conclude that the reasons for the problem are uncertain although no physical barriers that would prevent normal speech are evident. Reviewing the general role of stress and conflict in producing speech disorders may help the patient be more attuned to the effects of psychosocial factors in the future, although this will not necessarily be the outcome for people whose basic insight into their feelings is superficial.

3. When symptomatic therapy fails to produce any change in speech but the clinician believes that continuing therapy will be beneficial because of the patient's motivation to improve, then further sessions should be scheduled. When underlying psychological explanations for the problem have not been identified, it is also valuable to ask the patient to review in the interim current stresses and conflicts, especially those that were also active at the time the speech problem began. This review should be discussed during the next session.

4. When the patient has failed to improve and salient psychosocial issues have been identified, the need to pursue psychiatric or psychological evaluation and counseling should be addressed. Sometimes the issues are volatile, pervasive, and profound, and sometimes they were not apparent to the patient until they were revealed during the evaluation. Sometimes the patient has been aware of them but has minimized their importance until they affected physical well-being. These patients often accept a referral for counseling. Symptomatic therapy can be conducted concurrently with psychiatric counseling, but sometimes it should be deferred until counseling is underway and it is clear that speech is not improving.

5. When symptomatic therapy has not succeeded, when psychological difficulties are denied, and when the patient insists on the organicity of the problem, it is unlikely that a referral for psychiatric consultation will be accepted. Nonetheless, the clinician who is confident that the speech problem is not organic should explain to the patient that nonorganic factors may be at work and that discussing the psychological history of the problem with a specialist would work toward leaving no stone unturned in efforts to get to the bottom of the problem. Many of these patients are unlikely to respond to further symptomatic therapy until they accept of the possibility that causal organic (or nonorganic) factors are no longer active and that it may be possible to resolve the problem symptomatically.

SYMPTOMATIC TREATMENT OF SPECIFIC PSYCHOGENIC SPEECH DISORDERS

The general principles, guidelines, and techniques just discussed probably apply equally well to the broad range of symptoms that characterize psychogenic speech disorders. Differences in management probably vary more as a function of patients' past and current psychosocial and medical status and their insight, readiness, and manner of responding during evaluation and treatment than to differences in abnormal speech characteristics. The differences that do exist in management among "types" of psychogenic speech disorders seem to lie mostly in some of the symptomatic techniques that are used. In the remainder of this chapter, some techniques that have been reported as successful during symptomatic management of different types of psychogenic speech symptoms will be reviewed. This review, while neither exhaustive nor prescriptive, is meant to convey the theme that characterizes symptomatic treatment.

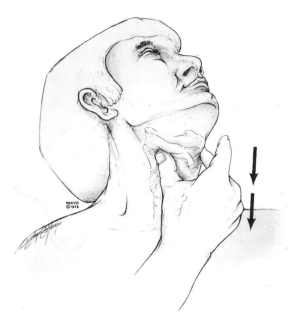

Figure 20–1 Placement of fingers in the thyrohyoid space for examination of musculoskeletal tension and for maneuvering the larynx to a lower position in the neck during symptomatic therapy. (From Aronson AE: Clinical voice disorders, New York, 1990, Thieme; with permission.)

Psychogenic voice disorders

Psychogenic voice disorders are usually characterized by aphonia, hoarseness, or spasmodic dysphonia. The theme that runs through the manner of voice production in these patients is one of *excessive musculoskeletal tension* or *vocal hyperfunction* (Aronson, 1990a). The goal of treatment is to reduce that tension because then the voice usually returns to normal. When the tension is not released psychologically or when psychological tension is no longer the factor that is maintaining the voice disorder, symptomatic reduction of musculoskeletal tension can be very effective. A general outline of steps that are useful in accomplishing this objective follows.*

1. People suspected of having a psychogenic voice disorder should be examined for laryngeal musculoskeletal tension, which is most readily detected by placing the thumb and index or middle finger in the thyrohyoid space and determining if that space is narrower than normal (Figure 20–1) or if the patient experiences discomfort or pain with digital pressure

---

*A more detailed description of this approach to treating psychogenic voice disorders can be found in Aronson (1990a), Case (1991), and Stemple (1993).

or gentle kneading in the area. Normal speakers and people without excessive musculoskeletal tension feel pressure but not discomfort or pain. Many patients with psychogenic voice disorders respond with pain or discomfort. Even when they do not, the steps that follow often are successful.

2. The patient can be told that discomfort reflects excessive musculoskeletal tension and that the tension is a significant contributor to an abnormal voice. If psychosocial explanations have already been uncovered and recognized, it may help to indicate that muscular tension represents a response to those factors. If not, it usually suffices to indicate that the tension does not represent an irreversible or uncontrollable muscular abnormality or that the tension represents the patient's great but misdirected physical effort to achieve normal voice.

3. With gentle kneading of the laryngeal muscles, the height of the larynx in the neck should lower (the thyrohyoid space should become less narrow) and the laryngeal cartilages should become looser. Patients sometimes protest because of the discomfort, but they should be reassured that it is temporary and a necessary step to relax muscles.

4. During efforts to reduce musculoskeletal tension, the patient should be asked to produce some lax vowels, a nasal /m/, or a gentle oral or nasal "uh huh." This is often done while manually lowering the thyroid cartilage (see Figure 20–1). Aphonic patients may be asked to clear the throat, grunt, cough gently, or briefly hum and then to attempt to prolong the act into a short vowel. The clinician should provide immediate feedback about positive changes in the quality of such productions because patients are not always aware of them. The patient needs to know that these traces of normal voice establish the capacity for normal phonation and show that no barrier is present to prevent further improvement. When voice is reliably achieved, the patient should attempt to produce the improved voice with reduced physical assistance from the clinician and eventually without any.

The goal of all of these efforts is to elicit even a brief trace of improved or normal voice so that it may be shaped toward normal quality or extended to lengthier utterances. These efforts sometimes succeed very rapidly, but they may take an extended period of time that is physically demanding of both clinician and patient. Much of the effort is trial and error and requires the clinician to take advantage of accidental or unplanned voice improvements;

the clinician should use whatever works during this step and drop whatever fails (Aronson, 1990a).

5. Once a brief but relatively normal voice can be achieved reliably, the patient should be asked to prolong a vowel or /m/ or to reflexively answer some yes-no questions with an appropriately inflected oral or nasal "uh huh" or "uh." Voiced phrases such as "one Monday morning" may then be attempted. Manual lowering of the larynx may continue or be reintroduced at this point, but with a goal of fading it as soon as possible. The patient should be asked to feel as well as listen to the voice and to note how much easier it is to produce voice under these conditions than with the degree of tension that they had been exhibiting.

6. Patients who are able to produce some short phrases or do some counting with the improved voice should be asked to read a paragraph. They should be stopped and assisted by verbal instruction or manual assistance in regaining normal voice if they slip back to their previous pattern. They can then be asked to "play with" the voice, as if reading to entertain. When successful, they should then be engaged in casual conversation that may begin with basic biographical and factual information, proceed to narratives, and finally to a discussion of their feelings about their improved voice, explanations for the improvement and causes for the problem, their prognosis, and so on. In most cases, the improved voice is maintained without effort and may improve further during conversation. This should be pointed out so that the patient recognizes control over the voice. Some patients comment about how much easier it is to speak; others note that it feels odd or that the neck is sore from laryngeal manipulation. They can be reassured that any soreness will subside in a short time, certainly within a day or two.

The rate of improvement in response to this kind of symptomatic therapy varies. If the problem has been due to musculoskeletal tension alone, if it has not been present for long, or if underlying psychological triggers are no longer active, normal voice is sometimes achieved in minutes. Stemple (1993) suggests that the average time for achieving normal voice is 30 to 45 minutes, but some patients may require a few sessions (Aronson, 1990a; Boone, 1977). Most who benefit go through various stages of dysphonia as improvement occurs, rather than making a sudden jump from baseline to normal voice.

Regarding efficacy, Aronson (1990a) notes that "the majority of patients can be helped considerably, if not completely, within that time [a single session]. Patients whose voices fail to improve . . . may not be ready to relinquish the abnormal voice because of musculoskeletal tension secondary to conversion reaction" (p. 315). Similarly, Boone (1977) indicates that symptomatic therapy is usually effective in restoring normal voice and that the normal voice usually remains.

The presence of neurologic disease does not preclude the effectiveness of symptomatic therapy. Sapir and Aronson (1985) reported two cases with aphonia and evidence of associated laryngeal musculoskeletal tension following closed head injury whose voices returned to normal in one or two sessions of symptomatic therapy. Similarly, Sapir and Aronson (1987) discussed one patient with a psychogenic strained voice, plus a unilateral upper motor neuron dysarthria from stroke, and another patient with a severely breathy voice that exceeded that expected for a postsurgical vocal cord paralysis, both of whose voices improved rapidly with symptomatic treatment. They also discussed two additional patients, one with organic voice tremor and hoarseness and another with myasthenia gravis and a strained dysphonia, whose voices improved markedly during discussion of psychosocial concerns and fears they had about physical illness. These cases highlight the role of psychological mechanisms in some dysphonias that develop in people with organic illness, as well as the responsiveness of at least some of these patients to methods that are effective for those with psychogenic voice disorders but no organic illness.

Chewing therapy, progressive relaxation, and biofeedback are other symptomatic treatments that may be used (Aronson, 1990a; Case, 1991; Sapir and Aronson, 1990). Some patients also may respond to methods of psychiatry that are sometimes effective for treating conversion and anxiety-induced disorders, such as counseling, minor tranquilizers, hypnosis and sodium amytal interview. Some have spontaneous remission of their symptoms (Sapir and Aronson, 1990; Stoudemire, 1988; Tomb, 1981).

Psychogenic stuttering

The speech characteristics of psychogenic stuttering (PS) are highly variable but usually include sound/syllable/word repetitions, prolongations, hesitations and blocking that are frequently accompanied by secondary struggle behavior such as facial grimacing. These and other characteristics were discussed in Chapter 14.

Relatively little is known about the management of PS. There are few reports in the literature that focus on its management. Nonetheless, enough is known to suggest that the general principles, guidelines, and techniques that already have been discussed probably apply quite well to the management of PS. It also appears that the symptomatic management of PS can be quite effective, possibly as often and as rapidly as it is for psychogenic voice disorders.

Similar to psychogenic voice disorders, the dysfluencies of PS are *often associated with excessive musculoskeletal tension in speech and sometimes nonspeech muscles.* An important and sometimes crucial goal of symptomatic therapy, therefore, is reduction of musculoskeletal tension, which often normalizes fluency. Therefore, many of the techniques that were described for reducing musculoskeletal tension in people with psychogenic voice disorders can be applied to people with PS. In fact, in some people with PS, the focus of tension reduction may also be on the larynx, in which case the same techniques may be applied. The following steps summarize some techniques that seem to be effective in the symptomatic treatment of PS.

1. People suspected of having PS should be observed for evidence of excessive musculoskeletal tension in speech and nonspeech muscles. When phonation is perceived as effortful, the larynx may be examined in the same way described for psychogenic voice disorders. The jaw, face, and eyes also should be observed for evidence of exaggerated movement or excessive contraction. Excessive neck flexion or extension may occur during speech, as may secondary movements or muscle tightness in the shoulders, torso, arms, or legs. If multiple loci of increased tension are apparent, those structures that can be manipulated by the clinician should be identified; they may become the initial focus of symptom reduction.

2. Patients often can be told that their dysfluencies at least partially reflect excessive musculoskeletal tension generated by their efforts to speak. They can also be told that this effort is actually preventing normal speech, that it does not represent an irreversible or uncontrollable abnormality, and that it can be brought under control.

3. The clinician should select a high-frequency and high-amplitude abnormal behavior for modification, preferably one associated with tension in muscles that can be touched or manipulated. The muscle tension during speech should be pointed out to the patient (for example, neck extension, lower face retraction, eye closing, arm movements). The patient should then be asked to identify the behavior when it occurs, with reinforcement provided for accurate identification. If laryngeal muscle ten-

sion is chosen, the steps outlined in the previous section for psychogenic voice disorders can then be followed.

4. The patient should be asked to speak without abnormal movement or excessive tension in the selected structure (that is, for example, without excessive lower face retraction, eye closing, or neck extension). It may be necessary to begin with the production of single sounds, such as vowel prolongation. It may help for the clinician to touch the structure of focus during these initial attempts in order to focus attention and provide a source of feedback. Patients may benefit from being told to do something different than what they have been doing, even if it is not part of normal motor behavior. For example, a patient who abnormally retracts the lips when speaking may be told to open the eyes widely instead; these alternative behaviors (that probably serve as distractors) usually can be faded quickly once the target behavior changes.

5. When a sound can be prolonged without excessive muscle tension, the patient should produce some single words, with reinforcement for doing so without tension in the target structure and without dysfluencies. Adopting a slow, prolonged rate may help patients whose dysfluencies are characterized by hesitation and repetition. The patient should be reminded frequently about their success in reducing muscle tension and modifying dysfluencies. Sentence repetition and reading then can be pursued with similar strategies.

Some patients who have difficulty reducing dysfluencies benefit from learning to be dysfluent in a different way. For example, if PS is characterized by repetitions, the patient may be asked instead to prolong all syllables, rather than repeat; if they hesitate before initiating each word or phrase, they can be told to "never stop" by using continuous voicing and not pausing at phrase boundaries. Once the pattern of baseline dysfluencies has been altered, these alternative abnormalities usually can be faded quickly.

6. When excessive tension, abnormal movements, and dysfluencies arising from a single structure have been modified, frequently all musculoskeletal tension and dysfluencies begin to decrease. When this is the case, it should be pointed out to the patient. When it is not the case, the remaining abnormalities should be attacked with the same strategies, although success tends to accelerate and steps often can be skipped. Any return of musculoskeletal tension or dysfluencies should be pointed out immediately and modified.

7. As dysfluencies are reduced, the patient may maintain a slow rate with flattened prosody. If so, they should be asked to "play with" their speech during reading, as if to entertain. When successful, the patient should then engage in conversation. Most patients who have moved rapidly to this point continue to improve during conversation.

Like psychogenic voice disorders, the rate of improvement varies. Many patients dramatically improve in less than an hour, and others require several sessions. Most go through a gradual reduction of dysfluency, rather than making a sudden jump from their baseline behavior to fluency.

A number of clinical reports provide support for the efficacy of behavioral management of PS in people without as well as those with neurologic disease. As discussed in Chapter 14, Baumgartner and Duffy's (1986) review of 49 cases with PS in the absence of neurologic disease established that of the 43% of the patients in the group who were treated symptomatically with methods similar to those just described, 47% improved to normal in one or two sessions, often during the diagnostic evaluation; another 28% improved nearly to normal, and 19% showed some improvement. Similarly, in their review of 20 cases with PS who did have evidence of neurologic disease, of the 55% of the cases who were treated, 45% improved to normal in one or two sessions, often during the diagnostic evaluation; another 18% improved nearly to normal, and 18% showed some improvement. Therefore, symptomatic treatment was quite successful, sometimes dramatically so, and success was often achieved rapidly, even in people with neurologic disease. However, these success rates may not be representative of the population of people with PS. They apply only to treatment provided to people seen in a large tertiary care center, and there may be features of such patients that could make treatment efficacy rates higher or lower for them than for the population as a whole. More important, perhaps, is the fact that only about half of the patients in Baumgartner and Duffy's review were treated; the reasons for not pursuing treatment in untreated cases were highly diverse or unclear, but sometimes were due to patient resistance to treatment or to the clinician's belief that treatment was inappropriate or unlikely to be effective. The rates of treatment success are, nonetheless, impressive.

Several case studies also illustrate the duration, specific techniques, and efficacy of symptomatic treatment. Mahr and Leith (1992) discussed four cases of adult-onset PS in which the mechanism was presumed to be conversion disorder. One person improved to normal after 9 months of twice-weekly sessions that focused on careful articulation and slow production of speech. Another improved within minutes when instructed to slow speech rate and articulate clearly. Another whose PS began during the process of divorce improved when instructed to speak slowly and finally normalized when the person was able to accept the marriage's termination. A fourth individual failed to improve after 30 months of three-times-weekly symptomatic therapy.

Duffy (1989) detailed a case of PS without neurologic disease whose speech became normal during the diagnostic encounter, in which a discussion of contributing psychosocial issues was combined with symptomatic treatment. The case study details the symptomatic technique but also emphasizes the importance and value of the psychosocial interview and discussion in management. It also highlights the value of interdisciplinary contributions to management; that is, follow-up psychiatric evaluation and completion of comprehensive neurologic and medical examinations also were important to the overall management of the patient's psychological difficulties.

Roth, Aronson, and Davis (1989) summarized in detail 12 cases of PS without neurologic disease (most of whom were included in Baumgartner and Duffy's 1986 retrospective review). Eleven of the 12 cases improved, five in response to symptomatic speech therapy, one during group psychotherapy, one during a discussion of events surrounding the onset of the problem, and four spontaneously. Symptomatic treatment included "traditional techniques" such as easy onset of voicing, light touch articulation, or bouncing during blocking or struggle. The authors noted that a clinician attitude of encouragement and optimism seemed to be an indispensable component of treatment.

Brookshire (1989) presented a case whose stuttering was considered at least partially psychogenic in origin, even though it began several months after a stroke. The patient did not improve significantly during 21 sessions of a commercially available relaxation program but responded dramatically within a single session to a behavior modification program that focused on decreasing the muscle tensing that preceded dysfluencies. The procedures are well described and provide a useful model for systematic behavioral management. Brookshire concluded that placing "consistent and inescapable contingencies" on behaviors that precede dysfluent speech can produce dramatic and durable effects. The patient remained fluent during 8 years of follow-up.

Two additional case reports suggest that PS may respond favorably to techniques that often modify developmental stuttering. Tippett and Siebens (1991) summarized speech therapy for a man with anoxic encephalopathy, weakness and spasticity, depression, and pseudoseizures (psychogenic seizures). His stuttering began to improve during an initial treatment session that emphasized rhythmic speaking techniques, became normally fluent without rhythmic speaking during two-weeks of therapy, and was maintained at three month follow-up. Deal (1982) reported on a patient whose dysfluencies began after a suicide attempt. He became increasingly fluent over the course of about seven weeks in a treatment program that initially used delayed auditory feedback; he also concurrently participated in group psychotherapy. Fluency was normal at follow-up two months later.

Other psychogenic speech disorders

As noted in Chapter 14, psychogenic speech disorders sometimes express themselves in ways that are less conventional than disturbances of voice or fluency. If the Mayo Clinic experience is an accurate reflection of the frequency with which such problems are encountered in speech pathology practices, however, they represent less than 10% of psychogenic speech disorders (see Table 14–1). These unusual problems most often reflect abnormalities in articulation, resonance, and prosody. The literature on their symptomatic management by speech pathologists is nearly nonexistent. The following guidelines for the management of these problems seem reasonable but are largely untested.

1. Psychogenic articulation, resonance, and prosodic disturbances probably reflect psychodynamic mechanisms that are very similar to those that lead to psychogenic voice and fluency disorders; that is, it is likely that underlying causal mechanisms are generally the same for all psychogenic speech disturbances, with different symptoms representing different routes of expression that may be influenced by factors such as somatic compliance, secondary gain, notions about and experiences with illness and speech disorders, and, possibly, differences in the symbolic meaning of various symptoms. If this is true, then the general principles, guidelines, and techniques for management that have already been discussed should apply to people with these unusual symptoms. Differences in management, therefore, are mostly related to specific symptomatic techniques.

2. When psychogenic articulation, resonance, or prosodic disorders are accompanied by excessive musculoskeletal tension, the reduction of such tension should be undertaken in a manner similar to that described for psychogenic voice and stuttering problems. However, *musculoskeletal tension may not be a primary feature of these disorders.*

3. Psychogenic articulation disorders often seem characterized by substitution or distortion of specific sounds (for example, w/r, w/l, all sounds produced with lingual retraction), rather than general imprecision. When this is the case, it seems reasonable to employ "traditional" articulation therapy techniques for their modification.

4. Psychogenic hypernasality, particularly when somatic compliance and conversion reaction mechanisms seem to be at work, may respond to "traditional" approaches to modifying articulation and resonance in people with organic velopharyngeal insufficiency.

5. Psychogenic prosodic disturbances can be quite variable. Because they may be accompanied by abnormalities in fluency, articulation, and even resonance, it may be best to focus on modification of fluency, articulation, or resonance because they are more easily localized to specific muscles and structures, making it simpler to focus symptomatic efforts. When the prosodic disturbance resembles that of a foreign accent, techniques for modifying foreign accent or neurogenic pseudoforeign accent (Chapter 19) may be appropriate. When the prosodic disturbance conveys an impression of infantile speech, it is often accompanied by abnormally high-pitch or "developmental" articulation errors that may be more modifiable than the abnormal prosodic pattern. Similarly, people with psychogenic stuttering sometimes also have infantile speech characteristics; modifying the dysfluencies often results in a simultaneous spontaneous resolution of the infantile pattern of articulation and prosody.

   When an infantile speech pattern is accompanied by prominent infantile affective behavior, the patient may deny any speech difficulty and be incapable of interacting as an adult. They are not likely to respond to symptomatic efforts to modify their speech pattern, at least without concurrent psychiatric treatment.

6. People with psychogenic (conversion) mutism are quite similar in personality traits and histories to those with conversion aphonia and dysphonias (Aronson, Peterson, and Litin, 1966) and may exhibit other psychogenic voice or fluency problems as they emerge from their mute state (Aronson, 1990a). In general, they seem to respond well to symptomatic treatment techniques that are effective for people with psychogenic aphonia and dysphonia, including the physical techniques that are effective in reducing musculoskeletal tension.

SUMMARY

1. People with psychogenic speech disorders that are associated with conversion disorder or responses to life stresses are often responsive to treatment provided by a speech pathologist. Symptom resolution with speech therapy can be achieved for some patients before psychiatric evaluation, and psychiatric referral is not always necessary. The prognosis for recovery from psychogenic speech disorders is generally good.

2. Management usually requires that speech symptoms as well as the explanations for their existence be addressed with the patient. In many cases, treatment can be initiated within the diagnostic session.

3. The clinician's attitude and manner of interacting with the patient are crucial to management. Empathy, compassion, respect, honesty, confidence, and assertiveness are as important to competent, effective, and caring treatment for people with psychogenic speech disorders as they are to the management of motor speech disorders.

4. When symptomatic therapy is successful, it is important to address the mechanisms that may explain the improvement as well as the possible need for psychiatric referral.

5. Not all people with psychogenic speech disorders wish or are ready to be helped, and not all can be helped by speech therapy.

6. Therapy is best conducted following completion of all relevant medical evaluations.

7. The psychosocial history is crucial to both diagnosis and management. Symptomatic treatment usually involves the identification of abnormal behaviors and the gradual behavioral shaping of more normal speech responses, with continuous explanation and reinforcement for change. Physical contact may be important to the success of symptomatic therapy.

8. Symptomatic therapy for psychogenic voice disorders (including mutism) and psychogenic stuttering very often involves efforts to reduce excessive musculoskeletal tension and the gradual shaping of normal phonation and fluency. A high proportion of patients with psychogenic voice disorders and stuttering respond

well to symptomatic therapy, many of them during the diagnostic encounter or within one or two treatment sessions.

9. Little is known about the symptomatic treatment of infrequently occurring psychogenic disorders of articulation, resonance, and prosody. It is likely that the principles, guidelines, and techniques that seem important to managing psychogenic voice and stuttering disorders are applicable to them. The need to reduce musculoskeletal tension may not be as pervasive in patients with them, however, and symptomatic therapy may employ traditional techniques for modifying articulation, resonance, and prosody.

REFERENCES

Aronson AE: Clinical voice disorders, New York, 1990a, Thieme.

Aronson AE: Importance of the psychosocial interview in the diagnosis and treatment of "functional" voice disorders, J Voice 4:287, 1990b.

Aronson AE, Peterson HW, and Litin EM: Psychiatric symptomatology in functional dysphonia and aphonia, J Speech Hear Disord 31:115, 1966.

Baker JHE and Silver JR: Hysterical paraplegia, J Neurol Neurosurg Psychiatry 50:375, 1987.

Baumgartner J and Duffy JR: Adult onset stuttering: psychogenic and/or neurologic. Miniseminar presented at American Speech-Language-Hearing Association Convention, Detroit, MI, November 1986.

Boone DR: The voice and voice therapy, Englewood Cliffs, NJ, 1977, Prentice-Hall.

Brookshire RH: A dramatic response to behavior modification by a patient with rapid onset of dysfluent speech. In Helm-Estabrooks N and Aten JL, editors: Difficult diagnoses in communication disorders, Boston, 1989, College-Hill Press.

Case JL: Clinical management of voice disorders, ed 2, Austin, TX, 1991, Pro-Ed.

Deal JL: Sudden onset of stuttering: a case report, J Speech Hear Disord 47:301, 1982.

Duffy JR: A puzzling case of adult onset stuttering. In Helm-Estabrooks N and Aten JL, editors: Difficult diagnoses in communication disorders, Boston, 1989, College-Hill.

Ford CV and Folks DG: Conversion disorders: an overview, Psychosomatics 26:371, 1985.

Head H: An address on the diagnosis of hysteria, BMJ, 1:827, 1922.

Lazare A: Current concepts in psychiatry: conversion symptoms, N Engl J Med 305:745, 1981.

Mahr G and Leith W: Psychogenic stuttering of adult onset, J Speech Hear Res 35:283, 1992.

Nemiah JC: Psychoneurotic disorders. In Nicholi AM, editor: The new Harvard guide to psychiatry, Cambridge, 1988, The Belknap Press of Harvard University Press.

Roth CR, Aronson AE, and Davis LJ: Clinical studies in psychogenic stuttering of adult onset, J Speech Hear Disord 54:634, 1989.

Sapir S and Aronson AE: Aphonia after closed head injury: aetiologic considerations, Br J Disord Commun 20:289, 1985.

Sapir S and Aronson AE: Coexisting psychogenic and neurogenic dysphonia: a source of diagnostic confusion, Br J Disord Commun 22:73, 1987.

Sapir S and Aronson AE: The relationship between psychopathology and speech and language disorders in neurologic patients, J Speech Hear Disord 55:503, 1990.

Stemple JC: Voice therapy: clinical studies, St Louis, MI, 1993, Mosby–Year Book.

Stoudemire GA: Somatoform disorders, factitious disorders, and malingering. In Talbott JA, Hales RE, and Yudofsky SC, editors: Textbook of psychiatry, Washington, DC, 1988, American Psychiatric Press.

Teitelbaum ML and McHugh PR: Psychiatric conditions presenting as neurologic disease. In Johnson RT, editor: Current therapy in neurologic disease, ed 3, Philadelphia, 1990, BC Decker.

Tippett DC and Siebens AA: Distinguishing psychogenic from neurogenic dysfluency when neurologic and psychologic factors coexist, J Fluency Disord, 16:3, 1991.

Tomb DA: Psychiatry for the house officer, Baltimore, 1981, Williams and Wilkins.

Index

Page numbers in italics indicate illustrations; *t* indicates tables; *n* indicates notes.